TISSUE RESPONSES TO ADDICTIVE DRUGS

Proceedings of a Workshop Session
for the International Society for Neuroendocrinology
Downstate Medical Center, State University of New York
June, 1975

TISSUE RESPONSES TO ADDICTIVE DRUGS

Edited by

Donald H. Ford, Ph.D.
Downstate Medical Center
State University of New York
Brooklyn, New York

and

Doris H. Clouet, Ph.D.
New York State Drug Abuse Control Commission
Brooklyn, New York

S P Books Division of
SPECTRUM PUBLICATIONS, INC.
New York

Distributed by Halsted Press
A Division of John Wiley & Sons

New York   Toronto   London   Sydney

SPECTRUM PUBLICATIONS, INC.
86-19 Sancho Street, Holliswood, N.Y. 11423

Distributed solely by the Halsted Press division of John Wiley & Sons, Inc., New York

Library of Congress Cataloging in Publication Data

Main entry under title:

Tissue responses to addictive drugs.

   Includes index.
   1. Narcotics--Physiological effect--Congresses.
2. Cells, Effect of drugs on--Congresses.
3. Drug receptors--Congresses. I. Ford, Donald
Herbert, 1921-   II. Clouet, Doris H.
III. International Society of Psychoneuroendocrinology. [DNLM: 1. Drug Dependence--Congresses.
2. Narcotics--Pharmacodynamics--Congresses.
3. Receptors, Drug--Congresses. QV80 T616 1975]
RM328.T57   615'.782   76-21325
ISBN 0-470-15192-7

Contributors

H. BEGLEITER
Department of Psychology
SUNY, Downstate Medical Center
Brooklyn, New York

BARRY A. BERKOWITZ
Roche Institute of Molecular Biology
Nutley, New Jersey

HEMENDRA N. BHARGAVA
Department of Pharmacolognosy
and Pharmacology
College of Pharmacy
University of Illinois at the
Medical Center
Chicago, Illinois

PHILIP B. BRADLEY
Department of Pharmacology
The Medical School
Birmingham, England

DAVID J. BRIGATI
Department of Pathology
SUNY, Downstate Medical Center
Brooklyn, New York

K. R. BRIZZEE
Delta Regional Primate
Research Center
Tulane University
Covington, Louisiana

CONSTANCE CARDASIS
Laboratory of Electron Microscopy
Wellesley College
Wellesley, Massachusetts

G. CASELLA
New York State Office of
Drug Abuse Services
Testing and Research Laboratory
Brooklyn, New York

H. CHESLAK
Department of Anatomy
SUNY, Downstate Medical Center
Brooklyn, New York

T.M. CHO
Langley Porter Neuropsychiatric
Institute and Department of
Pharmacology
University of California
San Francisco, California

J.L. CLAGHORN
Texas Research Institute of
Mental Sciences
Houston, Texas

DORIS H. CLOUET
New York State Drug Abuse
Control Commission
Testing and Research Laboratory
Brooklyn, New York

JOSEPH COCHIN
Department of Pharmacology
Boston University School of Medicine
Boston, Massachusetts

CONTRIBUTORS

R.W. COLBURN
Intramural Research Laboratory
Division of Research
National Institute on Drug Abuse
Rockville, Maryland

J. COMATY
New York State Research Institute
for Neurochemistry and Drug
Addiction
Ward's Island, New York

B.M. COX
Stanford University and
Addiction Research Foundation
Palo Alto, California

EVA B. CRAMER
Department of Anatomy
SUNY, Downstate Medical Center
Brooklyn, New York

GALE L. CRAVISO
Department of Pharmacology
New York University
School of Medicine
New York, New York

IAN CREESE
Departments of Pharmacology and
Experimental Therapeutics and
Psychiatry and the Behavioral
Sciences
Johns Hopkins University
School of Medicine
Baltimore, Maryland

MARSHA CROFFORD
Departments of Pharmacology
and Anatomy
New York Medical College
Valhalla, New York

WILLIAM L. DEWEY
Department of Pharmacology
Medical College of Virginia
Richmond, Virginia

IHSAN M. DIAB
Department of Pharmacological and
Physiological Sciences and the
Department of Psychiatry
The University of Chicago
Chicago, Illinois

ROBERT J. DINERSTEIN
Department of Pharmacological and
Physiological Sciences and the
Department of Psychiatry
The University of Chicago
Chicago, Illinois

EDWARD F. DOMINO
Department of Pharmacology
University of Michigan
Ann Arbor, Michigan

S. EHRENPREIS
New York State Research Institute
for Neurochemistry and Drug
Addiction
Ward's Island, New York

ELLEN FEINGOLD
Departments of Pediatrics and
Obstetrics and Gynecology
Cornell Medical College
New York, New York

JAMES FORBES
Department of Pharmacology
Medical College of Virginia
Richmond, Virginia

D. H. FORD
Department of Anatomy
SUNY, Downstate Medical Center
Brooklyn, New York

ROBERT GEORGE
Department of Pharmacology
and Brain Research Institute
University of California
Los Angeles, California

AVRAM GOLDSTEIN
Stanford University and
Addiction Research Foundation
Palo Alto, California

J. GREENBERG
New York State Research Institute
for Neurochemistry and Drug
Addiction
Ward's Island, New York

JOHANNA HAGEDOORN
Departments of Pharmacology and
Anatomy
New York Medical College
Valhalla, New York

RITA G. HARPER
Division of Perinatal Medicine
Departments of Pediatrics and
Obstetrics and Gynecology
North Shore University Hospital
Manhasset, New York

LOUIS S. HARRIS
Department of Pharmacology
Medical College of Virginia
Richmond, Virginia

J. M. HILLER
Department of Medicine
New York University
School of Medicine
New York, New York

ANDREW K.S. HO
Department of Basic Sciences
University of Illinois
Peoria School of Medicine
Peoria, Illinois

JONG S. HORNG
The Lilly Research Laboratories
Indianapolis, Indiana

FERDINAND HUI
Departments of Pharmacology and
Anatomy
New York Medical College
Valhalla, New York

S. HUROWITZ
Department of Psychology
SUNY, Downstate Medical Center
Brooklyn, New York

KATSUYA IWATSUBO
The University of Osaka
Dental School
Osaka, Japan

YASUKO F. JACQUET
New York State Research Institute
for Neurochemistry and Drug
Addiction
Ward's Island, New York

M. S. JOSHI
Department of Anatomy
SUNY, Downstate Medical Center
Brooklyn, New York

M.B. KAACK
Delta Regional Primate
Research Center
Tulane University
Covington, Louisiana

MICHAEL KARBOWSKI
Department of Pharmacology
Medical College of Virginia
Richmond, Virginia

BENJAMIN KISSIN
Division of Alcoholism and
Drug Abuse
Department of Psychiatry
SUNY, Downstate Medical Center
Brooklyn, New York

NORIO KOKKA
Department of Pharmacology and
Therapeutics
California College of Medicine
University of California
Irvine, California

MICHAEL J. KUHAR
Departments of Pharmacology and
Experimental Therapeutics and
Psychiatry and the Behavioral
Sciences
The Johns Hopkins University
School of Medicine
Baltimore, Maryland

CONTRIBUTORS

HARBANS LAL
Department of Pharmacology
and Toxicology
College of Pharmacy
University of Rhode Island
Kingston, Rhode Island

CHI HO LEE
Department of Pharmacology
Cornell Medical College
New York, New York

MICHAEL A. LEVI
Department of Anatomy
SUNY, Downstate Medical Center
Brooklyn, New York

HORACE H. LOH
Langley Porter Neuropsychiatric
Institute and Department of
Pharmacology
University of California
San Francisco, California

ISAAC MANIGAULT
New York State Research Institute
for Neurochemistry and Drug
Addiction
Ward's Island, New York

JACQUELINE F. MC GINTY
Department of Anatomy
SUNY, Downstate Medical Center
Brooklyn, New York

ANAND L. MISRA
New York State Drug Abuse
Control Commission
Testing and Research Laboratory
Brooklyn, New York

C. MONTESINOS
Department of Radiology
SUNY, Downstate Medical Center
Brooklyn, New York

S. J. MULÉ
New York State Office of Drug
Abuse Services
Testing and Research Laboratory
Brooklyn, New York

JOSE M. MUSACCHIO
Department of Pharmacology
New York University
School of Medicine
New York, New York

BARRY E. MUSHLIN
Department of Pharmacology
Boston University School of Medicine
Boston, Massachusetts

L.K. NG
Intramural Research Laboratory
Division of Research
National Institute on Drug Abuse
Rockville, Maryland

K.E. OPHEIM
Stanford University and
Addiction Research Foundation
Palo Alto, California

J. MARK ORDY
Delta Regional Primate
Research Center
Tulane University
Covington, Louisiana

C.N. PANG
Department of Anatomy and
Brain Research Institute
UCLA School of Medicine
Los Angeles, California

GAVRIL W. PASTERNAK
Departments of Pharmacology and
Experimental Therapeutics and
Psychiatry and Behavioral Sciences
Johns Hopkins University
School of Medicine
Baltimore, Maryland

NORMAN PEDIGO
Department of Pharmacology
Medical College of Virginia
Richmond, Virginia

CANDACE B. PERT
Departments of Pharmacology and
Experimental Therapeutics and
Psychiatry and the Behavioral
Sciences
The Johns Hopkins University
School of Medicine
Baltimore, Maryland

LOUIS P. PERTSCHUK
Department of Pathology
SUNY, Downstate Medical Center
Brooklyn, New York

B. PORJESZ
Department of Psychology
SUNY, Downstate Medical Center
Brooklyn, New York

SURENDRA PURI
Department of Pharmacology
and Toxicology
College of Pharmacy
University of Rhode Island
Kingston, Rhode Island

R.K. RHINES
Department of Anatomy
SUNY, Downstate Medical Center
Brooklyn, New York

LLOYD J. ROTH
Department of Pharmacological and
Physiological Sciences and the
Department of Psychiatry
The University of Chicago
Chicago, Illinois

HERBERT SCHUEL
Department of Biochemistry
SUNY, Downstate Medical Center
Brooklyn, New York

CHARLES R. SCHUSTER
Department of Pharmacological and
Physiological Sciences and the
Department of Psychiatry
The University of Chicago
Chicago, Illinois

JOANNA H. SHER
Department of Pathology
SUNY, Downstate Medical Center
Brooklyn, New York

RABI SIMANTOV
Departments of Pharmacology and
Experimental Therapeutics and
Psychiatry and Behavioral Sciences
John Hopkins University
School of Medicine
Baltimore, Maryland

H. SIMMONS
Department of Anatomy
SUNY, Downstate Medical Center
Brooklyn, New York

E.J. SIMON
Department of Medicine
New York University
School of Medicine
New York, New York

ALFRED A. SMITH
Departments of Pharmacology
and Anatomy
New York Medical College
Valhalla, New York

SOLOMON H. SNYDER
Departments of Pharmacology and
Experimental Therapeutics and
Psychiatry and Behavioral Sciences
Johns Hopkins University
School of Medicine
Baltimore, Maryland

GEORGE I. SOLISH
Department of Obstetrics
and Gynecology
SUNY, Downstate Medical Center
Brooklyn, New York

THEO SONDEREGGER
Department of Psychology
University of Nebraska
Lincoln, Nebraska

CONTRIBUTORS

SYDNEY SPECTOR
Roche Institute of Molecular Biology
Nutley, New Jersey

MICHAEL TENNER
Department of Radiology
SUNY, Downstate Medical Center
Brooklyn, New York

N.B. THOA
Intramural Research Laboratory
Division of Research
National Institute on Drug Abuse
Rockville, Maryland

J. TOTH
New York State Research Institute for
Neurochemistry and Drug
Addiction
Ward's Island, New York

MICHAEL R. VASKO
Department of Pharmacology
University of Michigan
Ann Arbor, Michigan

LADISLAV VOLICER
Department of Pharmacology
and Toxicology
College of Pharmacy
University of Rhode Island
Kingston, Rhode Island

ISABEL J. WAJDA
New York State Research Institute
for Neurochemistry and Drug
Addiction
Ward's Island, New York

MITSUTOSHI WATANABE
Department of Pharmacological
and Physiological Sciences and
the Department of Psychiatry
The University of Chicago
Chicago, Illinois

E. LEONG WAY
Department of Pharmacology
School of Medicine
University of California
San Francisco, California

ANN E. WILSON
Department of Pharmacology
University of Michigan
Ann Arbor, Michigan

G. WODRASKA
Department of Radiology
SUNY, Downstate Medical Center
Brooklyn, New York

DAVID T. WONG
The Lilly Research Laboratories
Indianapolis, Indiana

EMERY ZIMMERMANN
Department of Anatomy and
Brain Research Institute
UCLA School of Medicine
Los Angeles, California

Preface

In the past few years there has been an explosion in the rate of accumulation of information on the use of drugs of abuse, particularly the narcotic analgesic drugs. Many reports have dealt with sociological and legal problems arising from the use of dependence-producing drugs, especially by young people. As public concern about drug-related problems increased, so also has governmental support for studies on drug addiction, particularly studies of a basic or clinical nature. Today there are hundreds of investigators in the United States and abroad, examining various aspects of the abuse of drugs such as the opiate narcotics, depressants and stimulants. Fortunately, the growth of important new knowledge about drug abuse has paralleled the growth in numbers of investigators.

One basic aim of bio-medical studies of drug dependence is an understanding of the mechanisms of drug action in animals and man, and of the phenomena of tolerance and dependence. In considering the mechanisms of opiate actions, one may ask: where are the sites of drug accumulation, and how are these sites related to those associated with pharmacological activity of the drugs; are there specific receptors for opiates in the central nervous system and elsewhere, and are there nonspecific drug receptors which also can produce biological actions; can opiates be considered unnatural neurohormones for receptors for which natural ligands also exist? Many reports presented in this text have addressed these questions. Despite different methodologies, studies on the sites for specific anatomical accumulation and for pharmacological activity have resulted in general agreement that the sites are the same. Another area of general agreement is that there are specific receptors in nervous tissue for opiates. Evidence has been presented that there are naturally occurring ligands for the "opiate receptor," and that the ligands may be polypeptides. These findings have opened up a new area of research.

Another basic aspect of the mechanisms of drug action involves the reactions following the interaction of drug with receptor: transduction of the receptor and subsequent "second messenger" activity. Further evidence for the involvement of neurotransmitters and cyclic nucleotides in the secondary effects of opiates is presented in several chapters.

A bio-medical research area more directly related to the clinical situation is whether chronic use of the opioid, methadone, by pregnant females has any effect on their offspring. Since methadone maintenance therapy is the most popular method of treating heroin abuse, the results of such studies in man and animals can be put into clinical use directly.

The need for this conference on "Tissue Responses to Addictive Drugs" in addition to the many other symposia and conferences on drug dependence that were, or will be held during this year might be questioned. The rapidity with which new information about opiate action is evolving, however, demands many forums, both to disseminate current experimental results to the experienced investigators, and to acquaint newcomers with the state of the art. This conference represents such a forum because it brings together experienced investigators in bio-medical research on drug dependence with newcomers from the discipline of psychoneuroendocrinology and from the geographical area of the conference.

The organizers of this conference are indebted to several agencies for the successful operation of the conference: to the direct sponsor of the conference, the International Society for Psychoneuroendocrinology for encouragement; to the Department of Continuing Education of the Downstate Medical Center, SUNY, Brooklyn, for assistance in planning the Conference; and to the

Downstate Medical Center for providing the excellent facilities for holding the Conference. Financially, assistance was kindly provided by the National Institute on Drug Abuse, HEW (Grant DA-01211) and the National Science Foundation, as well as by Endo Laboratories, Garden City, N. Y., Eli Lilly, Indianapolis, Ind., Charles Pfizer & Co., New York, N. Y., Sandoz, Inc., Hanover, N. J., and Roche Laboratories, Nutley, N. J. Without such cooperation from public and private sources, the conference could not have been held. Both the organizers and the participants therefore wish to express their appreciation for this support.

Contents

CONTENTS

CONTENTS

CONTENTS

CONTENTS

Tissue Responses to Addictive Drugs
© 1976, Spectrum Publications, Inc.

Physiological Disposition of Some Narcotic Drugs in the Central Nervous System

ANAND L. MISRA

New York State Drug Abuse Control Commission
Testing and Research Laboratory
Brooklyn, New York

I. INTRODUCTION

In the last two decades the development of highly sensitive radio-isotopic, gas chromatographic-mass spectrometric, and radioimmunologic techniques for the assay of submicrogram quantities of drugs and their metabolites in biofluids and tissues has considerably extended the scope of many studies on drug dynamics and aided in the accumulation of important information on biological disposition of narcotic drugs. Regardless of the basic mechanism of action of narcotic drugs, they must reach their site of action in the central nervous system (CNS) in adequate concentration to elicit the pharmacologic effect. The intensity and duration of such an effect depends on the maintenance of adequate concentrations of these drugs at receptor sites in the CNS. The common overall structural features of narcotic drugs, the important role of stereochemical factors on potency, specificity of antagonism with

1

structurally related antagonists and the fact that analgesic doses (ED_{50}) of a variety of narcotic drugs are much lower after intraventricular and intracisternal than after systemic injection, provide evidence of specific receptors in the CNS. The concentration of narcotic drugs at receptor sites however cannot be conveniently determined, consequently the measurements of drug levels in the CNS or its selected anatomic areas have had to suffice.

The passage of drugs into the CNS and their exit therefrom depend on the properties of the blood-brain-cerebrospinal fluid (CSF) system and the physicochemical parameters of the drug. This chapter covers a general discussion of these areas and newer information on the physiological disposition and pharmacokinetics of some narcotic drugs in the CNS. Some earlier literature on biological disposition and metabolism of narcotic drugs cited in the reviews of Way and Adler (1962), Mellett and Woods (1963), Way (1968a), Mulé (1971), and Misra (1972) has been alluded to for the sake of continuity of discussion.

ANATOMIC BASIS OF BLOOD, BRAIN, AND CSF BARRIERS

Blood-brain barrier

Although brain accounts for only 2% of the body weight, it receives nearly 17% of the total cardiac output and consumes 20% of the oxygen used by the whole body at rest. The cerebral white matter has a much lower blood supply than the gray matter (Kety, 1960). Recent studies by Oldendorf and Davson (1967) and Levin et al. (1970) indicate that the CNS has an extracellular space of 10–20%, of the same order as the mean extracellular space of the entire body. The mechanism by which many substances carried in the bloodstream are excluded from the CNS is generally referrred to as the blood-brain barrier (BBB). Previous studies of Rall and Zubrod (1962), Rall (1971), and Oldendorf (1974a) have shown that the blood-brain barrier is based upon a continuous layer of tight junctioned endothelial cells which block intercellular passage of drugs. This and the absence of pinocytosis are two important structural features of the CNS capillaries (Crone and Thompson, 1970). A drug molecule must pass directly through the lumenal endothelial cell membrane, a thin layer of cytoplasm, and an outer cell membrane to gain access to the interstitial fluid (See Fig. 1). Permeation of these two membranes determines the permeability of BBB. The permeability characteristics of brain capillary endothelium is similar to those of cell membranes in other parts of the body. Biotransformation

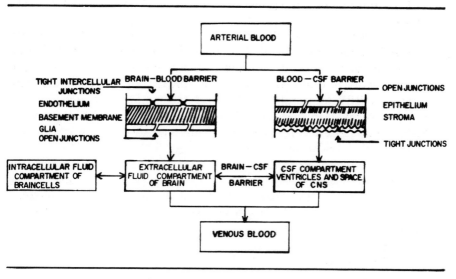

1 Structural and functional relationship of the blood supply, CSF, extracellular and intracellular fluid compartments of brain, and the pathways that a drug can take in the exchange between blood, brain, and CSF. (Adapted from Levine, 1973.)

of some drugs could occur in brain capillary endothelial cytoplasm before they enter the brain extracellular fluid (ECF). Some compounds, e.g., carbohydrates, amino acids, and short chain fatty acids have been reported by Oldendorf 1971) to penetrate BBB by specialized carrier-mediated transport mechanism. After a drug crosses the BBB and gains access to the ECF, it may penetrate various organs of the brain tissue at different rates. Myelin sheaths of nerve fibers in the white matter impede penetration of drugs. Regional differences in penetration of drugs in gray and white matter in the CNS are related to myeliniza-tion and relative vascularity of these areas (Roth and Barlow, 1961). Degree of myelinization, water content in various anatomic areas and biochemical organization in the CNS vary with the age of the animal. Autoradiographic techniques developed by Roth and Barlow (1961) provide important information about the routes of entry, differential dis-tribution, and binding of drugs to neuronal elements in the CNS. Localization of narcotic drugs in CNS and other tissues by auto-radiographic techniques has been studied by Miller and Elliott (1955), Mellett and Woods (1959), Hug and Mellett (1963), Teschemacher et al.

(1968), Matsumota and Takahashi (1970), and Appelgren and Terenius (1973).

A decrease in sensitivity to morphine analgesia and lethality which occurred in rats from about 2 to 4 weeks (Jóhannesson and Becker, 1973) and an increase in the ratio of morphine concentration in blood to brain with age (Kupferberg and Way, 1963) were due to the development of a BBB to morphine. The BBB to morphine reportedly (Way, 1968) developed 16 days after birth in rats. On the CNS side of the BBB, diffusional exchange occurred readily between various areas of the brain and the cerebrospinal fluid.

Nonspecific penetration of some narcotic drugs could also occur into potential sites which are without BBB (area postrema in the medulla or part of the floor of the hypothalamus) and some pharmacological effects may be mediated through this entry (Oldendorf 1974b).

Blood-CSF relationships

Most of the CSF is continuously secreted by the choroid plexus by a process of active secretion in which Na-K-ATPase plays an essential role. It is contained within the ventricles, flows into the subarachnoid spaces, and ultimately into the blood in the dural sinuses (see Fig. 2). It bathes the surfaces of the brain and the spinal cord and is thus a third fluid compartment within the brain, the other two being extracellular and intracellular fluid compartments. In man, the CSF forms at the rate of 0.3 ml/min and its total volume is 200 ml, so the rate of turnover is approximately 10% per hour (Welch and Friedman, 1960). Its pH is approximately 0.1 unit less than the plasma. It is essentially protein-free and has a lower concentration of K^+, Ca^{2+}, and PO_4^{3-} and a higher concentration of Cl^- as compared to the plasma. To enter CSF from blood, a drug can pass through the open junctions between capillary endothelial cells through the basement membrane and stroma and then directly through the continuous tight junctions of choroidal epithelial cells (see Fig. 1). Finally the drug entering by blood-CSF barrier must pass through an additional brain- CSF barrier in order to reach the extracellular fluid compartment of the brain. Many drugs such as N-methyl morphine, which cannot penetrate the BBB and have little effect on the CNS after systemic injection, produced striking pharmacological effects after intraventricular injection because drugs in CSF diffuse readily into brain interstitial ECF (Feldberg, 1963; Foster et al., 1967). The rate of entry into brain by such routes however depended on the molecular size (compounds with high molecular weight

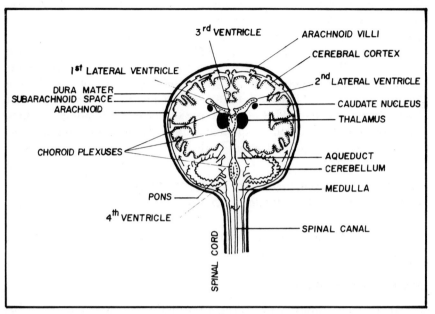

2

Pathways of CSF flow (indicated by arrows) from ventricles to cerebral and spinal subarachnoid space.

entered slowly), charge, lipid solubility, and regional differences in capillaries at different places.

Passage of drugs from CSF into blood was only partly dependent on molecular size or lipid solubility, and even compounds with low lipid solubility left the CSF almost as rapidly as those with high lipid solubility after intracisternal injection. Active transport of narcotic drugs by the choroid plexus may be responsible for the apparent blood- CSF barrier to these compounds and for their rapid disappearance from CSF when they are injected directly into this fluid. Maintenance of a low CSF concentration of morphine-like drugs would permit the CSF to act as a "sink" for diffusion of these drugs out of the brain tissue (Wang and Takemori, 1972; Asghar and Way, 1970). The CSF levels of morphine have been shown to be lower than those in brain or plasma (Mulé and Woods, 1962). Isolated choroid plexus tissue *in vitro* also accumulated narcotic drugs by active transport against a concentration gradient (Takemori and Stenwick, 1966; Hug, 1967; Huang and Takemori, 1975). This transport was not altered by chronic treatment of animals with morphine and it was concluded by Craig et al. (1971) that carrier-mediated transport systems for morphine in choroid plexus did not play a role in the development of tolerance to morphine. The choroid plexus does not transport morphine-3-glucuronide by an active process (Muraki, 1971).

Recent work (Kutter et al., 1970; Kayan et al., 1970; Seeman et al., 1972; Teller et al., 1974) has established that active transport, as previously described (Scrafani and Hug, 1968), is not involved in the uptake of morphine and its analogues into brain slices and that lipophilicity, passive diffusion, and physicochemical binding of these drugs to brain tissue could adequately explain the accumulation of drugs in tissue against a concentration gradient.

FACTORS DETERMINING THE RATE OF DRUG PENETRATION INTO BRAIN AND CSF

Various physicochemical parameters determine the rate of entry of a drug through the blood-brain barrier.

Degree of ionization

The rate of transfer of a drug from plasma to the brain is proportional to the concentration of the unionized lipid soluble form of the drug. Many drugs are either weak bases or weak acids, i.e., they are partly ionized at a physiological pH. The relative proportions of ionized and unionized forms of acidic or basic drugs can be calculated from the Henderson-Hasselbach equation, if the pH of the solution and the dissociation constant (pK_a) of the drug is known. For an acid,

$$pK_a = pH + \log \frac{[\text{unionized}]}{[\text{ionized}]}$$

and for a base,

$$pK_a = pH + \log \frac{[\text{ionized}]}{[\text{unionized}]}.$$

Drugs can undergo considerable change in ionization with the slight shift of blood pH generally encountered in respiratory and metabolic acid-base imbalances. The penetration of the CNS will therefore be increased for basic narcotic drugs at a slightly alkaline pH. An acidic pH will produce a higher concentration of ionized species of narcotic drugs and consequently a lower level in the CNS.

Lipid Solubility

Lipid solubility plays a major role in determining the rate of penetration of drugs into BBB and CSF. Apparent partition coefficients of narcotic drugs (or the rank order in a series of compounds) at 37°C in 1-octanol, heptane, benzene, and buffers of pH's which span the range of attainable human physiological pH values provide a good measure of lipid solubility (Misra et al., 1974c). An attempt was made in a recent study by Oldendorf (1974c) to correlate the lipid (olive oil)/ buffer partition coefficients of some drugs with their uptake in brain following carotid arterial injection. When this partition coefficient was greater than about 0.03, a substantial fraction of the drugs penetrated the BBB and for most drugs above this range, uptake was essentially complete. The highly lipophilic compound, heroin, easily passes the BBB; is deacetylated to 6-mono-acetyl morphine and to morphine in the brain, which mediates the pharmacological effects of heroin (Way, 1967).

The importance of lipid solubility for permeation of narcotic drugs into the brain has been outlined by Herz and Teschemacher (1971). Lipophilic compounds reached the brain in much higher concentrations than did hydrophilic ones. A good correlation also existed between duration of antinociceptive effect and lipid solubility of narcotic drugs when equipotent doses of drugs were administered intraventricularly. Morphine had a much longer action by this route compared to synthetic lipophilic narcotics such as methadone and pethidine (Herz and Teschemacher, 1971). This negative correlation could be explained by these authors on the basis of pharmacokinetic differences between two groups of compounds. Considerations of affinity and intrinsic activity of drugs at receptor sites therefore are more important determinants of pharmacological potency of narcotic drugs.

Protein binding

The rate of diffusion of drugs across the BBB is proportional to the concentration of the free drug. It is important therefore to ascertain the degree of binding of narcotic drugs at normal body temperature and plasma pH. Plasma protein and tissue binding of drugs has been covered in recent reviews by Mayer and Guttman (1968) and Gillette (1971, 1973). Although albumin is the major plasma protein which binds, drugs may also be bound to antibodies in the gamma globulin fraction. Thus, treatment of rabbits with morphine covalently bound to serum albumin has been shown by Spector and Parker (1970) and Spector (1971) to evoke the formation of antibodies that bind morphine and its analogues. The state of ionization of a drug can alter its affinity for plasma protein binding sites and competition for these sites may result in displacement of one drug by another, with consequent rise in

Table I. Binding of Some Narcotic Drugs with Plasma Proteins *In Vitro*

Drugs*	Mean percentage of drugs bound
[14C] Morphine[a]	34 – 37.5
Heroin[b]	20 – 39
[3H] Thebaine[c]	66.7
[3H] Methadone[d]	83.7 – 87.3
Pethidine[e]	40
Levorphanol[f]	50
[14C] Nalorphine[g]	57.3
[14C] Naloxone[g]	68.3

[a]Olsen, 1975, [b]Cohn et al., 1974, [c]Misra et al., 1974.

[d]Olsen, 1973, [e]Burns et al., 1955, [f]Shore et al, 1955.

[g]Misra et al., 1975c.

unbound concentration of the first drug in plasma and in the CNS (Christensen, 1959). Melanin granules in eyes and skin, nucleoproteins, adipose tissue, fat, phospholipids in intracellular organelles, and plasma membranes may also be responsible for accumulation of some drugs in certain tissues. Methadone has been shown by Robinson and Williams (1971) and Misra et al. (1973a, 1974a) to accumulate in a high concentration in the lungs of humans and experimental animals. Accumulation or peristence of certain narcotic drugs, e.g., morphine and methadone, in the brain reported by Misra et al. (1971) and Misra and Mulé (1972) implies an interaction between these drugs and some specific anatomic structure in the CNS or a metabolic conversion to a nonpermeable form of the drug. Binding of drugs to plasma or tissue proteins invariably increases the half-life of the drugs. It is also important to point out that tissue binding and active transport of drugs frequently have certain characteristics in common, e.g., saturability and competition among the analogues of drug.

A correlation has been observed between binding of drugs to proteins and their lipid solubility. The percentage of binding increased with the increase in lipid solubility (Höllt and Teschemacher, 1972) suggesting a hydrophobic interaction between drug and protein. (Data on plasma protein binding of some narcotic drugs are given in Table I.)

SPECIFIC FEATURES OF NARCOTIC DRUGS

Many narcotic drugs have certain specific features in common.

Basic nitrogen function

The majority of narcotic drugs have a tertiary nitrogen function although some pharmacologically active nor-metabolites of narcotic drugs have secondary and primary amine groups (methadone and LAAM metabolites). The pK_a of a number of narcotic drugs generally ranges between 7.8–9.6, which corresponds to the bases being 86–99.6% ionized as cations at pH 7.2. Narcotic drugs with a pK_a at the lower end of this range should be able to enter the CNS more readily than those with a pK_a near the upper limit. Extensive protonation of narcotic drugs at physiological pH permits formation of electrostatic bonds between the cationic center of a drug and the anionic center of the receptor. The degree of ionization of narcotic drug and the steric dimensions of the basic group therefore influence the affinity of these drugs for the receptor site (Beckett, 1956; Casy, 1973). Conceivably carboxylic acid groups (dibasic amino acids, pK_a 3.86–4.07), sulfhydryl groups or phosphatidic acids (pK_a 3.5–4.0) could fulfill the requirements of adequate negativity for attracting the cationic head of the narcotic drugs. Phosphatidic acids (phosphoinositide) have been proposed as carriers for Na^+ ions (Hokin and Hokin, 1958) and interaction of narcotic drugs with these groups could also disrupt normal Na^+ transport.

Aromatic features

All pharmacologically active narcotic drugs have at least one aromatic ring which permits the molecule to bind with the flat portion of the receptor surface comprising the amino acid residues of the protein by van der Waal forces (Casy, 1973).

Oxygen function

In polycyclic narcotic drugs, e.g., morphine, levorphanol, nalorphine, naloxone, etc., the presence of a phenolic group provides an additional binding site to the receptor surface through H bonding. Although in methadone and LAAM, this group is not an essential requirement, the presence of a secondary alcohol group in methadols permits formation of similar but somewhat weaker bonds with the receptor surface.

Stereochemical features

Narcotic drugs which exist as two or more optically active enantio-morphs are known to exert their pharmacological activity exclusively or preponderantly in one configuration, the levo isomers are more active than the dextro isomers. (Stereoselective differences observed by the author in the case of isomers of 3-hydroxy N-methyl morphinan and methadone will be described later in the text.)

Interesting topographical models (Beckett and Casy, 1954) and variants involving multiple uptake modes of interaction of known analgesics with hypothetical "opiate receptor" (Portoghese, 1965, 1966) have been proposed, but it is not known whether the receptor has (have) a rigid structure possessing high stereoselectivity or a confor-mationally labile structure (Mautner, 1967) capable of adapting to a variety of narcotic agonists or antagonists. Much effort is currently being expended on this challenging area of inquiry.

METABOLISM OF NARCOTIC DRUGS

The different metabolic pathways for narcotic drugs have been described in earlier reviews (Way and Adler, 1962; Way, 1968a; Misra, 1972). These could be summarized as follows:

  (a) Conjugation of phenolic and hydroxyl groups with glucuronic acid in several mammalian species, ethereal sulfate conjugation predominantly in cat and chicken;
  (b) N- and O- dealkylation to the corresponding nor-compounds;
  (c) Hydrolysis of ester groups (pethidine and heroin);
  (d) Hydroxylation (methadone, morphine, levallorphan);
  (e) Keto group reduction (methadone, naloxone, naltrexone);
  (f) N-oxidation (morphine, pethidine, and methadone); and
  (g) Acetylation of primary and secondary amine groups (bisnor-methadol).

EXCRETION OF NARCOTIC DRUGS

Detailed aspects on excretion of narcotic drugs have been covered in earlier reviews (Way and Adler, 1962; Way, 1968a; Misra, 1972). Renal and bilary excretion are prime pathways for several narcotic drugs. Pulmonary excretion and excretion via saliva and perspiration (of metha-done) are minor routes.

PHYSIOLOGICAL DISPOSITION OF NARCOTIC AGONISTS AND ANTAGONISTS IN THE CNS

Morphine

Previous studies on the biological disposition of morphine (pK_a, 8.05) in several species have been reviewed by Way and Adler (1962), Way (1968a), Misra (1972). Recent studies on rats by Abrams and Elliott (1974), Berkowitz et al. (1974a,b), Klutch (1974), and on man by Brunk and Delle (1974) and Yeh (1975) have provided additional information on metabolism and disposition of this drug.

There is general agreement that (a) tolerance to morphine develops with marked rapidity apparently with the very first dose (Martin and Fraser, 1961; Cochin and Kornetsky, 1964; Kornetsky and Bain, 1968, Lomax and Kirkpatrick, 1967); and (b) the cerebrospinal axis and the matrix of the central nervous system is critically involved in the genesis of tolerance to and physical dependence on morphine. Alterations of absorption, metabolism, and excretion could not be involved in tolerance development as even large intravenous doses of morphine will not produce death in tolerant persons. In view of the fact that neurons have high protein output and little mitotic activity, it is essential to know the acute effects of morphine which induce a biochemical or adaptive change in appropriate neuronal structure leading to a decreased sensitivity or response to the opiate. Our study on the kinetics of distribution of morphine-N-methyl-^{14}C (Misra et al., 1971) following an analgesic 10 mg/kg s.c. dose (See Fig. 3) in the rats showed that although the levels of free morphine and their decline ($T^{1/2}=1.2$ hr) could be correlated with duration of analgesia, there was consistently higher radioactivity in the brain than could be accounted for on the basis of free morphine alone. Measurable and significant amounts of the drug were present as polar conjugated drug. Part of this radioactivity was due to the pharmacologically inactive morphine-3-glucuronide and the rest due to a conjugate which was not hydrolyzable by relatively harsh chemical procedures. Studies with [^{3}H] morphine in our laboratory gave similar results. Repeated extractions of the brain of rats injected subcutaneously with a 10 mg/kg dose of [^{3}H] morphine by homogenization in 0.5 N HCl and basification to pH 9.5 with chloroform-isopropanol (3:1 v/v) removed all loosely bound morphine. A significant portion of radioactivity[*] however remained bound to the brain debris even after

[*]This bound radioactivity was gradually released on repeated treatment with aqueous Triton X-100 solution.

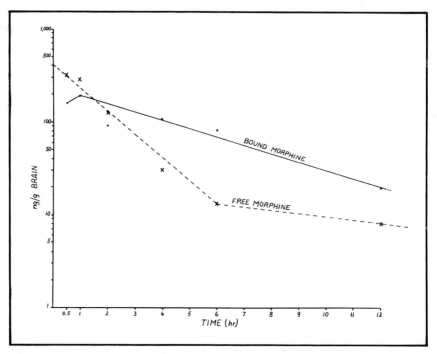

3 Uptake of morphine-N-methyl--^{14}C by rat brain at different times after a single 10 mg/kg subcutaneous injection. Dotted lines represent decay of free morphine and solid lines the decay of bound morphine (Data from Misra et al., 1971.)

repeated extractions or washouts with water, alcohol, and ether. Such a treatment would effectively remove all morphine bound to lipids or proteolipids. This persistent and firm association of radioactivity suggests a firm binding of morphine or its metabolite to some specific intracellular constituent in the brain (probably protein or glycoprotein of cell membrane). *In vitro* binding of morphine to brain and serum proteins is of the weak electrostatic type and easily dissociable with shifts of pH to the acidic side or on prolonged dialysis. Although the exact nature of this binding is not known, it is possible that a part of it could be covalent in nature. The possibilities of conjugation of morphine to a protein through sulfhydryl groups at (a) 7,8-position either by activation of 6-alcoholic group to a ketone (Misra and Woods, 1970) or through an intermediate epoxide formation at 7,8 double bond; (b) through intermediate quinone formation at 3-position; and (c) through the 2,3-catechol type of derivative have been suggested earlier (Misra

, et al., 1971). Coupling interactions of enzyme generated catechols or quinones and amino or -SH groups of proteins to form N- or S- catecholyl or quinonoid proteins have been reported (Mason, 1955) to take place easily.

Evidence has been presented recently for the formation *in vitro* of a 2,3-catechol type of metabolite of morphine by rat brain homogenates. Sequential oxidation of morphine by alkaline ferricyanide and hydrogen peroxide and copper ions has been shown to generate a zwitterionic 2, 3-morphine quinone (Misra et al., 1973c). This quinone possessed potent stimulant properties on intracisternal administration and in equal doses (0.5 mg/kg) could override the depressant effects of morphine injected by the same route (Misra et al., 1974e). Due to the highly polar character, the quinone was pharmacologically inactive by systemic routes of administration.

Persistent binding of morphine or its metabolite could bring about a biochemical alteration in structure and geometry of specific neuronal proteins in the CNS and could also produce hyperexcitability if the site of attachment happens to be one in which a neurotransmitter interaction is also involved. Dissociation of drug molecules from the specific protein would depend on its turnover in the CNS. The turnover of cerebral proteins differs with brain region but has a half-life of approximately 15 days in adult rats (Waelsch and Lajtha, 1961) compared to 2.2 days in young rats. Berkowitz et al. (1974a) have shown that brain and plasma levels of morphine in older rats were much higher than those in younger rats after i.v. injection. Persistence of morphine in the plasma of rats with a T½ of 7-9 days has also been observed by these workers after removal of a morphine pellet in chronic animals.

It is not yet clear whether (a) morphine itself is an inducer of changes in protein synthesis in the CNS; or (b) some other morphine effected change in state of postsynaptic membranes has inductive consequences, which changes the biochemical nature of membranes, making them hyperexcitable after chronic morphine treatment. Narcotic drugs have been reported to be localized in synaptic vesicles and nerve ending membranes in the CNS (Clouet and Williams, 1973; Terenius, 1973; Wong and Horng, 1973; Pert et al., 1974; Mulé et al., 1974), and although these synaptic structures are rich in sialic acids (which occur in these membranes as sialoglycolipids or sialoglycoproteins) no difference in whole brain sialic acid level in tolerant rates compared to the saline control group was observed in a recent study (Misra et al., 1974b). A significant increase in plasma sialic acid, however, occurred in tolerant rats, as compared to the acute animals Similarly no changes were observed in amount or rate of synthesis of specific proteins in tolerant mice brains (Hahn and Goldstein, 1971). Small changes in protein content of synaptic membranes in brain however cannot be ruled out.

Development of tolerance to morphine can be blocked by protein synthesis inhibitors (Way et al., 1968; Cox and Osman, 1970; Feinberg and Cochin, 1972). Recent work by Cox et al., (1975) showed a biphasic pattern of recovery of response to morphine analgesia in tolerant rats and mice, a fast phase and a slow phase with a mean T½ of 13.2 days in rats and 17.4 days in mice, the latter implying a reversal of the drug-induced metabolic disturbance. Studies on the inhibition of protein synthesis in rat liver by cycloheximide (Munro et al., 1968) have shown that the site of action presumably involved -SH sensitive or dependent enzyme transferase. This may indirectly suggest that the -SH groups of the target protein in the CNS are in someway involved in the inter-action with morphine. The modes of this interaction and nature of protein or peptide involved are not yet clear.

Although the presence of circulating antibodies to morphine in plasma of passively immunized mice has been reported (Berkowitz et al., 1974b) to lead to a decreased brain concentration of morphine and alteration in the disposition of this drug, the involvement of immune factors in the genesis of tolerance to morphine has yet to be established.

Several new approaches in the area of analgesia, tolerance, and dependence have yielded fascinating possibilities, but the precise mechanisms still remain obscure.

Heroin (3,6-diacetyl morphine)

Heroin (pK$_a$ 7.83) is rapidly hydrolyzed to 6-monoacetyl morphine (6 MAM) and to a lesser extent to morphine by tissue homogenates and blood of experimental animals in vitro and in vivo (Way et al., 1960, 1965). It probably survives as heroin only the 10–15 sec required to reach the CNS in humans after i.v. injection. Earlier studies of Way et al (1960, 1965) showed that following a 37.5 mg/kg dose by i.v. injection in the rat, levels of heroin, 6 MAM, and morphine in brain 2.5 min postinjection were 8.2, 23, and less than 2 μg/g, respectively. At 7.5 min, heroin was barely detectable in brain but morphine concentrations reached a peak level of 5 μg/g 15–30 min postinjection with a concomitant drop in levels of 6 MAM. It was concluded by Way (1967) that the pharmacological effects of heroin are mediated primarily by 6 MAM and morphine. Recent studies by Oldendorf et al. (1972) on the comparative uptake of some narcotic drugs after carotid injection in the rat showed a very rapid penetration of the BBB and an uptake by the brain of heroin, which probably became limited by the regional flow of blood within 10–20 sec after i.v. injection. This rapid entry into the brain was suggested to be a factor in "flush effect" and intractable addiction to this compound. Studies on the metabolism of heroin by continuous i.v. infusion in man (Elliott et al., 1971) showed that approximately 6 mg of heroin per hr could be metabolized by a 90 kg man. Comparative studies in heroin-treated and nontreated rats by Cohn et al. (1973) showed that treated animals maintained a relatively steady concentration of heroin 0–20 min postinjection while an immediate drop in heroin levels within 2 min occurred in nontreated control rats. In addition to free 6 MAM and morphine, conjugated morphine and 6 MAM, normorphine and conjugated normorphine have recently been shown to be the metabolites of heroin in man (Yeh et al., 1976).

Pethidine (meperidine)

Meperidine (pK$_a$ 8.72) is the most widely used obstetrical analgesic. Earlier studies of Way et al. (1949) showed peak levels of 17 μg/g in rat brain following 100 mg/kg s.c. injection. Plotnikoff et al. (1952) also observed a level of approximately 12 μg/g in the cerebrum following a 125 mg/kg dose of [N-methyl-^{14}C] meperidine. Burns et al. (1955) observed levels of 11.3 μg/g in brains of dogs administered a 20 mg/kg i.v. dose of the drug and in man peak plasma levels occurred 1–2 hr after a 150 mg dose. Meperidine is known to be metabolized to normeperidine, meperidinic acid, normeperidinic acid, and conjugates of these hydrolysis products (Way et al., 1949; Plotnikoff et al., 1952; Burns et al., 1955). N-oxidation of meperidine has recently been shown to be an additional route of metabolism (Mitchard et al., 1972). Normeperidine can penetrate the CNS and was shown to be more toxic than meperidine (Miller and Anderson, 1954) but none of the other metabolites had significant analgesic activity. No information is available on the pharmacokinetics of normeperidine which may contribute significantly to some pharmacological effects of meperidine. Increased capacity to inactivate meperidine was not a factor in tolerance development to this drug in man (Burns et al., 1955). Highly sensitive and specific gas chromatographic methods have recently been developed (Chan et al., 1974; Mather and Tucker, 1974) for the determination of meperidine and its metabolites in biological fluids and its distribution in maternal and fetal plasma (O'Donoghue, 1974). A good correlation between mean plasma levels of meperidine with response has been observed in women during labor following intramuscular injection. Plasma levels of meperidine after i.m. or i.v. injection in patients over 70 years of age were about twice those in patients under 30 years, and

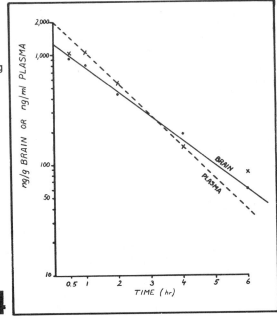

Distribution of thebaine in rat brain (solid line) and plasma (dotted line) following a 5 mg/kg (free base) dose of [³H] thebaine by s.c. injection. (Data from Misra et al., 1974c.)

the dosage of meperidine in elderly patients has to be reduced because of their higher sensitivity to the respiratory depressant effects of this drug. Increasing age was also associated with an increasing fraction of unbound meperidine in plasma (Mather et al., 1975). Increasing alcohol consumption was found to be associated with increasing volumes of distribution of meperidine (lower initial plasma levels); a result possibly related to the generalized vasodilatation as a result of alcohol intake, making these heavy drinkers more refractory to this CNS depressant (Mather et al., 1975). Metabolism of meperidine however was not shown to be impaired by chronic alcohol intake.

Thebaine

Thebaine (pK_a 8.15), a congener of morphine is primarily a CNS stimulant with only slightly depressant and analgesic activity in experimental animals. In higher doses, it produces strychnine-like convulsions in experimental animals while reportedly producing neither physical dependence nor tolerance to its convulsant effects (Seevers and Woods, 1953; Seevers, 1958).

Following a 5 mg/kg s.c. injection in the rat, peak concentrations of 937 ng/g occurred in brain at 0.5 hr (See Fig. 4) and brain to plasma ratio of mean concentrations was 0.92 (Misra et al., 1973b, 1974c). Peak levels of morphine and the brain to plasma ratio with an identical dose by the same route were 179 ng/g and 0.18, respectively (Jóhannesson and Woods, 1964). Greater lipid solubility of thebaine as compared to morphine gives rise to higher concentrations in the brain. Thebaine had a faster rate of penetration into and egression from the CNS than morphine and its levels were not sustained as long as those of morphine. It did not persist in brain for prolonged periods. The rise and fall of CNS levels of thebaine in brain coincided roughly with any change of levels in plasma and suggested three alternative possibilities: (a) thebaine was present in the CNS in the interstitial compartment; (b) its penetration and efflux out of the cell must be fast; and (c) any significant extra- or intracellular binding in the CNS must be freely reversible. With a 5 mg/kg s.c. dose of thebaine, minor metabolites of thebaine, e.g., norcodeine, normorphine, codeine, and morphine, were observed in rat brain 45 min after injection, but no significant persistence or accumulation of these metabolites was observed in pooled brain samples after 48 to 96 hr. Repeated administration of thebaine, however, could lead to some accumulation in the brain of these minor metabolites which may be responsible for the low grade dependence recently reported in the monkey (Yanagita, 1974).

Levorphanol and Dextrorphan

Earlier studies on the biological disposition of the levo isomer, levorphanol, have been reviewed by Way and Adler (1962) and Misra (1972).

Levorphanol (pK$_a$ 9.2) closely resembles morphine in its pharmacological action, respiratory effects, tolerance, and physical dependence liability. In contrast, the d-isomer, dextrorphan, is devoid of these properties and comparatively less toxic than the l-isomer. Although the l-isomer was reported to be N-dealkylated 2 to 3 times faster than the d-isomer (Axelrod, 1956), previous work on the metabolism and excretion of these isomers did not reveal significant differences (Fisher and Long, 1953; Shore et al., 1955). Our data (Misra et al., 1974d) on the comparative pharmacokinetic profiles of these two isomers in rat brain and plasma following a 5 mg/kg s.c. dose is shown in Figure 5. A reasonably good correlation existed between peak concentrations of the l-isomer in brain and analgesia. Plasma concentrations of l-isomer were consistently higher than those of the d-isomer. Small but detectable levels of levorphanol persisted in the rat brain for prolonged periods even though levels were not detectable in plasma 24 hr after injection. Dextrorphan initially attained higher levels than the l-isomer in brain

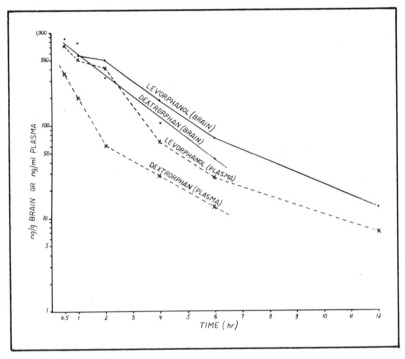

5 Comparative distribution of [³H] levorphanol and [N-Me-¹⁴C] dextrorphan in rat brain (solid lines) and plasma (dotted lines) after a single 5 mg/kg (free base) dose by s.c. injection. (Data from Misra et al., 1974d.)

(0.5 and 1 hr) but disappeared much more rapidly from the CNS at subsequent times. Brain to plasma ratios for dextrorphan were consistently higher than those of levorphanol, up to 4 hr, and the T½ of l- and d-isomer in the rat brain were 2.1 and 1.2 hr; that in plasma 1.2 and 0.6 hr, respectively. The T½ in rat plasma for levorphanol was close to the 1.2–1.5 hr value reported by Woods et al (1958) in the dog and monkey. The differences in T½ of l- and d-isomers suggested differential rates of metabolism for the two isomers. Earlier lower levels of the l-isomer in brain may be due to a slower absorption due to its profound pharmacological effects resulting in a possible decrease in blood flow and a slow rate of entry into the CNS. Slower efflux of l-isomer would give rise to its sustained levels and longer lasting effects. Levels of levorphanol in rat brain at peak times were approximately three times those of morphine with the same dose and route of injection. Significant differences were also observed (Misra et al., 1974d) in rates of elimination of the 2 isomers due to the faster metabolism of the d-isomer. Comparatively higher N-dealkylation of the l-isomer agreed with previous findings of Axelrod (1956), but there were no significant differences in plasma protein binding of the 2 isomers. Differential metabolic pathways and slower biotransformation of the l-isomer would account for its longer lasting effects. Higher toxicity of the l-isomer may possibly be due to retention of levorphanol and norlevorphanol in tissues on repeated administration. In contrast, rapid biotransformation and elimination of the d-isomer would not allow a critical accumulation in tissues.

Our studies also showed significant differences in affinity of binding of these 2-isomers *in vitro* with rat brain proteolipids, the binding with d-isomer being completely reversible; with levorphanol 5–10% of the radioactivity was firmly bound to the proteolipids. Recent studies of Richter and Goldstein (1970) have shown that brain tolerance to the l-isomer represented a decreased sensitivity to the drug at cellular and subcellular sites in the CNS. Furthermore, stereospecific binding of levorphanol to certain mouse brain fractions represented only 2% of total association of drug with this tissue, the rest being mostly nonspecific binding (Goldstein et al., 1971). Binding material according to these authors had the characteristics of a proteolipid. This binding with levorphanol remained intact even after 70% extraction of proteins with Triton X-100, but chloroform-methanol (2:1) broke down this binding. These studies (Pal et al., 1973) implied that the stereospecific binding material in brain represented "opiate receptors." Recent studies of Tremblay et al. (1974) have shown that cerebroside may be falsely identified as a soluble "brain specific protein," and other studies by Loh et al. (1974) have indicated similarities between cerebroside sulfate and the purified "opiate receptor" from the mouse brain reported earlier to have the characteristics of a proteolipid. Spectrospecific binding of narcotics to brain cerebroside sulfate (Loh et al., 1974) implies that endogenous glycolipids may play a role in narcotic drug-receptor interaction.

Methadone

Levo methadone

Earlier studies on methadone have been discussed in reviews of Way and Adler (1962), Way (1968a), and Misra (1972). Recently isolated substituted pyrrolidine and pyrroline metabolites of methadone (Beckett et al., 1968; Pohland et al., 1971; Beckett et al., 1971a,b; Robinson and Williams, 1971; Inturrisi and Verebely 1972; Sullivan and

Blake, 1972) have been found to be pharmacologically inactive. N-Oxidation (Beckett et al., 1972) and formation of hydroxylated pyrrolidine and pyrroline metabolites (Sullivan et al., 1972) have recently been identified as important metabolic pathways of methadone in both man and rat. Our studies (Misra et al., 1973a, 1974a) have provided evidence in addition for the presence of p-hydroxylated mono- and bis-normethadols and their conjugated metabolites in rat and dog.

The levo isomer of methadone (pK_a 8.25, 8.99) is approximately 20 times as potent as the d-isomer depending on the animal species and test employed. Levels of 1-methadone in rat brain at the time of peak analgesia, following 10 mg/kg s.c. injection were approximately 14 times that of morphine (324 ng/g) using the same dose and route, and the brain to plasma ratio of methadone 0.5 hr after injection was 2.15 compared to 0.18 with morphine (Misra et al., 1973a). These differences arose due to the greater lipid solubility of methadone as compared to morphine. Lower values of methadone were consistently observed in brain and plasma of methadone-tolerant as compared to nontolerant rats at all time periods after 10 mg/kg s.c. injections (See Fig. 6) and indicated a clear difference in the penetration and egression of drug from the CNS between the two groups. The lower T½ in brain and plasma of tolerant as compared to nontolerant rats reflected a higher rate of metabolism in tolerant animals and the differences in brain to plasma ratios suggested an altered distribution of drug in the two groups.

With a 50 mg/kg oral dose of methadone in rats, higher levels resulted in brain and plasma of tolerant animals at 0.5–1 hr, but these values dropped to levels lower than those in the nontolerant group at later times (Misra et al., 1973a), indicating a faster rate of egression of the drug from the tissues and plasma of tolerant rats.

Differences in the rates of egression of methadone from the plasma and CNS of rats and dogs indicated extensive intracellular distribution and binding of methadone in the CNS (Misra et al., 1973a; Misra et al., 1974a). In both species methadone persisted in the CNS long after it disappeared from the plasma. Significant amounts of the drug were present in the brain 3 weeks after a single injection in both rat and dog or after oral administration in the rat (Misra and Mulé 1972; Misra et al., 1974a). Persistence of drug in CNS was similar to that observed with morphine (Misra et al., 1971). In addition to methadone, evidence was obtained for the presence in brain of a p-hydroxylated bis-normethadol type of metabolite. Persistence of methadone in the CNS presumably involved, in addition to van der Waal's-London forces, association of the keto group of methadone with terminal amino groups of proteins. This persistence in the CNS is consistent with the postulate

Comparative distribution of
1-methadone-1-^{3}H in brain
and plasma of nontolerant
(white bar) and tolerant (black
bar) rats after subcutaneous
injection (10 mg/kg as free
base). (Data from Misra
et al., 1973a)

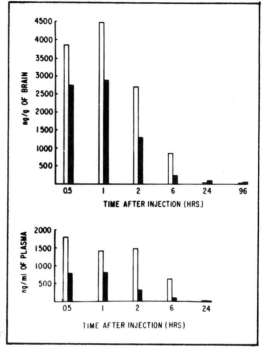

6

that methadone gains access to an intracellular neuronal site. The firm
attachment to some intracellular constituent results in its slow diffusion
out of the drug-sensitive cell lasting over a period of weeks. Prolonged
occupation of intracellular receptor sites by methadone and its metabolites could conceivably alter the biochemical nature of this site resulting in a reduced sensitivity of this target site to the drug. These studies
provided evidence that the pharmacological tolerance to methadone
arises due to: (a) decreased sensitivity of the target site in the CNS
(functional tolerance); and (b) accelerated metabolism in tolerant animals (dispositional tolerance) (Misra et al., 1973a, 1974a, 1975a; Masten
et al., 1975). Persistence of methadone and its metabolite in the brain
and prolonged occupation of target sites in the CNS may, in addition
have relevance to the mild withdrawal syndrome observed with methadone. Faster metabolism in tolerant dogs (Misra et al., 1975a) and
rats (Misra et al., 1973) did not allow accumulation of methadone in
the CNS despite its persistence in selected anatomic areas of the CNS.
No differences were observed in the plasma protein electrophoretic profiles of nontolerant and tolerant dogs and similar qualitative pattern of
metabolites was observed in two groups.

The mere presence and persistence of the low levels of methadone and its metabolites in selected areas of the CNS, however does not imply their pharmacological significance. EEG (Khazan and Roehrs, 1973) and single dose tolerance studies (Cochin and Kornetsky, 1964; Lomax and Kirkpatrick, 1967; Kornetsky and Bain, 1968; Jacob and Barthelemy, 1972) have provided evidence for long-lasting effects of opiates. Recent studies on specific binding of [³H] etorphine in synaptic membrane fractions (Mulé et al., 1974) have shown that the amount of etorphine specifically bound (8 X 10⁻¹¹ M) in the membrane fraction was less than 1% of the total etorphine present in brain 10 min after the injection of etorphine. The estimates of analgesic receptor density in rat brain (5 X 10¹⁰ per g.) provided by these studies were therefore markedly lower than the values of methadone persisting in the CNS of dog three weeks after a single administration.

Dextro methadone

Previous studies by Sung and Way (1953) showed that absorption, regional distribution, and metabolism of these two isomers was very similar. Our study on the comparative pharmacokinetics of these two isomers in the rat (Misra and Mulé, 1973) using identical 10 mg/kg s.c. doses suggested that: (1) the stereoselective N-demethylation pathway as previously postulated (Misra and Mulé, 1972) was a preferential route for the l-isomer; (2) significant differences (See Fig. 7) existed in the T½ of l- and d-isomers in the brain (2.4, 1.2 hr) and plasma (3.7, 1.5 hr), respectively; and (3) formation of an apparently active metabolite in the brain was observed with l-isomer but not with d-isomer. *In vitro* liver microsomal (Axelrod, 1956; Dann et al., 1971) and isomeric substrate studies (Beckett et al., 1971b) have shown the stereoselectivity of the N-dealkylation process.

1-α-Acetyl Methadol (LAAM)

Acetyl methadol (pK$_a$ 8.98) is somewhat less basic than methadone. Because of its property of longer duration of action and effective suppression of the opiate withdrawal syndrome for longer periods, LAAM has practical therapeutic advantages over methadone. A dose of 80 mg three times a week has been suggested as a substitute for 100 mg methadone daily. Previous (Sung and Way, 1954; McMahon et al., 1965) and recent studies (Billings et al., 1973, 1974; Nickander et al., 1974) have shown that acetyl normethadol (NAM) and acetyl bisnormethadol (NNAM), the metabolites of LAAM, were considerably

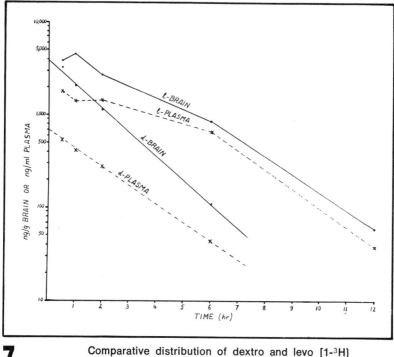

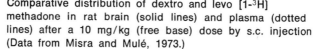

7 Comparative distribution of dextro and levo [1-³H] methadone in rat brain (solid lines) and plasma (dotted lines) after a 10 mg/kg (free base) dose by s.c. injection (Data from Misra and Mulé, 1973.)

more active than LAAM, had great affinity for tissues, and slowly declined in plasma. Methadol and normethadol have also been observed (Kaiko and Inturrisi, 1973) as metabolites of LAAM and possessed significant analgesic activity. N-acetylation of methadol metabolites occurred readily in the rat (Sullivan et al., 1973). Considerable variability in plasma levels of active metabolites of LAAM has been reported during LAAM therapy in addicts (Billings et al., 1974). The distribution of LAAM in the CNS has not been previously studied.

Our recent studies (Misra and Mulé, 1975; Misra et al., 1976) on the disposition of 1-α-[2-³H] acetyl methadol in the monkey have shown that peak plasma levels of the free drug 117–249 ng/ml occurred 1 hr post-injection of a 2 mg/kg s.c. dose, and that these values declined to 3–10 ng/ml after 48 hr. Major excretion of free LAAM occurred in feces and 38–46% of the dose was unaccounted for, probably due to sequestration and very gradual excretion over a prolonged period. Lower peak levels 73–79 ng/ml occurred in plasma 4–6 hr after 2 mg/kg oral administration and 45–55% of the dose was unaccounted for three to four weeks following oral administration. Noracetylmethadol, the N-acetyl derivative of acetyl bisnormethadol and p-hydroxy acetyl bisnormethadol were observed as metabolites in addition to unmetabolized LAAM. Methadol, normethadol, p-hydroxy acetyl bisnormethadol, and p-hydroxy acetyl methadol were present as conjugated metabolites, predominantly as glucuronides.

The levels of free drug (ng/g) in selected anatomic areas of the brain of the monkey 6 hr after administration of a 2 mg/kg oral dose were as follows: temporal cortex (gray) 191; temporal cortex (white) 156; cerebellum 157; spinal cord 119; hypothalamus 170; thalamus 163; medulla 126; pons 137; mesencephalon 150; caudate nucleus 187; and pituitary gland 1918. Adsorption chromatography (Amberlite XAD-2 resin, on monkey brain homogenates by the method previously described (Misra et al., 1973a), and thin layer chromatography (Misra et al., 1975b) provided evidence suggesting the presence in the brain of methadol, acetyl bisnormethadol, p-hydroxy acetyl bisnormethadol and acetyl normethadol in addition to unmetabolized LAAM.

Naloxone and Nalorphine

Naloxone (pK_a 7.94, 9.12) is a "pure opioid antagonist" which abolishes or prevents the pharmacological effects not only of narcotic agonists but also of mixed antagonists-agonists such as nalorphine (pK_a 7.88). Naloxone is about 10–20 times more active than nalorphine in the rat (Blumberg et al., 1961; Blumberg and Dayton, 1973). It has no abuse potential, and is well tolerated and accepted by humans without a tolerance or physical dependence liability. Some information is available on its metabolism and disposition in normal and narcotic-dependent humans (Fujimoto, 1970; Weinstein et al., 1971; Fishman et al., 1973) and experimental animals (Fujimoto, 1969; Ober and Fujimoto, 1972; Weinstein et al., 1973). No information, however, exists on its disposition in the CNS in any species. Earlier studies by Woods (1956), Woods and Muehlenbeck (1957), and Hug and Woods (1963) on nalorphine have provided extensive information on the pharmacokinetics and metabolism of this compound.

Data on the comparative uptake of [14C] naloxone and [14C] nalorphine in the rat brain and plasma after a single 1 or 10 mg/kg s.c. dose are given in Tables II and III (Misra et al., 1976). Rapid attainment of peak levels in brain and plasma occurred with both antagonists within 30 min and the decline (T½) was approximately 24 min for both

Table II. Distribution[a] of [allyl-1′, 3′-^{14}C] Naloxone and [allyl-1′, 3′-^{14}C] Nalorphine in Rat Brain, Plasma and Half-Lives after a 1 mg/kg (free base) Dose by Subcutaneous Injection

	0.25 hr	0.5 hr	1 hr	3 hr	6 hr	16 hr	Half-lives (hr)
[^{14}C] Naloxone							
Brain	506	252	110	17	4	0	0.4
Plasma	119	54	23	7	4	0	0.4
B/P[b]	4.3	4.7	4.8	2.4	1.0	—	—
Plasma (conjugated drug)	213	33	21	2	2	0	—
[^{14}C] Nalorphine							
Brain	212	125	62	8	4	0	0.4
Plasma	169	65	23	9	4	0	0.3
B/P[b]	1.3	1.9	2.7	0.9	1.0	—	—
Plasma (conjugated drug)	116	89	46	45	19	0	—

[a] Data represent mean values (ηg/g wet brain weight or ng/ml plasma) of four determinations from two animals at each time period.
[b] Ratio of mean brain to plasma concentrations.

Table III. Distribution[a] of [allyl-1', 3'-^{14}C] Naloxone and [allyl-1', 3'-^{14}C] Nalorphine in Rat Brain, Plasma and Half-Lives after a 10 mg/kg (free base) Dose by Subcutaneous Injection

	0.25 hr	0.5 hr	1 hr	2 hr	4 hr	6 hr	Half-lives (hr)
[^{14}C] Naloxone							
Brain	4.31 ± 0.73	3.58 ± 0.07	1.47 ± 0.06	0.20 ± 0.03	0.05 ± 0	0.03 ± 0	0.4
Plasma	1.27 ± 0.13	0.96 ± 0.05	0.44 ± 0.03	0.07 ± 0.01	0.02 ± 0	0.02 ± 0.01	0.4
B/P[b]	3.3	3.7	3.3	2.8	2.0	1.4	
Plasma (conjugated)	0.48 ± 0.17	1.30 ± 0.13	0.66 ± 0.05	0.16 ± 0.02	0.04 ± 0.01	0.05 ± 0	
[^{14}C] Nalorphine							
Brain	1.14 ± 0.07	1.35	0.97	0.11	0.03	0.02	0.4
Plasma	1.38 ± 0.13	0.85	0.47	0.05	0.03	0.02	0.4
B/P[b]	0.8	1.6	2.1	2.1	1.0	1.0	

[a]Data represent mean value ± S.E.M. (μg/g wet brain weight or μg/ml plasma) of six determinations from three animals at each time period for naloxone; for nalorphine three animals were used at 15 min and two at later times.

[b]Mean brain to plasma concentrations.

doses. At equivalent doses, levels of naloxone 1.5–3.7 times higher than nalorphine were attained in the brain but plasma values were only 0.7–1.4 times those of nalorphine. The values of naloxone in the brain at peak times were approximately 11 times those of morphine with the same dose (10 mg/kg) and route. The rate of disappearance of these antagonists was also faster than that of morphine (Misra et al., 1971). Naloxone and nalorphine persisted in the CNS and other tissues at a 10 mg/kg s.c. dose but not at a 1 mg/kg dose. Significant differences were observed in the brain to plasma ratios of these two antagonists, the naloxone values (3.4–4.8) being consistently higher than those with nalorphine (0.8–2.7), hence indicating an altered distribution for these two compounds.

Comparatively higher excretion of free nalorphine (13% of the dose) compared to naloxone (8%) and higher excretion of total radio-activity in urine and feces for naloxone (64.2% of the dose) compared to nalorphine (54.0%) was observed following a single 10 mg/kg s.c. injection in the rat. Data on comparative amounts of conjugated drugs in plasma suggested faster conjugation and excretion of naloxone as compared to nalorphine. The rapid metabolism and elimination rate of naloxone would appear to be important factors in its short duration of action.

Following a 1 or 10 mg/kg s.c. injection of [^{14}C] or [^{3}H] naloxone, 7, 8-dihydro-14-hydroxy-normorphinone and two other polar metabolites were shown to be present in brain along with free naloxone 0.5 hr after injection. These polar metabolites were also observed in the urine of rats and were different from naloxol, N-oxide or conjugated metabolites of naloxone previously reported by other workers. Tentative evidence has been obtained for dihydroxylation in the allyl side chain through the intermediate formation of an epoxide or hydroxylation at the 2-position of the aromatic nucleus. The ratio of metabolites to the free drug in the brain were lower for nalorphine than naloxone.

Several theories have been proposed to explain the agonistic and antagonistic actions of nalorphine and naloxone (Martin, 1967; Koster-litz and Watt, 1968; Takemori et al., 1969, 1972, 1973; Goldstein, 1974). Recent work (Simon et al., 1973; Lee et al., 1974; Wilson et al., 1975) has provided evidence that the distribution and characteristics of agonist and naloxone binding sites are different. It is conceivable therefore that the interaction of naloxone or its metabolites in the CNS to functional groups of a receptor at another site or a different receptor site could alter the affinity of agonists for the receptor in a noncompetitive manner. The relative proportions of polar metabolites to free antagonists in the CNS were significantly different for nalorphine and naloxone. Naloxone attained only 2–3 times higher levels than nalorphine in brain at 0.25–0.5 hr but was 20 times more active as an antagonist than nalorphine. Steric closeness of the 14-hydroxy group and the N atom in naloxone and the presence of vicinal hydroxy groups in its metabolite raise an alternative possibility of charge-transfer complexation and chelation with essential metal ions which maintain the receptor protein in its native or active configuration.

ACKNOWLEDGMENTS

The work reported here was supported in part by U.S. Public Health Service Grant MH-19004 and NIDA grant DA-00061 to Dr. S. J. Mulé, Director DACC Testing and Research Laboratory. The author wishes to thank Dr. Mulé, Mr. R. Bloch, Mr. R. B. Pontani, Mrs. J. Vardy, and Mr. N. L. Vadlamani for their contribution to the work.

REFERENCES

Abrams, L. S., and H. W. Elliott. 1974. Morphine metabolism *in vivo* and *in vitro* by homozygous Gunn rats. *J. Pharmacol. Exp. Ther.* 189: 285–292.

Appelgren, L. E., and L. Terenius. 1973. Differences in the autoradiographic localization of labeled morphine-like analgesics in the mouse. *Acta Physiol. Scand.* 88: 175–182.

Asghar, K., and E. L. Way, 1970. Active removal of morphine from the cerebral ventricles. *J. Pharmacol. Exp. Ther.* 175: 75–83.

Axelrod, J. 1956. The enzymatic N-demethylation of narcotic drugs, *J. Pharmacol. Exp. Ther.* 117: 322–330.

Beckett, A. H. 1956. Analgesics and their antagonists: Some steric and chemical considerations. I. Dissociation constants of some tertiary amines and synthetic analgesics: Conformations of methadone type compounds. *J. Pharm. Pharmacol.* 8: 848–589.

Beckett, A. H., and A. F. Casy. 1954. Synthetic analgesics: Stereochemical considerations. *J. Pharm. Pharmacol.* 6: 986–1001.

Beckett, A. H., J. F. Taylor, A. F. Casy, and M. M. A. Hassan. 1968. The biotransformation of methadone in man: Synthesis and identification of a major metabolite. *J. Pharm. Pharmacol.* 20: 754–762.

Beckett, A. H., M. Mitchard, and A. A. Shihab. 1971a. Identification and quantitative determination of some metabolites of methadone, isomethadone and normethadone. *J. Pharm. Pharmacol.* 23: 347–352.

Beckett, A. H., M. Mitchard, and A. A. Shihab. 1971b. The influence of methyl substitution on the N-demethylation and N-oxidation of normethadone in animal species. *J. Pharm. Pharmacol.* 23: 941–946.

Beckett, A. H., D. P. Vaughan, and E. E. Essien. 1972. N-oxidation—An important route in the metabolism of methadone in man. *J. Pharm. Pharmacol.* 24: 244.

Berkowitz, B. A., K. V. Cerreta, and S. Spector. 1974a. The influence of physiologic and pharmacologic factors on the disposition of morphine as determined by radioimmunoassay. *J. Pharmacol. Exp. Ther.* 191: 527–534.

Berkowitz, B. A., K. V. Cerreta, and S. Spector. 1974b. Influence of active and passive immunity on the disposition of dihydromorphine-^{3}H. *Life Sciences* 15: 1017–1028.

Billings, R. E., R. Booher, S. Smits, A. Pohland, and R. E. McMahon. 1973. Metabolism of acetylmethadol. A sensitive assay for noracetylmethadol and identification of a new metabolite. *J. Med. Chem.* 16: 305–306.

Billings, R. E., R. E. McMahon, and D. A. Blake. 1974. 1-Acetylmethadol (LAM) treatment of opiate dependence: Plasma and urine levels of two pharmacologically active metabolites. *Life Sciences* 14: 1437–1446.

Blumberg, H., H. B. Dayton, M. George, and D. N. Rapoport. 1961. N-allylnoroxymorphone—A potent narcotic antagonist. *Fed Proc.* 20: 311.

Blumberg, H., H. B. Dayton. 1973. Naloxone and related compounds. H. W. Kosterlitz, H.O.J. Collier and J. Villarreal, Eds. In *Agonist-Antagonists Actions of Narcotic Analgesic Drugs*. University Park Press, Baltimore, pp. 110–119.

Brunk, S. F. and M. Delle. 1974. Morphine metabolism in man. *Clin. Pharmacol. Ther.* 16: 51–57.

Burns, J. J., B. L. Berger, P. A. Lief, A. Wollack, E. M. Papper, and B. B. Brodie. 1955. The physiological disposition and fate of meperidine (demerol) in man and a method for its estimation in plasma. *J. Pharmacol. Exp. Ther.* 114: 289–295.

Casy, A. F. 1973. Analgesic receptors. R. M. Featherstone, Ed. In *A Guide to Molecular Pharmacology and Toxicology*, Part I. Marcel Dekker Inc., New York, pp. 217–278.

Chan, K., M. J. Kendall, and M. Mitchard. 1974. Quantitative gas-liquid chromatographic method for determination of pethidine, its metabolites norpethidine and pethidine N-oxide in human biological fluids. *J. Pharm. Pharmacol.* 89: 169–176.

Christensen, K. 1959. The metabolism of salicylates and other hydroxybenzoates. *Acta Pharmacol. Toxicol.* 16: 129–135.

Clouet, D. H., and N. Williams. 1973. Localization in brain particulate fractions of narcotic analgesic drugs administered intracisternally to rats. *Biochem. Pharmacol.* 22: 1283–1293.

Cochin, J. and C. Kornetsky. 1964. Development or loss of tolerance to morphine in the rat after single and multiple injections. *J. Pharmacol. Exp. Ther.* 145: 1–10.

Cohn, G. L., J. A. Cramer, and H. D. Klebber. 1973. Heroin metabolism in the rat. *Proc. Soc. Exp. Biol. Med.* 144: 351–355.

Cohn, G. L., J. A. Cramer, W. McBride, R. C. Brown, and H. D. Klebber. 1974. Heroin and morphine binding with human serum proteins and red blood cells. *Proc. Soc. Exp. Biol. Med.* 147: 664–666.

Cox, B. M., M. Ginsburg, and J. Willis. 1975. The offset of morphine tolerance in rats and mice. *Brit. J. Pharmacol.* 53: 383–391.

Cox, B. M., and O. H. Osman. 1970. Inhibition of development of tolerance to morphine in rats by drugs which inhibit ribonucleic acid and protein synthesis. *Brit. J. Pharmacol.* 38: 157–170.

Craig, A. L., R. F. O'Dea, and A. E. Takemori. 1971. The uptake of morphine by choroid plexus and cerebral cortical slices of animals chronically treated with morphine. *Neuropharmacology* 10: 709–714.

Crone, C. and A. M. Thompson. 1970. C. Crone and N. Lassen, Eds. *Capillary Permeability.* Academic Press, New York, pp. 447–453.

Dann, R. E., D. R. Feller, and J. F. Snell. 1971. The microsomal N-demethylation of the stereoisomers of ephedrine. *Europ. J. Pharmacol.* 16: 233–236.

Elliott, H. W., K. D. Parker, J. A. Wright, and N. Nomof. 1971. Actions and metabolism of heroin administered by continuous intravenous infusion in man. *Clin. Pharmacol. Ther.* 12: 806–814.

Feinberg, M. P. and J. Cochin. 1972. Inhibition of development of tolerance to morphine by cycloheximide. *Biochem. Pharmacol.* 21: 3082–3085.

Feldberg, W., 1963. A Pharmacologic Approach to the Brain from its Inner and Outer Surface, Williams and Wilkins Co. Baltimore.

Fisher, A. L. and J. P. Long. 1953. The absorption and excretion of Dromoran. *J. Pharmacol. Exp. Ther.* 107: 241–249.

Fishman, J., H. Roffwarg, and L. Hellman. 1973. Disposition of naloxone-7,8-^{3}H in normal and narcotic-dependent men. *J. Pharmacol. Exp. Ther.* 187: 575–580.

Foster, R. S., D. J. Jenden, and P. Lomax. 1967. A comparison of the physiological effect of morphine and N-methyl morphine. *J. Pharmacol. Exp. Ther.* 157: 185–195.

Fujimoto, J. M. 1969. Isolation of two different glucuronide metabolites of naloxone from urine of rabbit and chicken. *J. Pharmacol. Exp. Ther.* 168: 180–186.

Fujimoto, J. M. 1970. Isolation of naloxone-3-glucuronide from human urine. *Proc. Soc. Exp. Biol. Med.* 133: 317–319.

Gillette, J. R. 1971. Mathematical treatment of influence of different degrees of drug binding on drug elimination. *Ann. N. Y. Acad Sci.* 177: 43–66.

Gillette, J. R. 1973. Importance of tissue distribution in pharmacokinetics. *J. Pharmacokin. Biopharm.* 1: 497–520.

Goldstein, A. 1974. M. C. Braude, L. S. Harris, E. L. May, J. P. Smith, and J. E. Villarreal, Eds. *Narcotic Antagonists.* Raven Press, New York. *Advan. Biochem. Psychopharmacol.* 8: 471–481.

Goldstein, A., L. I. Lowney and B. K. Pal. 1971. Stereospecific and non-specific interactions of morphine congener levorphanol in subcellular fractions of mouse brain. *Proc. Nat. Acad. Sci.* (Washington) 68: 1742–1747.

Hahn, D. L. and A. Goldstein. 1971. Amounts and turnover rates of brain proteins in morphine-tolerant mice. *J. Neurochem.* 18: 1887–1893.

Herz, A. and H. J. Teschemacher. 1971. Activities and sites of antinociceptive action of morphine-like analgesics and kinetics of distribution following intravenous, intracerebral and intraventricular application. *Advan. Drug. Res.* 6: 79–119.

Hokin, L. E. and M. R. Hokin. 1958. Acetylcholine and the exchange of inositol and phosphate in brain phosphoinositide. *J. Biol. Chem.* 233: 818–821.

Höllt, V., and H. J. Teschemacher. 1972. Hydrophobic interaction effective in binding of morphine-like analgesics to albumin, plasma-proteins and tissue homogenates, *Naunyn Schmiedeberg Arch. Pharmakol.* (Suppl.) 274: R 53.

Huang, J. T., and A. E. Takemori. 1975. Accumulation of methadone by choroid plexus *in vitro*. *Neuropharmacology* 14: 241–246.

Hug, Jr., C. C. 1967. Transport of narcotic analgesics by choroid plexus and kidney tissue *in vitro*. *Biochem Pharmacol.* 16: 345–359.

Hug, Jr., C. C., and L. B. Mellett. 1963. Tritium-labeled dihydromorphine: An autoradiographic study of its tissue distribution in mice. *Univ. Mich. Med. Bull.* (Ann Arbor) 29: 165–173.

Hug, Jr., C. C., and L. A. Woods. 1963. Tritium-labeled nalorphine–Its CNS distribution and biological fate in the dog. *J. Pharmacol. Exp. Ther.* 142: 248–256.

Ingoglia, N. A. and V. P. Dole. 1970. Localization of d- and l-methadone after intraventricular injection into rat brains. *J. Pharmacol. Exp. Ther.* 175: 84–87.

Inturrisi, C. E. and K. Verebely. 1972. The levels of methadone in the plasma in methadone maintenance. *Clin Pharmacol. Ther.* 13: 633–637.

Jacob, J. C. and C. D. Barthelemy. 1972. Single dose and repeated dose tolerance to the antinociceptive effect of morphine in mice. *Minutes of the meeting of Committee on Problems of Drug Dependence NAS-NRC*, Ann Arbor, Mich., pp. 592–606.

Jóhannesson, T. and B. A. Becker. 1973. Morphine analgesia in rats at various ages. *Acta Pharmacol Toxicol.* 33: 429–441.

Jóhannesson, T. and L. A. Woods. 1964. Analgesic action and brain and plasma levels of morphine and codeine in morphine-tolerant, codeine-tolerant and nontolerant rats. *Acta Pharmacol. Toxicol.* 4: 381–396.

Kaiko, R. F., and C. E. Inturrisi. 1973. Gas-liquid chromatographic method for quantitative determination of acetylmethadol and its metabolites in human urine. *J. Chromat.* 82: 312–321.

Kayan, S., A. L. Misra, and L. A. Woods. 1970. Uptake of [7,8-³H] dihydromorphine by rat cerebral cortical slices and eye tissue. *J. Pharm. Pharmacol.* 22: 941–943.

Kety, S. S. 1960. The cerebral circulation. In J. Field, H. W. Magoun and V. E. Hall, Eds., *Handbook of physiology*. American Physiological Society, Washington, D. C., 3: Chapter 71.

Khazan, N. and T. Roehrs. 1973. EEG responses to morphine test dose in morphine and methadone-treated rats. *Pharmacologist* 15: 168.

Klutch, A. 1974. A chromatographic investigation of morphine metabolism in rats. Confirmation of N-demethylation of morphine and isolation of a new metabolite. *Drug. Metab. Disp.* 2: 23–30.

Kornetsky, C., and G. Bain. 1968. Morphine-single dose tolerance. *Science* 162: 1011–1012.

Kosterlitz, H. W., and A. J. Watt. 1968. Kinetic parameters of narcotic agonists and antagonists with particular reference to N-allylnoroxymorphone (naloxone). *Brit. J. Pharmacol.* 33: 266–276.

Kupferberg, H. J. and E. L. Way. 1963. Pharmacological basis for increased sensitivity of newborn rat to morphine. *J. Pharmacol. Exp. Ther.* 141: 105–112.

Kutter, E., A. Herz, H. J. Teschemacher, and R. Hess. 1970. Structure-activity correlations of morphine-like analgesics based on efficiencies following intravenous and intraventricular applications. *J. Med. Chem.* 13: 801–805.

Lee, C. Y., T. Akera, M. Nozaki, S. L. Stolman, and T. M. Brody. 1974. Specific binding sites for dihydromorphine and naloxone in rat brain particulate fractions. *Pharmacologist* 16: 269.

Levin, V. A., J. D. Fenstermacher, and C. Patlak. 1970. Sucrose and inulin space measurements of cerebral cortex in four mammalian species. *Amer. J. Physiol.* 219: 1528–1533.

Levine, R. R. 1973. *Pharmacology, Drug Actions and Reactions.* Little Brown & Co. Boston, p. 107.

Loh, H. H., T. M. Cho, Y. C. Wu, and E. L. Way. 1974. Spectrospecific binding of narcotics to brain cerebrosides. *Life Sciences,* 14: 2231–2245.

Lomax, P. and W. E. Kirkpatrick. 1967. The effect of N-allylnormorphine on the development of acute tolerance to analgesic and hypothermic effects of morphine in the rat. *Med. Pharmacol. Exp.* 16: 165–170.

Martin, W. R. 1967. Opioid antagonists. *Pharmacol. Rev.* 19: 463–521.

Martin, W. R., and H. F. Fraser. 1961. A comparative study of physiological and subjective effects of heroin and morphine administered intravenously in addicts. *J. Pharmacol. Exp. Ther.* 133: 388–399.

Mason, H. S. 1955. Reactions between quinones and proteins. *Nature* (London) 175: 771–772.

Masten, L. W., G. R. Peterson, A. Burkhalter, and E. L. Way. 1975. Microsomal enzyme induction by methadone and its implications on tolerance to methadone lethality. *Nature* (London) 253: 200–201.

Mather, L. E., and G. T. Tucker. 1974. Meperidine and other basic drugs: General method for determination in plasma. *J. Pharm. Sci.* 63: 306–307.

Mather, L. E., G. T. Tucker, A. E. Pflug, M. J. Lindop, and C. Wilkerson. 1975. Meperidine kinetics in man. *Clin. Pharmacol. Ther.* 17: 21–30.

Matsumota, S., and T. Takahashi. 1970 Cited from Y. Sato, Whole body autoradiography: Classification by the element and drug action. *Pharma-cometrics* 4: 535–559.

Mautner, H. G. 1967. The molecular basis of drug action. *Pharmacol. Rev.* 19: 107–144.

Mayer, M. E., and D. E. Guttman. 1968. Plasma protein binding of drugs. *J. Pharm. Sci.* 57: 895–918.

McMahon, R. E., H. W. Culp, and F. J. Marshall. 1965. The metabolism of α-dl-acetylmethadol in the rat—The identification of the probable active metabolite. *J. Pharmacol. Exp. Ther.* 149: 436–445.

Mellett, L. B., and L. A. Woods. The intracellular distribution of N-^{14}C-methyl levorphanol in brain, liver and kidney tissue of the rat. *J. Pharmacol. Exp. Ther.* 125: 97–104.

Mellett, L. B., and L. A. Woods. 1963. Analgesia and addiction. In E. Jücker, Ed., *Progress in Drug Research*. Birkhäuser Verlag, Basel, 5: 157–267.

Miller, J. W., and H. H. Anderson. 1954. The effect of N-demethylation on certain pharmacological actions of morphine, codeine and meperidine in the mouse. *J. Pharmacol. Exp. Ther.* 112: 191–196.

Miller, J. W., and H. W. Elliott. 1955. Rat tissue levels of carbon-14 labeled analgesics as related to pharmacological activity. *J. Pharmacol. Exp. Ther.* 113: 283–291.

Misra, A. L. 1972. Disposition and metabolism of drugs of dependence. In S. J. Mulé and H. Brill, Eds., *Chemical and biological aspects of drug dependence*. CRC Press, Cleveland, Ohio, pp. 219–276.

Misra, A. L., R. Bloch, and S. J. Mulé, 1975b. Estimation of 1-α-[2-^{3}H] acetylmethadol in biological materials and its separation from some metabolites and congeners on glass fibre sheets. *J. Chromat.* 106: 184–187.

Misra, A. L., R. Bloch, N. L. Vadlamani, and S. J. Mulé. 1974a. Physio-logical disposition and biotransformation of levo methadone-l-^{3}H in the dog. *J. Pharmacol. Exp. Ther.* 188: 34–44.

Misra, A. L., R. Bloch, N. L. Vadlamani, and S. J. Mulé. 1975a. Levo [1-^{3}H] methadone disposition in tolerant dogs. *Xenobiotica* 5: 237–244.

Misra, A. L., C. L. Mitchell, and L. A. Woods. 1971. Persistence of morphine in central nervous system of rats after a single injection and its bearing on tolerance. *Nature* (London) 232: 48–50.

Misra, A. L., and S. J. Mulé. 1972. Persistence of methadone-^{3}H and metabo-lite in rat brain after a single injection and its implications on pharma-cological tolerance. *Nature* (London) 238: 155–157.

Misra, A. L., and S. J. Mulé. 1973. Stereoselectivity and differential metabo-lism *in vivo* of dextro and levo methadone-1-^{3}H. *Nature* (London) 241: 281–283.

Misra, A. L., and S. J. Mulé. 1975. 1-α-Acetyl methadol (LAAM) Pharma-cokinetics and metabolism: Current Status. *Amer. J. Drug & Alcohol Abuse.* 2: 301–305.

Misra, A. L., S. J. Mulé, R. Bloch, and N. L. Vadlamani. 1973a. Physiological disposition and metabolism of levo methadone-1-³H in non-tolerant and tolerant rats. *J. Pharmacol. Exp. Ther.* 185: 287–299.

Misra, A. L., R. B. Pontani, and S. J. Mulé. 1973b. Relationship of pharmacokinetic and metabolic parameters to the absence of physical dependence liability with thebaine-³H, *Experientia* 29: 1108–1110.

Misra, A. L., R. B. Pontani, and S. J. Mulé. 1974b. Effect of morphine on brain and plasma sialic acid levels in the rat. *Res. Comm. Chem. Pathol. Pharmacol.* 9: 383–386.

Misra, A. L., R. B. Pontani, and S. J. Mulé. 1974c. Pharmacokinetics and metabolism of [³H] thebaine. *Xenobiotica* 4: 17–32.

Misra, A. L., R. B. Pontani, N. L. Vadlamani, and S. J. Mulé. 1976. Physiological disposition and biotransformation of [allyl-1′,3′-¹⁴C] naloxone in the rat and some comparative observations on nalorphine. *J. Pharmacol. Exp. Ther.* 196: 257–268.

Misra, A. L., N. L. Vadlamani, R. Bloch, and S. J. Mulé. 1974d. Differential pharmacokinetic and metabolic profiles of the stereoisomers of 3-hydroxy-N-methyl-morphinan. *Res. Comm. Chem. Pathol. Pharmacol.* 7: 1–16.

Misra, A. L., N. L. Vadlamani, R. B. Pontani, and S. J. Mulé. 1973c. Evidence for a new metabolite of morphine-N-methyl-¹⁴C in the rat. *Biochem. Pharmacol.* 22. 2129–2139.

Misra, A. L., N. L. Vadlamani, R. B. Pontani, and S. J. Mulé. 1974e. Some physiochemical and pharmacological properties of morphine-2,3-quinone, the morphine metabolite in the rat brain. *J. Pharm. Pharmacol.* 26: 990–992.

Misra, A. L., J. Vardy, R. Bloch, S. J. Mulé, and G. A. Deneau. 1976. Pharmacokinetics, metabolism of (-)-α-[2-³H]acetyl methadol (LAAM): evidence for a new metabolite. *J. Pharm. Pharmacol.* (In Press)

Misra, A. L., and L. A. Woods. 1970. Evidence for interaction *in vitro* of morphine with glutathione. *Nature* (London) 228: 1226–1227.

Mitchard, M., M. J. Kendall, and K. Chan. 1972. Pethidine N-oxide, a metabolite in human urine. *J. Pharm. Pharmacol.* 24: 915.

Mulé, S. J. 1971. Physiological disposition of narcotic agonists and antagonists. In D. H. Clouet, Ed., *Narcotic drugs, biochemical pharmacology.* Plenum Press, New York, pp. 99–121.

Mulé, S. J., G. Casella, and D. H. Clouet. 1974. Localization of narcotic analgesics in synaptic membranes of rat brain. *Res. Comm. Chem. Pathol. Pharmacol.* 9: 55–77.

Mulé, S. J., and L. A. Woods. 1962. Distribution of N-¹⁴C-methyl labeled morphine: I. In central nervous system of nontolerant and tolerant dogs. *J. Pharmacol. Exp. Ther.* 136: 232–241.

Munro, H. N., B. S. Baliga, and A. W. Pronczuk. 1968. *In vitro* inhibition of peptide synthesis and GTP hydrolysis by cycloheximide and reversal of inhibition by glutathione. *Nature* (London) 219: 944–946.

Muraki, T., 1971. Uptake of morphine-3-glucuronide by choroid plexus *in vitro. Europ. J. Pharmacol.* 15: 393–395.

Nickander, R., R. Booher, and H. Miles. 1974. α-1-Acetylmethadol and its N-demethylated metabolites have potent opiate action in the guinea pig ileum. *Life Sciences* 14: 2011–2017.

Ober, K. F. and J. M. Fujimoto. 1972. Isolation of naloxone-3-ethereal sulfate from the urine of the cat. *Proc. Soc. Exp. Biol. Med.* 139: 1068–1070.

O'Donoghue, S. E. F. 1974. Distribution of pethidine in maternal and fetal plasma following intramuscular administration during labour, *IRCS* 2: 1476.

Oldendorf, W. H. 1971. Brain uptake of radiolabeled amino acids, amines and hexoses after arterial injection. *Amer. J. Physiol.* 221: 1629–1639.

Oldendorf, W. H. 1974a. Blood-brain barrier permeability to drugs. *Ann Rev. Pharmacol.* 14: 239–248.

Oldendorf, W. H. 1974b. Drug penetration of the blood-brain barrier. In E. Zimmerman and R. George, Eds., *Narcotics and the Hypothalamus.* Raven Press, New York, pp. 213–221.

Oldendorf, W. H. 1974c. Lipid-solubility and drug penetration of the blood-brain barrier. *Proc. Soc. Exp. Biol. Med.* 147: 813–816.

Oldendorf, W. H., and H. Davson. 1967. Brain extracellular space and sink action of cerebrospinal fluid. Measurement of rabbit brain extracellular space using sucrose labeled with carbon-14. *Arch. Neurol.* 17: 196–205.

Oldendorf, W. H., S. Hyman, L. Braun, and S. Z. Oldendorf. 1972. Blood-brain barrier: Penetration of morphine, codeine, heroin and methadone after carotid injection. *Science* 178: 984–986.

Olsen, G. D. 1973. Methadone binding to human plasma proteins. *Clin Pharmacol. Ther.* 14: 338–343.

Olsen, G. D. 1975. Morphine binding to human plasma proteins. *Clin. Pharmacol. Ther.* 17: 31–35.

Pal, B. K., L. I. Lowney, and A. Goldstein. 1973. Further studies on the stereospecific binding of levorphanol by a membrane fraction from mouse brain. In H. W. Kosterlitz, H. O. J. Collier and J. Villarreal, Eds., *Agonist and Antagonist Actions of Narcotic Analgesic Drugs.* University Park Press, Baltimore, pp. 62–69.

Pert, C. B., A. M. Snowman, and S. H. Snyder. 1974. Localization of opiate receptor binding in synaptic membranes of rat brain. *Brain Res.* 70: 183–188.

Plotnikoff, N. P., H. W. Elliott, and E. L. Way. 1952. The metabolism of N-^{14}CH$_3$ labeled meperidine. *J. Pharmacol. Exp. Ther.* 104: 377–386.

Plotnikoff, N. P., E. L. Way, and H. W. Elliott. 1956. Biotransformation products of meperidine excreted in the urine of man. *J. Pharmacol. Exp. Ther.* 117: 414–419.

Pohland, A., H. E. Boaz, and H. R. Sullivan. 1971. Synthesis and identification of metabolites resulting from biotransformation of dl-methadone in man and in the rat. *J. Med. Chem.* 14: 194–197.

Portoghese, P. S. 1965. A new concept on the mode of interaction of narcotic analgesics with receptors. *J. Med. Chem.* 8: 609–616.

Portoghese, P. S. 1966. Stereochemical factors and receptor interactions associated with narcotic analgesics. *J. Pharm. Sci.* 55: 865–887.

Rall, D. P. 1971. Drug entry into brain and cerebrospinal fluid. In B. N. LaDu, H. G. Mandel and E. L. Way, Eds., *Fundamentals of Drug Metabolism and Drug Disposition.* Williams and Wilkins, Baltimore, pp. 76–87.

Rall. D. P. and C. G. Zubrod. 1962. Mechanism of drug absorption and excretion—Passage of drugs in and out of the central nervous system. *Ann. Rev. Pharmacol.* 2: 109–128.

Richter, J. A., and A. Goldstein. 1970. Tolerance to opioid narcotics. II. Cellular tolerance to levorphanol in mouse brain. *Proc. Natl. Acad. Sci.* (Washington), 66: 944–951.

Robinson, A. E., and F. M. Williams. 1971. The distribution of methadone in man. *J. Pharm. Pharmacol.* 23: 353–358.

Roth, L. J., and C. F. Barlow. 1961. Drugs in the brain. *Science* 134: 22–31.

Scrafani, J. T., and C. C. Hug. 1968. Active uptake of dihydromorphine and other narcotic analgesics by cerebral cortical slices. *Biochem. Pharmacol.* 17: 1557–1566.

Seeman, P., M. Chan-Wong, and S. Moyyen. 1972. The membrane binding of morphine, diphenylhydantoin and tetrahydrocannabinol. *Canad. J. Physiol. Pharmacol.* 50: 1193–1200.

Seevers, M. H. 1958. Termination of drug action by tolerance development. *Fed Proc.* 17: 1175–1181.

Seevers, M. H., and L. A. Woods. 1953. The phenomena of tolerance. *Amer. J. Med.* 14: 546–557.

Shore, P. A., J. Axelrod, C. A. M. Hogben, and B. B. Brodie. 1955. Observations on the fate of dromoran in the dog and its excretion into the gastric juice. *J. Pharmacol. Exp. Ther.* 113: 192–199.

Simon, E. J., J. M. Heller, and I. Edelman. 1973. Stereospecific binding of the potent narcotic analgesic [³H] etorphine to rat brain homogenate. *Proc. Natl. Acad. Sci* (Washington) 70: 1947–1949.

Smits, S. E. and H. R. Sullivan. 1971. Optical isomers of methadone: Analgesic activity and accumulation in blood and brain. *Pharmacologist* 13: 262.

Spector, S. 1971. Quantitative determination of morphine in serum by radioimmunoassay. *J. Pharmacol. Exp. Ther.* 178: 253–258.

Spector, S., and C. W. Parker. 1970. Morphine radioimmunoassay. *Science* 168: 1347–1348.

Sullivan, H. R., and D. A. Blake. 1972. Quantitative determination of methadone concentrations in human blood, plasma and urine by gas chromatography. *Res. Comm. Chem. Pathol. Pharmacol.* 3: 467–478.

Sullivan, H. R., S. L. Due, and R. E. McMahon. 1972. The identification of 3 new metabolites of methadone in man and the rat. *J. Amer. Chem. Soc.* 94: 4050–4051.

Sullivan, H. R., S. L. Due, and R. E. McMahon. 1973. Metabolism of α-1-methadol: N-acetylation a new metabolic pathway. *Res. Comm. Chem. Pathol. Pharmacol.* 6: 1072–1078.

Sung, C. Y., and E. L. Way. 1953. The metabolic fate of the optical isomers of methadone. *J. Pharmacol. Exp. Ther.* 190: 244–254.

- Sung, C. Y., and E. L. Way. 1954. The fate of the optical isomers of alpha acetyl methadol. *J. Pharmacol. Exp. Ther.* 110: 260–270.

Takemori, A. E., G. Hayashi, and S. E. Smith. 1972. Studies on the quantitative antagonism of analgesics by naloxone and diprenormorphine. *Europ. J. Pharmacol.* 20: 85–92.

Takemori, A. E., H. J. Kupferberg, and J. W. Miller, 1969. Quantitative studies on antagonism of morphine by nalorphine and naloxone. *J. Pharmacol. Exp. Ther.* 169: 39–45.

Takemori, A. E., T. Oka, and M. Nishiyama. 1973. Alteration of analgesic receptor-antagonist interaction induced by morphine. *J. Pharmacol. Exp. Ther.* 186: 261–265.

Takemori, A. E., and M. W. Stenwick, 1966. Studies on the uptake of morphine by choroid plexus *in vitro*. *J. Pharmacol. Exp. Ther.* 154: 586–594.

Teller, D. N., T. DeGuzman, and A. Lajtha. 1974. The mode of morphine uptake into brain slices. *Brain Research* 77: 121–136.

Terenius, L. 1973. Stereospecific interaction between narcotic analgesics and a synaptic plasma membrane fraction of the rat cerebral cortex. *Acta. Pharmacol. Toxicol.* 32: 317–320.

Teschemacher, H. J., P. Schubert, C. W. Kreutzberg, and A. Herz. 1968. Autoradiographische darstellung ^{14}C-markierten morphins nach intraventrikularer und intracerebraler injektion. *Arch. Exp. Pathol. Pharmakol.* 260: 211.

Tremblay, J., M. Simon, and S. H. Barondes. 1974. Cerebroside may be falsely identified as a soluble brain specific protein. *J. Neurochem.* 23: 315–318.

Waelsch, H., and A. Lajtha. 1961. Protein metabolism in the central nervous system. *Physiol. Rev.* 41: 709–815.

Wang, J. H., and A. E. Takemori. 1972. Transport of morphine out of the perfused ventricles of the rabbit. *J. Pharmacol. Exp. Ther.* 181: 46–52.

Way, E. L. 1967. Pharmacologic implications of some factors in influencing the brain uptake of morphine. *Arch. Biol. Med. Exp.* 4: 92–98.

Way, E. L. 1968a. A. Wikler, Ed., *The Addictive States*. Williams and Wilkins, Baltimore, pp. 13–31.

Way, E. L. 1968b. Infantile drug distribution. *Rep. Ross Pediat. Res. Conf.* 58: 66–70.

Way, E. L., and T. K. Adler. 1962. *The Biological Disposition of Morphine and its Surrogates*. World Health Organization, Geneva. pp. 1–114.

Way, E. L., A. I. Gimble, W. P. McKelway, H. Ross, C. Y. Sung, and H.

Ellsworth. 1949. The absorption, distribution and excretion of isonipecaine (demerol). *J. Pharmacol. Exp. Ther.* 96: 477–484.

Way, E. L., J. W. Kemp, J. M. Young, and D. R. Grassetti. 1960. The pharmacologic effects of heroin in relationship to its rate of biotransformation. *J. Pharmacol. Exp. Ther.* 129: 144–151.

Way, E. L., H. H. Loh, and Fu-Hsiung Shen. 1968. Morphine tolerance, physical dependence and synthesis of 5-hydroxy tryptamine. *Science* 162: 1290–1292.

Way, E. L., J. M. Young, and J. W. Kemp. 1965. Metabolism of heroin and its pharmacologic implications. *Bull. Narcotics.* (U. N.) 17: 25–33.

Weinstein, S. H., M. Pfeffer, J. M. Schor, L. Indindoli, and M. Mintz. 1971. Metabolism of naloxone in human urine. *J. Pharm. Sci.* 60: 1567–1568.

Weinstein, S. H., M. Pfeffer, J. M. Schor, L. Franklin, M. Mintz, and E. R. Tutko. 1973. Absorption and distribution of naloxone in rats after oral and intravenous administration. *J. Pharm. Sci.* 62: 1416–1420.

Welch, K., and V. Friedman. 1960. The cerebrospinal fluid valves. *Brain,* 83: 454–469.

Wilson, H. A., G. W. Pasternak, and S. H. Snyder. 1975. Differentiation of opiate agonist and antagonist receptor binding by protein modifying reagents. *Nature* (London) 253: 448–450.

Wong, D. T., and J. S. Horng. 1973. Stereospecific interaction of opiate narcotics in binding of [3H] dihydromorphine to membranes of rat brains. *Life Sciences* 13: 1543–1556.

Woods, L. A. 1956. The pharmacology of nalorphine (N-allyl normorphine). *Pharmacol. Rev.* 84: 175–198.

Woods, L. A., L. B. Mellett, and K. S. Anderson. 1958. The synthesis and estimation of N-14C-methyl labeled levorphanol and its biological disposition in the monkey, dog and the rat. *J. Pharmacol. Exp. Ther.* 124: 1–8.

Woods, L. A., and H. E. Muehlenbeck. 1957. Distribution and fate of nalorphine in the dog and the rat. *J. Pharmacol. Exp. Ther.* 120: 52–57.

Yanagita, T. 1974. An experimental framework for evaluation of dependence liability of various types of drugs in the monkey. *Bull. Narcotics* (U. N.) 25: 57–64.

Yeh, S. Y. 1975. Urinary excretion of morphine and its metabolites in morphine-dependent subjects. *J. Pharmacol. Exp. Ther.* 192: 201–210.

Yeh, S. Y., C. W. Gorodetzky and R. L. McQuinn. 1976. Urinary excretion of heroin and its metabolites in man. *J. Pharmacol. Exp. Ther.* 196: 249–256.

Tissue Responses to Addictive Drugs
© 1976, Spectrum Publications, Inc.

Immunofluorescent Localization of Methadone in the Central Nervous System of the Rat

LOUIS P. PERTSCHUK
DONALD H. FORD
DAVID J. BRIGATI
JOANNA H. SHER

Departments of Pathology and Anatomy
State University of New York
Downstate Medical Center
Brooklyn, New York

Fluorescent antibody procedures allow for the visual localization of antigens in tissue (Coons et al., 1942). When tissue containing an antigen is incubated with a specific antibody and then with a fluorochrome conjugated antiglobulin, the presence of the antigen is revealed in sections microscopically examined under ultraviolet light (Coons and Kaplan, 1950).

The successful production of an antibody to methadone by Liu and Adler (1973), although primarily designed for use in a hemagglutination-inhibition assay for detection of the drug in urine, suggested its trial in an immunofluorescence system in an attempt to identify and localize methadone in the tissues of experimental animals.

METHODS AND MATERIALS

Ten male Sprague-Dawley rats, weighing between 175 and 225 gm, were given dl-methadone subcutaneously over a four week period.

They were started on a dose of 2 mg/kg, which gradually increased to a dose of 18 to 21 mg/kg by the 21st day. This dose was maintained until the 28th day at which time each animal was overdosed with 63 mg/kg of methadone and decapitated within one hour of the final injection.

Five additional rats were given methadone in a dose of 2 mg/kg via an indwelling polyethylene cannula implanted into the left jugular vein, twice daily for four days, and were sacrificed shortly after receiving an overdose of 20 mg/kg on the fifth day.

The brains were quickly dissected and tissue blocks were frozen and stored in liquid nitrogen. Four micron-thick sections were cut from each block in a cryostat, fixed for five minutes in 97% ethanol, and then processed by standard indirect immunofluorescence technics.

The antimethadone serum was produced commercially (Technam, Inc., Park Forest South, Illinois) by injection into rabbits of a methadone congener coupled to bovine serum albumin (BSA) together with complete Freund's adjuvant. The congener was 4 dimethylamino -2, 2-diphenylpentanoic acid (DDA), a compound possessing hapten properties.

Tissue sections were washed in phosphate buffered saline (PBS), pH 7.11–7.18, for ten minutes. They were then overlaid with a 1:10 dilution of antimethadone serum for 30 minutes in a humidifying chamber at room temperature. The sections were then washed in PBS for 15 minutes and covered with a 1:10 dilution of fluorescein conjugated goat antirabbit immunoglobulins (Behring Diagnostics, Somerville, N. J.) for an additional 30 minutes. This conjugate had a molar fluorescein to protein ratio of 3.0 and contained 10 ± 3 mg/ml of protein in its conjugated gamma globulin fraction. Antiserum and conjugate dilutions were made with PBS containing 4% BSA.

Following a final 60 minute PBS wash, all sections were mounted in buffered glycerol, pH 7.0, and examined with a Zeiss Universal Research fluorescence microscope (Carl Zeiss, Oberkochen, West Germany) equipped for both incident light and transillumination. An Osram HBO 200 high pressure mercury vapor lamp, an FITC interference excitation filter, and a K 530 barrier filter were utilized.

Substrate controls consisted of rats given morphine and rats given a 0.9% NaCl solution. Serum controls included sections incubated with anti-barbiturate rabbit serum (Technam, Inc.) and antimethadone serum absorbed with DDA (1 mg/ml).

In addition, sections from each animal were also incubated with naloxone (Endo Laboratories, Inc., Garden City, New York) in a concentration of 0.02 mg/ml in PBS, pH 7.4, at 35°C for 30 minutes prior to processing.

Photomicrographs of fluorescent preparations were taken with a Zeiss C 35 camera on high speed Ektachrome film (EH 135). Low and

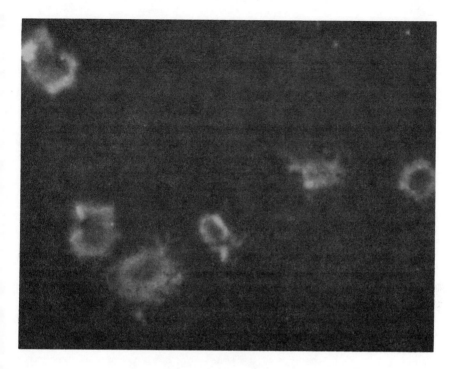

1 Dorsolateral thalamus showing bright perinuclear neuronal fluorescence. The cytoplasmic extensions give the cells a pinwheel appearance.
(Immunofluorescence microscopy x 500)

medium power photographs required a 30 second exposure and high power photomicrographs were exposed for one minute. Exposures were kept constant to allow for rough comparison of the intensity of fluorescence. Film was developed by Kodak's ESP-1 process for a final ASA rating of 400.

RESULTS

When brain tissue from the 28 day methadone-treated rats was examined with incident ultraviolet light, fluorescent neurons were easily visible at all magnifications in various regions of the brain. The number of fluorescent neurons varied from 1% to more than 50% of the total cell population in any given area and was not constant from rat to rat.

The patterns of fluorescence were variable and also were not constant in the same areas of different animals. The most common pattern seen was one of perinuclear staining with threadlike extensions radiating out into the cytoplasm, giving the neurons a pinwheel appearance (See Fig. 1). Occasional cells showed nuclear staining. Fluorescing cell

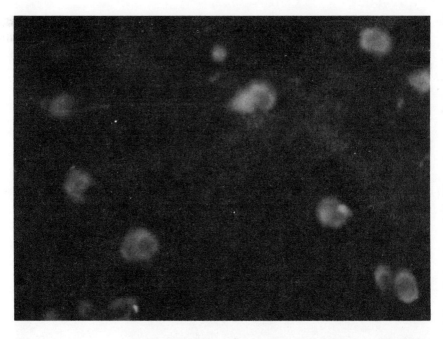

2 Pyramidal cells in the hippocampal formation. The two neurons at the upper right exhibit nuclear fluorescence. Fluorescing neuronal processes are visible at the center and lower right.
(Immunofluorescence microscopy x 500)

processes were not uncommon (See Fig. 2) and sometimes were brightly beaded. The neuropil was usually unstained and appeared dark. Fluorescent neurons were occasionally observed side by side with nonfluorescent neurons in the same microscopic field.

Fluorescent glial cells (arrows) were also observed (See Fig. 3) and showed a similar intracellular distribution of fluorescent material, i.e., perinuclear, as did the majority of neurons. Such glial cells were commonly seen in the dorsal columns of the spinal cord where neurons were absent. However, in the cord as a whole, the majority of fluorescing cells were neuronal.

The distribution of methadone by anatomical region in the 28-day-treated rats is shown in figure 4. Of the ten rats, nine showed fluorescent neurons in the pyramidal layer of the hippocampal formation. No positive cells were noted in the dentate gyrus. In eight animals, positive neurons were seen in the mammillary body, while the head of the caudate nucleus, medial reticular formation, median eminence-arcuate area, and the medial geniculate body were positive in seven rats.

The thalamus, sensory-motor cortex, cerebellar vermis, amygdaloid nucleus, superior colliculus, and the dorsal horns of the cervical spinal cord were less frequently positive. The spinal cord below the cervical level was not examined. The lateral geniculate body, olfactory bulb, putamen and globus pallidus, and the anterior horn cells of the cervical spinal cord were occasionally positive, although the inferior olive, olfactory tubercle and the preoptic area were rarely positive.

In general, areas most often positive showed a particularly large proportion of fluorescent neurons. Two exceptions were the sensory-motor cortex and the amygdaloid nucleus which, when positive, contained close to 50% of strongly fluorescent cells, and yet in almost half the animals were completely negative.

In the cerebellum, fluorescence was usually limited to the stellate

3 Dorsal columns of rat spinal cord. There is perinuclear fluorescence of the glial cells (arrows). The white matter in the background shows some nonspecific staining. (Immunofluorescence microscopy x 500)

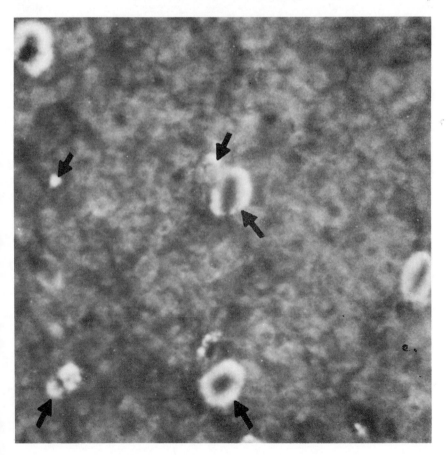

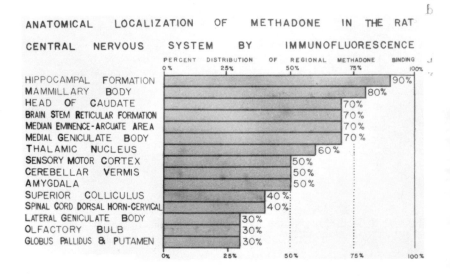

ANATOMICAL   LOCALIZATION   OF   METHADONE   IN   THE   RAT
CENTRAL   NERVOUS   SYSTEM   BY   IMMUNOFLUORESCENCE

PERCENT DISTRIBUTION OF REGIONAL METHADONE BINDING

	%
HIPPOCAMPAL FORMATION	90%
MAMMILLARY BODY	80%
HEAD OF CAUDATE	70%
BRAIN STEM RETICULAR FORMATION	70%
MEDIAN EMINENCE-ARCUATE AREA	70%
MEDIAL GENICULATE BODY	70%
THALAMIC NUCLEUS	60%
SENSORY MOTOR CORTEX	50%
CEREBELLAR VERMIS	50%
AMYGDALA	50%
SUPERIOR COLLICULUS	40%
SPINAL CORD DORSAL HORN-CERVICAL	40%
LATERAL GENICULATE BODY	30%
OLFACTORY BULB	30%
GLOBUS PALLIDUS & PUTAMEN	30%

4

cells of the cortex. No fluorescent Purkinje cells were seen, but in one animal the cells of the internal granular layer were focally positive.

No fluorescence was observed in the inferior colliculus, dorsal root ganglion, ganglion of the trigeminal nerve, the floor of the fourth ventricle, the pineal gland, the choroid plexus, or in either anterior or posterior lobe of the pituitary gland.

Sections from animals given morphine or 0.9% NaCl solution were negative. Control sections that had been reacted with antibarbiturate serum were negative. Absorption of the antimethadone serum with DDA prior to processing completely inhibited its antimethadone activity. Incubation of known positive tissue sections with naloxone resulted in marked diminution or abolition of the fluorescence.

Fluorescent cells were not seen in any section obtained from the nervous system of the 5-day-methadone-treated rats.

DISCUSSION

Apparently the immunofluorescence technique accurately identifies and localizes methadone in the cell bodies and processes of neurons, and occasionally glial cells in the central nervous system of 28-day-methadone-treated rats. Since these animals were given a mixture of - and l-methadone, it is not as yet proven that there is recognition of the stereospecific drug, even though prior incubation of the tissue sections with naloxone inhibited or abolished the reaction, presumably by displacement of the methadone. At present therefore, it is not clear whether the method distinguishes between opiate binding sites that are pharmacologically active or inactive. However, it appears highly unlikely that only the inactive binding sites are being visualized.

It is generally accepted that pharmacologically significant narcotic receptors are limited to the synaptosomal region (Scrafani et al., 1969; Hug and Oka, 1971; Terenius, 1973; Pert et al., 1974). However, significant uptake of opiates in nuclear, mitochondrial, and microsomal fractions obtained by differential ultracentrifugation, has also been shown (Mulé et al., 1967; Navon and Lajtha, 1970; Pert and Snyder, 1973). Furthermore, Goldstein et al. (1969) reporting on the stereospecific binding of levorphanol, found little, if any in synaptosomal membranes and showed that the major portion of the stereospecific binding was confined to membranes in the crude nuclear fraction. These latter findings are fully consistent with the patterns of fluorescence seen in this study.

Ehrenpreis and co-workers (1969) have emphasized that drug interaction with isolated receptors may be quite different than such interactions occurring *in situ*. Possibly therefore, the immunofluorescence method, performed on tissue much more intact morphologically than ultracentrifuged fragments, may be superior in pinpointing the site(s) of opiate binding.

The failure to demonstrate methadone by immunofluorescence in the central nervous system of rats given only a short course of the drug is of considerable interest. One might speculate that the brains of such rats, which would be only minimally tolerant, would contain amounts of methadone below the limits of sensitivity of the immunofluorescence procedure. Possibly in the animals treated longer (four weeks), binding sites may have been unmasked, perhaps by displacement of endogenous ligand, which permit accumulation of more narcotic. The term "opiate receptor" implies a surface binding site. Most investigators believe that these are of fixed number, although Collier (1965) has presented the hypothesis that tolerance is due to an increased number of receptors, many of which are pharmacologically ineffective. The binding we show, however, is principally intracellular, and is therefore of a different character. Nonetheless, it seems reasonable to assume that this phenomenon parallels and is possibly associated with the development of drug tolerance and dependence.

The distribution of methadone in rat brain as shown by immuno-fluorescence is in basic agreement with distribution studies of opiate in rat brain demonstrated by several different techniques (Pert and Snyder, 1973; Wei et al., 1973), in that most of the drug is found within the limbic system and regions closely associated with it. However, since other investigators used different drugs and widely varying experimental methods, comparison of results is difficult.

The results of the present and related experiments (Sher et al., 1976; Pertschuk and Sher, 1975, 1976) indicate that immunofluorescence should prove to be a valuable tool with which to study narcotic drugs and to gain insights into mechanisms of drug tolerance and dependence.

ACKNOWLEDGMENTS

We thank Ms. Evelyn Rainford for her expert technical assistance and Mr. Robert Simowitz for his help with the photomicrographs.

This study was supported, in part, by a grant from the United States Public Health Service, RO1 DA 0014-04.

REFERENCES

Collier, H. O. J. 1965. A general theory of the genesis of drug dependence by induction of receptors. *Nature* (London) 205: 181–182.

Coons, A. H., H. J. Creech, R. N. Jones, and E. Berliner. 1942. The demonstration of pneumococcal antigen in tissues by the use of fluorescent antibody. *J. Immunol.* 45: 159–170.

Coons, A. H., and M. H. Kaplan. 1950. Localization of antigen in tissue cells. II. Improvements in a method for the detection of antigen by means of fluorescent antibody. *J. Exp. Med.* 91: 1–13.

Ehrenpreis, S., J. H. Fleisch, and T. W. Mittag. 1969. Approaches to the molecular nature of pharmacological receptors. *Pharmacol. Rev.* 21: 131–181.

Goldstein, A., L. E. Lowney, and B. K. Pal. 1969. Stereospecific and non-specific interactions of the morphine congener levorphanol in subcellular fractions of mouse brain. *Proc. Nat. Acad. Sci.* 68: 1742–1747.

Hug, C. C. Jr., and T. Oka. 1971. Uptake of dihydromorphine-^{3}H by synaptosomes. *Life Sci.* 10: 201–213.

Liu, Chi-Tan, and F. L. Adler. 1973. Immunologic studies on drug addiction. I. Antibodies reactive with methadone and their use for detection of the drug. *J. Immunol.* 111: 201–213.

Mulé, S. J., C. H. Redman, and J. W. Flesher. 1967. Intracellular disposition of H^3 morphine in the brain and liver of non tolerant and tolerant guinea pigs. *J. Pharmacol. Exp. Ther.* 157: 459–471.

Navon, S., and A. Lajtha. 1970. Uptake of morphine in particulate fractions from rat brain. *Brain Res.* 24: 534–536.

Pert, C. B., A. M. Snowman, and S. H. Snyder. 1974. Localization of opiate receptor binding in synaptic membranes of rat brain. *Brain Res.* 70: 184–188.

Pert, C. B., and S. H. Snyder. 1973. Opiate receptor: Demonstration in nervous tissue. *Science* 179: 1011–1014.

Pertschuk, L. P., and J. H. Sher. 1975. Demonstration of methadone in the human brain by immunofluorescence. *Res. Commun. Chem. Pathol. Pharmacol.* 11: 319–322.

Pertschuk, L. P., and J. H. Sher. 1976. Immunofluorescent detection of narcotic drugs in human brain. (Abstract) *J. Neuropathol. Exp. Neurol.* 35: 111.

Scrafani, J. T., N. Williams, and D. H. Clouet. 1969. Binding of dihydromorphine to subcellular fractions of rat brain. *Pharamcologist* 11: 256.

Sher, J. H., L. P. Pertschuk, W. Kane, J. O'Connor, and M. Wald. 1976. Regional localization of methadone in human brain. In D. H. Ford and D. H. Clouet, Eds., *Tissue Responses to Addictive Drugs.* Spectrum Publications, Holliswood, New York.

Terenius, L. 1973. Stereospecific interaction between narcotic analgesics and a synaptic plasma membrane fraction of rat cerebral cortex. *Acta Pharmacol. Toxicol.* 32: 317–320.

Wei, E., H. H. Loh, and E. L. Way. 1973. Brain sites of precipitated abstinence in morphine-dependent rats. *J. Pharmacol. Exp. Ther.* 185: 108–115.

Tissue Responses to Addictive Drugs
© 1976, Spectrum Publications, Inc.

Regional Localization of Narcotic Drugs in Human Brain

JOANNA H. SHER
LOUIS P. PERTSCHUK
WALTER C. KANE
MILTON A. WALD
JOHN E. O'CONNOR

Department of Pathology
State University of New York
Downstate Medical Center
and the Office of the Chief Medical Examiner
of the City of New York

Investigation of opiate binding in monkey and human nervous system, by incubation of tissue homogenates with tritiated narcotic drugs, has demonstrated high density of opiate receptors in the limbic system and related areas (Kuhar et al., 1973, and Hiller et al., 1973). The use of tissue homogenates in these studies of the regional distribution of narcotics in the brain has the advantage of allowing determination of stereospecificity of drug receptors, but cannot show the cellular localization of receptor sites.

Recently, antisera to morphine and methadone have been produced for use in radioimmunoassay and in hemagglutination-inhibition assays for these drugs in urine (Spector and Parker, 1970; Liu and Adler, 1973). The availability of these antisera suggested their use with immunofluorescence techniques to detect and localize narcotics in tissue.

Table I. Characteristics of 20 Cases Studied

Age: 14–38 years	*Sex:* 17 male; 3 female

History: Methadone maintenance . . . . 10 cases

Prior Heroin addiction . . . . 6 cases

Alcoholism . . . . 4 cases

METHODS AND MATERIALS

Twenty brains were obtained at autopsy from patients who were known to have died from drug overdose. The brains were removed between 12 and 36 hours portmortem.

The characteristics of the cases included in this study are summarized in Table I. All but three were males, and most were in their twenties. In ten cases there were definite histories of methadone maintenance, for periods of six months to three years. The lack of a history of drug addiction in a few of the cases simply reflected the lack of information available to the medical examiner in those cases. In all cases, the circumstances of death together with the anatomical and toxicological findings at autopsy led to the diagnosis of death from drug overdose.

Table II summarizes the drugs identified at autopsy in these cases by routine toxicological analysis. Methadone was identified in a total of eighteen cases. Morphine was found, only in association with methadone, in two cases.

The method used was similar to that described by Pertschuk and Sher (1975), and is described in detail elsewhere in this volume (Pertschuk et al., 1976). Fresh tissue blocks were taken from many areas of cerebral cortex, diencephalon, brainstem, and cerebellum. Samples of choroid plexus, liver, and kidney were also taken. The tissue was rapidly frozen in liquid nitrogen, and frozen sections were cut at 4 microns. The sections were incubated with 1:20 antimethadone or antimorphine rabbit serum, washed, and then overlaid with 1:20 fluorescein conjugated rabbit immunoglobulin. They were examined by incident ultraviolet light with a Zeiss Universal Research microscope.

Serum controls were sections incubated with antisera which had been absorbed with morphine or methadone, and sections incubated with plain rabbit serum, and saline. Substrate controls, incubated the

**Table II. Drugs Detected at Autopsy by Routine
Toxicological Analysis in 20 Patients Dead
from Drug Overdose**

Methadone only	5 cases
Methadone plus	13 cases

Alcohol	3
Amitriptyline	3
Barbiturates	2
Morphine	2
Propoxyphene	3

Propoxyphene only	1 case
Propoxyphene, amitriptyline, phenothiazine	1 case

regular way, were human brain sections from autopsy cases known not to have received narcotics. All controls failed to show fluorescence.

RESULTS

Various patterns of neuronal fluorescence were observed in the addicts' brain sections which had been incubated with antinarcotic sera. These patterns were seen in all areas, so that with few exceptions no one pattern of staining was characteristic of any particular region. Definite staining of glial cells was not observed, although in some sections the possibility that a few glial cells were fluorescent could not be ruled out.

A pattern of diffuse neuronal fluoresence was commonly observed in sections from cortex, hippocampus, amygdala and hypothalamus (see Figure 1). Occasionally, cells staining diffusely showed small concentrations of granular fluorescence in areas adjacent to the nucleus or the cell membrane. Less commonly only the nuclei fluoresced, diffusely (see Figure 2). Perinuclear fluorescence, in a ringlike pattern, was frequently observed (see Figure 3). Often the perinuclear rings showed strands of fluorescence radiating outward from the nucleus, in a pinwheel pattern, similar to that described in the rat (Pertschuk et al., 1976). Rarely, fluorescent cell processes were demonstrated, sometimes containing small "beads" of fluorescent material (see Figure 3).

In general, between 1 and 20 per cent of neurons in a section showed fluorescence. Regional differences were noted, however, in the

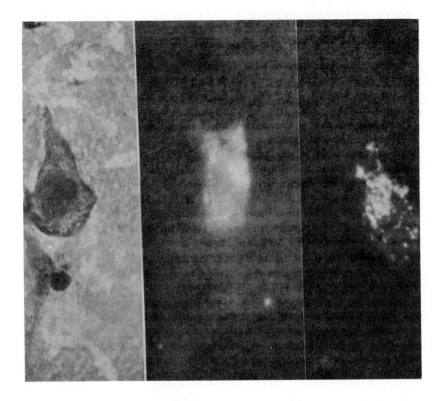

1 A cortical neuron showing diffuse fluorescence
with a small concentration of granular fluorescence adjacent
to the nucleus is shown in the center panel. On the left
is a neuron from the same area stained with hematoxylin
and eosin. On the right, negative neuron containing
autofluorescent lipofuscin granules. (Hematoxylin
and eosin, and immunofluorescence microscopy. Original
magnification, 500X).

large proportion of positive neurons in some areas, notably the hippocampus and thalamus. In some sections of the hippocampal formation,
most of the neurons of the dentate gyrus were fluorescent (see Figure
4). It is noteworthy that staining of dentate gyrus neurons was common
in the human material, whereas in the rat hippocampus only the cells
of the pyramidal layer stained (Pertschuk et al., 1976).

Fluorescence in the cerebellum was usually limited to the Purkinje
cells, which stained relatively diffusely (see Figure 5). By contrast, in
the rat cerebellum, the Purkinje cells did not stain, but positive stellate
cells were observed.

Figure 6 lists the various brain regions examined in this study, and shows the frequency of finding fluorescent neurons with antimethadone serum in these different areas. The regions most frequently positive, in over half the cases studied, were the amygdaloid nucleus, hypothalamus, motor cortex, centromedian nucleus of the thalamus, and postcentral cortex. The hippocampus, medial reticular formation of midbrain and medulla, preoptic area, cingulate gyrus, and mammillary bodies, showed fluorescent neurons in over 40% of cases. Cerebellum and caudate nuclei were positive in a third or more of cases examined. The supraoptic nucleus and frontal cortex showed positive neurons less frequently. Occipital cortex and choroid plexus, not shown here, were consistently negative. Sections of liver and kidney were also negative.

Table III summarizes the findings in a typical case, known to have been maintained on methadone for the three years prior to death.

2   Four diffusely fluorescent neuronal nuclei in a section of motor cortex are shown on the right. On the left, neurons from the same area stained with hematoxylin and eosin are shown for comparison. (Hematoxylin and eosin and immunofluorescence microscopy. Original magnification, 500X).

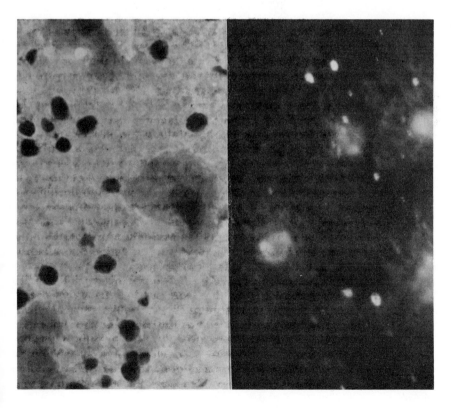

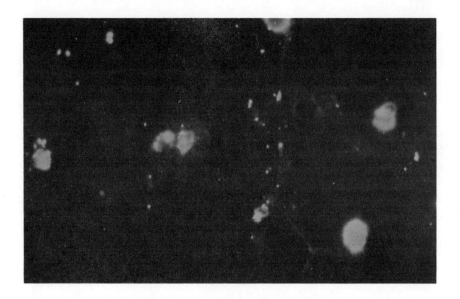

3

Sections of hypothalamus showing nuclear and perinuclear fluorescence, and a fluorescent cell process containing a "bead" of brightly fluorescent material. (Immunofluorescence microscopy. Original magnification, 500X).

4

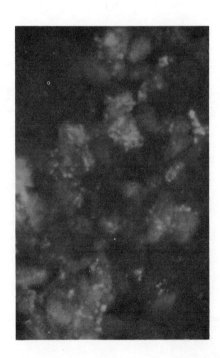

Dentate gyrus of hippocampus treated with antimethadone serum, showing a majority of positive neurons. (Immuno-fluorescence microscopy. Original magnification, 500X).

Numbers of fluorescent neurons in the different regions were quite variable from case to case, and no particular region showed fluorescent cells in every case.

In order to evaluate the usefulness of immunofluorescent techniques in the detection of opiates for forensic purposes, our results were compared with the results of the routine toxicological analysis done on each case by the laboratory of the office of the medical examiner. The results are shown in Table IV. In seventeen cases, methadone was detected by both immunofluoresence and toxicological analysis. In only one case was immunofluoresence negative for methadone and the toxicological analysis positive. No false positives were encountered with the immunofluorescent method. In two of our cases, both immunofluorescence and toxicological analysis detected morphine. However, in four cases which showed positive immunofluorescence with antimor-

5

A fluorescent Purkinje cell in a section of cerebellum from a methadone addict is shown on the right. On the left, a hematoxylin and eosin stain showing Purkinje cells in an adjacent section, for size comparison. (Hematoxylin and eosin, and immunofluorescence microscopy. Original magnification, 500X).

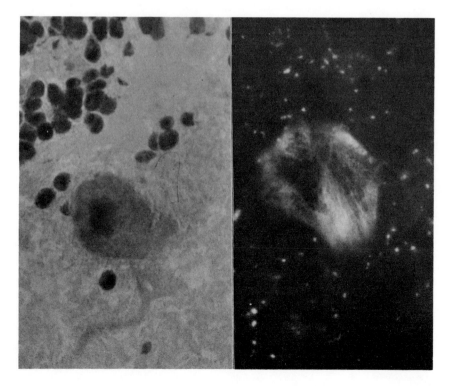

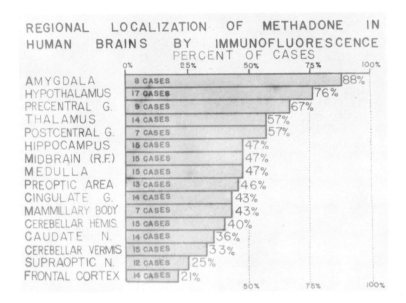

REGIONAL LOCALIZATION OF METHADONE IN HUMAN BRAINS BY IMMUNOFLUORESCENCE

6 Per cent of cases containing positive neurons in different regions shown by length of bars. Number of cases examined in each region is given at the left of each bar.

Table III. Immunofluorescent Detection of Methadone in Human Brain

(Subject: a 22 year old woman on methadone maintenance for a 3 year period.)

Frontal cortex	+	Thalamus	+
Cingulate cortex	0	Medial geniculate	++
Motor cortex	+	Lateral geniculate	++
Postcentral cortex	+++		
Preoptic area	0	Cerebellum	+
Supraoptic nucleus	++	(stellate cells)	
Hypothalamus	+		
Mammillary body	0		
Amygdala	+		
Hippocampus	+	Medial reticular	
Caudate (head)	++	formation (midbrain)	0

    0 — negative
    + — 1–5% of neurons fluorescent
  ++ — 6–10% of neurons fluorescent
+++ — 11–20% of neurons fluorescent

Table IV. Immunofluorescent (IF) Detection of Drugs in Brains of 20 Patients Dead from Drug Overdose

(Comparison with toxicological analysis)

IF and toxicological detection of methadone	17
Toxicological detection of methadone (negative IF)	1
IF and toxicological detection of morphine	2
Positive IF with morphine antiserum; toxicological detection of propoxyphene	4
Negative IF with morphine antiserum; toxicological detection of propoxyphene.	1

phine serum, chromatography detected propoxyphene. (This was not unexpected, as the serum is known to cross react with propoxyphene in urine assay.) In one case, immunofluorescence was negative, but toxicological analysis detected propoxyphene.

The distribution of morphine and propoxyphene in the few cases studied was similar to that of methadone (see Table V). Morphine was demonstrated in the hypothalamus, dentate gyrus of the hippocampal formation, and in the reticular formation. Propoxyphene was shown in those areas, and in cingulate gyrus and Purkinje cells.

DISCUSSION

Our observations on the regional distribution of methadone in human brain are in partial agreement with recent studies of opiate binding in brain homogenates, insofar as high binding was reported in the amygdala, hypothalamus, cingulate cortex, thalamus, caudate nucleus, and moderate binding in the hippocampus (Hiller et al., 1973; Kuhar et al., 1973). However, our relatively frequent observation of neuronal fluorescence in pre-and post-central cortex, and in the cerebellum is at variance with the results of the pharmacological studies.

Possible explanations for these differences are suggested by comparison of the methods used in these investigations. Our demonstration of drug in one cell type in a certain region, e.g. the Purkinje cells of the cerebellum, may reflect significant opiate binding which would not be apparent when diluted with a total homogenate of cerebellar tissue. For this reason the immunofluorescent method may provide a more

Table V. Distribution of Morphine and Propoxyphene in Brain

	Morphine (2 cases) (By Immuno-fluorescence)	Propoxyphene (4 cases) (Toxicological Assay)
Frontal cortex	0	0
Cingulate gyrus	0	+
Hypothalamus	+	+
Hippocampus	+	++
Brainstem (medial reticular formation)	+	+
Purkinje cells of Cerebellum	0	+

accurate indication of opiate binding in certain regions of brain which show low overall binding in studies using tissue homogenates.

Another important difference between our work and the pharmacological investigations using brain homogenates is that our studies were done on the brains of addicts, many with histories of long exposure to narcotic drugs, whereas the pharmacological determinations were done on naive brain tissue, from nonaddicted monkeys and humans. In this regard, it is of some interest to note that brain sections from several nonaddicts, who had received one or two doses of morphine prior to death, failed to show any fluorescence when stained with the anti-morphine serum. Therefore the possibility that the neuronal staining we have shown in addicts' brains is a phenomenon related to tolerance must be considered. The idea gains support from the experimental evidence set forth elsewhere in this volume (Pertschuk et al., 1976).

Difficulties arise in the attempt to relate our demonstration of narcotic in neurons to the elegant demonstrations of stereospecific opiate receptors in synaptic membranes (Pert et al., 1974). Certainly, with the immunofluorescent technique, stereospecificity of drug binding remains to be demonstrated. Two main possibilities suggest themselves for investigation. Significant opiate binding may occur in neurons as well as in synaptosomes perhaps with the addition of new neuronal binding sites occurring as tolerance develops. The theory of the formation of new receptors with tolerance has been put forward previously (Collier, 1965). Alternatively, the intraneuronal narcotic demonstrated by immunofluorescence may be functionally unrelated to the pharmacologically active, receptor-bound drug in the synaptic membrane. If that be the case, the drug in the nerve cell may be indicative of some other facet of opiate metabolism, developing only with chronic use.

SUMMARY

Methadone and morphine have been demonstrated in neurons of brains from human drug addicts by immunofluorescence. The method detects methadone accurately, but with the antimorphine serum used, cross reaction with propoxyphene was observed. Immunofluorescent detection of narcotics may prove valuable for forensic purposes, as well as for the study of opiate distribution in the nervous system. The significance of the demonstration of narcotics in addicts' neurons in relation to the metabolism and binding of opiates in nervous tissue remains to be investigated.

ACKNOWLEDGMENTS

We are grateful to Mrs. Carol Clapman and Mrs. Evelyn Rainford for expert secretarial and technical assistance, and to Mr. Robert Simowitz for help with the photomicrographs.

REFERENCES

Collier, H. O. J. 1965. A general theory of the genesis of drug dependence by induction of receptors. *Nature* (London) 205: 181–182.

Hiller, J. M., J. Pearson, and E. J. Simon. 1973. Distribution of stereospecific binding of the potent narcotic analgesic etorphine in the human brain: Predominance in the limbic system. *Res Commun. Chem. Pathol. Pharmacol.* 6: 1052–1061.

Kuhar, M. J., C. B. Pert, and S. H. Snyder. 1973. Regional distribution of opiate receptor binding in monkey and human brain. *Nature* (London) 245: 447–450.

Liu, Chi-Tan, and F. L. Adler. 1973. Immunologic studies on drug addiction. 1. Antibodies reactive with methadone and their use for detection of the drug. *J. Immunol.* 111: 201–213.

Pert, C. B., A. M. Snowman, and S. H. Snyder. 1974. Localization of opiate receptor binding in synaptic membranes of rat brain. *Brain Res.* 70: 184–188.

Pertschuk, L. P., D. H. Ford, D. J. Brigati, and J. H. Sher. 1976. Immunofluorescent localization of methadone in the central nervous system of the rat. In D. H. Ford, and D. H. Clouet, Eds., *Tissue Responses to Addictive Drugs*. Spectrum Publications, Holliswood, New York.

Pertschuk, L. P., and J. H. Sher. 1975. Demonstration of methadone in human brain by immunofluorescence. *Res. Commun. Chem. Pathol. and Pharmacol.* 11: 319–322.

Spector, S., and C. W. Parker. 1970. Morphine: Radioimmunoassay. *Science* 168: 1347–1348.

Tissue Responses to Addictive Drugs
© 1976, Spectrum Publications, Inc.

³H-Morphine Localization in Brain

MITSUTOSHI WATANABE
IHSAN M. DIAB
CHARLES R. SCHUSTER
LLOYD J. ROTH

*Department of Pharmacological and Physiological Sciences
and the Department of Psychiatry
The University of Chicago
Chicago, Illinois*

The opium alkaloids and their synthetic congeners elicit a multiplicity of pharmacological responses which have largely eluded attempts to define and characterize their sites and modes of action. No single paradigmatic approach seems likely to provide definitive answers to the perplexing problems posed by these drugs. The correlation of drug localization with pharmacological response and the identification and isolation of specific receptor sites are all of great interest.

Continued research on the pharmacology of morphine is centered on efforts to correlate sites of action with drug localization. Identification of potential receptor areas in the brain and the *in vitro* isolation of stereospecifically bound opiates from these areas is being vigorously pursued in several laboratories (Lowney et al., 1974; Pert et al., 1973; Teschemacher et al., 1972). Because precise *in vivo* anatomical localization and distribution of morphine may provide new clues to the mechanism and sites of action of the opiates we restudied this problem using a cellular autoradiographic procedure developed specifically for work with diffusible substances (Roth and Stumpf, 1965; Roth, 1971; Roth et al., 1974; Stumpf and Roth, 1965, 1966; Diab et al., 1971; Diab and Roth, 1972).

METHODS AND MATERIALS

Adult Sprague-Dawley rats (120-130 gms) and newborn rats (6-7 gms) were injected intraperitoneally with morphine (6-^{3}H) 5 μC/gm body weight equivalent to 10 mg/kg. The ^{3}H-morphine was checked for purity prior to injection by thin layer chromatography Silica Gel G with a solvent system of methanol, benzene, and water (75: 10:15 v/v/v/). It is also assumed in our study that ^{3}H-morphine in the brain is not metabolized due to short interval between injection and sacrifice. The animals were sacrificed 15 minutes after injection because whole body autoradiography demonstrated an absence of ^{3}H-morphine in the brain at 60 minutes after administration. Brain sections were processed for light microscope autoradiography by conventional, and by frozen freeze-dry histology.

RESULTS AND DISCUSSION

We found that a number of areas of the brain treated in the conventional manner for autoradiography were devoid of ^{3}H-morphine while autoradiograms from similar areas, in the same animal, prepared by the frozen freeze-dry section technique demonstrated the presence of ^{3}H-morphine. All the tissues tested, including the adult cerebral and cerebellar cortex, thalamus, and hypothalamus, choroid plexus, pituitary, adrenal gland and intestine, showed removal of radioactivity by conventional techniques. Blood vessels in tissue so treated were also devoid of radioactivity. Its retention by the dry technique demonstrates the necessity to consider morphine as a diffusible substance when studying its tissue distribution by autoradiography. Unless otherwise stated all results presented in this report were derived using the dry technique designed for diffiusible substances.

Blood vessels of the brain, regardless of size, contained a high concentration of ^{3}H-morphine (see Figures 1, 2). The silver grain density in the autoradiogram was distinctly higher than adjacent brain parenchyma with a blood to tissue ratio of about 25:1 in the adult rat. The high concentration of ^{3}H-morphine in adult cerebral blood vessels, surrounded by parenchyma of low concentration, is in contrast to the

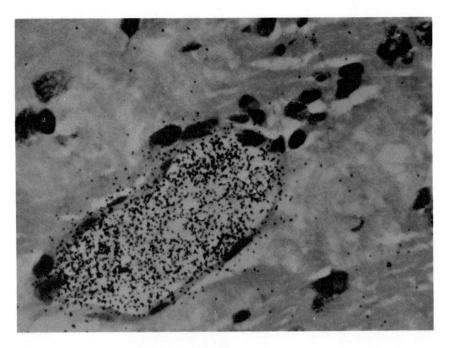

1 High concentration of ³H-morphine seen in blood vessels of adult cerebral cortex. Autoradiographic exposure, 180 days. ³H-morphine administered intraperitoneally and rats sacrificed at 15 minutes. All sections stained with methyl green pyronine. (Procedure identical for all figures.)

more equal concentration of morphine in the blood vessels and parenchyma of the newborn rat brain. However, in peripheral tissues such as muscle and intestine no such concentration difference was found between blood vessels and surrounding tissue. These autoradiograms support the concept of a specific blood brain barrier in the vasculature of the adult which is undeveloped in the newborn. For this reason, the increased pharmacological sensitivity to morphine of newborn rats may, in part, be attributed to an underdeveloped barrier (Kupferberg and Way, 1963). The high concentration of diffusible substances, such as ³H-morphine, in blood vessels of the brain poses a clear risk of false labeling for surrounding tissue when assaying for a mean concentration in such a heterogeneous system, by homogenation, or treatment of tissues by conventional histological techniques.

At the pia mater the silver grain density in autoradiograms of the cortex is high at the junction of the cortex and the pia mater. The density of silver grains in the autoradiogram over the tissue decreases progressively from the pia mater into the brain parenchyma. This

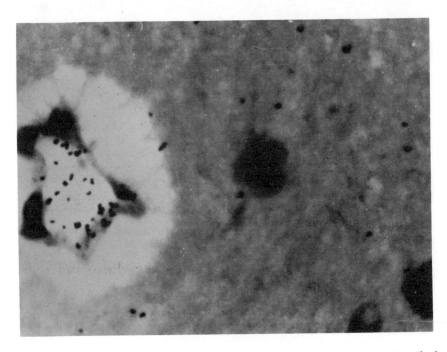

2   High activity of ³H-morphine in adult cerebral cortical capillary. Autoradiographic exposure, 88 days.

concentration gradient of ³H-morphine in the cortex suggests that the labeled drug in the subarachnoid space diffuses through the pia mater into the cortex from which it penetrates deeper into the brain parenchyma (see Figures 3, 4, and Table I).

An interesting distribution pattern of ³H-morphine in a nerve tract is illustrated in Figure 5 which shows high radioactivity in the tractus opticus lying in contact with the pia mater. Similar autoradiograms were obtained from additional sections in the same tract. The significance of this distribution pattern within the tractus opticus is not clear.

The localization of ³H-morphine in the adult rat choroid epithelium, as seen in the autoradiogram (see Figure 6), does not by itself permit a judgment concerning transport into or out of the cerebral spinal fluid. It should be noted, however, that a small concentration of ³H-morphine was seen in tissue abutting the ependymal layer of the ventricles with no apparent concentration gradient from the ependymal layer into the brain parenchyma.

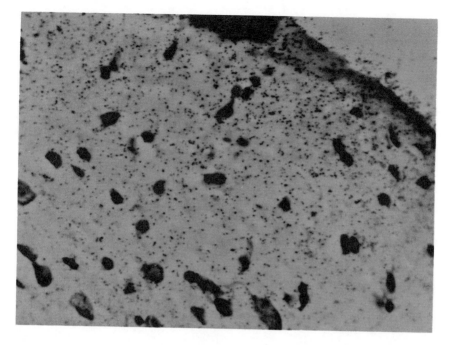

3

Pia mater labeled heavily with ^{3}H-morphine with concentration decreasing with distance from pia matter Autoradiographic exposure, 90 days.

4

Distribution gradient ^{3}H-morphine from pia mater. Autoradiographic exposure, 120 days.
(Siliver grain counting data in Table 1.)

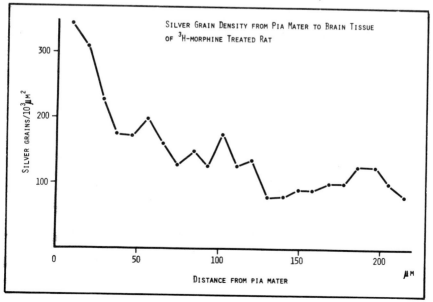

Silver Grain Density from Pia Mater to Brain Tissue in the Autoradiograms of ^{3}H-morphine

	1	2	3	4	5	6	7	8	9	10	11	12	13	14	15
Distance from pia mater (µm)	9.34	18.68	28.02	37.36	46.70	56.04	65.38	74.72	84.06	93.40	102.74	112.08	121.42	130.76	140.10
grains $/10^3 \mu m^2$	389 297 412	424 217 275	412 171 114	217 103 206	103 160 252	114 229 229	126 217 137	137 126 126	183 91 183	114 114 160	148 240 114	80 160 126	252 68 103	57 103 68	91 103 45
mean	366.0	305.3	171.7	190.7	160.0*	129.7	152.3*	129.3**	152.3	129.3**	167.3*	122.0**	141.0*	76.0**	79.7**
S.D.	60.9	106.8	75.2	66.4	49.7	6.4	53.1	26.6	65.2	26.6	65.2	40.1	97.7	24.0	30.6
S.E.	35.1	61.7	43.4	38.3	28.7	3.7	30.7	15.3	37.6	15.3	37.6	23.2	56.4	13.9	17.7

	16	17	18	19	20	21	22	23	24	25	26	27	28	29	30
Distance from pia mater (µm)	149.44	158.78	168.12	177.46	186.80	196.14	205.48	214.82	224.16	233.50	242.84	252.18	261.52	270.86	280.20
grains $/10^3 \mu m^2$	80 126 137	80 126 114	137 80 103	103 68 137	160 160 68	137 160 91	148 57 91	126 68 34	194 103 57	114 34 126	126 11 68	103 22 11	126 171 45	68 114 45	91 34 114
mean	114.3**	106.7**	106.7*	102.7*	129.3*	129.3*	98.7*	76.0**	118.0**	91.3**	68.3**	45.3**	114.0**	75.3**	79.7**
S.D.	30.2	23.9	28.7	34.5	53.1	35.1	46.0	46.5	69.7	50.0	57.5	50.2	63.9	35.1	41.2
S.E.	17.5	13.8	16.6	19.9	30.7	20.3	26.5	26.9	40.3	28.9	33.2	29.0	36.9	20.3	23.8

Each value was calculated from the number of the grains in 87.2 um^2 counted in 3 slides.

* Statistically significant at 5 percent level.

** Statistically significant at 1 percent level.

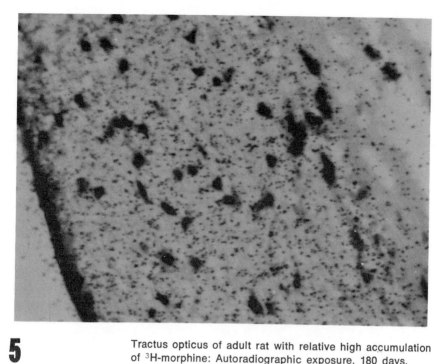

5   Tractus opticus of adult rat with relative high accumulation of ^{3}H-morphine: Autoradiographic exposure, 180 days.

6   Choroid plexus of lateral ventricle. Accumulation of ^{3}H-morphine predominant in epithelium. Autoradiographic exposure, 88 days.

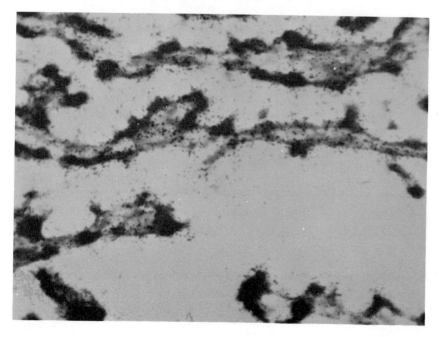

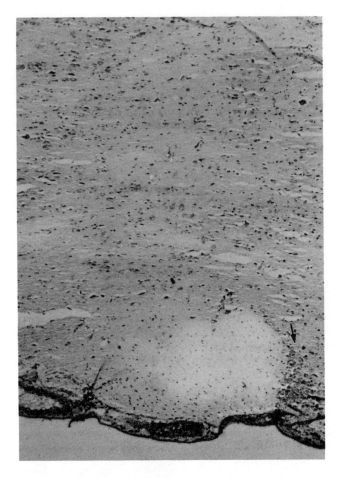

7

Distinct localization of ³H-morphine in ventromedial
hypothalamic nucleus. Autoradiographic exposure, 180 days.

A significant localization of ³H-morphine was found in the ventromedial hypothalamic nucleus (see Figures 7, 8), and the medial
thalamic nucleus (see Figures 9, 10). ³H-morphine in these areas could
be clearly distinguished from the generalized nonspecific, low level
distribution present in surrounding tissue. Scattered neurons throughout
the brain were labeled with ³H-morphine showing higher silver grain
concentration than adjacent tissue. These neurons were mostly present
in the cerebral cortex, caudate nucleus, medulla oblongata, and spinal
cord.

A generalized distribution of ³H-morphine was seen throughout
the anterior and posterior lobes of the pituitary while the medial lobe

contained distinctly lower activity. Within the pituitary, the stalk contained the highest concentration of morphine. In the adrenal gland ^{3}H-morphine was distributed in the cortex and the medulla with the latter containing the highest concentration (see Figure 11). The ganglionic cells in the adrenal medulla showed a specific cellular localization with cytoplasmic labeling being the most prominent (see Figure 12).

Morphine has been shown to stimulate the release of ADH by direct action on the posterior pituitary gland and on the adrenal medulla where it releases norepinephrine (George, 1971). These actions of morphine correlate with our autoradiographic distribution of ^{3}H-morphine in the above tissues. The possibility that morphine may have

 High magnification of ventromedial hypothalamic nucleus. Autoradiographic exposure, 120 days.

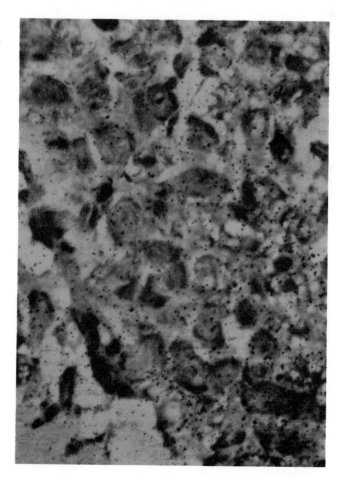

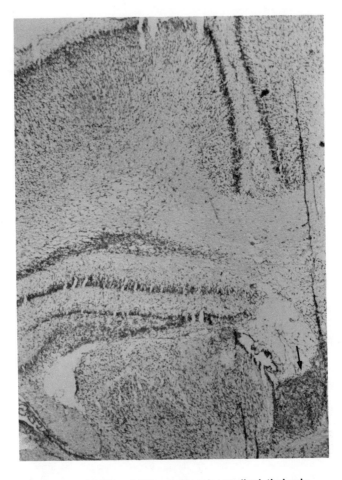

Distinct localization of ^{3}H-morphine in medical thalamic nucleus. Autoradiographic exposure, 120 days. (Newborn rat.)

a direct action on the anterior pituitary and on the adrenal cortex should be considered.

From these studies we found a nonspecific general distribution of ^{3}H-morphine throughout the brain with higher concentrations in cortical gray, medulla, spinal cord and areas beneath the pia mater. Except for the tractus opticus, other areas made up of tracts such as cortical white and the internal capsule, contained relatively low radioactivity. Such areas as the ventromedial hypothalamic nucleus, and the medial thalamic nucleus contained distinctly higher morphine concentrations than tissue surrounding these particular brain nuclei. This specific accumulation can not be attributed to artifact due to contamination from blood vessels or translocation of activity from surrounding tissue. Nonspecific general distribution of ³H-morphine was seen in the cortex, medulla, and spinal cord. The localization of ³H-morphine in ganglionic cells of the adrenal medulla is a new and significant finding although no pharmacological interpretation is advanced at this time. The high concentration of morphine relative to surrounding tissue, seen in blood vessels and capillaries of the brain, demonstrates the existence of a blood barrier in the brain vasculature. Autoradiographic evidence presented in this report suggests a new portal of entry for morphine located in the arachnoid space and the pia mater. Penetration from the arachnoid space may account for the presence of morphine in the spinal cord as well as brain. The significance of the subarachnoid space

10   High magnification of medial thalamic nucleus.
Autoradiographic exposure, 30 days.

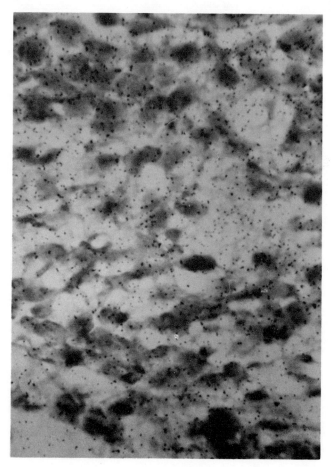

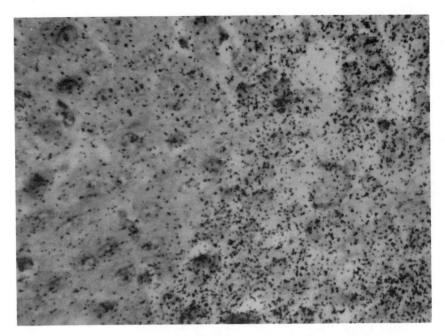

11 ³H-morphine in adrenal gland of rat. Activity in medulla higher than in cortex. Autoradiographic exposure, 50 days.

12 Autoradiogram of ganglion cells in adrenal medulla showing concentration of ³H-morphine in periphery of cells. Autoradiographic exposure, 90 days.

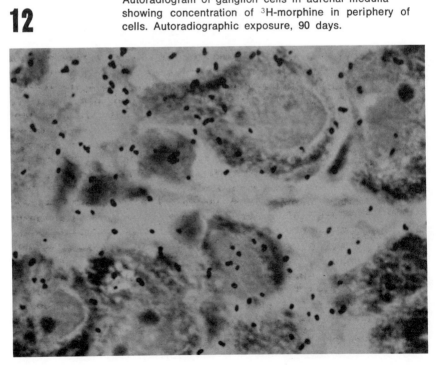

as a portal of entry for drugs has been emphasized by Feldberg (1963). We studied the distribution and localization, following parenteral injection, of ^{3}H-morphine in pharmacological dosage in rats. Its normal physiological entry into brain, and other areas, was determined autoradiographically. We have now shown that it is not necessary to use excessive doses and/or intraventricular injection to see the normal *in vivo* distribution of morphine in brain.

ACKNOWLEDGMENTS

This work was supported in part by Grants PHS 5-RO1 DA-00397-PHS 5-TO1 MH 07083 and PHS PO 1 DA-00250 from the United States Public Health Service.

We thank Zenaida Paragas for her technical assistance.

REFERENCES

Diab, I. M., D. X. Freedman and L. J. Roth. 1971. [^{3}H] Lysergic Acid Diethylamide: Cellular Autoradiographic Localization in Rat Brain. *Science* 173: 1022–1024.

Diab, I. M. and L. J. Roth. 1972. Cellular autoradiography of ^{3}H-LSD in brain, ^{3}H-thymidine in intestine, WR-2529-^{14}C in bone utilizing dry mounted, frozen, freeze-dried sections. *J. Microscopy*, 96: pt. 2, 155–164.

Feldberg, W., Ed. 1963. In *A Pharmacological Approach to the Brain from Its Inner and Outer Surface*. The Williams and Wilkins Company, Baltimore.

George, R. 1971. Hypothalamus: Anterior pituitary gland. In D. H. Clouet, Ed. *Narcotic Drugs Biochemical Pharmacology*. Plenum Press, New York, London, pp. 283–299.

Kupferberg, H. J. and E. L. Way. 1963. Pharmacologic basis for the increased sensitivity of the newborn rat to morphine. *J. Pharmacol. Exp. Therap.* 141: 105–112.

Lowney, L. I., K. Schulz, P. J. Lowery, and A. Goldstein. 1974. Partial purification of an opiate receptor from mouse brain. *Science*, 183: 749–753.

Pert, C. V., G. Pasternak, and S. H. Snyder. 1973. Opiate agonists and antagonists discriminated by receptor binding in brain. *Science* 182: 1359–1361.

Roth, L. J. 1971. The use of autoradiography in experimental pharmacology. In B. B. Brodie and J. Gillette, Eds. *Handbook of Experimental Pharmacology* (New Series). 28: #1, pp. 286–316.

Roth, L. J., I. M. Diab, M. Watanabe, and R. J. Dinerstein. 1974. A correlative radioautographic, fluorescent, and histochemical technique for cytopharmacology. *Mol. Pharmacol.* 10: 986–998.

Roth, L. J., and W. E. Stumpf, Eds. 1965. In *Autoradiography of Diffusible Substances*. Academic Press, New York.

Stumpf, W. E., and L. J. Roth. 1966. High resolution autoradiography with dry mounted, freeze-dried frozen sections. Comparative Study of Six Methods Using Two Diffusible Compounds ^{3}H-Estradiol and ^{3}H-Mesobilirubinogen. *J. of Histochem. and Cytochem.* 14: #3 274–287.

Stumpf, W. E., and L. J. Roth. 1967. Freeze-drying of small tissue samples and thin frozen sections below −60°C. A simple method of cryosorption pumping. *J. of Histochem. and Cytochem.* 15:4 243–251.

Teschemacher, H., P. Schubert, and A. Herz. 1973. Autoradiographic studies concerning the supraspinal site of the antinociceptive action of morphine when inhibiting the hindleg flexor reflex in rabbits. *Neuropharmacol.* 12: 123–131.

Tissue Responses to Addictive Drugs
© 1976, Spectrum Publications, Inc.

³H-Morphine in the Myenteric Plexus; Fluorescence and Autoradiographic Correlation

IHSAN M. DIAB
ROBERT J. DINERSTEIN
MITSUTOSHI WATANABE
LLOYD J. ROTH

*Department of Pharmacological and Physiological Sciences
and the Department of Psychiatry
The University of Chicago
Chicago, Illinois*

Opium alkaloids have been utilized as analgesics of choice for hundreds of years. However, their pharmacological mode of action, anatomical localization, and molecular receptor sites, remain elusive. In order to demonstrate that narcotic analgesics act at a specific pharmacological site, one must localize these compounds at or near the specific anatomical area involved and correlate such localization with various pharmacological, physiological and biochemical parameters. There is considerable evidence for pharmacological interaction of morphine with one or more putative neurotransmitters, but the available evidence regarding this interaction is often incomplete, confusing, and in some instances contradictory (Vogt, 1973). Acetylcholine, catecholamines and indolealealkylamines have all been implicated in one or another of the pharmacological actions of morphine (Lees et al., 1973; Way, 1973, Smith and Sheldon, 1973; and Ehrenpreis et al., 1972).

While the major pharmacological action of morphine is thought to take place in the central nervous system, the complexity of the brain and the number of neurotransmitters involved therein have made the discovery of the exact site of action of morphine a difficult task. In order to circumvent some of these problems associated with morphine in the brain, simpler peripheral systems have been proposed as models (Paton, 1955; Kosterlitz and Wallis, 1966). The isolated guinea pig ilium preparation containing the myenteric plexus is now an important tool for the study of narcotic drugs and antagonists. Such plexus preparations have demonstrated that morphine and other narcotic agonists result in inhibition of smooth muscle contractions induced by coaxial stimulation. This action is dose dependent, stereospecific, and the inhibition is reversed by narcotic antagonists (Paton, 1957; Kosterlitz and Watt, 1968; and Ehrenpreis, 1972). This preparation, which contains the myenteric plexus attached only to the longitudinal muscle layer, serves as a useful model for the central nervous system due to the presence of well defined neurons, glial cells and nerve fibers within its structure. Diffusion of drugs into this isolated preparation is facilitated by its large surface area. We have found this preparation to be ideally suited for cellular autoradiographic and fluorescence studies because of its thinness and well defined structure.

Using combined autoradiography, fluorescence microscopy and microspectrophotofluorometry we have studied the localization of ^{3}H-morphine in the myenteric plexus preparation to identify the cells labeled with ^{3}H-morphine and its binding to these cells. This preparation may also be used to demonstrate the presence of biogenic amines by fluorescence microscopy, their characterization by their excitation and emission spectra, and, to correlate the localization of morphine with a particular neurotransmitter within the same preparation.

MATERIALS AND METHODS

Female guinea pigs (150-200 gm) were starved for 24-48 hours prior to sacrifice. The ilia were cut 1-3 cm from the ceceum to a length of 20-30 cm, flushed 3 times with ice cold Tyrode's solution and divided into segments 4-5 cm in length. Each segment was then pulled over a delivery pipette for isolation of the longitudinal muscle layer only with the attached myenteric plexus of Auerbach. An initial separation of the external longitudinal muscle layer from the internal circular muscle layer was created at one end of the segment by gentle rubbing with a Q-tip wetted with Tyrode's solution. The separated longitudinal muscle end was grasped with a small tweezer and stripped free from the rest of the circular muscle along the entire length of the intestinal segment. The isolated longitudinal muscle strip with the myenteric plexus attached was placed in a petri dish containing ice cold Tyrode's solution for dissection of 4-6 mm sections, and examined for the presence of the plexus under the dissecting microscope. The presence of the myenteric plexus attached to the longitudinal muscle can be easily identified without staining by its honeycomb network appearance (see Figures 1a and 1b). The small sections of the myenteric plexus preparation are incubated in Tyrode's solution containing 0.1 μg/ml of ^{3}H-morphine (1 μc/ml) for 1 minute at 25°C, washed three times for one minute each in a nonradioactive Tyrode's solution and mounted directly on Formvar coated microscope slides without adhesive or mounting media. After blotting and air drying, the sections were stored over Drierite for at least 24 hours. Sections prepared in this manner may be coated directly with NTB-3 Kodak liquid emulsion for autoradiography alone. However, for correlative autoradiography, fluorescence microscopy, microspectrophotofluorometry and histochemistry (see Figure 2), the Formvar coated slide was cemented at one end to a dry coverslip (25 x 77 mm #0) previously coated with NTB-3 Kodak emulsion. Following 90 days of exposure at –15°C, the slide and coverslip were spaced apart in a manner permiting photographic development of the emulsion while the tissue remains uncontaminated by the developing solutions. The sections were then gassed with formaldehyde, generated from paraformaldehyde (previously equilibriated at 60% relative humidity) at 80°C for one hour, to induce the formation of fluorophore. The autoradiogram and "fluorogram" were photographed (Roth et al., 1974). Microphotofluorometric spectra of the fluorescence was performed on a Leitz Orthoplan microscope using Pleom vertical illumination through all quartz optics and grating monochrometers. A photon counter was used to maximize sensitivity, thereby minimizing fluorescence fading (Dinerstein et al., 1976). Finally, the sections were stained for histochemistry.

RESULTS

Autoradiograms of isolated myenteric plexus sections incubated with ^{3}H-morphine and then washed with Tyrode solution demonstrated specific localization on small glial satellite cells. Silver grains of the autoradiograms were present over these small cellular elements surrounding the ganglionic neurones as well as the cells within the nerve fibers network (see Figures 3a and 3b). The unwashed plexus prepara-

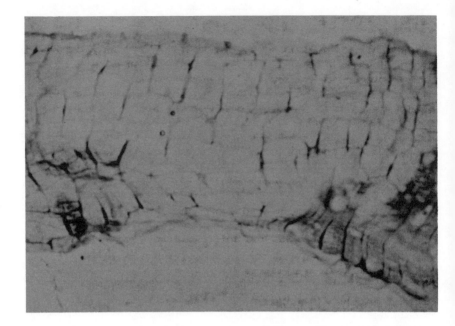

1a

b

Guinea pig ilium strip showing the myenteric plexus of Auerbach's overylaying the longitudinal muscle layer. Stained lightly with Toludine Blue 0.01%. (a) Low magnification, 10X, showing the plexus with its honeycomb appearance. (b) Higher magnification, 98X, showing the plexus junctions, its nerve fibers network and its ramification over the muscle layer.

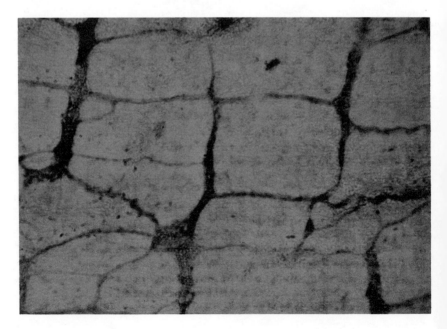

CORRELATIVE AUTORADIOGRAPHIC AND FLUORESCENCE MICROSCOPY

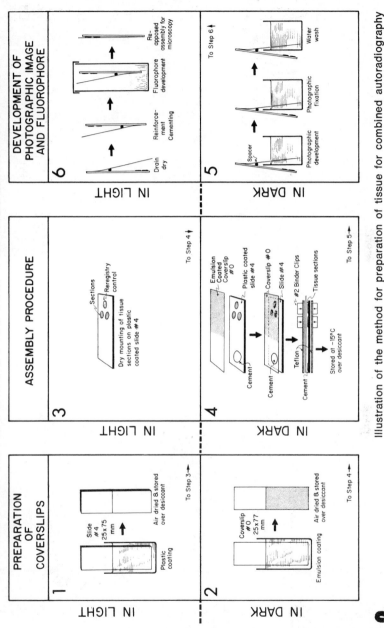

Illustration of the method for preparation of tissue for combined autoradiography and fluorescence microscopy.

79

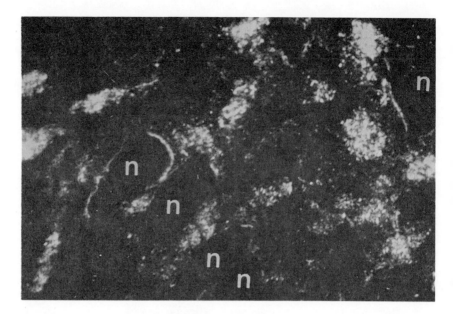

3a

Autoradiogram of guinea pig ilium myenteric plexus preparation incubated for one minute in ^{3}H-morphine (o.1 μg/ml) and exposed for 90 days. (a) Autoradiogram darkfield illumination showing silver grains as white dots. The silver grain activity is present over small cellular elements surrounding the ganglionic neurones (n) and within fiber tracts from one ganglionic junction to another. (640X.) (b) The similar autoradiogram photographed through brightfield illumination. Showing silver grains as black dots. (640X.)

b

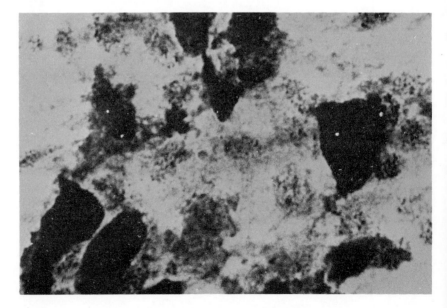

tion revealed high silver grains distribution throughout the entire myenteric plexus including the muscle and blood vessels in the preparation. The satellite cells "gliocytes," containing morphine activity, could be differentiated from other neuronal elements in the plexus by their small size, their spherical or oval shape, their location around the large ganglionic cells within the plexus junctions and the nerve fibers network, as well as their staining properties (De Castro, 1946).

The myenteric plexus preparation, when gassed with formaldehyde, exhibited specific green fluorescent varicosities characteristic of nerve endings. The fluorescing varicosities outline the fiber tracts of the plexus and their ramifications (see Figures 4a and 4b). The large ganglionic neurones at junctions in the plexus network did not exhibit fluorescence within them, however, they were surrounded by small green fluorescent varicosities. The type of biogenic amine present in these varicosities was shown to be norepinephrine by microphotofluorometric spectra. Norepinephrine and dopamine, when gassed with formaldehyde, each show the same fluorescence spectra with an excitation peak at 410 nm and emission peak at 490 nm. However, when the tissue sample is treated with HCl vapor, following formaldehyde gassing, a shift in the norepinephrine excitation peak from 410 nm to 390 nm occurs together with the appearance of a new peak at 320 nm while the emission peak remains unchanged (Bjorklund et al., 1972). The new excitation peak is identical with the observed spectra of a standard sample of norepinephrine treated in the same manner (see Figure 5). No such change in the excitation spectrum occurs with a standard sample of dopamine.

Some yellow fluorescing cells were observed in the myenteric plexus preparation following formaldehyde gassing. These yellow cells were present in the sections incubated with ^{3}H-morphine as well as those of nonincubated controls. A few of these fluorescing cells were identified as serotonin containing, primarily by microphotofluorometric spectra, and by the usual rapid disappearance of the yellow fluorescence upon exposure to uv light. The microphotofluorometric spectra of these cells showed an excitation peak 410 nm and emission peak at 525 nm (see Figures 6a and 6b). The spectrum is identical with standard sample of serotonin treated in the same manner. These serotonin containing cells are probably not neuronal in nature since they were observed on the longitudinal muscle layer outside the myenteric plexus proper. Most likely, these cells are mast cells or fibroblasts present within the intestinal wall. Pretreatment of animals with biogenic amine depleting agents, loading with 5-hydroxytryptophan and application of monoamine oxidase inhibitors (Ross and Gershon 1972; and Gershon

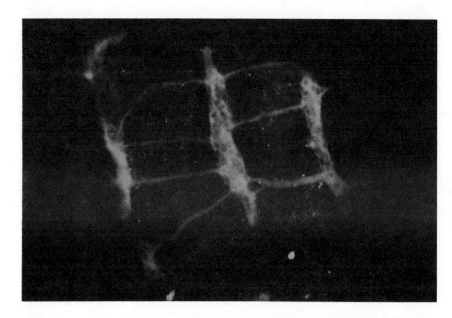

4a

A fluorogram of myenteric plexus preparation incubated with ^{3}H-morphine and gassed with formaldehyde for one hour at 80°C. (Photographed through Zeiss microscope illuminated with mercury H BO 200 W Lamp with Zeiss activation filter No. 1 and barrier filters 53 and 47.) The induced fluorescence observed was green. (a) Fluorogram showing nerve fibre fluorescent varicosities outlying the plexus. (63X). (b) Fluorogram at the junction of the plexus showing fluorescent nerve fiber varicosities surrounding ganglionic neurones. (250X).

b

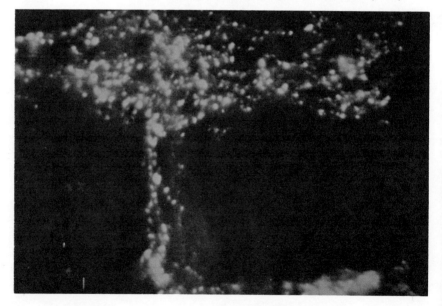

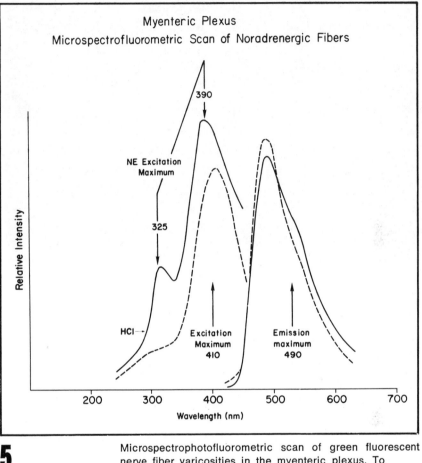

Myenteric Plexus
Microspectrofluorometric Scan of Noradrenergic Fibers

5

Microspectrophotofluorometric scan of green fluorescent nerve fiber varicosities in the myenteric plexus. To differentiate norepinephrine from dopamine the tissue was gassed with formaldehyde (broken lines - - - - -) and regassed with HCl (solid line ————). The relative intensity, uncorrected, and the spectra were compared with biogenic amine standards and were found to be consistent with norepinephrine.

and Dreyfus 1975) demonstrated the presence of serotonin in myenteric plexus. In this study we were unable to show the presence of serotonin in neuronal cells, nor, could we demonstrate a correlation between serotonin fluorescence and morphine. Other occasional cells adjacent to the myenteric plexus were observed to exhibit yellow-orange fluorescence upon exposure to formaldehyde gas which did not fade upon prolonged

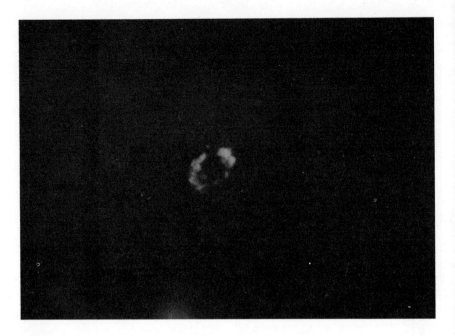

6a

exposure to uv light. These cells were present in both control and morphine incubated strips. The microphotofluorometric spectra of these cells showed an excitation peak at 350 nm and a broad emission maximum at 480-555 nm (see Figure 7). This yellow-orange fluorescence is consistent with autofluorescence or tryptophan rich protein breakdown products, but, not with biogenic amines (Smith and Kappers, 1975).

DISCUSSION

Localization of ^{3}H-morphine in specific neuronal elements in the myenteric plexus correlates with some of its pharmacological actions on the guinea pig ilium. The predominant autoradiographic localization and specific binding of morphine on the glial satellite cells or nerve endings impinging on these cells, suggests that the site of action of morphine in the myenteric plexus preparation may be associated with the glial elements rather than the larger ganglionic neurones of the plexus. By inference, the glial involvement in the myenteric plexus may also apply to the glial cells in the central nervous system. The large gangli-

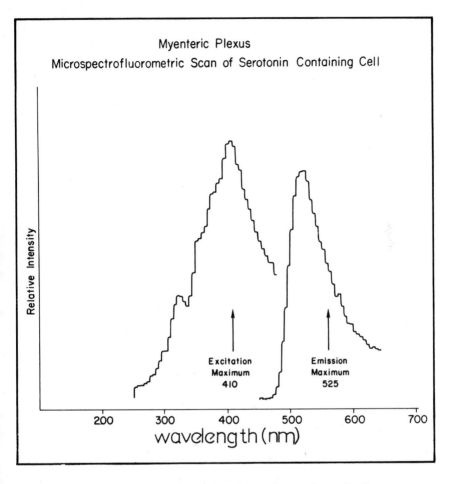

Myenteric Plexus
Microspectrofluorometric Scan of Serotonin Containing Cell

Relative Intensity

Excitation
Maximum
410

Emission
Maximum
525

wavelength (nm)

b

(a) Fluorogram of a yellow fluorescing cell after exposure
to formaldehyde gas for one hour at 80°C (viewed as in
Figure 4). This yellow fluorescence was identified as
serotonin tentatively by its rapid fading following exposure
to uv light and definitively by microspectrophotofluorometric
scan. (510X.) (b) Microspectrophotofluorometric scan of the
above yellow fluorescing cell. The low intensity and
fluorescence fading required spectral measurement 5 nm
and 4 seconds duration by photon counting, giving
staircase spectra. The relative intensity, uncorrected, and
the spectra were compared with biogenic amine standards
and were found to be consistent with serotonin.

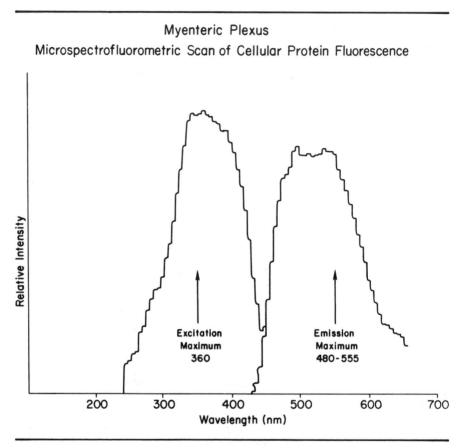

7 Microspectrophotofluorometric scan of yellow-orange fluorescing cells. The relative intensity uncorrected, the spectral comparison with biogenic amine standards, the resistance to uv bleaching, and the very broad emission maximum suggests this yelow-orange fluorescence is not due to biogenic amine but might be due to protein breakdown products rich in tryptophan.

onic neurones of the plexus showed neither morphine localization nor biogenic amine fluorescence. However, intense noradrenergic varicosities and labeled satellite cells surrounding these neurones suggest an indirect action of morphine and norepinephrine on the ganglionic neurones. The intense noradrenergic fluorescence associated with nerve fibers impinging on the "gliocytes" correlates the localization and binding of morphine with the presence of norepinephrine in these fibers.

The specific localization of morphine on the myenteric plexus, its binding to some neuronal elements within the plexus as well as its correlation with noradrenergic fibers, opens a new approach to the study of narcotic analgesic agents and their antagonists.

ACKNOWLEDGMENTS

This work was supported in part by Grants PHS 5-RO1 DA-00397-PHS 5-TO 1 MH 07083 and PHS PO 1 DA-00250 from the United States Public Health Service.
We thank Zenaida Paragas for her technical assistance.

REFERENCES

Bjorklund, A., B. Ehinger, and B. Falk. 1972. Analysis of fluorescence excitation peak ratios for cellular identification of noradrenaline, dopamine and their mixtures. *J. Histochem. and Cytochem.* 20: 56–64.

De Castro, F. 1946. Sobre el comportamineto y significacion de la oligodendroglia en la substancia gris central, y de los gliocitos en los ganglios nerviosos perifericos. *Archivos De Histologia Normal & Patologica* (Buenos Aires) 3: 317–343.

Dinerstein, R. J., A. Ferber, I. M. Diab, and L. J. Roth. 1976. (To be published)

Ehrenpreis, S., I. Light, and G. H. Schonbach. 1972. Use of the electrically stimulated guinea pig ileum to study potent analgesics. In J. M. Singh, L.I. Miller, and H. Lal, Eds. *Drug Addiction: Experimental Pharmacology.* Futura Publishing Co., New York, pp. 319–342.

Gershon, M. D., and C. F. Dreyfus. 1975. Serotonin in neurons of mammalian myentric plexus. Fed Proc. 34: Abstract number 3288, p. 801.

Kosterlitz, H. W., and D. I. Wallis. 1966. The effects of hexamethonium and morphine on transmission in the superior cervical ganglia of the rabbit. *Brit. J. of Pharmacol. & Chemotherap.* 26: 334–341.

Kosterlitz, H. W. and A. J. Watt. 1968. Kinetic parameters of narcotic agonists and antagonists. *Brit. J. Pharmacol. & Chemotherap.* 33: 266–276.

Lees, G. M., H. W. Kosterlitz, and A. A. Waterfield. 1973. Characteristics of morphine sensitive release of neurotransmitter substances. In H. W. Kosterlitz, H. O. J. Collier, and S. E. Villarreal, Eds. *Agonist and Antagonist Actions of Narcotic Analgesic Drugs.* University Park Press, Baltimore pp. 142–152.

Paton, W. D. 1955. The response of guinea-pig ileum to electrical stimulation by coaxial electrodes. *J. Physiol.* 127: 40–41.

Paton, W. D. 1957. The action of morphine and related substances on contraction and on acetylcholine output of coaxially stimulated guinea-pig ileum. *Brit. J. Pharmacol. & Chemotherap.* 12: 119–127.

Ross. L. L., and M. D. Gershon. 1972. Electron microscopic radioautographic and fluorescence localization of sites of 5-hydroxytrpytamine (5-HT) uptake in the myenteric plexus of the guinea pig ileum. *J. Cell. Biol.* 55: 220–439.

Roth, L. J., I. M. Diab, M. Watanabe, and R. J. Dinerstein. 1974. A correlative radioautographic fluorescence and histochemical technique for cytopharmacology. *Molecular Pharmacol.* 10: 986–998.

Smith, A. R. and J. A. Kappers. 1975. Effect of pinealectomy, gonadectomy, PCPA and pineal extracts on the rat parvocellular neurosecretory hypothalmic system; a fluorescence histochemical investigation. *Brain Res.* 86: 353–371.

Smith, C. B., and M. I. Sheldon. 1973. Effects of narcotic analgesics drugs on brain noredrenergic mechanisms. In H. W. Kosterlitz, et al., Eds. *Agonist and Antagonist Actions of Narcotic Analgesic Drugs.* University Park Press, Baltimore, pp. 164–175.

Vogt, M. 1973. Types of Neurons Involved in Analgesic Effect of Morphine. In H. W. Kosterlitz et al., Eds. *Agonist and Antagonist Actions of Narcotic Analgesic Drugs.* University Park Press, Baltimore, pp. 139–141.

Way, E. L. 1973. Reassessment of brain 5-hydroxytryptamine in morphine tolerance and physical dependence. In H. W. Kosterlitz et al., Eds. *Agonist and Antagonist Actions of Narcotic Analgesic Drugs.* University Park Press, Baltimore pp. 153–163.

Tissue Responses to Addictive Drugs
© 1976, Spectrum Publications, Inc.

Opiate Receptor Binding in Intact Animals

CANDACE B. PERT
SOLOMON H. SNYDER
MICHAEL J. KUHAR

*Departments of Pharmacology and Experimental Therapeutics
and Psychiatry and the Behavioral Sciences
The Johns Hopkins University School of Medicine
Baltimore, Maryland*

For some time it has been postulated that opiates must, first, combine with discrete tissue constituents termed "receptors" in order to exert their effects in the living animal (Dole, 1970; Golstein et al., 1968). Biochemical demonstration of these opiate receptors was accomplished using *in vitro* methods in which opiate binding unrelated to specific receptor sites could be washed away (Pert and Snyder, 1973a,b; Simon et al., 1973; Terenius, 1973).

While *in vitro* techniques for studying opiate receptors have been useful for many purposes, the development of a method for measuring opiate receptor sites in the living, intact animal became a desirable goal. Such techniques could conceivably reveal alterations in opiate receptors which are relevant to the development of tolerance and physical dependence. Thus far, *in vitro* methods have failed to reveal such changes (Klee and Streaty, 1974; Pert et al., 1973; Pert and Snyder, in press). However, if opiate tolerance and/or physical dependence is mediated by a shift in the equilibrium of opiate receptor conformations (Snyder, 1975; Pert, 1974), this subtle qualitative alteration would go undetected using *in vitro* methods since homogenization and tissue processing would disrupt the receptor environment.

While the distribution of opiate receptors in various regions of the mammalian brain has been studied by dissection and subsequent binding assay *in vitro* (Hiller et al., 1973; Pert et al., 1974a,b; Kuhar et al., 1973), this method is clearly inadequate for a detailed analysis. Autoradiographic visualization of fine receptor distribution in tissue sections requires a method for labeling opiate receptors with a tritiated ligand in the living animal. Unfortunately, opiate distribution *in vivo* is influenced primarily by blood flow, lipid soluability, degree of ionization, and other nonspecific effects. Under most conditions, the density of opiate receptors in a given brain region does not affect opiate distribution sufficiently to detect regional differences in drug distribution (Ingoglia and Dole, 1970; Chernov and Woods, 1965; Berkowitz and Way, 1971; Clouet and Williams, 1973).

[3]H-NALOXONE BINDING *IN VIVO*

We have recently described a method for measuring opiate receptor binding in intact animals using ^{3}H-naloxone (Pert and Snyder, 1975). When extremely low doses of ^{3}H-naloxone (.001 mg/kg) are injected intravenously into rats, about one-third of the drug is associated with opiate receptors 15 minutes after injection. Several lines of reasoning led to this conclusion. First, two-thirds of the ^{3}H-naloxone could be washed away, using rapid filtration and an ice cold buffer, from a brain homogenate, obtained within two minutes of the rat's decapitation. When the high affinity portion of tissue-bound naloxone which could not be washed away was analyzed, it was found to parallel the regional variations in opiate receptor density determined by *in vitro* methods. That is, the striatum displayed two or three times more binding than the hindbrain and about seven times more than the cerebellum. Moreover, bound ^{3}H-naloxone could be reduced by 63% by an injection of nonradioactive nalorphine (2 mg/kg, i.p.) five minutes prior to ^{3}H-naloxone injection. A 50-fold higher dose of morphine was required to obtain the same degree of inhibition. Grumbach and Chernov (1965) reported that nalorphine is at least 20 times more potent than morphine when they compete *in vivo*. The relative weakness of morphine compared to nalorphine in displacing ^{3}H-naloxone binding *in vivo* was also consistent with the nearly 30-fold greater potency of nalorphine in displacing *in vitro* ^{3}H-naloxone binding (Pert and Snyder, 1974) in the presence of sodium.

BINDING *IN VIVO* IN RATS PHYSICALLY DEPENDENT ON MORPHINE

As animals become more physically dependent on opiates, the dose of naloxone required to precipitate the same degree of withdrawal response decreases (Way, Loh and Shen, 1969). We therefore examined the binding of ^{3}H-naloxone *in vivo* in naive and morphine-dependent rats to determine whether enhanced binding could be detected in "addicted" rats, despite large quantities of morphine present from the addiction regimen. A number of different schedules were used for implanting rats with morphine pellets (75 mg) which resulted in varying degrees of physical dependence. In some experiments, the control rats were pretreated acutely with various doses of morphine in order to make their brain morphine levels more comparable to those of addicted rats. Despite these efforts, we could not demonstrate a difference in ^{3}H-naloxone binding between control and addicted animals (see Table I).

^{3}H-diprenorphine, a potent opiate antagonist, binds to receptors *in vivo* with such great affinity that one hour after injection, about 80% of the drug is associated with specific receptors (Pert, Kuhar and Snyder, 1975). Thus, it is possible to assay receptor binding *in vivo* with ^{3}H-Diprenorphine without washing brain tissue homogenates. Rats which had been subjected to a strenuous addiction regimen were injected with ^{3}H-diprenorphine (13 Ci/mmole), killed, and their brains dissected into four regions: corpus striatum, midbrain, hindbrain, and cerebellum. The striatum contained nine times more radioactivity than the cerebellum on a per weight basis and the midbrain and hindbrain contained, respectively, seven to eight, and three times more radioactivity than the cerebellum, in good agreement with the relative enrichment in opiate receptors in these regions, as assessed by *in vitro* methods (Pert and Snyder, 1973b). However, we could detect no significant difference in ^{3}H-diprenorphine content between the "addict" and control rats in any region examined (see Table I). Since this procedure was truly "*in vivo*," with no manipulations of homogenates, our failure to detect alterations in the receptor binding of diprenorphine constitutes fairly strong evidence against the notion that receptor alterations in binding mediate opiate tolerance and physical dependence.

Table I. Binding of ^{3}H-Opiates *In Vivo* in Control and "Addicted" Rats
(Values are the mean from groups of 4-6 rats)

Addiction Regimen*	^{3}H-Opiate Dose (µCi)	Morphine Dose mg/kg	Injection Time Relative to ^{3}H-Naloxone Injection (min)	Specific Radioactivity (CPM) Bound Control/Addict
^{3}H-Naloxone				
1., 5.., 7...9	20	None		505/496
1., 3	20	None		423/511
1., 6..., 8.., 13	5	None		177/122+
1., 5	20	None		448/439
1., 4...7...,11	20	10, i.v.	30-PRE	130/119+
1., 4...7...,13	20	40, i.p.	15-PRE	244/234
1., 4	30	20, i.p.	60-PRE	412/578
1., 5	30	20, i.p.	60-PRE	698/731

1.,3.,4..,7	30	20, i.p.	60-PRE	820/716
1.,3	20	20, i.p.	30-PRE	309/380
1.,2..,5	20	15, i.p.	30-PRE	583/403
1.,6..,10	20	15, i.p.	3-POST	407/414
1.,4...6	20	10, i.v.	10-POST	451/332
[3]H-Levallorphan	100	None		463/481
[3]H-Diprenorphine	60	None		320/359 (Striatum)
				114/158 (Hindbrain)
				260/282 (Midbrain)
				36/36 (Cerebellum)

Rats were decapitated 15 minutes after ^{3}H-naloxone injection. Cerebella and the rest of brain were rapidly homogenized in 150 volumes of cold TRIS-HCl buffer (pH 7.4 at 25°C) containing 100 mM NaCl (unless marked with +), filtered and washed as described. Specific radioactivity bound in 2 ml of homogenate is obtained by subtracting cerebellar binding from that of the rest of the brain (see Pert and Snyder, 1975).

For ^{3}H-Diprenorphine, 1 ml of the *unwashed* homogenate was counted.

*Each period represents the implantation of a 75 mg morphine pellet on the given day. The last number is the day of sacrifice.

FAILURE TO DETECT BINDING OF
RADIOLABELED AGONISTS *IN VIVO*

We investigated the ability of a number of ^{3}H-opiate agonists to assess receptor binding *in vivo* by comparing the relative radioactivity content of the cerebellum and the rest of the brain at 15, 30 and 60 minutes after intravenous injection. Over a wide range of doses employed (2–100 uCi), we were unable to demonstrate a differential accumulation of either ^{3}H-dihydromorphine (55 Ci/mmole), ^{3}H-oxymorphone (1 Ci/mmole), ^{3}H-levorphanol (5 Ci/mmole), ^{3}H-heroin (34 Ci/mmole), or ^{3}H-etorphine (41 Ci/mmole) in rat cerebellum (which is devoid of opiate receptors) and in the rest of the brain. In the presence of sodium ion, agonists have reduced affinity for the opiate receptor which is due to a more rapid dissociation from the receptor (Pert and Snyder, 1974). Our failure to detect binding of ^{3}H-opiates *in vivo* is probably due to their reduced affinity in the sodium-rich cellular environment.

AUTORADIOGRAPHIC VISUALIZATION OF
OPIATE RECEPTOR DISTRIBUTION

^{3}H-diprenorphine is able to label opiate receptors *in vivo* with only about 20% of the total radioactivity content attributable to unbound, nonspecificially distributed drug, presumably due to its high affinity for opiate receptors (K_D = 1-2 x 10^{-10}) (Pert et al., 1975). However, the reversible nature of its binding to receptors requires that special methods be utilized during tissue processing for autoradiography in order to prevent diffusion away from receptor sites (Appleton, 1964). One hour after intravenous injection of ^{3}H-diprenorphine, the rat brain was carefully mounted on a brass chuck and lowered into liquid nitrogen. After bringing coronal tissue sections gradually up to $-20°$C, extremely thin (4 micron) sections were transferred by thawing onto precoated emulsion-covered slides in the dark by briefly touching the room temperature slide to the frozen section lying on the cold microtome blade. Slides were stored for five weeks for exposure in a low humidity box and then developed and viewed (Pert et al., 1975) (see Figure 1).

A number of small areas, inaccessible by dissection techniques, showed an extremely high density of autoradiographic grains which was six to ten times above "background." The zona compacta of the substantia nigra which contains the cell bodies of the nigral-striatal dopamine pathway was among these (see Figure 2). Interestingly, the adjacent zona reticulata had grain counts only two to three times above

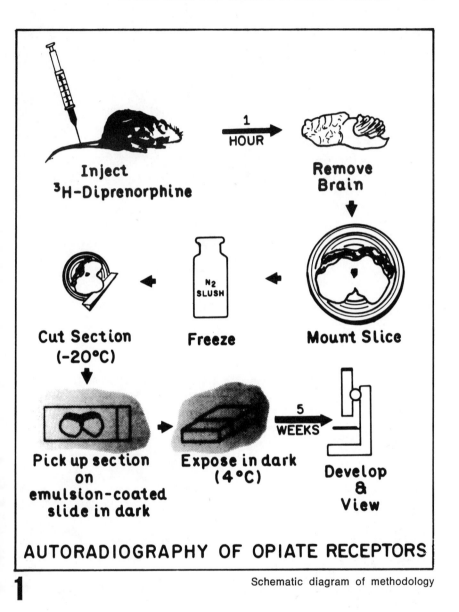

AUTORADIOGRAPHY OF OPIATE RECEPTORS

1

Schematic diagram of methodology

"background." The locus coeruleus, which contains the cell bodies of the ascending noradrenergic pathway, was also found to be highly enriched in grains (see Figure 3). The lateral edge of the medial habenula, which contains cell bodies of cholinergic neurons which terminate in the interpeduncular nucleus, was another of these high density grain

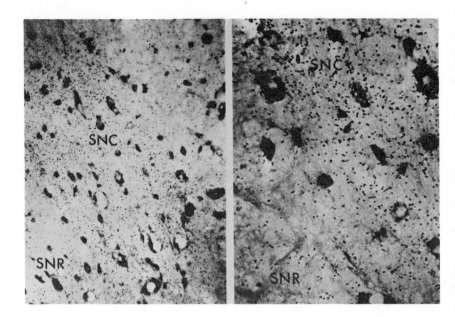

2

Coronal section through the substantia nigra. SNC=zona compacta, SNR=zona reticulata. (Left 200X; right 500X.) The large dark areas are cell bodies, while the small black spots are autoradiographic grains.

3

Coronal section through rat locus coeruleus. (Left 200X; right 500X.) Autoradiographic grains are clearly visible only at higher magnification.

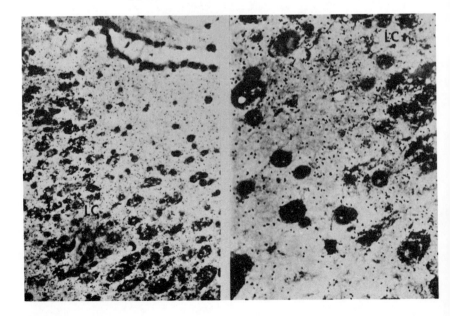

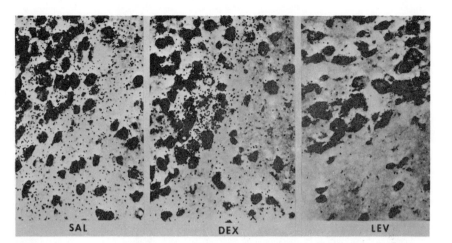

4

Distribution of ³H-diprenorphine in the lateral edge of medial habenula visualized by autoradiography (500X). The large dark areas are cell bodies, while the small black spots are autoradiographic grains. Rats were injected with saline (SAL), levallorphan (LEV), or "dextrallorphan" (DEX) (5 mg/kg i.v.), and ³H-diprenorphine (.008 mg/kg) one hour before sacrifice. Levallorphan, a potent opiate antagonist, reduces the grain count to background levels in all brain areas examined, while "dextrallorphan," its pharmacologically-inert enantiomer, produces no significant difference in grain distribution from saline.

areas (see Figure 4). While our analysis of all receptor-dense areas has not yet been completed, our present findings already suggest possible anatomical substrates for opiate effects which have been observed on catecholamine and cholinergic neurochemistry (Clouet, 1971).

While dissection and *in vitro* binding assay had previously revealed that the rat corpus striatum was enriched in opiate receptors, autoradiographic methods show that receptors are distributed strikingly heterogeneously within the caudate (see Figure 5). A high density "streak" of grains was consistently observed in a narrow band just ventral to the corpus callosum, perhaps coinciding with the stratum subcallosum, a thalamo-fronto fiber bundle (see Figure 5a). Within the caudate, irregularly distributed "patches" of grains were observed which often encircled, but never appeared directly over the fibers of the internal capsule (see Figure 5b). While the quality of tissue sections varied

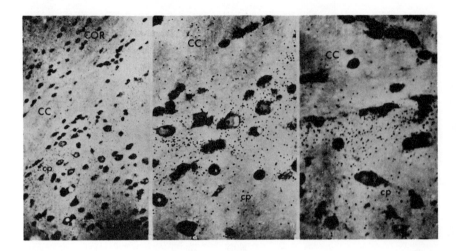

5a

A "streak" of densely distributed autoradiographic grains was observed in the caudate-putamen (CP) just ventral to and completely outlining the corpus callosum (CC).

b

"Patches" of high density autoradiographic grains occur irregularly over the caudate-putamen (CP) but never encroach on the fibers of the internal capsule (IC).

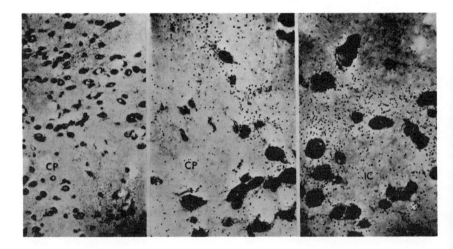

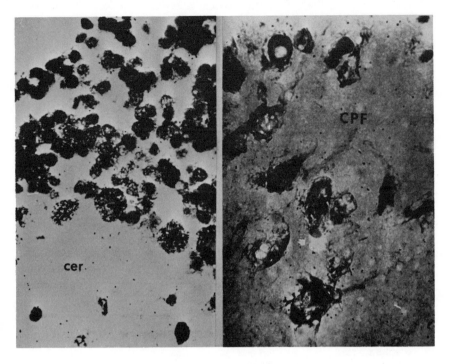

6

The cerebellum (CER) and pyriform cortex (CPF) contain only very low, "background" levels of autoradiographic grains (0.8 - 1.1 grains per 100 microns^2). Shown here (at 660X magnification), grains are sparse and barely visible. Rat cerebellum is devoid of opiate receptors as examined by *in vitro* methods (Pert and Snyder, 1973a).

from one rat to another, the distribution of autoradiographic grains was highly reproducible and was confirmed by ten slides in each area from three to five rats.

"Background" levels of autoradiographic grains (about one grain per 100 square microns) were observed over all regions of the cerebellum and pyriform cortex (see Figure 6). In addition, grain counts over cell bodies (large dark solid circles in these high contrast exposures) were very low and never exceeded 20% of the surrounding area, even in grain-rich areas. This is consistent with our suggestion that opiate receptors are located on the membranes of the synaptic junction (Pert, Snowman, and Snyder, 1974), and is additional evidence that diffusion has been minimized by our methodology.

Through continued investigation into the autoradiographic distribution of opiate receptors, we hope to enumerate potential "target areas" for electrophysiological and lesioning studies. It is not unlikely that "opiate receptors" represent post-synaptic neurotransmitter receptors for a previously undescribed peptide (Hughes, 1975; see Pasternak et al. in this volume). If that proves to be the case, autoradiographic maps of receptor-dense areas would represent areas where synaptic contact between "opaminergic" neurons and other neurons occur, as well as areas of potential importance in the mechanism of opiate action.

REFERENCES

Appleton, T. 1964. Autoradiography of soluble, labeled compounds. *J. Royal Microsc. Soc.* 83: 277–281.

Berkowitz, B., and W. Way. 1971. Analgesic activity and central nervous system distribution of the optical isomers of pentazocine in the rat. *J. Pharmacol. Exp. Ther.* 177: 500–508.

Chernov, H., and L. Woods. 1965. Central nervous system distribution and metabolism of C^{14}-morphine during morphine induced feline mania. *J. Pharmacol. Exp. Ther.* 149: 146–155.

Clouet, D. 1971. *Narcotic Drugs: Biochemical Pharmacology.* New York: Plenum Press.

Clouet, D., and N. Williams. 1973. Localization in brain particulate fractions of narcotic analgesic drugs administered intracisternally to rats. *Biochem. Pharmacol.* 22: 1283–1293.

Dole, V. 1970. Biochemistry of addiction. *Ann. Rev. Biochem.* 39: 821–840.

Goldstein, G., L. Aronow, and S. Kalman. 1968. In *Principles of Drug Action.* New York: Harper & Row, p. 50.

Grumbach, L., and H. Chernov. 1965. The analgesic effect of opiate-opiate antagonist combinations in the rat. *J. Pharmacol. Exp. Ther.* 149: 385–396.

Hiller, J., J. Pearson, and E. Simon. 1973. Distribution of stereospecific binding of the potent narcotic analgesic etorphine in the human brain: Predominance in the limbic system. *Res. Comm. Chem. Path. Pharmacol.* 6: 1052–1062.

Hughes, J. 1975. An endogenous ligand for the morphine receptor. *Brain Res.* 295–308.

Ingoglia, N., and V. Dole. 1970. Localization of d- and l-methadone after intraventricular injection into rat brains. *J. Pharmacol. Exp. Ther.* 175: 84–87.

Klee, W., and R. Streaty. 1974. Narcotic receptor sites in morphine-dependent rats. *Nature* (London) 248: 61–63.

Kuhar, M., C. Pert, and S. Snyder. 1973. Regional distribution of opiate receptor binding in monkey and human brain. *Nature* (London) 245: 447–450.

Pert, C. B. 1974. The opiate receptor: its demonstration, distribution and properties. Doctoral Dissertation: The Johns Hopkins University.

Pert, C., E. Aposhian, and S. Snyder. 1974. Phylogenetic distribution of opiate receptor binding. *Brain Res.* 75: 356–361.

Pert, C., M. Kuhar, and S. Snyder. 1975. Autoradiographic localization of the opiate receptor in rat brain. *Life Sci.* 16: 1849–1854.

Pert, C., G. Pasternak, and S. Snyder. 1973. Opiate antagonists and antagonists discriminated by receptor binding in brain. *Science* 182: 1359–1361.

Pert, C., A. Snowman, and S. Snyder. 1974. Localization of opiate receptor binding in synaptic membranes of rat brain. *Brain Res.* 70: 184–188.

Pert, C., and S. Snyder. 1973a. Opiate receptor: Demonstration in nervous tissue. *Science* 179: 1011–1014.

Pert, C., and S. Snyder. 1973b. Properties of opiate-receptor binding in rat brain. *Proc. Nat. Acad. Sci., USA,* 70: 2243–2247.

Pert, C., and S. Snyder. 1974. Opiate receptor binding of agonists and antagonists affected differentially by sodium. *Molec. Pharmacol.* 10: 868.

Pert, C., and S. Snyder. 1975. Identification of opiate receptor binding in intact animals. *Life Sci.* 16: 1322.

Snyder, S. H. 1975. A model of opiate receptor function with implications for a theory of addiction. In *Opiate Receptor Mechanisms, Neurosciences Research Program Bulletin* 13: 137–141.

Simon, E., J. Hiller, and I. Edelman. 1973. Stereospecific binding of the patent narcotic analgesic (^{3}H) etorphine to rat brain homogenate. *Proc. Nat. Acad. Sci., USA.* 70: 1947–1949.

Terenius, L. 1973. Characteristics of the "receptor" for narcotic analgesics in synaptic plasma membrane fraction from rat brain. *Acta Pharmacol. et Toxicol.* 33: 377–384.

Way. E., H. Loh, and F. Shen. 1969. Simultaneous quantitative assessment of morphine tolerance and physical dependence. *J. Pharmacol. Exp. Ther.* 167: 1–8.

Tissue Responses to Addictive Drugs
© 1976, Spectrum Publications, Inc.

An Endogenous Morphine-like Factor

GAVRIL W. PASTERNAK
RABI SIMANTOV
SOLOMON H. SNYDER

*Departments of Pharmacology and Experimental Therapeutics
and Psychiatry and Behavioral Sciences
Johns Hopkins University School of Medicine
Baltimore, Maryland*

The highly selective interactions of opiate receptor binding (Pert and Snyder, 1973; Simon et al., 1973; Terenius, 1973), its distinctive regional localization in the brain (Kuhar et al., 1973; Hiller et al., 1973), and its association with pain pathways (Pert and Yaksh, 1974; LaMotte, Pert and Snyder, in preparation) suggest that some normally occurring substance serves as an endogenous ligand for the opiate receptor (Collier, 1972), possibly a neurotransmitter. Hughes (1975a, b, c) has identified a morphine-like factor (MLF) in pig brain which mimics the ability of morphine to inhibit electrically induced contractions of the mouse vas deferens. The actions of the substance described by Hughes are antagonized by low concentrations of the opiate antagonist naloxone and its regional distribution in pig brain parallels the distribution of the opiate receptor in rat and monkey brain (Kuhar et al., 1973; Hiller et al., 1973). Independently, Terenius (1975; Terenius and Wahl-strom, 1974, 1975) has also found an endogenous inhibitor of ^{3}H-opiate binding in rat brains and human cerebral spinal fluid which has the same characteristics as the material described by Hughes. Previously we observed that incubation of brain extracts released a substance which inhibits opiate receptor binding, possesses a regional distribution in rat brain resembling that of the opiate receptor, and is destroyed by carboxypeptidase A but not trypsin (Pasternak, Wilson and Snyder, 1975; Pasternak, Goodman and Snyder, 1975; Pasternak and Snyder, 1975c). More recently, Teschemacher et al. (1975) have reported the presence of a material from rat pituitary which has somewhat different characteristics from the substance described by Hughes, Terenius and Pasternak. In this chapter we describe the characteristics of a morphine-like factor (MLF) in rat and calf brain, its interactions with the receptor and a hypothetical molecular mechanism of action.

Hughes et al. (1975) have recently established the structure of the two pentapeptides comprising *enkephalin* or morphine-like factor in pig brain (methionine enkephalin: Tyr-Gly-Gly-Phe-Met-OH; and leu-cine enkephalin: H-Tyr-Gly-Gly-Phe-Leu-OH) and have formally named them enkephalin. The terms "enkephalin" and "morphine-like factor" are interchangeable. The structures were confirmed in bovine brain by Simantov and Snyder (1976), although the bovine brain has a different ratio of leucine to methionine enkephalin than the pig brain. Through-out this article the term "morphine-like factor" or "MLF" will be used.

METHODS

Morphine-like factor (MLF) extracts were prepared from synaptoso-mal preparations as previously described (Pasternak, Wilson and Snyder, 1975; Pasternak, Goodman and Snyder, 1975; Pasternak and Snyder, 1975c). Activity of preparations was determined by their ability to inhibit stereospecific opiate receptor binding in a standard binding assay (Pasternak, Wilson and Snyder, 1975). Since inhibition of bind-ing is not a linear function of concentration, MLF activity is defined in terms of 50% receptor occupancy, determined according to Col-quhoun (1973), assuming classical binding interactions. All binding values were determined in triplicate which varied less than 10% and represent specific opiate binding. All experiments described were repli-cated at least three times, unless stated otherwise.

Table I. Effect of Preincubation on ^{3}H-Naloxone Binding

Rat brains, minus cerebella, were homogenized, centrifuged and the pellets resuspended in 100 volumes standard buffer. Aliquots were preincubated for the appropriate amount of time at 37°C and assayed in the presence and absence of 100 mM NaCl with ^{3}H-naloxone (1 nM). (Data are the mean of triplicate determinations which varied less than 10%. The experiment was replicated twice.)

Preincubation Time (min)	Specific ^{3}H-Naloxone Binding (cpm)	
	Assayed with NaCl	Assayed without NaCl
0	2207	1533
5	2811	1887
15	3442	—
30	3350	3520
45	—	3413
60	3319	3380

Specificity of MLF Inhibition

Incubation of brain membranes results in a time and temperature dependent doubling of ^{3}H-naloxone binding (see Table I; Pasternak, Wilson and Snyder, 1975). This effect is due to an increase in the number of binding sites and is seen for all tritiated agonists and antagonists tested. Since we felt it unlikely that new receptors were being synthesized, we felt this increase might be explained by the dissociation of an endogenous ligand from the opiate receptor. Accordingly, we tested the supernatants after centrifuging incubated membranes and found an inhibitor of opiate receptor binding (MLF). The appearance of this inhibitor correlates extremely well with the appearance of new opiate receptor binding with regard to both time and temperature of incubation.

To make certain that the inhibition of ^{3}H-opiate binding by MLF is a general effect, we examined its ability to inhibit a series of tritiated opiate agonists and antagonists (see Table II). MLF inhibits binding of all opiates equally well. The apparent differences for levorphanol and levallorphan are due to the relatively high concentrations used in the assay. This was necessary because of their low specific activity. When detailed dose-response experiments were performed with ^{3}H-dihydro-

Table II. Inhibition of ^{3}H-Opiate Binding by a Morphine-Like Factor (MLF)

Rat brains were prepared and assayed as previously described (Pasternak, Wilson, and Snyder, 1975). Assays were performed with 1 mM $MnCl_2$, MLF from 50 mg calf caudate, and the following amounts of ^{3}H-opiates: naloxone, 50,000; dihydromorphine, 66,000; levorphanol, 39,000; levallorphan, 39,000; and diprenorphine, 4,000. (Specific binding was determined from triplicate samples which varied less than 10% and inhibition calculated from specific binding in the presence and absence of MLF. The experiment was replicated three times.)

^{3}H-Opiate	MLF Inhibition of ^{3}H-Opiate Binding (%)
Naloxone	81
Diprenorphine	60
Dihydromorphine	71
Levorphanol	42
Levallorphan	37

morphine and ^{3}H-naloxone, 50% inhibition of binding for both tritiated opiates was seen with the same concentration of MLF (see Figure 1).

Localization of MLF

If MLF were associated with the opiate receptor, it should have a regional distribution of MLF corresponding to that of opiate receptor binding. There is an excellent correlation between regional variations in binding and MLF concentrations in both the calf and the rat (see Table III). The highest regions are the caudate nucleus and the hypothalamus, while the cerebellum and corpus callosum have minimal, if any, enkephalin. Similar results were found with extensive regional studies on monkey brains (Simantov et al., 1976).

If MLF is a modulator of synaptic activity in the brain, it should be localized to nerve terminals. Homogenizing the brain in 0.32 M sucrose with a loosely fitting Teflon pestle (Potter-Elvehjem) results in the formation of synaptosomes, or pinched-off nerve terminals (Gray and Whittaker, 1962). Differential centrifugation of this homogenate shows the highest levels of MLF in the P_2 fraction (see Table IV), consistent with a synaptosomal localization. Preliminary work on discontinuous gradients which yield more precise information confirm this synaptosomal localization (Simantov, Snowman, and Snyder, 1976).

Synaptosomes are osmotically sensitive and can be easily disrupted

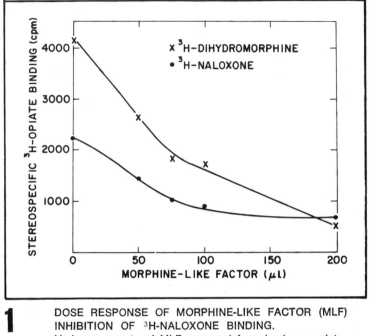

1

DOSE RESPONSE OF MORPHINE-LIKE FACTOR (MLF)
INHIBITION OF ³H-NALOXONE BINDING.
Various amounts of MLF prepared from bovine caudate
were included in a standard binding assay with ³H-naloxone
(40,000 cpm/ml) and 1 mM $MnCl_2$. All values represent
opiate specific binding. Triplicates varied by less than
10%. (The experiment was repeated three times.)

by hypotonic lysis and sonification, which will release their constituents into the supernatant fluid. When the brain is extensively disrupted by Polytron treatment, synaptosomes are not formed and potential synaptosomal constituents are also released into the supernatant fluid. When a synaptosome-containing Potter-Elvehjem pellet is subjected to hypotonic lysis and sonification, about 60% of the recovered MLF is released into the supernatant fluid while only 40% remains bound to the residual pellet (see Table IV). Pellets from homogenates subjected to Polytron treatment contain only a third as much MLF as the Potter-Elvehjem pellet after lysis. This residual amount might be due to MLF which is bound to the receptor and thus pelleted. Thus, MLF appears to be associated with synaptosomes and is stored in an osmotically sensitive compartment.

Table III. Regional Localization of a Morphine-Like Factor (MLF) and Opiate Receptor Binding

Region	MLF Distribution			Opiate Receptor Binding
	^{3}H-Naloxone Binding (cpm)	Calculated Amount MLF (Units)	MLF/mg Protein (Units)	cpm/mg Protein
BOVINE				
Control	2865 ± 188	0	0	
Caudate			480	3197
50 μl	1250 ± 69	5.4		
100 μl	820 ± 119	11.0		
200 μl	400 ± 58	28		
Hypothalamus			250	2820
50 μl	1655 ± 73	2.8		
100 μl	1265 ± 74	5.2		
200 μl	700 ± 70	13.6		
Spinal Cord			140	2050
50 μl	1990 ± 120	1.52		
100 μl	1490 ± 120	3.8		
200 μl	1125 ± 75	6.6		
Pons			135	2310
50 μl	2107 ± 90	1.2		
100 μl	1650 ± 46	2.8		
200 μl	1250 ± 80	2.7		
Parietal Cerebral Cortex			80	1735
50 μl	2110 ± 105	1.2		
100 μl	1780 ± 95	2.4		
200 μl	1340 ± 60	4.6		

Thalamus				
50 µl	2315 ± 140	0.6	75	1795
100 µl	1990 ± 75	1.6		
200 µl	1430 ± 65	4.0		
Cerebellum				
50 µl	2330 ± 75	0.6	50	860
100 µl	2070 ± 70	1.2		
200 µl	1670 ± 85	2.8		
Medulla-Oblongata				
50 µl	2170 ± 70	1.0	50	885
100 µl	1900 ± 70	1.8		
100 µl	1920 ± 160	1.8		
Corpus Callosum				
50 µl	2340 ± 75	0.5	10	610
100 µl	2621 ± 120	0.1		
200 µl	2500 ± 55	0.1		
RAT				
Caudate	1730	4.8		
Brainstem	2430	1.4		
Cortex	2640	0.8		
Cerebellum	2860	0		

Various bovine regions were dissected, homogenized and centrifuged as previously described. Aliquots were tested for ^{3}H-naloxone binding and the remainder used to isolate MLF. Rat brain regions were tested the same way. The assay for MLF activity was performed with ^{3}H-naloxone and 1 mM $MnCl_2$. Rat brain fractions were prepared similarly but their MLF was assayed without $MnCl_2$. All values represent opiate specific binding.' (The experiment was repeated three times.)

Table IV. Subcellular Localization of Rat Morphine-Like Factor (MLF)

Rat brains were either Polytroned in 10 volumes 50 mM Tris buffer or homogenized with a Potter-Elvehjem homogenizer (Teflon pestle and glass tube) in 10 volumes of 0.32 M sucrose and centrifuged at 100,000 g for 60 min. MLF was then extracted from the pellets. A Potter-Elvehjem pellet was lysed by resuspension in 58 M Tris and sonication and then centrifuged 50,000 x g for 30 min. The pellet was extracted for MLF and supernatant tested directly. A Potter-Elvehjem homogenate was subjected to differential centrifugation and the pellets extracted for MLF. Fractions were assayed with ^{3}H-naloxone and 1 mM $MnCl_2$. (The experiment was repeated three times.)

	MLF (Units)
Polytron Pellet	2.2
Potter-Elvehjem Pellet	6.8
Lysed Potter-Elvehjem Pellet	2.4
Supernatant from Lysed Potter-Elvehjem Pellet	3.2
P_1 (crude nuclear)	0.45
P_2 (crude mitochondrial)	2.7
P_3 (crude microsomal)	1.8
S_3 (supernatant)	0.87

Biochemical Characteristics of MLF

In an effort to estimate the molecular weight, we performed gel chromatography on Biogel P2 (200–400 mesh), a high resolution molecular sieve with an exclusion limit of 2,000 daltons. The column was calibrated with proteins of known molecular weight after which MLF was applied to the column and run at 4°C. The MLF was eluted in a sharp peak with

$$K_{av} = 0.23 \quad (K_{av} = (V_e\text{-}V_o) (V_t\text{-}V_o)^{-1}$$

which corresponds to a molecular weight of 1,000 daltons. This low molecular weight is consistent with the observation that MLF is stable to heating in a boiling water bath for fifteen minutes. Large proteins would be expected either to denature or precipitate. The peptide nature of MLF can be established by reacting the MLF with proteolytic enzymes (see Table V).

Leucine aminopeptidase and carboxypeptidase A are effective in destroying the ability of MLF to inhibit opiate binding. These enzymes cleave amino acids off the amino and carboxy ends of peptides respectively. When carboxypeptidase A is examined more closely (see Figure

Table V. Enzyme Effects on a Morphine-Like Factor (MLF)

Rat and calf MLF were prepared and reacted with trypsin (1 mg/ml), chymotrypsin (1 mg/ml), carboxypeptidase A (40 U/ml), leucine aminopeptidase (448 U/ml), neuraminidase (50 μg/ml) or nothing at 37°C for 30 min. The enzymes were inactivated by boiling (trypsin also had soybean trypsin inhibitor added; 4 mg/ml) and the mixtures tested in a binding assay with 1 mM MnCl$_2$ and ^{3}H-naloxone. (The experiment was repeated three times.)

Treatment	Sensitivity of MLF to Enzymes Inhibition of Binding	
	Calf	Rat
None	49%	69%
Trypsin	50%	72%
Chymotrypsin	41%	44%
Leucine aminopeptidase	12%	38%
Carboxypeptidase A	25%	40%
Neuraminidase	49%	70%

2), a dose-dependent destruction of MLF is observed. Trypsin, a highly specific endopeptidase which cleaves only after arginine or lysine, is totally without effect on either the rat or the calf MLF, as was neuroaminidase. Chymotrypsin influences are not as easy to interpret. In several experiments, chymotrypsin decreased the ability of calf MLF to inhibit binding, but not nearly as much as it destroyed the rat MLF. This discrepancy might be explained by species differences in the amino acid composition. These differences, however, are probably not major since both rat and calf MLF inhibit ^{3}H-opiate binding to rat or calf membranes with identical potency (Pasternak, Simantov and Snyder, 1976). Extreme care was taken in all enzyme experiments to totally inactivate the enzymes before testing with a binding assay since the enzymes themselves have marked effects (Pasternak and Snyder, 1974, 1975a).

Molecular Pharmacology of the Opiate Receptor and Its Interactions with MLF

The biochemical criteria for agonist and antagonist binding to the opiate receptor differ markedly. The first difference which we observed was the ability of physiological concentrations of sodium ions to pro-

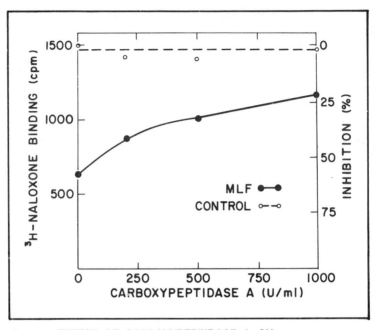

2 EFFECT OF CARBOXYPEPTIDASE A ON
THE MORPHINE-LIKE FACTOR (MLF).
MLF, prepared from bovine caudate, was incubated at
37°C for 45 min with the appropriate amount of
carboxypeptidase A, the enzymes inactivated and tested
in a standard binding assay with [³H]naloxone (25,000
cpm/ml) and 1 mM MnC1$_2$. All values represent opiate
specific binding. (Reacted MLF fractions are represented
by [●]; reacted controls containing the appropriate amount
of enzyme but no MLF by [O].)

portionately enhance antagonist binding and reduce agonist binding
(Pert, Pasternak, and Snyder, 1973). These findings, in addition to the
discovery of two different affinity binding sites for agonists and antagonists (Pasternak and Snyder, 1975b), suggest a model in which the
receptor is postulated to exist in two interconvertible forms, one in the
presence of sodium, which binds antagonists preferentially, and one in
the absence of sodium, which has preferential affinity for agonists
(Pasternak and Snyder, 1975b; Pert and Snyder, 1974). The differential
effects of sodium on a series of tritiated agonists and antagonists is illustrated in Table VI. All three agonists show significant inhibition while

Table VI. Effects of Sodium on Binding of ^{3}H-Labeled Opiate
Agonists and Antagonists

Stereospecific binding of tritiated opiates was determined in a standard binding assay. Concentrations of labeled opiates were 1 to 40 nM. (Values represent triplicate determinations from a typical experiment that was replicated three times.)

^{3}H-Labeled Drug	Control Stereo-Specific Binding (count/min)	Binding in 100 mM NaCl (% of control)
AGONISTS		
Dihydromorphine	2256 ± 113	30
Oxymorphone	669 ± 32	56
Levorphanol	1292 ± 61	72
ANTAGONISTS		
Nalorphine	408 ± 22	145
Naloxone	1582 ± 80	241
Levallorphan	2861 ± 123	129

the binding all three antagonists is markedly enhanced. When unlabeled opiates are used to displace ^{3}H-naloxone binding, the concentration of unlabeled agonist necessary to displace 50% of the binding is substantially increased, while the concentration of antagonist needed is unchanged. Mixed agonist-antagonists show intermediate effects (Pert, Pasternak, and Snyder, 1973). Thus, by measuring the potency of a drug to displace ^{3}H-naloxone binding in the presence and absence of sodium, one is able to establish its agonist and antagonist character.

Subsequently, we have shown that modification of the receptor with a series of protein modifying reagents is also able to differentiate the binding of agonists and antagonists (Pasternak, Wilson, and Snyder, 1975; Wilson, Pasternak and Snyder, 1975). Table VII shows the ability of iodoacetamide treatment to differentiate between the binding of a series of tritiated agonists and antagonists. In addition to iodoacetamide, agonist and antagonist binding is differentiated by the following reagents: dithionitrobenzoic acid, N-ethylmaleimide, mercuriacetate, mersalyl acid, glutathione, N-bromosuccinimide, iodine, 2-methoxy-5-nitrobenzyl bromide, 2-hydroxy-5-nitrobenzyl bromide, p-aminophenylmercuric acetate, p-chloromercuribenzoate, and 1-ethyl-3-(3-dimethylaminopropyl) carbodiimide. Reagent treated receptors can also be used to deter-

Table VII.   Effect of Iodoacetamide on Receptor Binding of ^{3}H-Opiate Agonists and Antagonists

Rat brains were homogenized in 20 volumes of standard Tris buffer and centrifuged at 50,000 g for 15 min. The pellet was resuspended in 100 volumes of standard Tris buffer and equal volumes were incubated in the presence and absence of 20 mM iodoacetamide for 20 min at 25°C. The homogenates were then centrifuged as before, resuspended in their original volumes and assayed with either (+)-3-hydroxy-N-allylmorphinan or (−)-3-hydroxy-N-allylmorphinan (levallorphan) at 200 nM and the appropriate ^{3}H-opiate. Samples were filtered and counted. The following concentrations of ^{3}H-opiates were used: 1.7 nM ^{3}H-naloxone, 2.8 nM ^{3}H-levallorphan, 3.7 nM ^{3}H-oxymorphone; 4 nM ^{3}H-levorphanol and 0.7 nM ^{3}H-dihydromorphine (from Wilson, Pasternak, and Snyder, 1975).

| | Stereospecific Opiate Binding (cpm) | | |
| | | Iodoacetamide | |
Opiate	Control	Treated	% Change
Antagonists			
^{3}H-naloxone	1040	1092	+ 5
^{3}H-levallorphan	1551	1672	+ 8
Agonists			
^{3}H-oxymorphone	719	401	− 44
^{3}H-levorphanol	1288	827	− 36
^{3}H-dihydromorphine	1871	878	− 53

mine the agonist and antagonist character of unknown compounds in a manner similar to using sodium ions (Pasternak, Wilson, and Snyder, 1975).

In addition to sodium ions and reagents, extremely low concentrations of trypsin, chymotrypsin, and phospholipase A destroy agonist binding to a much greater extent than antagonist binding (Pasternak and Snyder, 1975a). (This effect is illustrated in Figure 3). As with the other treatments, reaction of receptors with enzymes provides an additional method of determining the agonist and antagonist character of unknown compounds.

All the treatments described selectively decrease the binding of agonists. Recently we have been able to increase the binding of agonists without any effect on antagonists (Pasternak and Snyder, 1975c; Pasternak, Snowman and Snyder, 1975; Pasternak, Goodman and Snyder, 1975). One compound used is manganese chloride. Table VIII shows the effects of 1 mM manganese chloride on the binding of a series of tritiated agonists and antagonists. This striking increase in agonist binding is due to an increase in the number of binding sites. Manganese

3

EFFECT OF TRYPSIN, CHYMOTRYPSIN and PHOSPHOLIPASE A ON THE BINDING OF ^{3}H-DIHYDROMORPHINE AND ^{3}H-NALOXONE. Assays in the presence of 100 mM NaCl were performed as previously described (Pasternak, Wilson, and Snyder, 1975) with tissue reacted with (a) trypsin, trypsin and a four-fold excess of soybean inhibitor (b) chymotrypsin, or (c) boiled phospholipase A and 5 mM CaC1$_2$ for 30 min at 25°C. The specific binding of the treated homogenate was compared to the specific binding of the control, all assayed in the presence of sodium chloride. All values are based on the means of triplicate determinations and represent specific binding. All experiments were replicated at least three times. The ability of phospholipase A to differentiate between agonists and antagonists was dependent on calcium and unaffected by boiling (Pasternak and Snyder, 1975a).

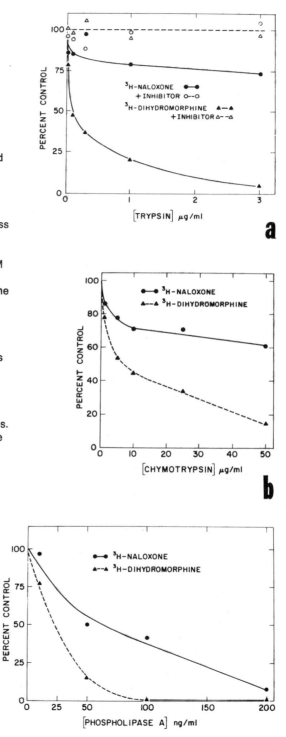

Table VIII. Effects of MnCl$_2$ on ^{3}H-Opiate Binding

Rat brain homogenate was prepared and assayed in the presence of 100 mM NaCl and in the presence and absence of 1 mM MnCl$_2$ and 1 μM levallorphan. The following amounts of ^{3}H-opiate were used per tube: naloxone, 49,000 cpm; levallorphan 40,000 cpm; diprenorphine, 4300 cpm, dihydromorphine, 66,000 cpm; and levorphanol, 39,000 cpm. [Binding values are the mean of triplicate determinations which varied less than 15% and represent specific opiate binding. The experiment was replicated three times (Pasternak, Snowman, and Snyder, 1975.)]

^{3}H-Opiate	Binding (cpm)		
	No MnCl$_2$	1 mM MnCl$_2$	% Change
Naloxone	2300	2400	+ 4
Levallorphan	1900	2200	+ 16
Diprenorphine	1600	1400	− 13
Dihydromorphine	1850	3300	+ 78
Levorphanol	700	1150	+ 64

also increases the ability of nonradioactive agonists to displace ^{3}H-naloxone while having relatively no effects on antagonists' ability to displace the binding (Table IX, Pasternak, Snowman and Snyder, 1975). Thus, by employing sodium and certain divalent cations, protein reagents and enzymes to alter receptor function, we are able to determine the agonist or antagonist character of an unknown drug.

Using these techniques, we have shown that endogenous MLF is an agonist (Pasternak, Goodman, and Snyder, 1975; Pasternak and Snyder, 1975c), which agrees with the findings of Hughes (1975a, b, c). The effects of ions on the ability of MLF to inhibit the binding of ^{3}H-naloxone are shown in Table X. Manganese chloride (1 mM) markedly enhances the ability of MLF to inhibit the binding of ^{3}H-naloxone while very low concentrations of sodium chloride almost abolish MLF inhibition. To ensure that the effect of sodium is specific, potassium was also tested and was ineffective in affecting the inhibition at concentrations as high as 100 mM.

The agonist character of MLF on reagent and enzyme-treated receptors is shown in Table XI. Extreme care was taken to remove all reagents and enzymes before adding the MLF to ensure that the effects are entirely due to modification of the receptor and not MLF. All treatments significantly lowered the MLF inhibition, as would be expected with an agonist.

Table IX. Effect of Manganese Ions on the ID_{50} of Unlabeled Opiates

Rat brain membranes were prepared and assayed with ^{3}H-naloxone in triplicate with five concentrations of the appropriate opiates. ^{3}H-Naloxone was present at 1 nM and control binding was 3000 cpm, 3400 cpm in the presence of 1 mM $MnCl_2$, 3400 cpm in the presence of 100 mM NaCl and 3400 cpm in the presence of both 1 mM $MnCl_2$ and 100 mM NaCl. ID_{50}'s were determined by log-probit analysis. (The experiment was repeated three times.) (From Pasternak, Snowman, and Snyder, 1975.)

ASSAY CONDITIONS	ID_{50} (nM)				$\dfrac{ID_{50}NaCl}{ID_{50}NaCl + MnCl_2}$
	Absence of Sodium		Presence of Sodium (100 mM)		
	Control	$MnCl_2$	Control	$MnCl_2$	
Methadone	4.5	1.9	65	11	5.9
Oxymorphone	2.0	1.0	19	4.2	4.5
Morphine	2.5	0.6	29	7	4.1
Levorphanol	0.9	0.5	6.4	2.5	2.7
Pentazocine	16	18	95	35	2.7
Nalorphine	3.9	2.2	11	6.6	1.7
Levallorphan	0.75	0.57	1.5	1.2	1.2

Table X. Effect of Ions on Inhibition by a Morphine-Like Factor (MLF)
of ^{3}H-Naloxone Binding

Calf MLF was assayed with ^{3}H-naloxone (35,000 cpm/ml) and the appropriate addition. MLF inhibition was determined by the binding remaining in samples with MLF and the addition to samples with only the addition. Thus, the inhibition is due to only MLF, not to the additions used. (The experiment was repeated twice.)

	Inhibition (%)
None	67
NaCl	
5 mM	11
45 mM	15
100 mM	21
KCl	
5 mM	70
15 mM	43
100 mM	56
MnCl$_2$	
1 mM	84

DISCUSSION

These studies show the presence of endogenously occurring, agonistlike peptides of molecular weight 1000, which bind specifically to the opiate receptor. While the exact function is not known, their presence in synaptosomes and release by osmotic lysis suggests a neurotransmitter role. Pharmacologically, MLF behaves like an agonist and thus would be expected to have analgesic properties. Interestingly, electrical stimulation of specific areas of the brain in rats and cats corresponding very closely to areas of morphine sensitivity (Pert and Yaksh, 1974) and opiate binding (Kuhar et al., 1974) can induce analgesia (Mayer et al., 1971; Liebeskind et al., 1974). In addition, electrical stimulation analgesia can be reversed by naloxone and results in tolerance (Akil et al., 1972). These effects might be expected if there were a naturally occurring morphine-like material which was released by electrical stimulation.

Thus, it is tempting to propose a hypothetical molecular model for opiate receptor function based on the presence of an endogenous agonist and our knowledge of opiate receptor binding. This model is

**Table XI. Inhibition by a Morphine-Like Factor of ^{3}H-Naloxone
Binding in Membranes Treated with Enzymes and Reagents**

Rat brain membranes were prepared and treated with trypsin (0.5 μg/ml), chymotrypsin (50 μg/ml), N-ethylmaleimide (10 μM), iodoacetamide (5 mM), and p-chloromercuribenzoate (10 μM), for 20 min at 25°C and the reagents or enzymes washed out by centrifugation. Aliquots of the tissue were then assayed with ^{3}H-naloxone and 1 mM MnCl$_2$ in the presence and absence of calf MLF (100 γ). (The experiment has been repeated three times.)

Treatment	MLF Inhibition
None	53%
Trypsin	20%
Chymotrypsin	30%
N-Ethylmaleimide	30%
Iodoacetamide	27%
p-Chloromercuribenzoate	34%

very similar to the one presented previously (Pert and Snyder, 1974; Pasternak and Snyder, 1975b). The major additions have been the introduction of a polarity of the receptor within the membrane and the addition of a manganese binding site (see Figure 4). The receptor might exist in either a high affinity agonist binding site induced by manganese and antagonized by sodium or a low affinity agonist binding site induced by sodium and antagonized by manganese. Morphine-like factor or agonist binding to the high affinity agonist site might then induce an increase in the sodium ion conductance (g_{Na}) and a partial depolarization of the cell, perhaps by inhibiting adenylate cyclase. The increased concentration of intracellular sodium, especially in the vicinity of the receptor, might then convert the receptor to the low affinity agonist state (or antagonist state) through a conformational change. Transformation of the receptor would terminate the agonist's actions and markedly increase the dissociation of the agonist from the receptor, permitting rapid onset and offset of agonist action. If the receptor has a presynaptic location, a partial depolarization by sodium would result in an inhibition of transmitter release, presynaptic inhibition. Antagonists might work by stabilizing the low affinity agonist (high affinity antagonist) state of the receptor. Placing the sodium binding site within the cell might explain the presence of a high affinity agonist binding site under normal

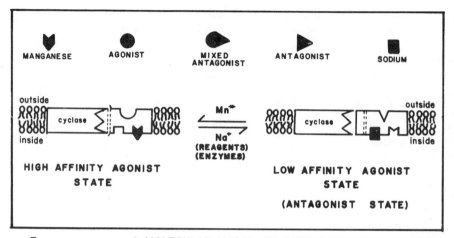

4

A MOLECULAR MODEL OF OPIATE RECEPTOR ACTION
Binding of an agonist to the receptor results in an effect
on cyclase activity and an increase in sodium conductance.
This increase in conductance raises the concentration
of intracellular sodium which converts the receptors into
the low affinity agonist conformation, turns off the receptor
and markedly increases the rate dissociation of the
agonist from the receptor. Antagonists work by stabilizing
the low affinity agonist binding state; mixed agonist-
antagonists bind to both states.

physiological conditions and provides a rapid feedback mechanism for
rapidly turning the receptor both on and off.

ACKNOWLEDGMENTS

This research was supported by United States Public Health Service
Grant DA 00266. Gavril W. Pasternak is a recipient of an Insurance Medical
Scientist Scholarship through the Mutual of Omaha and United Benefit of
Omaha Insurance Companies and Drug Abuse Center Research Fellowship
1 F22–DA 01646–01. Solomon H. Snyder is a recipient of Research Scien-
tist Development Award MH 33128.
We thank Adele Snowman for her excellent technical assistance.

REFERENCES

Akil, H., Mayer, D. J., and J. C. Liebeskind. 1972. Comparison chez le rat
entre l'analgésie induite par stimulation de la substance gris péri-
aqeducale et l'analgesie morphanique. *C.R. Acad. Sci.* 274: 3603–3605.

Collier, H. O. J. 1972. Pharmacological mechanisms of drug dependence. In J. Cochin, Karger, and Basel, Eds. *Pharmacology and the Future of Man.* pp. 65–76.

Colquhoun, D. 1973. The relation between classical and cooperative models for drug action. In H. P. Rang, Ed. *Drug Receptors.* University Park Press, Baltimore, pp. 149–182.

Gray, E. G., and V. P. Whittaker. 1962. The isolation of nerve endings from brain: An electron-microscopic study of cell fragments derived from homogenization and centrifugation. *J. Anat.* 96: 79–86.

Hiller, J. N., J. Pearson, and E. J. Simon. 1973. Distribution of stereospecific binding of the potent narcotic analgesic etorphine in the human brain: Predominance in the limbic system. *Res. Comm. Chem. Path.* 6: 1052–1061.

Hughes, J. 1975a. Isolation of an endogenous compound from the brain with pharmacological properties similar to morphine. *Brain Research* 88: 295–308.

Hughes, J. 1975b. Assay and nature of the endogenous ligand (enkephaline) for the opiate receptor. *Life Sciences.* 16: 1753–1758.

Hughes, J. 1975c. Search for the endogenous ligand of the opiate receptor. *Neurosciences Research Prog. Bull.* 13 (No. 1): 55–58.

Hughes, J., Smith, T., Kosterlitz, H. W., Fothergill, L. A., Morgan, B. A. and Morris, H. R. 1975. Identification of two related pentapeptides from the brain with potent opiate agonist activity. *Nature* 258: 577–579.

Kuhar, M., C. B. Pert, and S. H. Snyder. 1973. Regional distribution of opiate receptor binding in monkey and human brain. *Nature* (London) 245: 447–451.

Liebeskind, J. C., D. J. Mayer, and H. Akil. 1974. Central mechanisms of pain inhibition: Studies of analgesia from focal brain stimulation. In J. J. Bonica, Ed. *Advances in Neurology*, Vol. 4. (International Symposium on Pain.) New York, Raven Press, pp. 261–268.

Mayer, D. J., T. L. Wolfe, H. Akil, B. Carder, and J. C. Liebeskind. 1971. Analgesia from electrical stimulation in the brainstem of the rat. *Science* 174: 1351–1354.

Pasternak, G. W., R. Goodman, and S. H. Snyder. 1975. An endogenous morphine-like factor in mammalian brain. *Life Sciences.* 16: 1765–1769.

Pasternak, G. W., Simantov, R., and Snyder, S. H. 1976. Characterization of an endogenous morphine-like factor (enkephalin) in mammalian brain. *Molec. Pharmacol.* (In Press)

Pasternak, G. W., A. Snowman, and S. H. Snyder. 1975. Selective enhancement of ^{3}H-opiate agonist binding by divalent cations. *Molec. Pharmacol.* 11: 735–744.

Pasternak, G. W., and S. H. Snyder. 1974. Opiate receptor binding: Effects of enzymatic treatments. *Molec. Pharmacol.* 10: 183–193.

Pasternak, G. W., and S. H. Snyder. 1975a. Opiate receptor binding: Enzymatic treatments discriminate between agonist and antagonist interactions. *Molec. Pharmacol.* 11: 478–484.

Pasternak, G. W., and S. H. Snyder. 1975b. Identification of novel high affinity opiate receptor binding in rat brain. *Nature* (London) 253: 563–565.

Pasternak, G. W., and S. H. Snyder. 1975c. Opiate receptor mechanisms. *Neurosciences Res. Prog. Bull.* 13 (No. 1): 59.

Pasternak, G. W., H. A. Wilson, and S. H. Snyder. 1975. Differential effects of protein modifying reagents on receptor binding of opiate agonists and antagonists. *Molec. Pharmacol.* 11: 340–351.

Pert, C. B., G. W. Pasternak, and S. H. Snyder. 1973. Opiate agonists and antagonists discriminated by receptor binding in brain. *Science* 182: 1359–1361.

Pert, C. B. and S. H. Snyder. 1973. Opiate receptor: Demonstration in nervous tissue. *Science* 179: 1011–1014.

Pert, C. B. and S. H. Snyder. 1974. Opiate receptor binding of agonists and antagonists affected differentially by sodium. *Molec. Pharmacol.* 10: 868–879.

Pert, A., and T. Yaksh. 1974. Sites of morphine induced analgesia in the primate brain: Relation to pain pathways. *Brain Research* 88: 135–140.

Simantov, R., A. M. Snowman, and S. H. Snyder. 1976. A morphine-like factor "enkephalin" in rat brain: Subcellular localization. *Brain Res.* (In press)

Simantov, R., Kuhar, M., Pasternak, G. W., and Snyder, S. H. 1976. The regional distribution of a morphine-like factor "enkephalin" in monkey brain. *Brain Res.* (In press)

Simantov, R., and Snyder, S. H. 1976. A morphine-like peptide "enkephalin" in mammalian brain: Isolation, structure elucidation, and interactions with the opiate receptor. *Proc. Nat. Acad. Sci. U.S.A.* (In press)

Simon, E. J., J. M. Hiller, and J. Edelman. 1973. Stereospecific binding of the potent narcotic analgesic ^{3}H-etorphine to rat brain homogenate. *Proc. Nat. Acad. Sci. USA* 70: 1947–1949.

Terenius, L. 1973. Stereospecific interaction between narcotic analgesics and a synaptic plasma membrane fraction of rat cerebral cortex. *Acta Pharmacol. Toxicol.* 32: 317–320.

Terenius, L. 1975. Narcotic receptors in guinea pig ileum and rat brain. *Neurosciences Res. Prog. Bull* 13 (No. 1): 39–42.

Terenius, L. and A. Wahlstrom. 1974. Inhibitor of narcotic receptor binding in brain extracts and cerebrospinal fluid. *Acta Pharmacol. Toxicol.* 34: 55 (Abstract)

Terenius, L., and A. Wahlstrom. 1975. Morphine-like ligand for opiate receptors in human CSF. *Life Sci.* 16: 1759–1764.

Teschemacher, H., K. Opheim, B. M. Cox, and A. Goldstein. 1975. A peptide-like substance from pituitary that acts like morphine. *Life Sciences.* 16: 1771–1776.

Wilson, H. A., G. W. Pasternak, and S. H. Snyder. 1975. Differentiation of opiate agonist and antagonist receptor binding by protein modifying reagents. *Nature* (London) 253: 448–450.

Tissue Responses to Addictive Drugs
© 1976, Spectrum Publications, Inc.

Opiate Effects at CNS Sites in the Rat

YASUKO F. JACQUET

*New York State Research Institute for
Neurochemistry and Drug Addiction
Ward's Island, New York, N.Y.*

Many of morphine's pharmacological effects appear to be mediated by the central nervous system (CNS). There is now increasing evidence that discrete, separate sites in the CNS mediate different effects of morphine, that is, there are morphine-induced "analgesic," "hypothermic," "toxic," "hyper-glycemic," "hyper-reactive," sites, etc. In this chapter, we will focus our interest on CNS sites which appear to mediate morphine analgesia.

Until recently, there was little agreement on the question of which CNS sites mediated morphine analgesia. For example, Herz and Metys (1968), on the basis of preliminary results, reported that analgesia resulted from morphine injections in thalamic and septal structures. Buxbaum et al. (1970) observed analgesia following morphine injections (0.1 and 2.0 μg) in the anterior thalamus. Herz, et al. (1970) subsequently reported that marked analgesia occurred following morphine injections (40 μg) in the hypothalamus, subthalamus and the mesencephalon, but that only moderate analgesia occurred following morphine administration in the third ventricle. Lotti, et al. (1965, 1966) observed analgesia following 50 μg of morphine injected into areas throughout the hypothalamus, while Foster, et al. (1967) observed analgesia following 25 μg of morphine injected into the periventricular region of the rostral hypothalamus. Tsou and Jang (1964) reported that injections of morphine (10 and 20 μg) in the periventricular area of the third ventricle resulted in analgesia. Recently, Vogt (1974) and Dey and Feldberg (1975) have suggested that the ventral surface of the brain stem mediates morphine analgesia.

On the other hand, there was some agreement as to which CNS sites were *not* involved in morphine analgesia. There were the caudate (Tsou and Jang, 1964; Buxbaum et al., 1970; Jacquet and Lajtha, 1973; Pert and Yaksh, 1975), hippocampus (Tsou and Jang, 1964; Herz et al., 1970; Jacquet and Lajtha, 1973), somatosensory cortex (Tsou and Jang, 1964; Pert and Yaksh, 1975), and reticular formation (Tsou and Jang, 1964; Buxbaum et al., 1970).

Recently there has been an increasing convergence of experimental evidence (Tsou and Jang, 1964; Jacquet and Lajtha, 1973, 1974; Pert and Yaksh, 1975), indicating that the periventricular-periaqueductal gray axis is involved in morphine analgesia. In the following pages, we will discuss results from our laboratory which bear on this question.

METHOD

Following the method of the earlier workers, we have been injecting morphine solutions into various CNS sites in the rat brain, and observing their effects. The intracerebral microinjection technique has the advantage of allowing precise quantities of drug to be injected into a CNS site while bypassing the blood-brain barrier. (Systemically-administered morphine does not pass the blood-brain barrier readily (Oldendorf et al., 1972); it has been estimated that as little as 1% of the systemically-injected dose gains access to the CNS (Mulé, 1971). The intracerebral microinjection technique, however, has several potential pitfalls. We attempted to eliminate the various possible sources of error inherent in this method by several modifications of this technique. These were: (1) use of finer-gauge cannula to minimize damage to the injection site; (2) injecting 1 mm beyond the outer cannula tip to minimize backwash and diffusion to other sites; and (3) slow injection of a small volume to avoid tissue damage and minimize drug diffusion. In addition, all experimental animals received histological follow-up to ascertain the site of microinjection.

Intracerebral cannula implantation and microinjection

For the surgical implantation, rats were anesthetized with chloral hydrate (380 mg/kg), mounted on a Baltimore stereotaxic instrument (with ear plugs to guard against damage to the inner ear), and with standard techniques (e.g., Myers, 1971), implanted with cannulae aimed at bilateral sites. The body weights of the animals ranged from 200 to 280 gms at the time of surgery. The 2 cannulae were mounted in parallel on a single pedestal with a 1.0 to 1.5 mm separation; the pedestal was secured to the skull by means of four mounting screws inserted about 0.5 mm in the skull (without penetrating the dura) with an overlay of dental cement which covered the screws and the base of the pedestal. Each cannula was made of 30-gauge (o.d. = 0.30 mm) stainless steel tubing of 17.5 mm length. A 35-gauge (o.d. = 0.13 mm) stainless steel wire stylet of 18.5 mm length, extending 1 mm beyond the outer cannula tip, was positioned in each cannula at all times to prevent cannula clogging, being removed only for injections. The injection needle, of 35-gauge stainless steel tubing, was also of 18.5 mm length. In this way, only the smaller diameter stylet or injection needle extended into the intended site, minimizing damage to the site. The injection was performed slowly, at a rate of 0.1 μl/15 sec, using a Hamilton microliter syringe connected to the injection needle by a length of PE-10 tubing. Injection volume was 0.5 μl. Movement of an air pocket in the transparent tubing provided a check on whether the drug solution moved into brain tissue without obstruction. (This sometimes occurred due to clogging of the small needle.) The needle was kept in place for another 45 sec after the drug was delivered to prevent the drug from being drawn back into the shaft of the cannula. The cannula and injection system have been described in detail elsewhere (Jacquet, 1975).

Analgesia testing

The analgesia test consisted of a battery of tests which could be applied quickly and with minimal damage to the rat. This has also been described in detail elsewhere (Jacquet and Lajtha, 1974). In brief, it consisted of: (1) a pinch test (pinch applied by a plastic hemostat to the ears, four limbs and tail); (2) a pin-prick test (pin pricks applied to the ventral quadrants of the body); (3) a hot plate test, with the fore- and hind-limbs placed separately on the 55°C hot plate, for a maximum period of 10 sec (an analgesic response being a lack of limb withdrawal during this period); and (4) a cold test, the animal being placed in 1–2 cm deep ice water for a maximum period of 60 sec (an analgesic response being a lack of escape attempts during this period). The maximum possible score was 19 points. Testing was carried out at 15 and 60 min after microinjection, and an average of the two scores served as the subject's analgesic score. Extensive pilot studies indicated that this analgesic test battery yielded dose-dependent scores following either intraperitoneal, or intracerebral (periaqueductal gray) injections of morphine. An intraperitoneal injection of 20 mg/kg yielded a test score of approximately 12 points, which was comparable to the analgesia score obtained following an intracerebral injection of 10 μg of morphine bilaterally in the periaqueductal gray. We avoided the use of more sensitive tests, such as the tail-flick test, which may give differences in response latencies in the milliseconds. We felt that an analgesic response should be viewed as a lack of response, rather than as small changes in response latencies to painful stimuli. In our earlier study, we used the flinch-jump test, varying the current level of scrambled electric shock to the grid floor as the graduated aversive stimuli. Unfortunately, this test can give false positives in the case in which the administered drug elevates the level of locomotor activity, as opiates frequently do, following injections into certain CNS sites. We therefore switched to the use of the present analgesia test battery which is unaffected by small changes in response latency or by changes in locomotor activity level. An added advantage of our analgesia test was that it included mechanical, punctate, and thermal stimulation (since we frequently observed that an animal may be "analgesic" in one stimulus mode and not in another).

RESULTS AND DISCUSSION

In our first study (Jacquet and Lajtha, 1973), we found, using the flinch-jump test, that morphine injections into the third ventricle, and the posterior hypothalamus (adjacent to the third ventricle) resulted in significant analgesia (see Figure 1). In our next study (Jacquet and Lajtha, 1974), we found that morphine injections in the periaqueductal gray, which we had previously observed to result in "hyperalgesia" also simultaneously resulted in analgesia to other painful stimuli. These paradoxical effects were due to a dual action of morphine in the periaqueductal gray: increasing reactivity to visual, auditory and light touch stimulation,[1] while at the same time, decreasing reactivity to normally painful stimuli, such as strong pinch, pinpricks, and thermal stimulation. Both effects (hyper-reactivity and analgesia) were dose-dependent (see Figure 2). In the majority of cases, the analgesia following 10 μg (or greater) morphine injections into this site was quite pronounced.

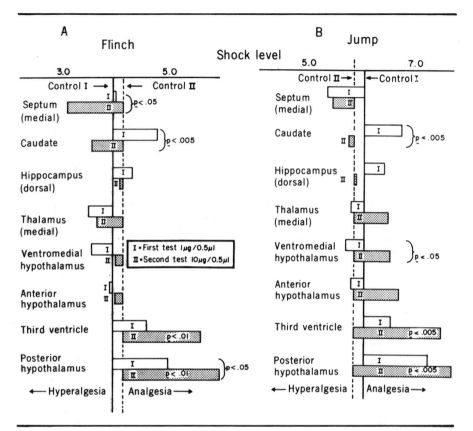

1 Flinch and jump thresholds of eight experimental groups and one control group (total n = 78). The baselines for the control group are shown by the center vertical lines, the solid line for the first day (I) and the broken line for the second day (II). The open bars are data representing the first day (I μg morphine); the stippled bars are data for the second day (10 μg). The bars to the left of the baseline represent hyperalgesia, while those to the right represent analgesia. Probability (p) values within bars represent significant differences from the control; those outside of bars represent significant differences between doses (that is, between tests I and II). (From Jacquet and Lajtha, 1973)

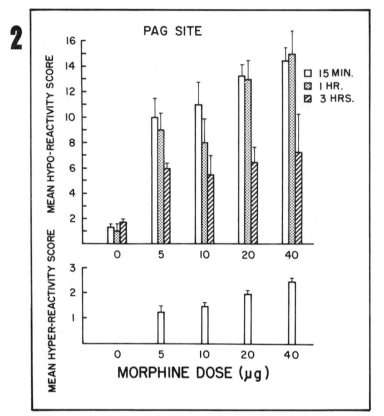

Dose-related scores of hyper- and hypo-reactivity (i.e., analgesia) of periaqueductal gray (PAG) animals after intracerebral doses of morphine. The hyperreactivity was rated on a 3 point rating scale at 5, 10 and 15 min after intracerebral administration, and the highest score achieved was assigned to the animal. The hypo-reactivity (analgesia) was measured at 15, 60 and 180 min after intracerebral administration. (Separate groups are shown at each morphine dose, each group consisting of four to six rats.) (From Jacquet and Lajtha, 1974)

For example, we were able to excise a small tumor from the dorsal area of the neck in a conscious rat without eliciting any sign of pain after bilateral microinjections of 20 μg of morphine in the PAG.

In order to provide further evidence that the PAG is a site mediating morphine analgesia and the development of analgesic tolerance, two additional groups of studies were conducted. These studies were concerned with ascertaining whether analgesic cross tolerance would occur between intraperitoneal (i.p.) and intracerebral (i.c.) morphine administrations, and whether this cross tolerance would be 2-way or 1-way (i.c to ip., and i.p. to i.c. analgesic cross tolerance).

Analgesic cross tolerance

i.p.→i.c. cross tolerance

When rats are pretreated and made tolerant to i.p. administrations of morphine, would they exhibit analgesic tolerance to a test dose of intracerebral (i.c) morphine in the PAG? Three separate studies were conducted. In Experiment 1, 24 cannulae-implanted rats were randomly assigned to either the experimental or control group. During the pretreatment phase, the experimental group received i.p. morphine once per day starting from a dose of 10 mg/kg, and gradually going up to a final level of 200 mg/kg (over 20 days), while controls received i.p. saline in an equivalent volume (1.0 cc/200 gm body weight) once per day during the same period.[2] In Experiment 2, 20 cannula-implanted rats were randomly assigned to either the experimental or control group. During pretreatment, the experimental group received morphine injections twice a day, starting from a dose of 10 mg/kg, and going up to a final level of 350 mg/kg over 11 days, while the control group received saline injections twice a day during the same period.[3] In Experiment 3, 25 cannula-implanted rats were randomly assigned to either the experimental or control group. During the pretreatment phase, the experimental group received morphine injections once per day starting from 10 mg/kg, and going up to a final level of 500 mg/kg over 26 days, while the control group received saline injections once per day during the same period.[4] On the final day of i.p. pretreatment, both experimentals and controls in the three experiments were tested with the analgesia test battery (with the exception of the control group in Experiment 1 due to an oversight). All groups showed a low to moderate level of analgesia, indicating that the i.p. morphine-pretreated groups had developed tolerance to the analgesic action of morphine administered intraperitoneally (see Figure 3). (There were no significant differences between morphine-treated experimentals and saline-treated controls in Experiments 2 and 3). One day following the final day of i.p. pretreatment, both experimental and control groups were tested with an i.c. administration of 10 μg of morphine administered bilaterally in the PAG. While the morphine-pretreated group in Experiment 1 did not show a significant reduction in analgesia from its saline-pretreated control group, the other two groups (i.e., morphine-pretreated groups in Experiments 2 and 3) did differ significantly from their saline-pretreated controls. From these

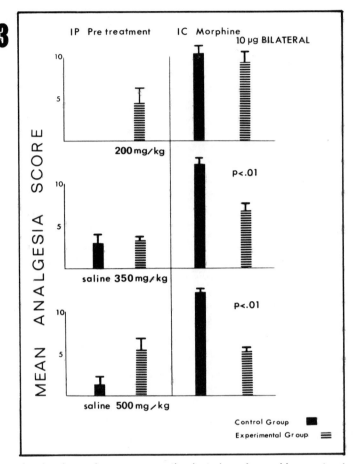

Mean analgesia shown by groups on the last day of morphine pretreatment (left panels) and following their first intracerebral morphine microinjection (10 μg/0.5 μl Ringer's bilaterally) the following day (right panels). Top row represents data from Experiment I where the morphine pretreatment reached a final level of 200 mg/kg; middle row represents data from Experiment 2 where the morphine pretreatment reached a final level of 350 mg/kg; bottom row is from Experiment 3 where the morphine pretreatment reached a final level of 500 mg/kg. Saline-pretreated groups in all three experiments show comparable high levels of analgesia following an i.c. administration of morphine in the PAG, while morphine-pretreated groups all show a reduction in analgesia (when compared with their saline-pretreated controls), indicating the development of analgesic cross tolerance from i.p. to i.c. (right panels). However, the difference between the experimental and control groups was not significant in Experiment I. The differences between experimental and control groups in Experiments 2 and 3 were highly significant (p less than .01). (Plotted points represent means and S.E.'s.)

results, we conclude that analgesic tolerance developed in the PAG during the pretreatment period in which the animals were given morphine intraperitoneally, but that the level of i.p. morphine pretreatment had to exceed 200 mg/kg in order for the analgesic tolerance to develop in the PAG.

i.c.→i.p. cross tolerance

If rats are pretreated with i.c. administrations of morphine in the PAG, would they exhibit analgesic tolerance to a test dose of intraperitoneal morphine? Four experimental groups (a total of 16 rats, with 4 in each group) received i.c. injections of morphine (10 μg bilaterally) in the PAG either 1,2,4 or 8 times, spaced 2 days apart during the pretreatment phase. Four control groups (a total of 15 rats, with 4 in each group except for C Gp $PAG_{ring\ 8}$ (which had 3 rats) were run in this study. These were: (1) C Gp_0, with no cannula (no i.c. or i.p. injections during pretreatment); (2) C Gp $SN_{morph\ 8}$, with cannula implanted in the substantia nigra, which received i.c. injections of morphine 8 times, spaced 2 days apart (a control to ascertain whether analgesic tolerance would develop following repeated morphine administrations in a CNS site which previously had never resulted in analgesia); (3) C Gp $PAG_{ring\ 8}$, with cannulae implanted in the PAG which received control injections of the vehicle alone (Ringer's) 8 times (to see if injections of the vehicle alone carried out 8 times in the PAG would result in analgesic tolerance, or a diminution of analgesia, due to nonspecific damage to the site); and (4) C Gp $PAG_{ring\ 1}$, with cannulae implanted in the PAG which received a control injection of the vehicle alone once in the PAG. Two days following the last day of pretreatment, all groups, both experimental and control, were tested with an i.p. injection of 20 mg/kg of morphine. On the final day of i.c. pretreatment, the control groups (with the exception of C Gp_0 which received no pretreatment) all showed a low level of analgesia as would be expected, while the four experimental groups showed high to moderate levels of analgesia, depending on the number of prior i.c. morphine administrations (see Figure 4). Following the test dose of i.p. morphine of 20 mg/kg, the converse occurred, i.e., all four controls showing high levels of analgesia, while the experimental groups showed lower levels of analgesia. All the experimental groups, with the exception of X Gp_1, differed significantly from the control group (C Gp $PAG_{ring\ 1}$). This indicates that analgesic tolerance developed during pretreatment of the experimental groups (excluding X Gp_1) with i.c. morphine administrations in the PAG. Thus, these results confirm that the PAG is involved in morphine analgesia and the development of analgesic tolerance.

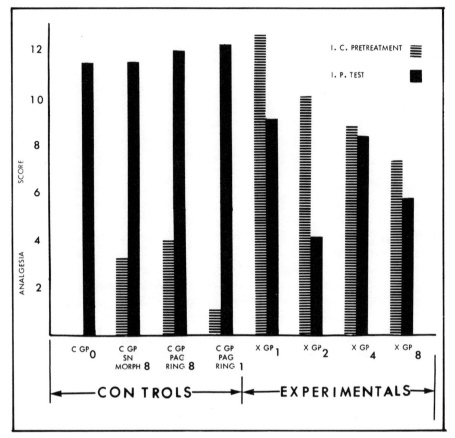

4 Mean analgesia shown by groups on the last day of i.c. pretreatment (horizontal striped bars) and following the i.p. test of 20 mg/kg of morphine (solid bars) two days later. Control groups (on left) show a low level of analgesia following their last i.c. pretreatment of either morphine into a nonanalgesic site (Substantia Nigra) or Ringer's into the PAG, while experimental groups (on right), following their last i.c. morphine injection into the PAG, show high to moderate levels of analgesia, depending on number of prior i.c. morphine administrations. Following the i.p. test dose of 20 mg/kg of morphine, the control groups show high levels of analgesia, while the experimental groups show lower levels of analgesia (all experimental groups, with the exception of $\times$ Gp$_1$, differed significantly from the control group, indicating the development of analgesic cross tolerance from i.c. to i.p. during repeated microinjections of morphine in the PAG. (Plotted points represent means.)

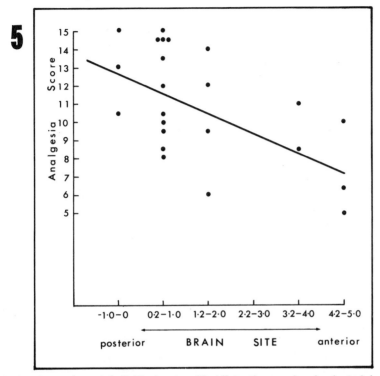

Analgesia scores of individual rats with bilateral cannulae implanted in periventricular-periaqueductal gray sites ranging from −1.0 to +5.0 AP (de Groot coordinates). A tendency for the analgesia to decrease with the more anterior placements was seen, although there was considerable overlap.

Next, we were interested in ascertaining which sites along the periventricular-periaqueductal gray axis produced optimal analgesic following morphine microinjection. This has been a matter of some dispute. For example, Tsou and Jang (1964) reported that morphine administered in the periventricular gray area surrounding the third ventricle resulted in the strongest analgesia, while Herz, et al. (1970) observed that the floor of the fourth ventricle was the site producing optimal analgesia following morphine administration.

Rats were implanted with bilateral cannulae aimed at bilateral sites along the periventricular-periaqueductal gray, ranging from A–P + 5.0 to −1.0 (de Groot coordinates). In general, there was a tendency for the analgesia to increase with the more posterior placements, although there was considerable overlap (see Figure 5).

Our results on analgesic cross tolerance indicate that tolerance development is a central phenomenon, and is not due to changes in the blood-brain barrier nor due to changes in metabolic factors. These findings are somewhat at variance with those of Kerr (1974) who found that rats made tolerant to toxic doses (100 mg twice daily) of systemic morphine succumbed to a toxic dose of intraventricular morphine (1 to 2 mg of morphine); Kerr concluded that tolerance was due to increasing effectiveness of the blood-brain barrier rather than to changes occurring in the neurons themselves. However, the lack of tolerance to the intraventricular morphine may have been due to a *loss* of tolerance following the surgery (which intervened between the development of tolerance to systemically-administered morphine and the intraventricular administration of morphine) to implant the intracerebral cannula. There have been some reports (e.g., Kerr and Pozuelo, 1972) that opiate tolerance is lost following cerebral insult.

The relative analgesic potencies of other analgesics injected into the PAG were found to differ from that following systemic administration. Etorphine at a dose of 0.2 μg, levorphanol at a dose of 80 μg, and methadone at a dose of 80 μg, were found to produce only weak to moderate analgesia following microinjection into the PAG. By the systemic (intravenous) route, it has been estimated (Kutter, et al., 1970) that etorphine has 5,000 times the analgesic potency of morphine; similarly, levorphanol and methadone have 11 and 5 times, respectively, the analgesic potency of morphine. However, following intraventricular injection, etorphine, levorphanol and methadone were reported to have 34 times, 1/14th and 1/33, respectively, the potency of morphine. Our results confirm that the analgesic potencies of opiates differ depending on route of administration. Levorphanol and methadone were more potent than morphine when administered systemically, but less potent than morphine when administered directly into the PAG, bypassing the blood-brain barrier. Etorphine remained more potent than morphine when administered directly into the PAG, but by a factor of only approximately 20 (i.e., 2 μg of etorphine in the PAG resulted in maximal analgesia). Undoubtedly, characteristics of the drug which influence its passage across the blood-brain barrier, such as lipophilicity, play a role in determining potency of action when drugs are administered systemically; this is minimized when analgesics are administered directly into the analgesic site.

Recently, interest has focused on the existence of an "opiate receptor." However the regional distribution of the "receptors" in the rat (Pert and Snyder, 1973), monkey (Kuhar, et al., 1973) and human (Hiller, et al., 1973) brain do not show good agreement with the CNS sites in the rat (Jacquet and Lajtha, 1973, 1974) and monkey brain (Pert and Yaksh, 1975) found to mediate morphine analgesia. For example, the caudate was found to have high "opiate receptor" binding (Pert and Snyder, 1973), but morphine microinjections into this site did not result in analgesia (Jacquet and Lajtha, 1973; Pert and Yaksh, 1975).

We conclude from the results of our studies that the PAG is involved in morphine analgesia. The question of whether this is the only pathway, or whether other pathways are involved, remains to be explored.

ACKNOWLEDGMENTS

This project was supported by NIDA Grant 00367.

FOOTNOTES

[1]It is not clear whether the significantly lowered flinch-jump thresholds were due to the rats reacting to the noise of the scrambler, despite the presence of masking white noise in the animal chamber (since it was observed that morphine injected into the PAG rendered the rats hypersensitive to auditory stimuli) or due to electrical stimulation of the foot pads.

[2]Due primarily to rats losing their cannula (the cannula assembly becoming loose on their skulls) or drug overdose, losses occurred in both groups during pretreatment, and the final number which reached the testing phase was: experimental = 8, control = 6. Of these, only half were tested initially with the standard dose of 10 μg bilaterally, while the others were tested with a higher dose. Thus, data for only the former are presented, i.e., experimental = 4, control = 3.

[3]During the pretreatment phase, 5 rats were lost due to drug overdose, and 1 due to cannula loss, leaving 6 experimental and 8 control animals for the test phase (i.e., intracerebral morphine injection).

[4]The final numbers which reached testing were: experimental = 4, control = 5. Most of the losses during pretreatment were due to cannula loss.

REFERENCES

Buxbaum, D. M., G. G. Yarbrough, and M. E. Carter. 1970. Dose-dependent behavioral and analgesic effects produced by microinjections of morphine sulfate into the anterior thalamic nuclei. The Pharmacologist 12: 210.

Dey, P. K., and W. Feldberg. 1975. Hyperglycaemia produced by drugs with analgesic properties introduced into the cerebral ventricles of cats. Br. J. Pharmac. 54: 163–170.

Foster, R. S., D. J. Jenden, and P. Lomax. 1967. A comparison of the pharmacologic effects of morphine and N-methyl morphine. J. Pharmacol. Exp. Ther. 157: 185–195.

Herz, A., K. Albus, J. Metys, P. Schubert, and H. Teschemacher. 1970. On the central sites for the antinociceptive action of morphine and fentanyl. *Neuropharmacology* 9: 539–551.

Herz, A., and J. Metys. 1968. Inhibition of nociceptive responses by substances acting on central cholinoceptive systems. In A. Soulairac, J. Cahn, and J. Charpentier, Eds. *Pain*. Academic Press, London and New York, pp. 321–333.

Hiller, J. M., J. Pearson, and E. J. Simon. 1973. Distribution of stereospecific binding of the potent narcotic analgesic etorphine in human brain: Predominance in the limbic system. *Res. Commun. Chem Pathol. Pharmacol.* 6: 1052–1062.

Jacquet, Y. F. 1975. Intracerebral administration of opiates. In S. Ehrenpreis, and A. Neidle, Eds. *Methods of Narcotics Research*. Dekker, New York, pp. 33–57.

Jacquet, Y. F., and A. Lajtha. 1973. Morphine action at central nervous system sites in rat: Analgesia or hyperalgesia depending on site and dose. *Science* 182: 490–492.

Jacquet, Y. F., and A. Lajtha. 1974. Paradoxical effects after microinjection of morphine in the periaqueductal gray matter in the rat. *Science* 185: 1055–1057.

Kerr, F. W. L. 1974. Tolerance to morphine and blood-brain CSF barrier. *Fed. Proc.* 33: 528.

Kerr, F. W. L., and J. Pozuelo. 1972. Suppression of physical dependence and induction of hypersensitivity to morphine by stereotaxic hypothalamic lesions in addicted rats and a new theory of addiction. In J. M. Singh, L. H. Miller and H. Lal, Eds. *Drug Addiction, Vol. I, Experimental Pharmacology*. Futura Publishing Co., New York, pp. 343–364.

Kuhar, M. J., C. B. Pert, and S. H. Snyder. 1973. Regional distribution of opiate receptor binding in monkey and human brain. *Nature* (London) 245: 447–450.

Kutter, E., A. Herz, H. J. Teschemacher, and R. Hess. 1970. Structure-activity correlations of morphine-like analgetics based on efficiencies following intravenous and intraventricular application. *J. Med. Chem.* 13: 801–805.

Lotti, V. J., P. Lomax, and R. George. 1965. Temperature responses in the rat following intracerebral microinjection of morphine. *J. Pharmacol.* 150: 135–139.

Lotti, V. J., P. Lomax, and R. George. 1966. Acute tolerance to morphine following systemic and intracerebral injection in the rat. *Int. J. Neuropharmacol.* 5: 35–42.

Mulé, S. J. 1971. Physiological disposition of narcotic agonists and antagonists. In D. H. Clouet. Ed. *Narcotic Drugs: Biochemical Pharmacology*. Plenum Press, New York, pp. 190–215.

Myers, R. D. 1971. Methods for chemical stimulation. In R. D. Myers, Ed. *Methods in Psychobiology*. Academic Press, London and New York, pp. 281–299.

Oldendorf, W. H., S. Hyman, L. Braun, and S. C. Oldendorf. 1972. Blood-brain barrier: Penetration of morphine, codeine, heroin, and methadone after carotid injection. *Science*. 178: 984–986.

Pert, C. B., and S. H. Snyder. 1973. Opiate receptor: Demonstration in nervous tissue. *Science* 179: 1011–1014.

Pert, A., and T. L. Yaksh. 1975. Localization of the anti-nociceptive action of morphine in primate brain. *Pharmacol. Biochem. Behav.* 3: 133–138.

Tsou, K., and C. S. Jang. 1964. Studies on the site of analgesic action of morphine by intracerebral micro-injection. *Sci. Sinica* 13: 1099–1109.

Vogt, M. 1974. The effect of lowering the 5-hydroxytryptamine content of the rat spinal cord on analgesia produced by morphine. *J. Physiol.* 236: 483–498.

Tissue Responses to Addictive Drugs
© 1976, Spectrum Publications, Inc.

Mechanisms of Narcotic Antagonist and Narcotic Antagonist Analgesic Action

BARRY A. BERKOWITZ
SYDNEY SPECTOR

Roche Institute of Molecular Biology
Nutley, New Jersey

CHI HO LEE

Department of Pharmacology
Cornell University Medical College
New York, New York

One of the newer classes of drugs is the narcotic antagonists. Two of the most frequently used drugs of this group are naloxone and pentazocine. Naloxone is usually considered a pure narcotic antagonist and is used in the treatment of narcotic overdose. This agent has also been explored for prevention of narcotic abuse. Pentazocine is a widely used analgesic with weak narcotic antagonist activity. This chapter will illustrate two approaches to the understanding of these drugs: their disposition and effects on neurotransmitters.

DISPOSITION

When considering the tissue responses of drugs, it is important to be aware of the disposition of the agent under study. For example, if two analgesics differ in their responses, by understanding their dispo-

139

sition one can differentiate between mechanisms which alter the ability of the drugs to reach and remain at their sites of action and other factors such as differences in their neurochemical sequelae.

Pentazocine

The metabolism and excretion of pentazocine has been extensively studied and reviewed (Berkowitz, 1971; Mitchard, 1971, Brogden et al., 1973). In man only 3–13% of the administered dose is excreted unchanged (Berkowitz and Way, 1969; Beckett et al., 1970) whereas 13–28% is excreted as the glucuronide conjugate (Berkowitz and Way, 1969). Hydroxylation of the dimethylallyl side chain is also a major metabolic pathway with one of the alcohols oxidized further to the carboxylic acid (Pittman, 1970). Of the oral dose, 11% is excreted as the cis alcohol, and 41% as the trans acid. These latter values include both free and conjugated metabolites.

Because little free pentazocine is excreted and the metabolites have little or no pharmacologic activity, the metabolism and distribution of pentazocine are the major factors which can limit its actions. In a study of normal volunteers, those with the most pronounced side effects (sweating, dizziness and nausea) excreted the most pentazocine and the least amount of metabolite (Berkowitz and Way, 1969). The inter subject variation in the metabolism of pentazocine was confirmed and studied further by Beckett et al. (1970) under conditions of controlled urinary pH. Vaughan and Beckett (1974) reported that the individual variations in pentazocine oxidation were directly responsible for the variations in the urinary excretion rate.

Blood levels of drugs are being measured with increased frequency to obtain objective correlates of drug intensity and duration of action. The assumption that blood levels reflect target organ levels is strengthened if the relationship between blood levels and pharmacologic response can be established. For pentazocine, the plasma half life was about 2 hours (Berkowitz et al., 1969, Agurell et al., 1974) in patients. There was a correlation between plasma levels and analgesia following intramuscular pentazocine (Berkowitz et al., 1969) and this suggests that at least for this class of drugs, analysis of plasma levels does in fact offer an objective method of correlating and predicting pharmacologic responses. In man, pentazocine rapidly enters the brain and by utilizing mass fragmentography Agurell et al. (1974) observed that maximal CSF levels occurred within 30 minutes after an i.v. administration.

In comparison with morphine, pentazocine has a faster onset but shorter duration of action. One explanation for this is that pentazocine enters the brain rapidly but also egresses rapidly (Berkowitz and Way,

1971, Medzihradsky and Ahmad, 1971) whereas the brain levels of morphine are more sustained (Miller and Elliot, 1955, Kupferberg and Way, 1963). A second interesting aspect of pentazocine distribution is the high brain-plasma ratio which is achieved by this class of drugs. For example the brain-plasma ratio for pentazocine, 30 minutes after s.c. administration is 5 (Berkowitz and Way, 1971) whereas for morphine it is less than 1 (Johannesson and Becker, 1973).

Naloxone

The major metabolic pathways of naloxone are glucuronide conjugation, N-dealkylation, and reduction of the 6-ketone group (Fujimoto, 1969a, 1969b and Weinstein et al., 1971, 1973) with the former the most prominent. The serum and brain disposition of morphine and naloxone were compared in the rat in an attempt to understand the reason for the short action of naloxone (see Figure 1). Following 5 mg/kg s.c. of either drug, the peak serum concentration, time to peak serum concentration and half life (40 minutes) were similar. Misra et al (1974) also reported a serum half life of about half an hour for naloxone in rat plasma.

Naloxone achieves a markedly higher (15 fold) brain to serum ratio than morphine. Peak brain levels of naloxone occurred within 15 minutes and had declined by 50% within 1 hour whereas the peak brain levels of morphine were sustained for up to 2 hours. We suggest the high brain-serum ratio of naloxone contribute to its potency whereas the rapid egress from the brain is important in its short duration of action (Evans et al., 1974).

Naltrexone is a congener of naloxone, with a longer duration of action (Resnick et al., 1974). This prolonged action might be explained by either a longer retention of naltrexone in the brain or the formation of pharmacologically active metabolites (Cone et al., 1974). The serum and brain concentrations of naloxone and naltrexone in the rat were compared following a 5 mg/kg dose (see Figure 2). There was no major difference between the serum or brain profile of these drugs. Thus the possibility that naltrexone produces pharmacologically active metabolites should be studied further.

EFFECTS ON SEROTONIN AND CATECHOLAMINES

Pentazocine

The putative neurotransmitters which have been most extensively studied biochemically for their role in the pharmacologic effects of

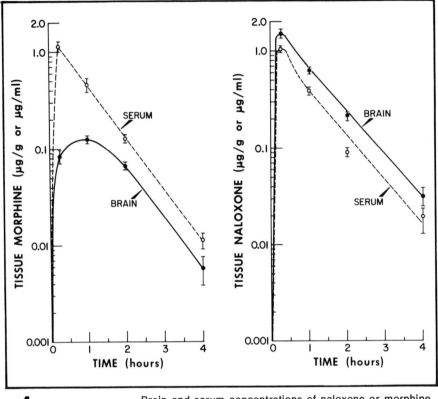

1   Brain and serum concentrations of naloxone or morphine in rats following 5 mg/kg s.c. (Results are the average ± standard error of 3-5 rats at each time interval.)

pentazocine are serotonin, norepinephrine and dopamine. In the rat, pentazocine itself has little or no effect on serotonin and does not alter the increased brain serotonin concentration produced by the monoamine oxidase inhibitor pargyline (Holtzman and Jewett, 1972, Berkowitz, 1974). Thus there is no evidence at present to indicate that serotonin mediates any of the central nervous system effects of pentazocine. This is not the case for norepinephrine or dopamine since pentazocine has pronounced effects on these brain catecholamines.

There is some agreement that pentazocine lowers the concentration of norepinephrine in the rat brain (Holtzman and Jewett, 1972; Berkowitz, 1974; and Paalzow et al., 1974) with both the dextrorotary and levorotary isomers of pentazocine able to deplete brain norepinephrine (Berkowitz, 1974). The ability of pentazocine to alter brain norepineph-

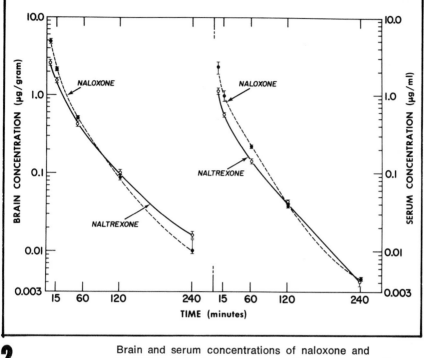

2 Brain and serum concentrations of naloxone and naltrexone following 5 mg/kg i.v. (Naloxone and naltrexone were measured by a radioimmunoassay (Berkowitz et al., 1975)).

rine content may vary with the route of administration since depletion was observed by the above investigators following i.v. or s.c. injection but not after i.p. administration (Sugrue, 1974). The brain monoamine system which has most recently been suggested to be involved in the action of narcotics and antagonists is that of dopamine. Sasame and Perez-Cruet (1972) proposed that methadone blocks dopamine receptors in the brain and they and Clouet and Ratner (1970) observed that narcotics increased the synthesis of dopamine in the brain. The highest concentration of narcotic antagonist receptors were found in the striatum, an area rich in dopamine (Pert and Snyder, 1973). Pentazocine lowers the concentration of brain dopamine (Hotzman and Jewett, 1972; Berkowitz, 1974; Paalzow et al., 1974; Sugrue, 1974) and the levorotary isomer of pentazocine was more potent than the dextrorotary isomer (Berkowitz, 1974). The specific mechanisms whereby pentazocine elicits these alterations in catecholamine disposition have been explored.

Table I. Effect of Narcotic Antagonists on Tyrosine Hydroxylase Activity[1]

Drug	% Inhibition	
	Rat	Guinea Pig
l-cyclazocine	11 ± 22[†]	16
d-cyclazocine	2 ± 5	3
1-pentazocine	12 ± 2[†]	25
l-pentazocine	6 ± 1[*]	14
Naloxone	(↑)4 ± 8	—
Naltrexone	5 ± 2	—
Norepinephrine	74 ± 10[††]	—
α-methyl tyrosine	52 ± 3[††]	78

[1]The results are the mean $\pm$ S.E., expressed as % inhibition for three determinations in rats and the average of two determinations in the guinea pig. Tyrosine hydroxylase activity was determined in adrenal gland homogenates by the method of Nagatsu et al. (1964), and all drugs were tested at 10^{-3}M. In rats, control enzyme activity was 1924 ± 28 CPM per assay, and in guinea pig 6871 ± 100 CPM/assay.

[*]Significantly differs from control $P < 0.05$, [†]$P < 0.01$, [††]$P < 0.001$.

The reduced levels of catecholamines in brain are not due to decreased synthesis. Pentazocine neither inhibits the activity of tyrosine hydroxylase, the rate limiting enzyme of catecholamine synthesis, nor reduces the conversion of tyrosine to norepinephrine (Berkowitz, 1974). In fact none of the narcotic antagonists or narcotic antagonist analgesics are potent inhibitors of tyrosine hydroxylase. As seen in Table I, tyrosine hydroxylase was inhibited only 25% or less by these drugs at concentrations of 10^{-3}M, whereas norepinephrine and α-methyl tyrosine, known inhibitors, decreased activity 52–78%.

The release of catecholamines is apparently increased by pentazocine. Indeed, in man, pentazocine raised the concentration of circulating catecholamines (Tommisto et al., 1971). When release and utilization of catecholamines are accelerated by a drug the depletion of these amines should be increased even further after synthesis is prevented. Following inhibition of tyrosine hydroxylase or dopamine-β-hydroxylase, pentazocine administration results in an increased depletion of norepinephrine and dopamine (Berkowitz, 1974; Paalzow et al., 1974; Sugrue, 1974). Undoubtedly when pentazocine alone is administered any release of catecholamines and reduction of neuronal catecholamine concentration should be sufficient to accelerate synthesis by reducing feedback inhibition of tyrosine hydroxylase. The conversion of tyrosine to dopamine and norepinephrine is increased in the brain following pentazocine (Berkowitz, 1974) and the concentration of catecholamine metabolites is elevated (Ahtee and Kaariainen, 1973). However, in addition to reduced end product inhibition of synthesis, other mechanisms should be considered. For example, a reflex increase in presynaptic catecholamine neural activity secondary to a postsynaptic blockade has not been ruled out as a contributor to the accelerated synthesis and turnover of these amines.

If the effects of pentazocine on brain amines are critical for the mediation of any of its pharmacologic responses these should be altered by drugs which influence catecholamine metabolism. With respect to behavioral effects, Holtzman and Jewett (1972) observed that pentazocine increased the locomotor activity in the rat and that this activity was blocked by inhibiting catecholamine synthesis. Pentazocine analgesia can also be altered by drugs which influence catecholamine disposition. Using vocalization after discharge (squeaking after cessation of noxious stimuli) as an index of analgesia, Paalzow et al. (1974) found that inhibition of either tyrosine hydroxylase or dopamine-β-hydroxylase reduced the analgesia of pentazocine in rats. Reserpine (Hoffmeister, 1968) administration also antagonized pentazocine analgesia. On the other hand methamphetamine, a sympathomimetic, potentiated pentazocine analgesia (Evans and Bergner, 1964; Hoffmeister, 1968). Many investigators have explored and speculated upon the neuroanatomical pathways influenced by analgesics. The evidence suggesting a role for the catecholamines in the analgesia of pentazocine fits well with the hypothesis of Shiomi and Takagi (1974). They observed that both morphine and pentazocine increased norepinephrine release in the spinal cord of rats as measured by an increase in normetanephrine content. It was proposed that this effect on the bulbospinal noradrenergic system inhibits the transmission in the pain pathways of the spinal cord.

Naloxone

In low doses naloxone has not been observed to significantly alter brain catecholamine neurochemistry. In doses of about 20 mg/kg catecholamine synthesis was increased (Costa et al., 1973).

MOLECULAR MECHANISMS IN MODEL SYSTEMS

Given the complexities of the central nervous system, it is not surprising that appreciable progress in understanding analgesic action and neurotransmitter mechanisms has been derived from model systems such as the isolated intestinal smooth muscle and rodent lens (see Weinstock, 1971 for review). Recently Hughes et al. (1975) examined the effects of narcotics and narcotic antagonists on the mouse vas deferens. One of the simplest of the in vitro model systems is the helically cut aortic strip (Furchgott and Bhadrakom, 1953; Fleisch, 1974). In our studies we wished to first focus on post-synaptic or receptor effects of pentazocine and naloxone and utilized the rat aortic strip which is poorly innervated with adrenergic fibers (Fleisch, 1974; Berkowitz et al., 1971).

Alpha receptors have been suggested to play a role in the action of analgesics. Paazlow (1974) reported that clonidine, an alpha receptor agonist, produced analgesia whereas Cicero et al. (1974) observed analgesia and enhancement of morphine analgesia with alpha adrenergic blocking agents. If pentazocine or naloxone interacted with alpha receptors it was expected that this action would be apparent on the aortic strip. Pentazocine, cyclazocine and levallorphan all contracted the aortic strip (see Figure 3). The levorotary isomer of pentazocine was the most potent with maximum contraction at 1×10^{-5}M. In fact, the levorotary isomers of all three drugs were at least 5 times more potent than their dextrorotary isomers in contracting the strip. Morphine also contracts this preparation with the maximal effect achieved at 1×10^{-4}M. Naloxone caused no significant contraction. The contractile effect of pentazocine and other drugs was not blocked by the α-receptor antagonist dibenamine. The data, therefore, indicate that these drugs are not α-receptor agonists at least in the aorta, that they can elicit a stereoselective contraction and that this is a direct effect. One aspect of these data of particular interest is that pentazocine, the most potent aortic contractile agonist, has been reported to have the side effect of increasing blood pressure following i.v. injection (for review see Brogden et al., 1973) in patients.

Calcium is a critical ion for vascular smooth muscle regulation and in order to assess the role of this ion on pentazocine induced vascular contraction a comparison was made with potassium and norepinephrine. Potassium mediated vascular contraction is highly dependent on extracellular calcium whereas norepinephrine mediated vascular contraction depends primarily on intracellular calcium, (Hiraoka et al., 1968; Hudgins and Weiss, 1968; and Greenberg et al., 1973). In Figure 4 it can be seen that as the calcium ion concentration was decreased all three agents exhibited a reduced ability to contract the aorta. However, there were clear differences among the drugs with their order of dependency on extracellular calcium concentration as follows: pentazocine > potassium > norepinephrine.

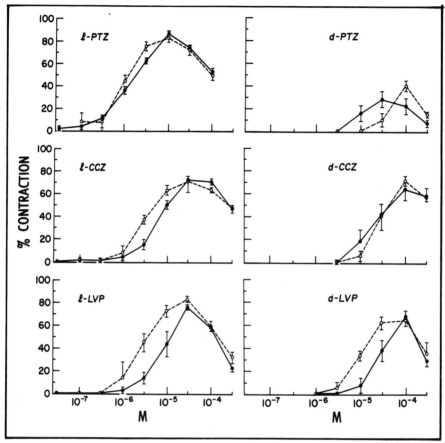

3

Dose—response curves of the l- and d- isomers of pentazocine (PTZ), cyclazocine (CLZ) and Levallorphan (LVP) in isolated rat thoracic aortic strips prepared as previously described (Cohen and Berkowitz, 1974). (Contractions for each strip were determined with 1 x 10^{-7}M norepinephrine and response to drugs was expressed as a percent of this value.) Dotted line denotes the dose response after pretreatment of 5 x 10^{-6}M Dibenamine, a dose which abolished the norepinephrine response.

Pentazocine may influence the aortic membrane, possibly by depolarization, to allow the movement of calcium into the muscle cells with the resultant effect of contraction. Moreover, we hypothesize that a similar pentazocine mediated influx of calcium into catecholamine neurons could contribute to its marked ability to deplete or release

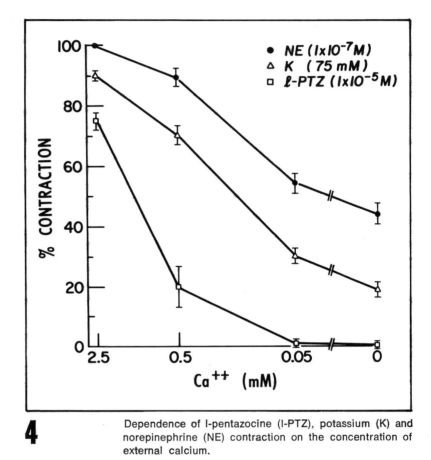

4 Dependence of l-pentazocine (l-PTZ), potassium (K) and norepinephrine (NE) contraction on the concentration of external calcium.

catecholamines. Perhaps a link between these two findings is that muscle like contractile proteins have in fact been isolated from brain synaptosomes (Blitz and Fine, 1974) and evidence has been presented suggesting their involvement in neurotransmitter release (Thoa et al., 1972).

The ability and specificity of naloxone to alter the aortic contractile effects of pentazocine was determined (see Figure 5). Naloxone (1×10^{-3}M) blocked completely pentazocine's contraction. However, at this dose naloxone reduced norepinephrine contraction 20% and potassium contraction 70% and thus naloxone cannot be considered an entirely specific blocker of pentazocine. The order of naloxone's inhibition of contraction was pentazocine > potassium > norepinephrine. This order of blockade is exactly the same for these drugs as their order of dependency on external calcium concentration for contraction. One

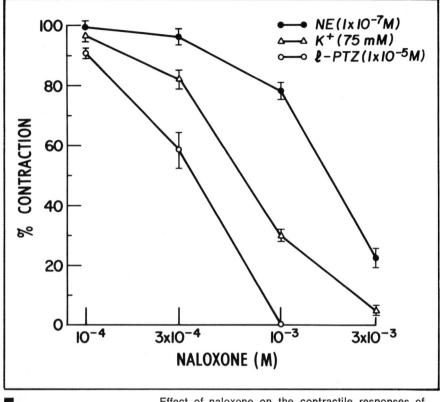

5 Effect of naloxone on the contractile responses of l-pentazocine, potassium and norepinephrine.

explanation of this data is that naloxone may be blocking calcium influx. If this were the case, naloxone should reduce the responses of drugs which are calcium dependent. Two studies may be cited in support of this hypothesis and both deal with release and utilization of norepinephrine which is dependent on calcium. Naloxone can prevent the release or depletion of brain dopamine elicited by pentazocine (Holtzman, 1974; Sugrue, 1974). This data could of course also be explained by a specific effect of naloxone to compete with pentazocine for a specific receptor. However, naloxone (30 mg/kg) can also antagonize the increase loco- motor activity produced in rats by the nonopioid amphetamine (Holtz- man, 1974). The locomotor effects of amphetamine appears to require catecholamine synthesis and release (Weissman et al., 1966).

In summary it is suggested that the catecholamine releasing effects of pentazocine may be mediated partially by its effects on calcium movement and that naloxone should be studied further for its effects on calcium mobility in order to better understand its action.

REFERENCES

Agurell, S., L. O. Boreus, E. Gorden, J. E. Lindgren, M. Ehrnebo, and U. Lonroth. 1974. Plasma and cerebrospinal fluid concentrations of pentazocine in patients assay by mass fragmentography. *J. Pharm. Pharmacol.* 26: 1–8.

Ahtee, L., and I. Kaariainen. 1973. Effect of narcotic analgesics on the homovanillic acid content of rat nucleus caudatus. *Eur. J. Pharm.* 22: 206–208.

Beckett, A. H., J. F. Taylor, and P. Kourounakis. 1970. The absorption, distribution and excretion of pentazocine in man after oral and intravenous administration. *J. Pharm. and Pharmacol.* 22: 123–128.

Berkowitz, B. A. 1971. Influence of plasma levels and metabolism on pharmacological activity: Pentazocine. *Annals N. Y. Acad. Sciences* 179: 269–281.

Berkowitz, B. A. 1974. Effects of the optical isomers of the narcotic antagonist analgesic pentazocine on brain and heart biogenic amines. *Europ. J. Pharm.* 26: 359–365.

Berkowitz, B. A., J. H. Asling, S. M. Shnider, and E. L. Way. 1969. Relationship of pentazocine plasma levels to pharmacological activity in man. *Clin. Pharm. and Therap.* 10: 320–328.

Berkowitz, B. A., S. H. Ngai, J. Hempstead, and S. Spector. 1975. Disposition of naloxone: Use of a new radioimmunoassay. *J. Pharm. Exp. Ther.* 195: 499–504.

Berkowitz, B. A., J. H. Tarver, and S. Spector. 1971. Norepinephrine in blood vessels: Concentration, binding, uptake and depletion. *J. Pharm. Exp. Therap.* 177: 119–126.

Berkowitz, B. A., and E. L. Way. 1969. Metabolism and excretion of pentazocine in man. *Clin. Pharm. Exp. Therap.* 10: 681–689.

Berkowitz, B. A. and E. L. Way. 1971. Analgesic activity and central nervous system distribution of the optical isomers of pentazocine in the rat. *J. Pharm. Exp. Therap.* 177: 500–508.

Blitz, A. L., and R. E. Fine. 1974. Muscle like contractile proteins and tubulin in synaptosomes. *Proc. Nat. Acad. Sci.* 71: 4472–4476.

Brogden, R. N., T. M. Speight, and G. S. Avery. 1973. Pentazocine: A review of its pharmacological properties, therapeutic efficacy and dependence liability. *Drugs.* 5: 6–91.

Cicero, T. J., E. R. Meyer, and B. R. Smithloff. 1974. Alpha adrenergic blocking agents: Antinociceptive activity and enhancement of morphine-induced analgesia. *J. Pharm. Exp. Therap.* 189: 72–82.

Clouet, D. H., and M. Ratner. 1970. Catecholamine biosynthesis in brain of rats treated with morphine. *Science* 168: 854–856.

Cohen, M. L., and B. A. Berkowitz. 1974. Age related changes in vascular responsiveness to cyclic nucleotides and contractile agonists. *J. Pharm. Exp. Therap.* 191: 147–155.

Cone, E. J., C. W. Gorodetzky, and S. Y. Yeh. 1974. The urinary excretion profile of naltrexone and metabolites in man. *Drug Metab. and Disp.* 2: 506–512.

Costa, E., A. Carenzi, A. Guidott, and A. Revuelta. 1973. Narcotic analgesics and the regulation of neuronal catecholamine stores. In E. Usdin and S. Snyder, Eds. *Frontiers in Catecholamine Research.* Pergamon Press, N. Y. pp. 1003–1010.

Evans, J. M., M. Hogg, J. Lunn, and M. Rosen. 1974. Degree and duration of reversal by naloxone of effects of morphine in conscious subjects. *Br. Med. J.* 2: 589–591.

Evans, W. O., and B. A. Bergner. 1964. A comparison of the analgesic potencies of morphine, pentazocine and a mixture of methamphetamine and pentazocine in the rat. *J. of New Drugs* 4: 82–85.

Fleisch, J. H. 1974. Pharmacology of the aorta—A brief review. *Blood Vessels* 11: 193–211.

Fuiimoto, J. M. 1969a. Isolation of naloxone-3-glucuronide from human urine. *Proc. Soc. Exp. Biol. Med.* 133: 317–319.

Fuiimoto, J. M. 1969b. Isolation of two different metabolites of naloxone from the urine of rabbit and chicken. *J. Pharm. Exp. Therap.* 168: 180–186.

Furchgott, R. F. and S. Bhadrakom. 1953. Reactions of strips of rabbit aorta to epinephrine, isopropyl arterenol, sodium nitrite and other drugs. *J. Pharm. Exp. Therap.* 108: 129–143.

Greenberg, S., J. P. Long, and F. P. J. Diecke. 1973. Differentiation of calcium pools utilized in the contractile response of canine arterial and venous smooth muscle to norepinephrine. *J. Pharm. Exp. Therap.* 185: 493–504.

Hiraoka, M., S. Yamagishi, and T. Sano. 1968. Role of calcium ions in the contraction of vascular smooth muscle. *Am. J. Physiol.* 214: 1084–1089.

Hoffmeister, F. 1968. On the possible relations between postganglionic adrenergic and cholinergic neurone blockade demonstrable in the peripheral autonomous nervous system and central analgesia. In *Pain.* Academic Press, N. Y. pp. 281–296.

Holtzman, S. G. 1974. Behavioral effects of separate and combined administration of naloxone and d-amphetamine. *J. Pharm. Exp. Therap.* 189. 51–60.

Holtzman, S. 1974. Interactions of pentazocine and naloxone on the monoamine content of discrete regions of the rat brain. *Biochem. Pharm.* 23: 3029–3035.

Holtzman, S. S., and R. E. Jewett. 1972. Some actions of pentazocine on behavior and brain monoamines in the rat. *J. Pharm. Exp. Therap.* 181: 346–365.

Hudgins, P. M., and G. B. Weiss. 1968. Differential effects of calcium removal upon vascular smooth muscle contraction induced by norepinephrine histamine and potassium. *J. Pharm. Exp. Ther.* 159: 91–97.

Hughes, J., H. W. Kosterlitz, and F. M. Leslie. 1975. Effect of morphine on adrenergic transmission in the mouse vas deferens assessment of agonist and antagonist potencies of narcotic analgesics. *Br. J. Pharm.* 53: 371–381.

Johannesson, T., and B. A. Becker. 1973. Morphine analgesia in rats at various ages. *Acta Pharm. Toxicol.* 33: 429–441.

Kupferberg, H., and E. L. Way. 1963. Pharmacologic basis for the increased sensitivity of the newborn rat to morphine. *J. Pharm. Exp. Therap.* 141: 105–112.

Medzihradsky, F., and K. Ahmad. 1971. The uptake of pentazocine into brain. *Life Sciences* 10: 711–720.

Miller, J., and H. Elliot. 1955. Rat tissue levels of carbon 14 labelled analgetics as related to pharmacological activity. *J. Pharm. Exp. Therap.* 113: 283–291.

Misra, A. L., R. B. Potani, and S. J. Mulé. 1974. Physiologic disposition and biotransformation of ^{14}C-naloxone in the rat. *Pharmacologist* 16 (2): 225.

Mitchard, M. 1971. Pharmacokinetics studies on pentazocine. *Acta Pharm. et. Tox.* 29: 171–180.

Nagatsu, T., M. Levitt, and S. Udenfriend. 1964. Tyrosine hydroxylase: The initial step in norepinephrine biosynthesis. *J. Biol. Chem.* 238: 2910–2917.

Paalzow, G., L. Paalzow, and B. Stalby. 1974. Pentazocine analgesia and regional rat brain catecholamine. *Europ J. Pharm.* 27: 78–88.

Paalzow, L. 1974. Analgesia produced by clonidine in mice and rats. *J. Pharm. Pharmacol.* 26: 361–363.

Pert, C. B., and S. H. Snyder. 1973. Opiate receptor: Demonstration in nervous tissue. *Science* 179: 1011–1014.

Pittman, K. A. 1970. Human metabolism of orally administered pentazocine. *Bichem. Pharm.* 19: 1833–1836.

Resnick, R. B., J. Valavka, A. M. Freedman, and M. Thomas. 1974. Studies of EN–1639A Naltrexone: A new narcotic antagonist. *Am. J. Psychiatry* 13: 646–650.

Sasame, H. A., and J. Perex-Cruet. 1972. Evidence that methadone blocks dopamine receptors in the brain. *J. Neurochem.* 19: 1953–1957.

Shiomi, H., and H. Takagi. 1974. Morphine analgesia and the bulbospinal noradrenergic system: Increase in the concentration of normetanephrine in the spinal cord of the rat caused by analgesics. *Br. J. Pharm.* 52: 519–526.

Sugrue, M. F. 1974. The effects of acutely administered analgesics on the turnover of noradrenaline and dopamine in various regions of the rat brain. *Br. J. Pharm.* 52: 159–165.

Thoa, N. B., G. F. Wooten, J. Axelrod, and F. J. Kopin. 1972. Inhibition of release of dopamine-β-hydroxylase and norepinephrine from sympathetic nerves by colchicine, vinblastine cytochalasin-B. *Proc. Nat'l Acad. Sci.* 69: 520–522.

Tommisto, T., A. Jaatella, P. Nikki, and S. Takki. 1971. Effect of pentazocine and pethidine on plasma catecholamine levels. *Ann. Clin. Res.* 3: 22–25.

Vaughan, D. P., and A. H. Beckett. 1974. An analysis of the inter-subject variations in the metabolism of pentazocine. *J. Pharm. Pharmacol.* 26: 789–798.

Weinstein, S. H., M. Pfeffer, J. M. Schor, L. Indindoli, and M. Mirtz. 1971. Metabolites of naloxone in human urine. *J. Pharm. Sciences* 60: 1567–1568.

Weinstein, S. H., P. N. Pfeffer, J. M. Schor, L. Franklin, M. Mintz, and E. R. Totko. 1973. Absorption and distribution of naloxone in rats after oral and intravenous administration. *J. Pharmac. Sciences* 62: 1416–1419.

Weinstock, M. 1971. Sites of action of narcotic analgesic drugs: Peripheral tissues. In D. H. Clouet, Ed. *Narcotic Drugs.* Plenum Press, N. Y. pp. 394–407.

Weissman, A., K. B. Koe, and S. S. Tenen. 1966. Anti-amphetamine effects following inhibition of tyrosine hydroxylase. *J. Pharmacol. Exp. Ther.* 151: 339–352.

Tissue Responses to Addictive Drugs
© 1976, Spectrum Publications, Inc.

Inhibition of Opiate Stereospecific Binding by Nonnarcotic Drugs

JOSÉ M. MUSACCHIO
GALE L. CRAVISO

Department of Pharmacology
New York University School of Medicine
New York, New York

Stereospecific opiate binding sites have been described in brain and other tissues (Pert and Snyder, 1973a; Terenius, 1973; Simon et al., 1973) of several species, including man (Hiller et al., 1973; Kuhar et al., 1973; Pert et al., 1974). The pharmacological relevance of these opiate binding sites is indicated by the close correlation between the pharmacological potency of various drugs and their affinity for the brain binding sites (Pert and Snyder, 1973b; Terenius, 1974). Apparent discrepancies in this correlation can be explained by the different degrees of penetration through the blood brain barrier and by the fact that some narcotic drugs (codeine, for example) are administered as precursors and have to be metabolized *in vivo* to the active compound (Snyder et al., 1974). The pharmacological relevance of the opiate binding sites is also well illustrated by the almost perfect correlation between the pharmacological activities of opioids on the guinea pig ileum and their binding to the myenteric plexus (Creese and Snyder, 1975). It has recently been

155

described that there is also good correlation between the regional brain distribution of the opiate binding sites and the endogenous morphine-like factor (Hughes et al., 1975; Pasternak et al., 1975).

Considerable evidence indicates that sodium decreases the binding of opiate agonists and increases the binding of antagonists (Simon et al., 1973; Pert and Snyder, 1974). The effects of sodium on the binding of opiate agonists and antagonists have been shown to be mediated through an allosteric effect (Simon et al., 1975). This allosteric interaction suggests that the opiate receptor may be involved in the control of sodium movements through membranes (Snyder, 1975; Craviso and Musacchio, 1975). This consideration prompted us to look at stereospecific opiate binding in the presence of several drugs and toxins that are known to interfere with the movement of sodium through biological membranes. This chapter is the continuation of our previous report (Craviso and Musacchio, 1975).

METHODS AND MATERIALS

Male Swiss-Webster mice (24-30 g) were sacrificed by cervical dislocation and the brains were removed. The cortex was dissected free and homogenized in 150 vol of 0.05 M Tris-Cl, pH 7.4, using a polytron homogenizer. Homogenate aliquots of 1.9 ml were preincubated for 10 min at 25°C with 10^{-7}M dextrorphan or levorphanol and the appropriate test drug. Each sample was then incubated for 30 min after the addition of the labelled naltrexone or etorphine. The incubation was terminated by cooling the samples to 0° in an ice water bath. Filtration of each sample was carried out on GF/B glass fiber filter paper as described by Pert and Snyder (1973a). After treatment of each filter with 1 ml NCS solubilizer, the amount of radioactivity was determined by liquid scintillation spectrometry at a counting efficiency of 40%.

Drugs used in this study were donated by the following companies: Abbott (pramoxine HCl); Astra (lidocaine HCl, prilocaine HCl, 6211, W49085); Ayerst (d- and l-propranolol HCl, pronethalol HCl, practolol HCl); Boehringer Sohn (dipyridamole); Lilly (piperocaine HCl); Roche (RO 20-1724); Smith, Kline and French (chlorpromazine, chlorpromazine sulfoxide, methochlorpromazine); Squibb (procainamide HCl); Winthrop (mepivacaine HCl). All other drugs were obtained from commercial sources. Etorphine-15-16-^{3}H (21 Ci/mmole) and naltrexone-15, 16-^{3}H (16.3 Ci/mmole) were obtained from the National Institute of Drug Abuse and they were used at the original specific activities.

Table I. Effect of Various Drugs on the Stereospecific
Binding of ^{3}H-Naltrexone[1]

(Experiments were carried out as described in METHODS with 1 nM ^{3}H-naltrexone.
Values represent the mean of duplicate determinations.

	Concentration (mM)	% Inhibition
Amiloride	0.001	0
Tetrodotoxin	0.001	0
Procaine	5.0	87
Diphenylhydantoin	0.8	29
Phenobarbital	5.0	3

[1]Appeared in Craviso and Musacchio. 1975. *Life Sci.* 16:1803-1808. (Permission to use granted.)

RESULTS

The effects of several drugs on opiate stereospecific binding were studied using concentrations similar to or slightly higher than those which have been reported to interfere with the movement of sodium through biological membranes (see Table I). The results of Table I indicate that only procaine, a well known local anesthetic, produces a significant inhibition of the stereospecific binding of ^{3}H-naltrexone. In order to establish whether the ability of procaine to compete with naltrexone binding is a characteristic unique to procaine or a property of local anesthetics in general, several other local anesthetics were tested. All the local anesthetics examined had the ability to decrease naltrexone stereospecific binding. A log probit analysis of the inhibition of stereospecific naltrexone binding by several local anesthetics was compared with that of naloxone and found to be parallel, indicating that the opiate ligand and the local anesthetics compete for the same population of binding sites (see Figure 1). Similar results were obtained when the log probit analysis of the local anesthetics was compared with that of levorphanol, an opiate agonist.

In order to study the nature of the interaction between local anesthetics and opiates on opiate binding sites, experiments were designed that could be analyzed with the aid of Klotz double reciprocal plots (Klotz, 1953). These experiments demonstrate that the interaction between cationic local anesthetics and opiates is competitive in nature.

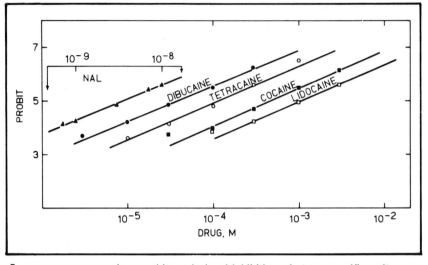

1 Log probit analysis of inhibition of stereospecific naltrexone binding by naloxone (NAL) and several local anesthetics. Experiment was carried out as described in METHODS with 1 nM ^{3}H-naltrexone and with the concentrations of the different drugs as indicated on the abscissa. Values represent the mean of duplicate determinations. (Appeared in Craviso and Musacchio. 1975. *Life Sci* 16: 1803-1808. Permission to use granted.)

The results are illustrated (see Figure 2) where the interaction between tetracaine on one side, and naltrexone and etorphine on the other side was studied. In contrast to the results obtained with the cationic local anesthetics, benzocaine and thymol, local anesthetics of a different class that do not carry a positive charge, inhibited the opiate binding in a noncompetitive fashion, producing a marked decrease in the number of binding sites and insignificant changes in the affinity for naltrexone (see Figure 3). The K_i's for the different local anesthetics were calculated from the slopes and constants obtained from the regression lines of the Klotz plots (see Table II).

Since several local anesthetics are known to have antiarrhythmic properties, the effects of some antiarrhythmic agents on the opiate stereospecific binding were also tested. These agents also decreased ^{3}H-naltrexone stereospecific binding. The log probit analysis of the effect of several antiarrhythmic agents is illustrated in Figure 4. It is evident from this experiment that quinidine is the most effective compound of the series in displacing ^{3}H-naltrexone and that *d-* and *l-*pro-

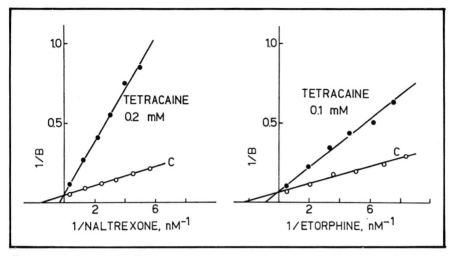

2 Effect of 0.2 mM tetracaine on ^{3}H-naltrexone stereospecific binding (left), and effect of 0.1 mM tetracaine on ^{3}H-etorphine stereospecific binding (right). All experiments were carried out as described in METHODS section and each point represents the mean of duplicate determinations. B: pmoles of stereospecifically bound labelled naltrexone or etorphine per g of brain cortex.

pranolol are equally effective. The effects of quinine as well as other compounds related to propranolol (such as β-blocking agents) are shown in Table III. Kinetic analysis indicates that quinidine and l-propranolol are both competitive inhibitors of naltrexone stereospecific binding (see Figure 5) with K_i's of 0.73 μM for quinidine and 19.0 μM for l-propranolol.

In addition to the drugs used specifically for local anesthesia, we tested a few drugs classified pharmacologically as antihistamines and neuroleptics since it has been shown that these compounds possess local anesthetic activity. Three different kinds of antihistamines were found to inhibit the stereospecific binding of naltrexone (Table IV). The nature of the competition (as shown in Figure 6 for diphenhydramine) is competitive with a K_i of 24 μM. The neuroleptic chlorpromazine and chlorpromazine sulfoxide (see Table V) also inhibited ^{3}H-naltrexone stereospecific binding. The kinetics of this competition were also found to be competitive (see Figure 6).

The report that the anticholinesterase agent eserine competes with naloxone for narcotic binding sites in the rat brain (Klee and Streaty,

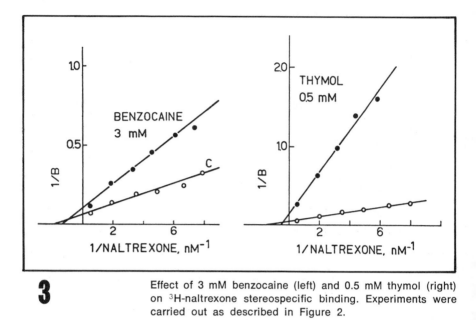

3 Effect of 3 mM benzocaine (left) and 0.5 mM thymol (right) on ³H-naltrexone stereospecific binding. Experiments were carried out as described in Figure 2.

1974), prompted us to test this and other anticholinesterases on mouse brain homogenates. The results of Table IV indicate that neostigmine is inactive, paraoxon very weakly active, and that eserine is active in this system as in the rat brain. Further kinetic analysis of this effect indicates that eserine is a competitive antagonist of naltrexone binding (see Figure 7) and that it has a K_i of 4 μM.

Since there are indications that narcotics interact in some systems with cAMP and adenyl cyclase (Ho et al., 1973a,b; Collier and Roy, 1974; Sharma et al., 1975), we investigated the possibility that some phosphodiesterase inhibitors could interact with stereospecific opiate binding. Of all the compounds tested, papaverine is the only one that shows some activity (see Table IV). A kinetic analysis of this interaction (see Figure 7) indicated that papaverine is a competitive antagonist of naltrexone binding with a K_i of 32 μM.

In order to determine whether the substitution of the tertiary nitrogen by a quaternary nitrogen produces any change in the affinity for the opiate binding site, the activities of lidocaine and chlorpromazine were compared with that of their quaternary derivatives and found to be essentially similar (see Table V). A kinetic analysis of the effects

Table II. Kᵢ (mM) of Some Local Anesthetics for the Inhibition of ^{3}H-Naltrexone Stereospecific Binding

(The Kᵢ's for the different local anesthetics were calculated from the slopes and constants obtained from the regression lines of Klotz plots.)

Dibucaine	0.02	Procaine	0.17
Piperocaine	0.03	Mepivacaine	0.24
Tetracaine	0.04	Procainamide	0.37
Pramoxine	0.12	Lidocaine	0.52
Cocaine	0.15	6211 (Astra)	0.85
Prilocaine	0.16	Benzocaine	2.21

of chlorpromazine and methochlorpromazine indicates that both compounds are competitive inhibitors of naltrexone stereospecific binding with Kᵢ's of 9 and 22 μM respectively.

DISCUSSION

The allosteric interactions between sodium and narcotic agonists and antagonists could be an indication that the narcotic receptor is involved in the control of sodium movements across nerve membranes. This idea led us to explore a possible interaction between drugs that modify the permeability of sodium through different kinds of cell membranes and the binding of opiates to the narcotic receptor. One of the most effective drugs which block sodium movements is tetrodotoxin (TTX), a very powerful nonprotein poison. TTX blocks the sodium ionic current across nerve membranes by occluding the external opening of the sodium channel (Kao and Nishiyama, 1965; Narahashi et al., 1967). The binding of TTX is so specific that it has been used to determine the number of sodium channels in different nerves (Colquhoun et al., 1972). TTX has no effect on naltrexone binding (see Table I) and similar experiments not described in this paper also demonstrate that it does not interfere with the binding of etorphine nor with the sodium effect on naltrexone binding. The lack of interaction between TTX and opiate binding may indicate that either the narcotic receptor does not have any TTX binding site or, that if it has one, it does not interact with the opiate binding site. Equally negative results were obtained with amiloride, a diuretic that binds to sodium channels

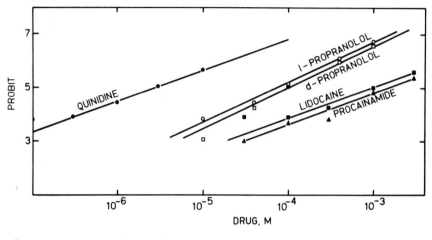

4

Log probit analysis of inhibition of stereospecific naltrexone binding by several antiarrhythmic agents. Experiment was carried out as described in Figure 1.

(Cuthbert and Shum, 1974) and with diphenylhydantion and pheno-barbital, drugs that are known to interfere with sodium conductance in some neurophysiological preparations (Barker and Gainer, 1973).

In contrast to the previous results, procaine and all the other local anesthetics tested were found to block the stereospecific binding of naltrexone and etorphine to the opiate receptor. Local anesthetics are a very heterogeneous group of compounds that block nerve impulses by blocking the sodium conductance (Taylor, 1959; Hille, 1966). The most widely used local anesthetics have certain structural similarities: they have a lipophilic or aromatic residue, an intermediate chain and an amino group. In order to exert its anesthetic action, the local anesthetic has to penetrate through the nerve membrane in an unionized form, ionize to an ammonium form inside the nerve, and then block a specific receptor from the axoplasmic side of the nerve membrane (Ritchie and Greengard, 1966; Narahashi and Frazier, 1971). There are indications that these local anesthetic receptors are located inside the sodium channels (Strichartz, 1973).

Hitzemann and Loh (1975) have shown that the opiate receptor is located on the external surface of the nerve membrane. Since the local anesthetic receptor is located inside the sodium channel and is accessible only from the axoplasmic side of the membrane, the mechanism by which the local anesthetics block the opiate binding is not immediately

Table III. Effect of Antiarrhythmic and β-Blocking Agents (β) on ^{3}H-Naltrexone Stereospecific Binding

(Experiments were carried out as described in Table I.)

	Concentration (mM)	% Inhibition
l-Propranolol (β)	0.1	55
d-Propranolol	0.1	52
Practolol (β)	0.5	52
Pronethalol (β)	0.2	87
Quinidine	0.01	77
Quinine	0.05	80

apparent. One possibility is that the opiate receptor has a sodium channel, the permeability of which is allosterically controlled by the binding of a narcotic agonist. If the conformation of the sodium channel is tightly coupled with the conformation of the opiate binding site, conceivably the binding of a local anesthetic to the sodium channel could produce conformational changes in the narcotic binding site that would change its affinity for the opiate agonist. However, it is quite unlikely that such a complicated allosteric mechanism would have the simple competitive antagonism that we have found and, moreover, that it would be identical for both narcotic agonists and antagonists.

The other possibility is that the local anesthetics compete for the same binding sites as the opiates. If this is the case, then local anesthetics should have some structural characteristics enabling them to bind to the narcotic receptor. Beckett and Casy (1954) have postulated the structural requirements of the opiate receptor surface: a) a flat surface for an aromatic ring; b) an anionic site for the amino group; and c) a cavity for ^{15}C and ^{16}C. Obviously the lipophilic or aromatic portion of the local anesthetic could fit on the flat surface of the opiate receptor and the amino group on the anionic site. The distance between the flat surface and the anionic site on the narcotic receptor should be identical to the distance between the aromatic residue and the amino group of the local anesthetic. In order to get a better insight into the possibility that local anesthetics could fit on the opiate receptor, we constructed molecular models of morphine and several local anesthetics. Upon inspection of these models, the distance observed between the aromatic ring and the amino group was longer in the local anesthetic models

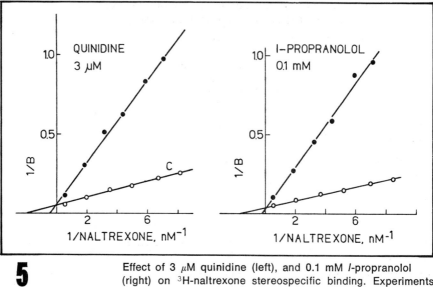

5   Effect of 3 μM quinidine (left), and 0.1 mM *l*-propranolol (right) on ³H-naltrexone stereospecific binding. Experiments were carried out as described in Figure 2.

Table IV. Effect of Various Drugs on the Stereospecific Binding of ³H-Naltrexone

(Experiments were carried out as described in Table I.)

	Concentration (mM)	% Inhibition
ANTIHISTAMINES:		
Diphenhydramine	2.0	97
Tripelennamine	1.0	95
Cyclizine	0.33	89
CHOLINESTERASE INHIBITORS:		
Eserine	0.005	34
Paraoxon	0.2	16
Neostigmine	0.05	0
PHOSPHODIESTERASE INHIBITORS:		
Theophylline	0.5	23
Papaverine	0.1	75
Dipyridamole	0.1	20
RO 20-1724	0.1	5

**Table V. Effects of Various Drugs on the Stereospecific Binding of
^{3}H-Naltrexone**

(Experiments were carried out as described in Table I.)

	Concentration (mM)	% Inhibition
Chlorpromazine	0.1	97
Chlorpromazine sulfoxide	0.1	76
Methochlorpromazine	0.1	76
Lidocaine	0.1	8.0
QX-222 (W49085)	0.1	9.2

than in the morphine model. However, also apparent was that, due to the large mobility of the intermediate chain on the local anesthetics, the aromatic and the amino group could be positioned in the same spacial configuration as the narcotic homologous structures. Our results and all these considerations strongly suggest that the cationic local anesthetics inhibit the opiate stereospecific binding by direct competition for the narcotic receptor.

In contrast to the cationic local anesthetics, benzocaine and thymol produced a noncompetitive inhibition of stereospecific opiate binding. These compounds belong to a different class of local anesthetics and act by a receptor-independent mechanism (Takman, 1975). The nerve blocking activity of the noncationic local anesthetics is well correlated with their membrane/buffer partition coefficient (Seeman, 1972). That the penetration of these compounds into the nerve membrane disorganizes its structure and impairs nerve function is generally accepted. Conceivably the noncationic local anesthetics also disrupt the organization of the narcotic receptor and therefore inhibit stereospecific binding. The noncompetitive type of inhibition that we have found for this class of compounds is consistent with this interpretation.

There is a large variety of other drugs which, in addition to their specific actions, have local anesthetic properties. Typical representatives of these other groups of drugs are antiarrhythmic agents, β-blockers, antihistamines and neuroleptics. As expected from structure-activity considerations, all the representative compounds of these groups that we tested were found to be competitive inhibitors of opiate stereospecific binding. Propranolol has previously been described as an inhibitor of stereospecific opiate binding and its effects have been attributed to its β-blocking properties (Charalampous and Askew, 1974). However, our

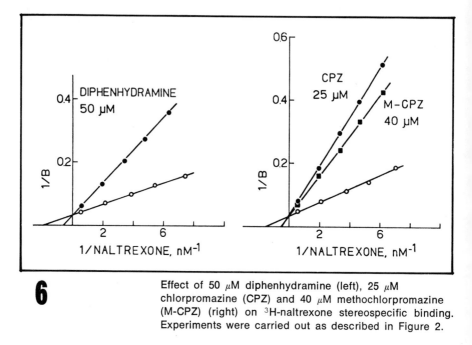

6

Effect of 50 μM diphenhydramine (left), 25 μM chlorpromazine (CPZ) and 40 μM methochlorpromazine (M-CPZ) (right) on ³H-naltrexone stereospecific binding. Experiments were carried out as described in Figure 2.

results demonstrate that the inhibition of opiate binding by propranolol is independent of its β-blocking properties as indicated by the finding that the *d* and *l* isomers are equally effective in blocking stereospecific binding while the *l* isomer is the only one with β-blocking activity. Propranolol has the structural requirements for local anesthetic activity and it has been described as inhibiting the peak transient sodium conductance on squid axon membranes (Wu and Narahashi, 1973). All these considerations indicate that the effects of propranolol on this system are due to its local anestheticlike effects and not to its β-blocking properties.

The report by Klee and Streaty (1974) that eserine inhibits ³H-dihydromorphine binding to rat brain homogenates prompted us to study the effects of several anticholinesterases in our system. Our results confirm their report that eserine can inhibit the opiate stereospecific binding to the narcotic receptor. In addition, our results indicate that this is not a general property of cholinesterase inhibitors since paraoxon and neostigmine were not effective.

CONCLUSIONS

What we have shown is that several nonnarcotic drugs can inhibit the stereospecific opiate binding to the narcotic receptor. However,

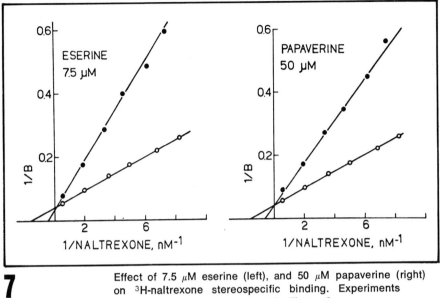

7

Effect of 7.5 μM eserine (left), and 50 μM papaverine (right) on ³H-naltrexone stereospecific binding. Experiments were carried out as described in Figure 2.

since the affinity of most of these nonnarcotic drugs for the opiate receptor is several orders of magnitude lower than the affinity of the most active opiates, one may question the relevance of the interactions that we have described. First of all, it should be pointed out that meperidine, a widely used synthetic narcotic, has an affinity for the receptor which is three orders of magnitude lower than that of morphine (Pert and Snyder, 1974) and almost identical to the one that we have found for quinidine. Secondly, it should be noted that many of the nonnarcotic drugs that we have tested are used *in vivo* and *in vitro* at concentrations at which they have been shown to compete effectively with opiates for the narcotic receptor. This consideration suggests that some of the interactions between narcotic and nonnarcotic drugs believed to occur at neurophysiological or biochemical levels may in fact occur at the opiate receptor level.

SUMMARY

Cationic local anesthetics and several other drugs with a similar general structure inhibit competitively the stereospecific binding of opiates to the mouse brain narcotic receptor. It is thought that the aromatic portion of these drugs fits on the flat surface of the narcotic receptor and the amino group on the anionic site. In contrast to these drugs, noncationic local anesthetics produce a noncompetitive inhibition of opiate binding, presumably by disrupting the structure of the opiate receptor.

Some of the nonnarcotic drugs tested are used *in vivo* and *in vitro* in concentrations that were found to compete effectively with opiates for the narcotic receptor. It is suggested that some of the interactions between narcotic and nonnarcotic drugs which are thought to occur at a neurophysiological or biochemical level may in fact occur at the opiate receptor level.

ACKNOWLEDGMENTS

These studies were supported by PHS Grant No. DA–00351, and José Musacchio was awarded Research Scientist Grant No. 1–K5-MH–17785.

REFERENCES

Barker, J. L., and H. Gainer. 1973. Phenobarbital: Selective depression of excitatory postsynaptic potentials. *Science* 182: 720–722.

Beckett, A. H., and A. F. Casy. 1954. Synthetic analgesics: Stereochemical considerations. *J. Pharm. Pharmacol.* 6: 986–1001.

Charalampous, K. D., and W. E. Askew. 1974. Effect of non-opiate antagonists on stereospecific opiate receptor binding of tritiated naloxone. *Res. Commun. Chem. Pathol. Pharmacol.* 8: 615–622.

Collier, H. O. J., and A. C. Roy. 1974. Morphine-like drugs inhibit the stimulation by E prostaglandins of cyclic AMP formation by rat brain homogenate. *Nature* (London) 248: 24–27.

Colquhoun, D., R. Henderson, and J. M. Ritchie. 1972. The binding of labeled tetrodotoxin to non-myelinated nerve fibers. *J. Physiol.* 227: 95–126.

Craviso, G. L., and J. M. Musacchio. 1975. Competitive inhibition of stereospecific opiate binding by local anesthetics in mouse brain. *Life Sci.* 16: 1803–1808.

Cresse, I., and S. H. Snyder. 1975. Receptor binding and pharmacological activity in the guinea pig intestine. *J. Pharmacol. Exp. Ther.* 194: 205–219.

Cuthbert, A. W., and W. K. Shum. 1974. Binding of amiloride to sodium channels in frog skin. *Mol. Pharmacol.* 10: 880–891.

Hille, B. 1966. Common mode of action of three agents that decrease the transient charge in sodium permeability in nerves. *Nature* 210: 1220–1222.

Hiller, J. M., J. Pearson, and E. J. Simon. 1973. Distribution of stereospecific binding of the potent narcotic analgesic etorphine in the human brain: Predominance in the limbic system. *Res. Commun. Pathol. Pharmacol.* 6: 1052–1062.

Hitzemann, R. J., and H. H. Loh. 1975. On the use of tryptic digestion to localize narcotic binding material. *Life Sci.* 16: 1809–1810.

Ho, I. K., H. H. Loh, and E. L. Way. 1973a. Cyclic adenosine monophosphate antagonism of morphine analgesia. *J. Pharmacol. Exp. Ther.* 185: 336–346.

Ho, I. K., H. H. Loh, and E. L. Way. 1973b. Effects of cyclic 3'5'-adenosine monophosphate on morphine tolerance and physical dependence. *J. Pharmacol. Exp. Ther.* 185: 347–357.

Hughes, J., T. Smith, B. Morgan, and L. Fothergill. 1975. Purification and properties of enkephalin—the possible endogenous ligand for the morphine receptor. *Life Sci.* 16: 1753–1758.

Kao, C. Y., and A. Nishiyama. 1965. Actions of saxitoxin on peripheral neuromuscular systems. *J. Physiol.* 180: 50–66.

Klee, W. A., and R. A. Streaty. 1974. Narcotic receptor sites in morphine-dependent rats. *Nature* 248: 61–63.

Klotz, I. M. 1953. Protein interactions. In H. Neurath and K. Bailey, Eds. *The Proteins.* Academic Press, New York, pp. 727–806.

Kuhar, M. J., C. B. Pert, and S. H. Snyder. 1973. Regional distribution of opiate receptor binding in monkey and human brain. *Nature.* 245: 447–450.

Narahashi, T., N. C. Anderson, and J. W. Moore. 1967. Comparison of tetrodotoxin and procaine in internally perfused squid giant axons. *J. Gen. Physiol.* 50: 1413–1428.

Narahashi, T., and D. T. Frazier. 1971. Site of action and active form of local anesthetics. *Neurosci. Res.* 4: 65–99.

Pasternak, G. W., R. Goodman, and S. H. Snyder. 1975. An endogenous morphine-like factor in mammalian brain. *Life Sci.* 16: 1765–1769.

Pert, C. B., D. Aposhian, and S. H. Snyder. 1974. Phylogenetic distribution of opiate receptor binding. *Brain Res.* 75: 365–361.

Pert, C. B., and S. H. Snyder. 1973a. Opiate receptor: Demonstration in nervous tissue. *Science* 179: 1011–1014.

Pert, C. B., and S. H. Snyder. 1973b. Properties of opiate-receptor binding in rat brain. *Proc. Nat. Acad. Sci. U.S.A.* 70: 2243–2247.

Pert, C. B., and S. H. Snyder. 1974. Opiate receptor binding of agonists and antagonists affected differentially by sodium. *Mol. Pharmacol.* 10: 868–879.

Ritchie, J. M., and P. Greengard. 1966. On the mode of action of local anesthetics. *Ann. Rev. Pharmacol.* 6: 405–430.

Seeman, P. 1972. The membrane actions of anesthetics and tranquilizers. *Pharmacol. Rev.* 24: 583–655.

Sharma, S. K., M. Nirenberg, and W. A. Klee. 1975. Morphine receptors as regulators of adenylate cyclase activity. *Proc. Nat. Acad. Sci. U.S.A.* 72: 590–594.

Simon, E. J., J. M. Hiller, and I. Edelman. 1973. Stereospecific binding of the potent narcotic analgesic ^{3}H-etorphine to rat brain homogenate. *Proc. Nat. Acad. Sci. U.S.A.* 70: 1947–1949.

Simon, E. J., J. M. Hiller, J. Groth, and I. Edelman. 1975. Further properties of stereospecific opiate binding sites in rat brain: On the nature of the sodium effect. *J. Pharmacol. Exp. Ther.* 192: 531–537.

Snyder, S. H. 1975. A model of opiate receptor function with implications for a theory of addiction. *Neurosci. Res. Prog. Bull.* 13: 137–141.

Snyder, S. H., C. B. Pert, and G. W. Pasternak. 1974. The opiate receptor. *Ann. Int. Med.* 81: 534–540.

Strichartz, G. R. 1973. The inhibition of sodium currents in myelinated nerve by quarternary derivatives of lidocaine. *J. Gen. Physiol.* 62: 37–57.

Takman, B. H. 1975. The chemistry of local anaesthetic agents: Classification of blocking agents. *Br. J. Anaesth.* 47: 183–190.

Taylor, R. E. 1959. Effect of procaine on electrical properties of squid axon membrane. *Amer. J. Physiol.* 196: 1071–1078.

Terenius, L. 1973. Stereospecific interaction between narcotic analgesics and a synaptic membrane fraction of rat cerebral cortex. *Acta Pharmacol. Toxicol.* 32: 317–320.

Terenius, L. 1974. A rapid assay of affinity for the narcotic receptor in rat brain: Application to methadone analogues. *Acta Pharmacol. Toxicol.* 34: 88–91.

Wu, C. H., and T. Narahashi. 1973. Mechanism of action of propranolol on squid axon membranes. *J. Pharmacol. Exp. Ther.* 184: 155–162.

Tissue Responses to Addictive Drugs
© 1976, Spectrum Publications, Inc.

Dopaminergic and Cholinergic Transmission in the Striatum and the Effect of Narcotic Drugs

ISABEL J. WAJDA
ISAAC MANIGAULT

*New York State Research Institute
for Neurochemistry and Drug Addiction
Ward's Island, New York, N.Y.*

Corpus striatum, which represents predominantly the cholinergic and dopaminergic center of integration in the central nervous system, cannot be easily implicated in the analgesic action of opiates. There are, however, other effects of narcotic drugs that can directly relate to the physiological function of striatum. A comparatively large body in rats, the corpus striatum includes the globus pallidus, putamen, and caudate nucleus. Functionally, especially in rodents, striatum represents an old, important motor center, with an inhibitory influence on motor activity, particularly when subjected to low frequency stimulation (Stille and Sayers, 1967). Signs of inhibitory phenomena, such as akinesia, arrest response, and catalepsy, can also be triggered by a number of cataleptogenic drugs, among them morphine.

Changes in neuronal transmission in the striatum could involve other parts of the brain, as striatal connections with many other parts of the CNS are known to exist. They could also influence the response of animals to painful stimuli, producing motor depression, which in the case of opiates or neuroleptic drugs reaches the levels of catalepsy; in man, it could be involved in euphoria or other emotional states. Cholinergic synapses in the caudate nucleus were studied by McLennan and York (1966), who found that both excitatory and inhibitory effects can be obtained by applying acetylcholine to single neurons. Both effects were inhibited by atropine, a response characterizing them as muscarinic in function. Regional distribution of muscarinic receptors in the CNS of rats showed predominance in the caudate nucleus and hippocampus (Yamamura et al., 1974). The muscarinic receptors in the central and peripheral nervous systems were claimed to be identical (Beld et al., 1975).

Studies of changes in the content of the two main neurotransmitters acetylcholine and dopamine or of the activity of enzymes involved in their biosynthesis, occurring after administration of narcotic drugs, during development of tolerance, or during the withdrawal period, might give clues as to the central action of those drugs. Equally important could be changes in the permeability of neuronal membranes resulting in either a leakage of enzymes or neurohormones, or a blockade of release, and also changes in the uptake of precursors.

Some of these problems were examined and are reported in the background of previous studies from other laboratories.

METHODS

Cholinergic system

Acetylcholine (ACh), choline acetyltransferase (Ch AT) (EC 2.3.1.6).

Acetylcholine

The levels of ACh increase in the brain (Giarman and Pepeu, 1962) and also in the striatum (Datta and Wajda, 1972) soon after administration of morphine. The increase, as analyzed by Crossland and Slater (1968), occurs in the "bound" and "total" ACh, with simultaneous reduction in the "free" form of the transmitter. Only the first challenge with morphine increases ACh levels, whereas during prolonged administration ACh content remains at the normal levels (Hano et al., 1964; Datta and Wajda, 1972; Large and Milton, 1970). Morphine-induced accumulation of ACh within the cholinergic nerve endings is changed to an excessive release of ACh during withdrawal (Crossland,

1970). Similar results were obtained by Large and Milton (1970). In our experiments (Datta et al., 1972) the increase in ACh levels occurred after only one injection of morphine, returned to normal during prolonged morphine treatment, and did not increase excessively either during the abstinence period (48 and 72 hours) or during withdrawal produced by injection of naloxone. Similar results were obtained by Hano et al. (1964). The turnover of ACh seems to be enhanced during different stages of morphine action, especially during the withdrawal period. (Domino and Wilson, 1973).

Accumulation of ACh after morphine is explained as a reduction in the normal, quantal release of ACh. Evidence was presented by Schaumann (1957) and Paton (1957) using intestinal strip, also by Beleslin and Polak (1965) in a perfused rat brain, and more recently by Matthews et al. (1973) in rat neocortex. The evidence, therefore, that narcotic drugs increase total brain acetylcholine is well established, and the reason for it is undoubtedly the inhibition of ACh release from central or peripheral cholinergic neurons. As shown by Jhamandas et al. (1971), and Matthews et al. (1973), the blocking action on the release of ACh is shared by many narcotic agonists, and mixed agonist-antagonists such as nalorphine, while a pure antagonist (naloxone) not only is devoid of this property but also antagonizes the effect of agonists.

The fact that the levels of ACh in the CNS were influenced by narcotic drugs initiated further research on drugs that influence the cholinergic transmission. Atropine, a muscarinic blocker which also depletes neuronal depots of ACh, was found to suppress the autonomic signs of withdrawal from morphine; it proved to be useful in clinical management of human abstinence syndrome (Crossland, 1970). On the other hand, physostigmine, a potent cholinesterase inhibitor, which increases the levels of acetylcholine, intensified the signs of withdrawal (Jhamandas et al., 1973).

Most of the work quoted here was performed on either the total brain or cerebral cortex of experimental animals. Our interest was concentrated on basal ganglia, and corpus striatum of rats served as the experimental material. In comparative studies we used also cortical and hypothalamic areas. Table I gives percent of ACh change in the striatum of rats injected S.C. with 30 mg/kg of morphine. The levels of total acetylcholine content assayed 15 minutes after injection were already increased, with the highest levels recorded 1 hour after injection. ACh was assayed using frog rectus (Datta et al., 1972).

In analyzing the effects of morphine on the release of ACh, one has to take into account different reactions to morphine observed in different animals. It is known that cats respond to opiates with excite-

Table I. Changes in the Acetylcholine Content of Rat Corpus Striatum after Morphine

Time after injection	% change from normal value	Number of experiments
15 min	+ 6	2
30 min	+ 39	6
1 hour	+ 42	5
5 hours	+ 30	3
24 hours	− 20	2

30 mg/kg of morphine was administered by subcutaneous route. Total ACh content was assayed using frog rectus abdominis preparation. ACh content in rats injected with saline was 28.5 nmoles of ACh per g of wet weight. Standard deviation in 16 experiments was: ± 4.5. (Two animals were used for each assay, and the estimations were performed in triplicates.)

ment and increased locomotor activity bordering on maniacal behavior. Therefore it is not surprising that Phillis et al. (1973) found in non-anesthetized cats an increase in the rate of release of ACh. Anesthetized cats responded to morphine with greatly reduced ACh release; moreover, naloxone alone produced a small increase in ACh release, and restored the reduction of ACh release produced by narcotic analgesics (Jhamandas et al., 1971). Changes in ACh levels are easily detectable in the whole brain of rats treated with morphine; they should be more obvious when assayed in the striatum, where ACh levels are more than twice higher. We recorded values for total content of ACh in the striatum of rats after one injection of morphine, after prolonged administration, during withdrawal period (72 hours), and also after administration of naloxone to morphine-treated rats. We also assayed ACh levels after levorphanol and its inert isomer dextrorphan. Table II presents the results obtained after a single dose of morphine, where an increase of more than 20% over the normal values was recorded. Naloxone, which by itself did not change the levels of ACh, but when administered together with morphine abolished the morphine-induced increase. Not shown are negative results obtained after prolonged administration of morphine and after an abstinence period of 72 hours in rats chronically treated with morphine.

We also examined the levels of ACh after atropine. This drug is known to reduce the levels of ACh in the brain, and indeed we found a 50% decrease in ACh levels after atropine (Table II). The fall in the levels of ACh after atropine is due to an increase in the release of the

Table II. The Effect of Narcotic and Cholinergic Drugs on the Levels of Acetylcholine in the Striatum of Rats

Drug and treatment	Dose in mg/kg	Time after the last injection	Total ACh content in nmoles of ACh/g of wet weight	
			Control	Experimental
Morphine	30.0	1 hour	28.5 ± 1.3	36.5 ± 4.5*
Morphine and Naloxone	30.0 4.0	1 hour 30 min.	28.8 ± 2.9	30.9 ± 2.7
Atropine	80.0	70 min.	29.3 ± 2.4	16.3 ± 1.9*
Morphine plus Atropine	30.0 80.0	1 hour 70 min.	28.5 ± 1.5	28.0 ± 4.6
Physostigmine	0.75	1 hour	28.1 ± 4.3	43.2 ± 4.4*
Morphine[†] Physostigmine	30 - 80 0.75	1 hour 1 hour	28.1 ± 2.9	37.8 ± 2.5*
Levorphanol	10.0	1 hour	28.8 ± 2.6	34.5 ± 3.5*
Dextrorphan	10.0	1 hour	28.8 ± 2.6	28.5 ± 2.6
Naloxone	4.0	30 min.	29.0 ± 1.3	30.5 ± 3.5

(Means of 6-12 experiments ± S.D.)

*Significant difference from the control P $<$ 0.001.

[†] Daily injections during 18-25 days.

Drugs were administered by subcutaneous injections, except for physostigmine which was given intraperitoneally. Experimental procedure the same as that described in Table I. Variations are expressed as S.D. (standard deviations) and the statistical analysis according to Student's test. * = significant difference from the control, P $<$ 0.001; [†] = Daily injections of morphine during 18-25 days. Means of 6 - 12 experiments.

transmitter. We have found also that atropine cancelled the blocking action of morphine, resulting in normal levels of ACh; this suggests an antagonistic effect of those drugs.

The effects of cholinesterase inhibition by eserine resulted, as expected, in accumulation of ACh. However, when physostigmine was given together with morphine, the increase in ACh levels was smaller than that produced by physostigmine alone. These results suggest that a ceiling effect is in operation; therefore it is difficult to posit synergistic action when the drugs are given simultaneously.

Changes in the cholinergic striatal system must, therefore, be included in analyzing the action of morphine on central neurotransmission. Crossland (1970) demonstrated that abstinence syndromes are attenuated by atropine and intensified by physostigmine. Therefore, centrally acting cholinergic drugs might possibly be of use in the treatment of human addiction.

Choline acetyltransferase (ChAT), (E.C. 2.3.1.6)

High ACh levels in the striatum of morphine-treated animals directed research in many laboratories toward investigations of the enzymatic processes involved in ACh biosynthesis and metabolism. Although the synthesis of ACh is dependent on several enzyme systems in intact brain tissue, ChAT activity is of particular interest because of the high concentrations of this enzyme at the nerve terminals. It is also believed that the levels of ACh in the brain are generally well correlated with the activity of the neurons (Giarman and Pepeu, 1964).

Similar to the distribution of ACh in the brain, corpus striatum contains highest activity of ChAT. At the time we began experiments with levels of ChAT in the striatum of morphine-treated rats, Kaita and Goldberg (1969) examined the effects of acetylcholine on ChAT and found an inhibitory action of the transmitter, suggesting a feedback inhibition by acetylcholine. In certain strains of rats we were able to demonstrate *in vivo* inhibition of ChAT after a single dose of morphine (Thal and Wajda, 1969). This effect disappeared in chronically treated animals. Further study of this effect (Datta et al., 1971) showed changes in conformation of the enzyme molecule induced by morphine (Datta and Wajda, 1972). It was shown by Malthe-Sörenssen and Fonnum (1972) that the ChAT from rat brain is present in three different molecular forms with isoelectric points at pH 7.4-7.6, 7.7-7.9, and 8.3. Prempeh and Prince (1974) examined the concentration of those three forms in corpora striata of control rats and found a 1:4:4 ratio. When similar extracts were prepared from morphine-treated rats (single dose), the ratio was changed to 4:4:0.5; however, normal distribution was found in extracts prepared from rats treated for a total of 5 days with morphine. The depression of the most basic ChAT and the increase in the most acidic form might also influence findings in different species of rats, related to the lowering of the total ChAT noticed after a single dose of morphine (Datta et al., 1971).

It is difficult to claim that these effects of morphine on the enzyme involved in the biosynthesis of ACh are either responsible for the central action of opiates or are involved in the process of tolerance or addiction. But the fact remains that the molecular conformation of ChAT and some of the forms of the rat brain enzyme are affected by morphine; this might be an effect of morphine presence, but it is not necessarily responsible for morphine central action.

Dopaminergic system

Dopamine (DA) and tyrosine hydroxylase (TH) EC 1.14.16.2.

Comparative studies of the distribution of DA in the brain show that striatum contains about ten times as much DA as other parts of the brain, with the exception of the olfactory tubercle, which shows half of the striatal content of DA. Dopamine plays an independent role in the striatal neural transmission, apart from being the precursor of norepinephrine; the major metabolite of DA in this region of the brain appears to be homovanillic acid (HVA, 4-hydroxy 3-methoxy phenylacetic acid).

Many studies on the effects of narcotic drugs included investigations of changes in the dopaminergic system. Increased incorporation of ^{14}C-tyrosine into ^{14}C-dopamine after administration of morphine indicated that narcotic drugs stimulate the synthesis and increase the turnover of DA (Clouet and Ratner, 1970; Smith et al., 1972; Costa et al., 1973; Gauchy et al., 1973). The general agreement that acute administration of morphine increases the turnover of DA did not, however, apply to studies on the content of DA. Tagaki and Nakama (1966) reported reduction of brain DA content, Kuschinsky (1973) found normal levels of DA, and Gauchy et al. (1973) reported increased levels of dopamine in the striatum of rats one hour after the administration of morphine. Johnson and Clouet (1973) reported normal levels of DA in the striatum after acute morphine, but they later published that an increase was noticed within 1 or 2 hours after morphine. (Johnson et al., 1974).

Activity of striatal tyrosine hydroxylase after acute and prolonged administration of morphine was found to remain at normal levels by Clouet and Ratner (1970), but Reis et al. (1970) concluded that significant changes in TH activity could be demonstrated after chronic treatment with morphine.

As far as the metabolism of DA is concerned, the results from different laboratories seem to agree that the levels of HVA, the major metabolite of DA in the striatum, increase after narcotic drugs. In experiments reported by Kuschinsky and Hornykiewicz (1972), the peak of catalepsy in rats injected with morphine occurred 40 minutes after injection. The levels of HVA rose between 90 and 150 minutes after injection.

"Cataleptic" behavior, which occurs in rats after acute morphine administration was described carefully by Buxbaum et al. (1973). According to those authors, catalepsy consists of a hypoactive phase, with essentially no spontaneous activity, a decrease in respiratory rate,

**Table III. Effect of Morphine Administration on the Levels of
Dopamine in the Striatum of Rats**

Time after injection	Dopamine Levels in μg/g of wet weight	
	Saline	Morphine
30 minutes	8.19 ± 1.60*	8.19 ± 1.40 (6)
1 hour	7.74 ± 1.07	8.26 ± 1.54 (17)
2 hours	7.27 ± 1.52	10.43 ± 1.12[†] (8)
4 hours	7.38 ± 1.21	10.22 ± 1.79[†] (18)
16 hours	7.98 ± 1.64	8.17 ± 1.23 (4)

*Standard deviation
[†]P value <0.001.

Numbers in parenthesis refer to number of experiments. *S.D. (standard deviation).
[†] = P value < 0.001; experimental conditions same as those described in Table I. Dopamine was assayed according to procedure described in text. (All experiments were done in duplicates.)

and hyperreactivity to various stimuli (noise, touch). Such motor behavior was considered to provide more fruitful framework for assessing the role of putative transmitters in narcotic effects than analgesia.

In view of the controversial results on the content of DA after acute administration of morphine, we examined the levels of striatal DA during a longer time period following injection of morphine. The procedure used was that described by Shellenberger and Gordon (1971), and the results are summarized in Table III. After administration of 30 mg/kg of morphine, the content of DA in the striatum was found to remain at normal levels 1 hour after the injection. After 2 and 4 hours the levels of DA rose significantly above the normal values. The activity of tyrosine hydroxylase was also examined using the method of Kuczenski and Segal (1974). In agreement with results published previously from other laboratories, we did not observe any significant changes in the activity of TH. The time-course study of dopamine, acetylcholine, and norepinephrine levels in the striatum after acute administration of morphine is presented in graphic form in Figure 1. It includes estimation of norepinephrine levels, which were depleted after morphine to about 40% of normal values. However, the decrease showed also large individual variations. Acetylcholine levels were already increased 15 minutes after morphine; this was also the time when cataleptic behavior appeared. The peak of such locomotor abnormality

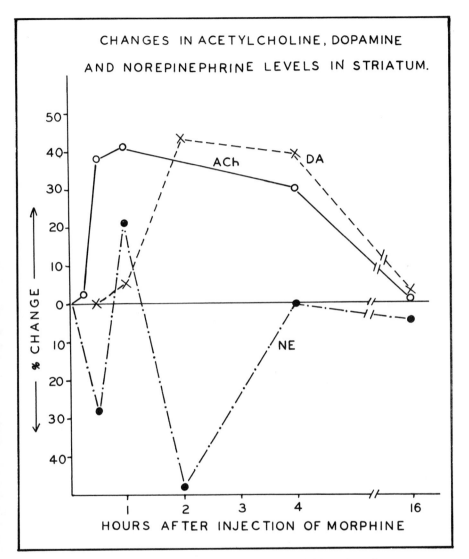

1

Effect of a single subcutaneous administration of
30 mg/kg of morphine sulfate on the levels of dopamine
(DA), acetylcholine (ACh) and norepinephrine (NE),
assayed in the striatum of rats. Each point represents
the mean values calculated as per cent change from controls.

coincided with the highest levels of ACh. At the time that high DA levels were observed (2 hours) the rats were moving without observable locomotor abnormalities.

DISCUSSION

A close relationship exists between the cholinergic and adrenergic neural transmission in the peripheral nervous system. In the CNS such relationship is more difficult to prove and its existence is often demonstrated by the effects of cholinergic and adrenergic drugs. Acetylcholine-dopamine balance in the striatum is essential for the normal physiological functioning of this part of the brain, and it can be changed by the action of drugs. Neuroleptic and narcotic drugs are among the substances able to change this internal balance and produce at the same time catalepsy or stereotyped behavior. Changes in the content, metabolism, or turnover of those two neurotransmitters could explain the mechanism of action of those potent centrally acting drugs.

Direct influence of the cholinergic system on dopaminergic transmission was demonstrated in several laboratories. O'Keeffe et al. (1970) found an increase in homovanillic acid in the striatum after neuroleptic drugs. This effect was interpreted as an increase in the turnover of dopamine. Although without effect on DA concentration, atropine was able to counteract this rise of HVA in the striatum. Smelik and Ernst (1966) produced stereotyped behavior in rats by implanting crystals of physostigmine in the substantia nigra, demonstrating activation of dopaminergic pathways by acetylcholine. Similar gnawing response was produced by implantation of DOPA. Striatal function and the turnover of striatal dopamine was shown to be influenced by centrally active anticholinergic drugs, among them scopolamine, atropine, and Diran (Anden and Bedard, 1971). Also, the turnover of cerebral dopamine was decreased without changing DA content, after peripheral administration of atropine (Bartholini and Pletscher, 1971). According to Bartholini and Pletscher (1972) the cholinergic input might influence the activity of the nigro-striatal neurons; they postulate two cholinergic systems, one inhibitory, and other other excitatory, both involved in the regulation of DA turnover in the nigrostriatal neurons. They based their conclusions on the opposite effects of atropine on the content of HVA in the striatum, according to the mode of administration.

The suggestions as to which of the two systems plays the primary role differ, although the cholinergic mechanism is considered to have an important influence. Sethy and Van Woert (1974) determined ACh

content in the striatum after a number of dopamine receptors antagonists, and agonists; they suggested that since dopamine receptors are
located on cholinergic neurons, and the concentrations of ACh in the
striatum may be regulated by dopamine receptors, the action of neuroleptic drugs may be mediated through a cholinergic mechanism. On the
other hand, Hull et al. (1974) minimize the influence of the dopaminergic system. Studying the spontaneous firing pattern of brain
neurons, they question a simple relation between dopamine and the
regulation of striatal neuronal activity, but they do not rule out the
importance of either acetylcholine or gamma-aminobutyric acid, both of
which are present in high concentrations in the striatum. Haubrich
and Goldberg (1975) measured the concentration of homovanillic acid
in the striatum after cholinomimetic and anticholinergic drugs and
came to a conclusion that the effects of those drugs on the metabolism
of dopamine are mediated through muscarinic receptors of the brain.
It is probably important to mention at this point that the so-called
"cholinergic link" postulated by Burn (1971) for the peripheral postganglionic sympathetic impulses may also be operating in the central
nervous system, involving dopamine and acetylcholine neural systems
in the striatum.

The influence of narcotic drugs was also investigated, and Ahtee
and Kaariainen (1973) showed that not only morphine and methadone
but many other narcotic analgesics increase HVA levels in the striatum.
They also observed behavior and muscle tone; after piminodine and
oripavine (M99) there was marked rigidity of muscles and strong catalepsy starting within a few minutes after injection. Less potent in that
respect and acting slightly later were methadone and morphine. The
correlation of catalepsy and HVA levels was very high with some
drugs (methadone), but not as high with others (piminodine). Naloxone antagonized the cataleptic effects and also the increase in HVA.
Morphine catalepsy and its relation to striatal HVA as studied by
Kuschinsky and Hornykiewicz (1972) occurred 40 min after injection
of morphine, while the peak of striatal HVA level was noticed 90 to 150
min after morphine.

More recently, involvement of the cholinergic mechanism in morphine dependence was investigated by Frederikson and Pinsky (1975),
who questioned the role of catecholamines in development of drug
dependence, and suggested that the cholinergic mechanism may play a
role in development of dependence as well as in its manifestations. They
based their conclusion on the study of cholinergic, anticholinergic drugs
and partial cholinergic agonists on the development and expression of
physical dependence on morphine in the rat. They reported that choline

chloride effectively reduced overall withdrawal severity and weight loss. From this and other similar experiments they concluded that derangement of cholinergic function is a factor in morphine abstinence syndrome.

Based on our own, and on the results of others, we thought it likely that since changes in ACh levels occur earlier, and can be correlated more closely with the disturbances in locomotor activities observed after morphine administration, the cholinergic system plays a monitoring role in activating other neural activities in the striatum.

It should be mentioned at this point that Bartholini et al. (1973) in their study of neuroleptic drugs on dopaminergic and cholinergic striatal systems, came to a conclusion that the two systems are interdependent and the DA system is activated by cholinergic neurons, whereas the cholinergic mechanism is under the influence of a tonic dopaminergic inhibitory input. Such a link and mutual regulation between DA and ACh systems seem to be specific for the neurostriatum. His study deals mainly with neuroleptic drugs, and it is probable that in morphine action on the striatum, such interregulation of the two systems is also in operation.

ACKNOWLEDGMENTS

This work was assisted in part by the Grant DA 00130 from the National Institute of Drug Abuse. We would like to express our gratitude to Dr. K. Datta, Dr. L. Thal, Dr. J. P. Hudick and Mrs. E. Toth for cooperation and assistance.

REFERENCES

Ahtee, L., and I. Kaariainen. 1973. The effect of narcotic analgesics on the homovanillic acid content of rat nucleus caudatus. *Europ. J. Pharmacol.* 22: 206–208.

Anden, N. E., and P. Bedard. 1971. Influences of cholinergic mechanisms on the function and turnover of brain dopamine. *J. Pharm. Pharmacol.* 23: 460–462.

Bartholini, G., and A. Pletscher. 1971. Atropine-induced changes in cerebral dopamine turnover. *Experientia* 27: 1302–1303.

Bartholini, G., and A. Pletscher. 1972. Drugs affecting monoamines in the basal ganglia. In E. Costa, Ed. *Advances in Biochemical Psychopharmacology.* 6: 135–148.

Bartholini, G., H. Stadler, and K. G. Lloyd. 1973. Cholinergic-dopaminergic relation in different brain structures. *Biochem. Pharmacol.* Suppl. (Part 2) 610–614.

Beld, A. G., S. Van Den Hoven, A. C. Wouterse, and M. A. P. Zegers. 1975. Are the muscarinic receptors in the central and peripheral nervous system different? *Europ. J. Pharmacol.* 30: 360–363.

Beleslin, D., and R. L. Polak. 1965. Repression by morphine and chloralose of acetylcholine release from cat's brain. *J. Physiol.* (London), 177: 411–419.

Burn, J. H. 1971. Release of noradrenaline from sympathetic endings. *Nature* (London) 231: 237.

Buxbaum, D. M., G. G. Yarbrough, and M. E. Carter. 1973. Biogenic amines and narcotic effects. Modification of morphine-induced analgesia and motor activity after alteration of cerebral amine levels. *J. Pharmacol. Exp. Ther.* 185: 317–327.

Clouet, D. H., and M. Ratner. 1970. Catecholamine biosynthesis in brains of morphine treated rats. *Science* 168: 854–855.

Costa, E., A. Crenzi, A. Guidotti, and A. Revuelta. 1973. Narcotic analgesics and the regulation of neuronal catecholamine stores. *Biochem. Pharmacol.* (Suppl. 2) 833–840.

Crossland, J. 1970. Acetylcholine and morphine abstinence syndrome. In E. Heilbronn, and A. Winter, Eds. *Drugs anl Cholinergic Mechanisms in the CNS.* F. Forksningsanstalt, Stockholm, pp. 355–357.

Crossland J., and P. Slater. 1968. The effect of some drugs on the "free" and "bound" acetylcholine content of rat brain. *Brit. J. Pharmacol.* 33: 42–47.

Datta, K., L. Thal, and I. J. Wajda. 1971. Effects of morphine on choline acetyltransferase levels in the caudate nucleus of the rat. *Brit J. Pharmacol.* 41: 84–93.

Datta, K., and I. J. Wajda. 1972. Morphine-induced alterations of choline acetyltranferase of rat caudate nucleus. *Brit. J. Pharmacol.* 44: 732–741.

Domino, E. F., and A. F. Wilson. 1973. Enhanced utilization of brain acetylcholine during morphine withdrawal in the rat. *Nature* (London) 243: 285–286.

Frederickson, R. C. A., and C. Pinsky. 1975. Effects of cholinergic and anticholinergic drugs and partial agonists on the development and expression of physical dependence on morphine in rat. *J. Pharmacol. Exp. Therap.* 193: 44–55.

Gauchy, C., Y. Agid, J. Glowinski, and A. Cheramy. 1973. Acute effect of morphine on dopamine synthesis and release and tyrosine metabolism in the rat striatum. *Europ. J. Pharmacol.* 22: 311–319.

Giarman, H. J., and G. Pepeu. 1962. Drug induced changes in brain aceytlcholine. *Brit. J. Pharmacol.* 19: 226–234.

Giarman, J. J., and G. Pepeu. 1964. The influence of centrally acting cholinolytic drugs on brain ACh levels. *Brit. J. Pharmacol.* 23: 123–130.

Hano, K., H. Kaneto, T. Kakunaga, and N. Moribayashi. 1964. Pharmacological studies of analgesics. *Biochem. Pharmacol.* 13: 441–447.

Haubrich, D. R., and M. E. Goldberg. 1975. Homovanillic acid concentration in rat brain: Effect of a choline acetyltransferase inhibitor and comparison with cholinergic and dopaminergic agents. *Neuropharmacol.* 14: 211–214.

Hull, C. D., M. S. Levine, N. A. Buchwald, A. Heller, and R. A. Browning. 1974. The spontaneous firing pattern of the brain neurons. I. The effects of dopamine and nondopamine depleting lesions on caudate unit firing patterns. *Brain Res.* 73: 241–262.

Jhamandas, K., C. Pinsky, and J. W. Phillis. 1971. Effects of morphine and its antagonists on the release of acetycholine *in vivo* from the cerebral cortex of the cat. *Bri. J. Pharmacol.* 43: 53–66.

Jhamandas, K., M. Sutak, and S. Bell. 1973. Modification of precipitiated morphine withdrawal syndrome by drugs affecting cholinergic mechanism. *Europ. J. Pharmacol.* 24: 296–305.

Johnson, J. C., and D. H. Clouet. 1973. Studies on the effect of acute and chronic morphine treatment on catecholamines levels and turnover in discrete brain areas of rats. *Fed. Proc.* 32: 757.

Johnson, J. C., M. Ratner, G. J. Gold, and D. H. Clouet. 1974. Morphine effects on the levels and turnover of catecholamines in rat brain. *Res. Comm. Chem. Path. Pharmacol.* 9: 41–53.

Kaita, A. A., and A. M. Goldberg. 1969. Control of acetylcholine synthesis—the inhibition of choline acetyltransferase by acetylcholine. *J. Neurochem.* 16: 1185–1191.

Kuczenski, R., and D. S. Segal. 1974. Intrasynaptosomal conversion of tyrosine to dopamine as an index of brain catecholamine biosynthetic activity. *J. Neurochem.* 22: 1039–1044.

Kuschinsky, K. 1973. Evidence that morphine increases dopamine utilization in corpora striata of rats. *Experientia* 15: 1565–1566.

Kuschinsky, K., and O. Hornykiewicz. Morphine catalepsy in the rat; relation to striatal dopamine metabolism. *Europ. J. Pharmacol.* 19: 119–122.

Large, W. A., and A. S. Milton. 1970. The effect of acute and chronic morphine treatment on brain acetylcholine levels in the rat. *Brit. J. Pharmacol.* 38: 451–452.

Malthe-Sörenssen, and F. Fonnum. 1972. Multiple forms of choline acetyltransferase in several species demonstrated by isoelectric focusing. *Biochem. J.* 127: 229–236.

Matthews, J. D., G. Labrecque, and E. F. Domino. 1973. Effects of morphine, nalorphine and naloxone on neocortical release of acetylcholine in the rat. *Psychopharmacol.* (Berlin) 29: 113–120.

McLennan, H., and D. H. York. 1966. Cholinergic mechanism in the caudate nucleus. *J. Physiol.* (London) 187: 163–175.

O'Keeffe, R., D. F. Sharman, and M. Vogt. 1970. Effect of drugs used in psychoses on cerebral dopamine metabolism. *Brit. J. Pharmacol.* 38: 287–304.

Paton, W. D. M. 1957. The action of morphine and related substances on contraction and on acetylcholine output of co-axially stimulated guinea-pig intestine. *Brit. J. Phamracol.* 12: 119–127.

Phillis, J. W., W. J. Mullin, and C. Pinsky. 1973. Morphine enhancement of acetylcholine release into lateral ventricle and from the cerebral cortex of unanesthetized cats. *Comp. General Pharmacol.* 4: 189–200.

Prempeh, A. B. A., and A. K. Prince. 1974. The effect of morphine on choline acetyltransferase population in rat caudate nucleus. *Brit. J. Pharmacol.* 50: 447p.

Reis, D. J., P. Hess, and E. C. Azmitia. 1970. Changes in enzymes subserving catecholamine metabolism in morphine tolerance and withdrawal in rat. *Brain Res.* 20: 309–312.

Schaumann, W. 1957. Inhibition by morphine of the release of acetylcholine from the intestine of the guinea-pig. *Brit. J. Pharmacol.* 12: 115–118.

Shellenberger, M. K., and J. H. Gordon. 1971. A rapid simplified procedure for simultaneous assay of norepineprine, dopamine, and 5-hydroxy-tryptamine from discrete brain areas. *Anal. Biochem.* 39: 356–372.

Sethy, V. H., and M. H. Van Woert. 1974. Modification of striatal acetyl-choline concentration by dopamine receptor agonists and antagonists. *Res. Comm. Chem. Path. Pharmacol.* 8: 13–27.

Smelik, P. G., and A. M. Ernst. 1966. Role of nigro-neostriatal dopaminergic fibers in compulsive gnawing behavior in rats. *Life Sci.* (Oxford) 5: 1485–1488.

Smith, C. B., M. J. Sheldon, J. H. Bednarczyk, and J. E. Villarreal. 1972. Morphine-induced increases in the incorporation of ^{14}C-tyrosine into ^{14}C-dopamine and ^{14}C-norepinephrine in the mouse brain. *J. Pharmacol. Exp. Ther.* 180: 547–557.

Stille, G., and A. Sayers. 1967. Concerning the effects of bulbocapnine on the caudate loop. *Experientia* 23: 1028–1029.

Tagaki, H., and M. Nakama. 1966. Effect of morphine and nalorphine on the content of dopamine in mouse brain. *Jap. J. Pharmacol.* 61: 483–492.

Thal, L. and I. J. Wajda. 1969. The effect of morphine on choline acetyltrans-ferase levels in the caudate nucleus of the rat. *Fed. Proc.* 28: 261.

Yamamura, H. I., M. J. Kuhar, and S. H. Snyder. 1974. In vivo identification of muscarinic cholinergic receptor binding in rat brain. *Brain Res.* 80: 170–176.

Tissue Responses to Addictive Drugs
© 1976, Spectrum Publications, Inc.

A Comparison between Narcotics and Neuroleptics: Effects on Striatal Dopamine Turnover, Cyclic AMP, and Adenylate Cyclase

HARBANS LAL
SURENDRA K. PURI
LADISLAV VOLICER

Dept. of Pharmacology and Toxicology
College of Pharmacy
University of Rhode Island
Kingston, Rhode Island

and

Dept. of Pharmacology and Experimental Therapeutics
Boston University School of Medicine
Boston, Mass.

There are many lines of evidence which suggest that brain neuro-transmitters are involved in the actions of narcotic analgesics. (Clouet and Iwatsubo, 1975; Lal, 1975). However, it has been difficult to obtain direct evidence for the neurotransmitter hypothesis of narcotic actions. From among the indirect approaches available, we chose to compare the actions of narcotic drugs with those of non-narcotic drugs having known mechanisms of action. Haloperidol is a prototype non-narcotic drug which blocks dopamine receptors, and many of haloperidol's actions are believed to be associated with this mechanism (Snyder et al., 1975). In this chapter we compare neurochemical actions of haloperidol with similarly measured neurochemical actions of morphine and other narcotic analgesics. A similar comparison of those two classes of drugs on

187

Table I. Effect of morphine and haloperidol on striatal
dopamine content

Drug[1]	Dose (µmole/kg)	N	Dopamine (nmole/g)	
			Mean	S.E.
Saline	1 ml/kg	16	44.9	1.35
Morphine	9.9	3	49.3	2.14
	19.8	3	49.7	2.49
	39.5	6	47.4	1.80
	79.0	8	46.6	0.83
	158.0	3	48.0	1.07
Haloperidol	0.21	3	42.2	1.44
	0.42	6	46.4	1.01
	0.84	3	43.2	0.74
	1.66	3	46.9	3.61
	3.32	7	47.5	3.35
	6.65	9	44.8	2.26

[1]Morphine sulfate was injected one hour before sacrifice, haloperidol two hours before sacrifice. Saline was injected at one hour (in 6 rats) or two hours (in 10 rats) before sacrifice.

appropriate behavioral measures has been recently presented elsewhere (Lal et al., 1975a). We hope that these comparisons provide certain insight into the role of dopaminergic mechanisms underlying narcotic actions and narcotic dependence.

METHODS, RESULTS AND DISCUSSION

Acute Actions

Effects of morphine and haloperidol on striatal dopamine

Morphine sulfate injected in a 15-fold dosage range and haloperidol injected in a 30-fold dosage range did not alter steady state concentrations of dopamine in the rat striatum (Table I). However, both morphine and haloperidol increased the rate of dopamine depletion after inhibition of its synthesis by alpha methyl-para-tyrosine (AMPT) (Table II). In the absence of changes in the steady state levels, an alteration in the depletion rates of a neurotransmitter can be considered as a measure of changes in the turnover rate of that transmitter (Costa and Neff, 1966). A comparison of dopamine turnover rates thus obtained is given in Figure 1. Both, morphine and haloperidol, produced a dose

Table II. Effect of morphine and haloperidol on depletion of striatal
dopamine after synthesis inhibition

Drug	Dose (μmol/kg)	N	Dopamine depletion[1] (nmole/g)
Saline	——	7	22 ± 0.79
Morphine	3.75	4	24 ± 0.96
	7.5	3	25 ± 0.21
	15.0	3	27 ± 1.91
	30.0	9	32 ± 1.43
Saline	——	6	21 ± 0.67
Haloperidol	0.08	4	20 ± 1.02
	0.16	4	23 ± 1.31
	0.33	4	30 ± 0.71
	0.63	4	32 ± 0.66
	1.25	3	33 ± 0.16
	2.5	5	34 ± 1.84

[1] Difference between 0 time and 2 hrs. after AMPT (250 mg/kg) injected I.P.

dependent increase in the striatal dopamine turnover. However, haloperidol was considerably more potent and its action achieved a higher
maximum. The increase in striatal dopamine turnover caused by morphine and haloperidol can also be demonstrated by their effect on a
dopamine metabolite, homovanillic acid. Data (Drawbaugh, Reddy, and
Lal, unpublished data) given in Table III show that both morphine
and haloperidol given in usual pharmacological doses cause a significant increase in striatal homovanillic acid. The action of morphine on
striatal dopamine-turnover was narcotic-specific as it was blocked by
naloxone which did not affect the similar action of haloperidol (see
Table IV).

It may be pointed out that the effects of morphine and haloperidol
in causing stimulation of dopamine turnover coincides with their effect
on catalepsy. As has been reported recently (Lal et al., 1975a), both
morphine and haloperidol cause dose-dependent catalepsy and, whereas
naloxone treatment is ineffective in haloperidol catalepsy, it readily
reverses the cataleptic action of morphine (Wauquier et al., 1974).

In order to estimate the precise location of the site of action for
each drug, we investigated the effects of morphine and haloperidol on
striatal dopamine turnover when these drugs were administered together. For this purpose, we combined a subthreshold dose and a maximally effective dose of haloperidol with an ED_{50} dose of morphine. The

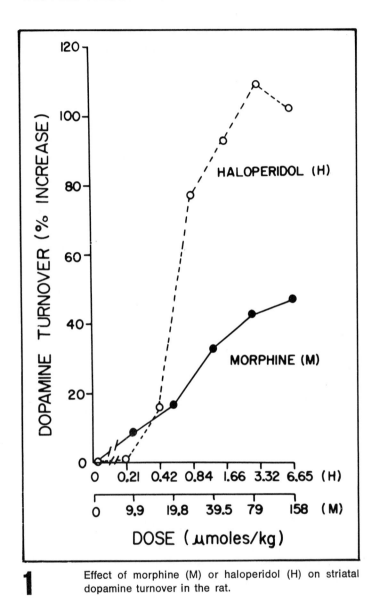

1 Effect of morphine (M) or haloperidol (H) on striatal dopamine turnover in the rat.

lower dose of haloperidol was below threshold in inducing catalepsy and did not produce an unequivocal effect on striatal dopamine turnover. As previously demonstrated with catalepsy (Lal et al., 1975a), there was an important interaction between haloperidol and morphine in causing an elevation of dopamine turnover. The subthreshold dose

Table III. Effects of morphine and haloperidol on striatal homovanillic acid in the rat striatum

Drug[1]	mg/kg	Homovanillic Acid ($\mu g/g$)
Saline	--	0.45 ± 0.03 (5)
Morphine	10	0.73 ± 0.05 (5)
	100	0.85 ± 0.08 (5)
Haloperidol	0.16	0.91 ± 0.06 (3)
	0.63	1.31 ± 0.08 (11)
	1.25	2.29 ± 0.06 (6)

[1] Morphine sulfate was injected 30 min, and haloperidol 120 min, before sacrifice.

of haloperidol (0.42 umole/kg) caused a significant increase in the effect of morphine so that an ED_{50} of morphine produced as great an effect as was produced by maximally effective dose. Addition of maximally effective dose of morphine to the maximally effective dose of haloperidol produced an increase in striatal dopamine turnover equivalent to that which was obtained by haloperidol alone (see Table V).

Effect of apomorphine and benztropine on dopamine turnover as affected by morphine and haloperidol

Apomorphine is known to directly stimulate dopamine receptors (Anden et al., 1967; Ernst, 1967; Costell and Baylor, 1973) and thereby to reduce dopamine turnover by a negative feedback mechanism (Puri et al., 1973). If the actions of morphine and haloperidol involve blockade of dopamine receptors, then apomorphine might reverse the actions of both drugs by stimulating the same receptor. Similarly, it has been known for sometime that anticholinergic type antiparkinsonian drugs interact with dopamine containing neurons in the central nervous system (CNS) and thereby alter the activity of neuroleptics. Therefore, if certain actions of morphine overlap with those of haloperidol then benztropine may interact with both drugs in a similar manner. As expected, both apomorphine (see Figure 2) and benztropine (see Figure 3) produced inhibition of dopamine turnover in a dose-dependent manner. To study the interaction between these drugs and morphine, ED_{50} doses of morphine and haloperidol were combined with a maximally effective doses of apomorphine and benztropine. The maximally effective doses were selected from the linear portions of dose-response curves. (The results of these drug interactions are summarized in Table VI). Treatment with morphine or haloperidol caused a significant increase in

Table IV. Effect of naloxone on stimulation of striatal dopamine turnover induced by morphine and haloperidol. (Data are mean ± S.E.)

Treatment[1] (μmol/kg)	N[2]	n mol Dopamine/g Steady State	Post AMPT[3]	Rate Constant[4]	Turnover (nmol/g/hr)
Saline	12	46.9 ± 1.48	26.3 ± 0.29	0.296	14.04 ± 0.26
Naloxone (14)	6	47.6 ± 2.20	26.1 ± 0.61	0.303	14.37 ± 0.64
Morphine (39.5)	12	47.4 ± 1.80	21.5 ± 1.00	0.399	18.95 ± 1.09
Naloxone + Morphine	6	47.5 ± 1.10	28.1 ± 0.54	0.263	12.49 ± 0.47
Haloperidol (3.32)	14	47.5 ± 2.34	19.7 ± 0.89	0.445	21.06 ± 1.03
Naloxone + Haloperidol	6	47.7 ± 3.95	20.1 ± 1.01	0.430	20.39 ± 1.21

[1] Dose of each drug is given in ( ). Dopamine concentration, taken as steady state, was determined 30 min after naloxone, 60 min after morphine, or 120 min after haloperidol.

[2] One-half of animals were killed at 0 time while other half at 2 hr after AMPT.

[3] Dopamine concentration 2 hrs after AMPT.

[4] Rate constant and turnover rates were calculated.

Table V. Catalepsy and striatal dopamine turnover in rats

Dose (μmole/kg)		Catalepsy	Dopamine, Mean $\pm$ S.E. (N)	
Haloperidol	Morphine	% (N)	Steady State,[1] nmole/g	Turnover,[2] nmole/g/hr
0	0	0 (10)	44.6 $\pm$ 2.72 (13)	14.19 $\pm$ 0.55 (13)
0	20	45 (20)	49.7 $\pm$ 2.14 (3)	17.93 $\pm$ 0.20 (3)
0	79	100 (10)	46.6 $\pm$ 0.83 (9)	21.52 $\pm$ 1.18 (9)
0.42	0	0 (10)	44.1 $\pm$ 1.18 (3)	15.62 $\pm$ 1.62 (3)
0.42	20	100 (20)	45.1 $\pm$ 3.84 (3)	23.52 $\pm$ 1.52 (3)
6.65	0	100 (10)	44.8 $\pm$ 2.26 (9)	32.60 $\pm$ 3.22 (3)
6.65	79	100 (10)	43.9 $\pm$ 1.91 (3)	29.35 $\pm$ 1.27 (3)

[1] Animals were sacrificed for determination of steady state levels 2 hr after haloperidol and 1 hr after morphine injection.

[2] See "Methods" for procedure.

Number in ( ) indicates number of animals employed.

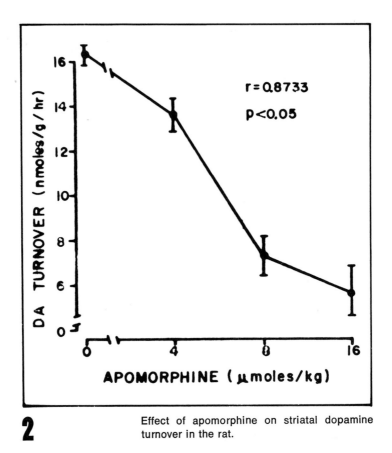

2 Effect of apomorphine on striatal dopamine turnover in the rat.

striatal dopamine turnover. In contrast, apomorphine and benztropine reduced the dopamine turnover. Apomorphine or benztropine when preceded by an injection of morphine or haloperidol reversed the elevation of dopamine turnover. An interaction, similar to that seen with dopamine turnover, was also seen with catalepsy. Neither apomorphine nor benztropine caused catalepsy on their own. However, either drug was effective in antagonizing catalepsy produced by haloperidol or morphine.

Effect of morphine on striatal dopamine turnover after nigrostriatal lesioning

Haloperidol-induced elevation of striatal dopamine turnover is markedly diminished after lesioning of the nigrostriatal tract in the lateral hypothalamus. To provide a comparison with haloperidol, we

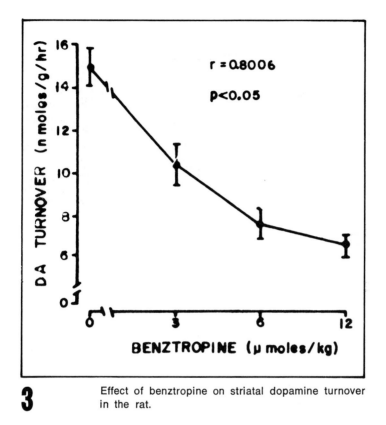

3   Effect of benztropine on striatal dopamine turnover
          in the rat.

lesioned the nigrostriatal tract 24 hr before the administration of morphine sulfate. Unilateral lesioning of nigrostriatal tract increased the
dopamine content of the striatum (see Table VII). This effect has
been previously reported (Hynes et al., 1975). In comparison to saline
effect, the morphine injection still caused an elevation of dopamine turnover but the magnitude of this elevation was smaller than that in the
intact side. When bilateral lesioning was performed, the effect of morphine on striatal dopamine turnover was completely eliminated (see
Table VIII).

Effect of morphine on adenylate cyclase and phosphodiesterase

Earlier studies have suggested that many actions of the catecholamines may be mediated by cyclic AMP (Greengard and Kebabian,
1974). An adenylate cyclase activated by low concentrations of dopamine
has been found in homogenates of rat caudate nucleus. This enzyme

Table VI. Effect of apomorphine, benztropine, morphine and haloperidol
given in combination on catalepsy and striatal
dopamine turnover

Drug[1] (μmole/kg)	Catalepsy, % (N)	Dopamine[2], mean ± S.E. (N)	
		Steady State, (nmole/g)	Turnover nmole/g/hr
Saline	0 (20)	45.8 ± 0.55 (15)	15.53 ± 0.49 (15)
Apomorphine (8)	0 (10)	46.5 ± 1.03 (6)	7.13 ± 1.02 (7)
Benztropine (6)	0 (10)	47.5 ± 1.87 (7)	9.17 ± 1.25 (6)
Morphine (39.5)	100 (10)	47.4 ± 1.80 (6)	17.94 ± 0.83 (6)
Haloperidol (1.66)	70 (10)	47.5 ± 2.35 (7)	19.66 ± 0.87 (6)
Morphine + Apomorphine	0 (6)	45.4 ± 0.94 (3)	12.75 ± 0.60 (3)
Morphine + Benztropine	0 (6)	43.5 ± 2.55 (3)	16.07 ± 0.25 (3)
Haloperidol + Apomorphine	0 (6)	46.6 ± 0.88 (3)	16.53 ± 1.43 (3)
Haloperidol + Benztropine	0 (6)	46.7 ± 2.32 (3)	17.03 ± 0.36 (3)

[1]Determined 2 hr after haloperidol, 1 hr after morphine, 30 min after apomorphine and 2 hr after benztropine.

[2]See "Method" for procedure.
Number in (   ) indicates number of rats employed.

is stimulated both by dopamine and l-norepinephrine, the maximal stimulation achieved by norepinephrine is equal to that observed with dopamine. In the presence of optimal amounts of either dopamine or norepinephrine, no further increase in adenylate cyclase activity can be obtained by the addition of the other catecholamine. Like dopamine and norepinephrine, morphine sulfate added to the homogenate of the rat striatum also increased the formation of cyclic AMP. However, the morphine stimulation of adenylate cyclase was not antagonized by naloxone (see Figure 4). The maximal stimulation of adenylate cyclase by either morphine or dopamine was about the same (Puri et al., 1975). When submaximally effective concentrations of dopamine were combined with morphine, there was an additive effect. However, in the presence of an optimal concentration of either dopamine or morphine, no further increase in adenylate cyclase activity could be obtained by

Table VII. Effect of unilateral lesioning of nigrostriatal bundle
on morphine-induced elevation in striatal
dopamine turnover

Treatment	Dopamine Level (μmole/g)	Turnover Rate (μmole/g/h)
	mean $\pm$ S.E.[1]	
	Intact Side	
Saline	43.2 ± 2.12	14.4 ± 0.34
Morphine[2]	46.1 ± 2.59	25.0 ± 1.09[†]
	Lesioned Side	
Saline	54.4 ± 2.67*	11.4 ± 1.19
Morphine[2]	56.2 ± 1.47*	16.0 ± 2.12[†]

[1]Based upon 3 rats in each group, 24 hr after lesioning.

[2]Morphine sulfate, 30 mg/kg, injected 1P, 60 min before sacrifice.

*Significantly different (P $<$ 0.05) from intact side.

[†]Significantly different (P $<$ 0.05) from saline treatment.

the addition of the other agent (see Table IX). Preliminary experiments also show that the *in vitro* effect of morphine is not stereospecific and also a similar effect can be observed with naloxone.

Intraperitoneal administration of morphine also caused an increase in the striatal adenylate cyclase activity but this effect was very weak and significant only at high doses (see Table X). Addition of dopamine to the striatal homogenates prepared from the rats systematically treated with morphine produced the usual increase in the cyclase activity but an increase in the enzyme activity due to morphine treatment was only marginal.

The effect of morphine on the striatal phosphodiesterase activity in the crude homogenates of rat striatum was also measured. The *in vitro* addition of morphine inhibited the phosphodiesterase activity only when the highest of the concentrations of cAMP was used (see Figure 5). Similarly, the *in vivo* administration of morphine also inhibited phosphodiesterase activity when the highest of the three cAMP concentrations was used as a substrate (see Table XI). The substrate-dependent sensitivity of the enzyme may indicate that a specific iso-enzyme form of the cyclase is inhibited by morphine.

Table VIII. Effect of bilateral lesioning of nigrostriatal bundle on morphine-induced elevation in striatal dopamine turnover

	mean ± S.E.[1]	
Treatment	Dopamine Level (μmole/g)	Turnover Rate (μmole/g/h)
Saline	46.7 ± 1.09	15.2 ± 1.08
Lesion + Saline	46.8 ± 1.88	9.2 ± 1.75*
Lesion + Morphine[2]	45.9 ± 2.57	7.8 ± 1.76*

[1]Based upon 4 rats in each group, 24 h after lesioning.

[2]Morphine sulfate (30 mg/kg) injected 1P, 60 min before sacrifice.

*Significantly different (P < 0.05) from saline treated.

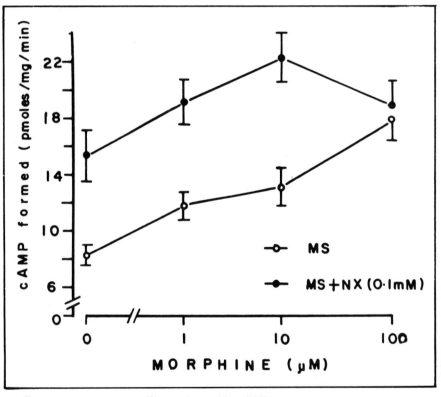

4   Effect of morphine (MS) and naloxone (NX) on adenylate cyclase activity in the rat striatum.

Table IX. Interaction of morphine and dopamine in the stimulation of adenylate cyclase in rat striatum

Drug (μMoles)		Adenylate Cyclase Activity[1] (mean ± S.E.)
Dopamine	Morphine	
0	0	6.07 ± 0.47
1	0	7.58 ± 1.17
10	0	11.55 ± 1.55
100	0	18.37 ± 1.21
0	1	9.64 ± 1.52
0	100	18.37 ± 1.21
1	1	11.81 ± 0.71
1	100	21.34 ± 1.82
10	1	23.46 ± 1.36
10	100	22.44 ± 1.53
100	100	21.76 ± 1.90

[1]Picomoles of cAMP/mg protein/min. based upon 4 samples in each group.

Chronic Actions

In order to compare the withdrawal effects of the two drugs, we chronically administered increasing doses of haloperidol and morphine in two groups of rats. The morphine was increased to 405 mg/kg/day and haloperidol was increased to 20 mg/kg/day as has been described previously (Gianutsos et al., 1974a; Puri and Lal, 1974). The animals were maintained at those maintenance doses for 3–7 days and then withdrawn. The withdrawal signs observed in these animals have alrseady been described (Gianutsos et al., 1974b; Lal et al., 1975). The neurochemical changes due to the chronic treatment are described below.

Dopamine turnover

The rates of dopamine turnover were computed from the rate of dopamine depletion after administration of AMPT as described by Costa and Neff (1966). (These data are summarized in Table XII). Unlike its effect in naive rats, an acute injection of morphine failed to produce an increase in the striatal dopamine turnover of morphine dependent rats. In these rats, the dopamine turnover was markedly lower than that ob-

Table X. Effect of morphine sulfate administration on dopamine (DA) and sodium fluoride induced stimulation of adenylate cyclase activity

Morphine[1] (mg/kg)	Adenylate Cyclase Activity (% of Control)		
	Basal	DA (0.1 mM)	NaF (10 mM)
0	100 ± 8	159 ± 16	701 ± 35
7.5	114 ± 4	167 ± 7	710 ± 61
15	121 ± 10	186 ± 9	715 ± 103
30	129 ± 11*	173 ± 12	636 ± 101

[1]Injection 60 min before sacrifice.
*Statistically significant from control (0 group) values.

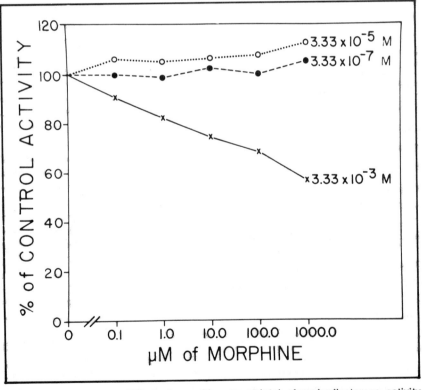

5   Effect of morphine on striatal phosphodiesterase activity at three different substrate concentrations.

Table XI. Effect of morphine sulfate administration on phosphodiesterase activity in the rat striatum

Morphine (mg/kg)	Phosphodiesterase Activity (%) (Mean ± S.E.)		
	Cyclic AMP Concentration (M)		
	3.33×10^{-3}	3.33×10^{-5}	3.33×10^{-7}
0	100 ± 3.46	100 ± 8.90	100 ± 6.25
7.5	76.49 ± 7.60	92.36 ± 6.55	96.87 ± 4.66
15	64.41 ± 10.98	89.17 ± 5.00	90.63 ± 3.44
30	49.08 ± 5.71	86.99 ± 2.22	80.14 ± 8.33

tained in naive rats or rats treated with haloperidol. Similarly, an acute dose of haloperidol, which caused an increase in the striatal dopamine turnover both in the naive rats and in the rats chronically treated with haloperidol, was only marginally effective in the morphine dependent rats. Similar to the observations on the dopamine turnover, we also observed tolerance to the cataleptic action of both haloperidol and morphine in the morphine dependent rats but not in the chronically haloperidol treated rats. It is interesting to note that while there was a definite tolerance to the behavioral and neurochemical actions of both haloperidol and morphine in the morphine dependent rats, such a tolerance was not seen in rats chronically treated with haloperidol.

Sensitivity to apomorphine and benztropine

It has been previously demonstrated that there develops a supersensitivity to the aggression-eliciting effects of apomorphine in rats withdrawn from chronic morphine or chronic haloperidol (Puri and Lal, 1973; Gianutsos et al., 1974b; Lal et al., 1975a). In similar experiments we also observed that after chronic morphine there is a supersensitivity developed to apomorphine's effect on striatal dopamine turnover. Doses of apomorphine which were previously ineffective in naive rats causing inhibition of striatal dopamine turnover, caused marked inhibition of striatal dopamine turnover in the rats withdrawn from either chronic morphine or haloperidol (see Figure 6). These neurochemical data are similar to those obtained in the behavioral experiments. In contrast to marked increase in the sensitivity to apomorphine, there was only a

Table XII. Effect of morphine or haloperidol on striatal dopamine turnover and catalepsy in chronically treated rats[1]

Measurement	Treatment	Saline	Morphine	Haloperidol
Dopamine Turnover (mean ± S.E.)	Naive	14.9 ± 0.72	17.1 ± 0.69	27.5 ± 2.20
(nmoles/g/hr)	Morphine Withdrawn	14.0 ± 0.73	10.1 ± 0.76	18.6 ± 1.15
	Haloperidol Withdrawn	15.7 ± 1.65	17.3 ± 0.13	25.9 ± 3.09
Catalepsy (%)	Naive	0	100	100
	Morphine Withdrawn	0	0	0
	Haloperidol Withdrawn	0	80	90

[1]See text for treatment procedure.

marginal increase in the sensitivity to benztropine in the morphine dependent rats (see Table XII).

Adenylate cyclase activity

In the morphine dependent rats, there was a significant increase in the basal levels of adenylate cyclase activity. The increase was seen from 1–72 hours after the last injection of morphine and therefore not related to the acute effect of morphine. However, these elevated levels of adenylate cyclase activity could not be further stimulated by *in vitro* addition of dopamine (see Table XIV).

CONCLUSIONS

Recently, based upon several different measures of behavior it was concluded that the actions of narcotic drugs sufficiently resemble the actions of neuroleptics so that the narcotic drugs can be considered to be antidopaminergic (Lal et al., 1975a). The present paper reviews corresponding neurochemical measurements taken from animals treated with narcotics and neuroleptics. Striatal dopamine turnover measured by three different methods showed that both narcotics and neuroleptics increase the turnover rate. The mechanism underlying the stimulatory action of neuroleptics on dopamine turnover is believed to be the

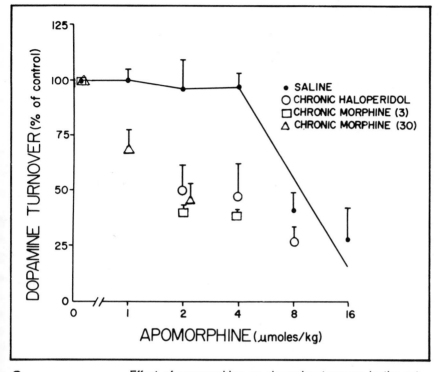

6 Effect of apomorphine on dopamine turnover in the rat striatium after chromic treatment with morphine or haloperidol. Number in ( ) in front of morphine show days of withdrawal. Haloperidol was withdrawn for 7 days.

blockade of dopamine receptors. We propose that the mechanism underlying the stimulatory action of narcotics on dopamine turnover is the same. The conclusion is supported by the observation that the stimulatory action of both morphine and haloperidol is blocked by apomorphine, benztropine, and lesioning of the nigrostrial nerve tract. It is also proposed that chronic treatment with narcotics increases the sensitivity of dopamine receptors to their agonists. In the narcotic-dependent animals, the effects of apomorphine on striatal dopamine turnover is enhanced. A similar enhancement of the behavioral effects of apomorphine in the narcotic dependent animals has been previously reported (Gianutsos et al., 1974a; Lal et al., 1975a). It is believed that the supersensitivity of dopamine receptors, caused by chronic narcotic administration, is due to adaptive changes to counteract the prolonged reduction in the dopamine receptor activity.

Table XIII. Effect of benztropine on dopamine turnover in
morphine dependent rats

Striatal Dopamine	Mean ± S.E. (N)	
	Saline	Benztropine
	Non-Dependent Rats	
Concentration (nmole/g)	46.1 ± 1.57 (3)	45.0 ± 2.71 (3)
Turnover (nmole/g/hr)	14.4 ± 0.66 (3)	9.79 ± 0.98 (3)
	Morphine-Dependent Rats[1]	
Concentration	47.8 ± 1.15 (3)	46.5 ± 1.09
Turnover	14.6 ± 0.77 (3)	8.04 ± 0.73 (8)

[1]24-72 hr after last morphine injection.

Although there is an overt resemblance between the dopaminergic actions of narcotics and neuroleptics, the cellular site of action differs in each case. Whereas, narcotic actions are blocked by naloxone and not by anticholinergic drugs (Lal, 1975), many actions of neuroleptics are blocked by anticholinergics (Wauquier et al., 1974; Lal, 1975; Singh and Ray, 1975) but not by naloxone. Also, the maximal stimulation of striatal dopamine turnover by narcotics is lower than the maximum stimulation achieved by neuroleptics and the maximum effect produced by narcotics can be further increased by additional doses of neuroleptics. These observations suggest that narcotics and neuroleptics act at different sites but the final outcome with respect to their effects on dopaminergic systems is similar. An expanded version of this view has been recently presented elsewhere (Lal, 1975).

It may be pointed out that information available, to date, on both behavioral and neurochemical measures of the relationship between dopaminergic systems and narcotic action as well as narcotic dependence is indirect. Experiments providing direct evidence are lacking. Initial experiments with single cell recording showed that, like the action of haloperidol, systemic administration of morphine increases the firing of dopamine sensitive cells of the zona compacta of the substantia nigra (Bunney, personal communication). Effects of narcotic drugs on dopamine sensitive adenylate cyclase activity are conflicting. Data obtained from in vitro experiments utilizing caudate homogenates as the enzyme source showed that high concentrations of narcotic drugs, their pharmacologically inactive stereoisomers, and naloxone, all stimulate the adenyl-

Table XIV. Striatal adenylate cyclase activity after morphine dependence

Hours after Last Morphine Injection	Adenylate Cyclase Activity, %			
	Dopamine Concentration (μMole)			
	0	0.5	5	50
	Non-Dependent Control Rats			
1	100 ± 8	140 ± 5	186 ± 3	260 ± 8
	Morphine-Dependent Rats			
1	171 ± 5	171 ± 6	179 ± 8	198 ± 8
24	162 ± 7	171 ± 6	81 ± 19	101 ± 16
48	152 ± 10	158 ± 9	131 ± 7	108 ± 7
72	173 ± 8	162 ± 15	195 ± 7	191 ± 8

ate cyclase. However, chronic treatment of the rat with morphine causes an increase in the basal levels of the adenylate cyclase activity in the caudate. Because, the homogenate preparations contain nerve ending, nerve cells, and glia, all of which contain adenylate cyclase, these data should be interpreted with caution. Recently, Iwatsubo and Clouet (1975) showed in *in vitro* studies that narcotic drugs do not affect activity of adenylate cyclase in mitochondrial-synaptosomal preparation derived from the caudate. When systemically injected in high doses, both morphine and haloperidol stimulate the adenylate cyclase activity. Chronic administration of narcotics significantly increases the response of adenylate cyclase activity to the stimulating potency of dopamine.

In conclusion, there is ample evidence existing to suggest that acute treatment with narcotics inhibit the central dopaminergic activity and chronic treatments with narcotics cause latent dopamine receptor supersensitivity.

REFERENCES

Anden, N. E., A. Rubenson, K. Fuxe, and T. Hokfelt. 1967. Evidence for receptor stimulation by apomorphine. *J. Pharmacol.* 19: 627–629.

Clouet, D. H., and K. Iwatsubo. 1975. Mechanisms of tolerance to and dependence on narcotic and analgesic drugs. *Ann. Rev. Pharmacol.* 15: 49–71.

Costa, E., and N. H. Neff. 1966. Isotopic and non-isotopic measurements of catecholamine biosynthesis. In E. Costa, L. Cote, and M. P. Yahr, Eds. *Biochemistry and Pharmacology of Basal Ganglia*. Raven Press, New York, 1966, p. 141.

Costell, B., and R. J. Baylor. 1973. The role of telencephalic dopaminergic systems in the mediation of apomorphine stereotyped behavior. *Europ. J. Pharmacol.* 24: 8–24.

Coyle, J. T., and S. H. Snyder. 1969. Antiparkinsonian drugs: Inhibition of dopamine uptake in the corpus striatum as a possible mechanism of action. *Science* 166: 899–901.

Ernst, A. M. 1967. Mode of action of apomorphine and dexamphetamine on gnawing compulsion in rats. *Psychopharmacologia* (Berlin) 10: 316–323.

Gianutsos, G., R. B. Drawbaugh, M. D. Hynes, and H. Lal. 1974a. Behavioral evidence for dopaminergic supersensitivity after chronic haloperidol. *Life Sci.* 14: 887–898.

Gianutsos, G., et al. 1974b. Effect of apomorphine and nigrostriatal lesions on aggression and striatal dopamine turnover during morphine withdrawal: Evidence for dopaminergic supersensitivity in protracted abstinence. *Psychopharmacologia.* (Berlin) 34: 37–44.

Greengard, P., and J. W. Kebbian. 1974. Role of cyclic Amp in synaptic transmission in the mammalian peripheral nervous system. *Fed. Proc.* 37: 1059–1067.

Hynes, M. D., C. D. Anderson, G. Gianutsos, and H. Lal. 1975. Effects of haloperidol, methyltyrosine and morphine on recovery from lesions of lateral hypothalamus. *Pharmacol. Biochem. Behav.* (In press)

Iwatsubo, K., and D. H. Clouet. 1975. Dopamine-sensitive adenylate cyclase of the caudate nucleus of rats treated with morphine or haloperidol. *Biochem. Pharmacol.* 24: 1499–1503.

Lal, H. 1975. Narcotic dependence, narcotic action and dopamine receptors. *Life Sci.* 17, 483–496.

Lal, H., G. Gianutsos, and S. Puri. 1975a. A comparison of narcotic analgesics with neuroleptics on behavioral measures of dopaminergic activity. *Life Sci.* 17: 29–34.

Lal, H., A. Wauquier, and C. Niemegeers. 1975b. Characteristics of narcotic dependence by oral ingestion of fantenyl solution. *Pharmacologist* 17: 237.

Puri, S. K., J. Cochin, and L. Volicer. 1975. Effect of morphine sulfate and adenylate cyclase and phosphodiesterase activities in rat corpus striatum. *Life Sci.* 16: 759–768.

Puri, S. K., and H. Lal. 1973. Effect of dopaminergic stimulation or blockade on morphine-withdrawal aggression. *Psychopharmacologia* 32: 113–120.

Puri, S. K., and H. Lal. 1974. Tolerance to behavioral and neurochemical effects of haloperidol and morphine in rats chronically treated with morphine or haloperidol. *Arch. Pharmacol.* 282: 115–170.

Puri, S. K., C. R. Reddy, and H. Lal. 1973. Blockade of central dopaminergic receptors by morphine: Effects of haloperidol, apormorphine or benztropine. *Res. Comm. Chem. Path. Pharmacol.* 5: 389–401.

Singh, M. M., and S. R. Ray. 1975. Therapeutic reversed into benztropine in schizophrenic. *J. Ner. Men. Dis.* 160: 258–266.

Snyder, S. H., S. P. Banerjel, H. L. Yamamure, and D. Greenberg. 1975. Drugs, neurotransmitters, and schizophrenia. *Science* 184: 1243–1253.

Wauquier, A., C. J. E. Niemegeers, and H. Lal. 1974. Differential antagonism by naloxone of inhibitory effects of haloperidol and morphine on brain self stimulation. *Psychopharmacologia* 37: 303–310.

Tissue Responses to Addictive Drugs
© 1976, Spectrum Publications, Inc.

In Vitro Interactions on Synaptosomal Uptake of Morphine and Biogenic Amines

Department of Basic Sciences
Peoria School of Medicine
University of Illinois
Peoria, Illinois

A.K.S. HO
L.K. NG
N.B. THOA
R.W. COLBURN

Intramural Research Laboratory
Division of Research
National Institute on Drug Abuse
Rockville, Maryland

Laboratory of Clinical Science
National Institute of Mental Health
Bethesda, Maryland

The interaction between morphine and catecholamines in the central nervous system (CNS) has been implicated as a possible mechanism in the production of morphine analgesia (Lee and Fennessy, 1970). It has been shown that following an analgesic dose, morphine depletes catecholamines in the brains of dogs, cats, and rats (Vogt, 1954; Gunne, 1963; and Reis et al., 1969). Moreover, the uptake of ^{14}C-tyrosine, as well as its incorporation into brain catecholamines, appears to be enhanced by morphine, which suggests depletion and derepression (Clouet and Ratner, 1970; and Smith et al., 1972). Reserpine, an indole alkaloid well-known for its effects on catecholamine depletion, has been reported to antagonize morphine analgesia (Schneider, 1954; Sigg et al., 1958; Medakovic and Banic, 1964; and Tagaki and Nakama, 1968). Although the localization of the subcellular sites through which morphine interacts with the adrenergic effector cells are not known, it is likely that nerve terminals or synaptosomes and storage vesicles containing putative neurotransmitters may be involved. Morphine and other potent analgesics have been shown to block active transport of a variety of amino acids at various sites (Teller et al., 1971). These findings suggest that the inhibition of uptake of putative neurotransmitters into nerve terminals may be a possible mechanism by which morphine exerts its central effects.

In this chapter, we report *in vitro* findings on the inhibitory effects of morphine on the uptake of radio-labelled putative neurotransmitters and their precursors into synaptosomes, as well as on the combined effects of morphine and reserpine on the uptake of ^{3}H-NE.

MATERIALS AND METHODS

Male Sprague-Dawley rats (200–150 g) were killed by decapitation. Their brains were dissected out immediately, chilled, weighed, and homogenized in 10 volumes of ice-cold 0.32M sucrose, as described by Whittaker et al. (1964). After centrifugation of the homogenate for 10 minutes at 1000 g and 4°C, the pellet which consists of nuclei and broken cells (P_1) was discarded. The supernatant fraction (S_1) was layered directly on a discontinuous sucrose gradient containing 10 ml layers of 1.2M and 0.8M sucrose and centrifuged at 50,000 g for 90 min. The myelin above the 0.8M layer was removed by aspiration and the synaptosomes above the 1.2 layer were transferred by pipet and diluted with incubation media to 50 mg initial whole brain tissue per 5 ml sample in 6 ml cellulose nitrate centrifuge tubes. The incubation medium contained 118 mM sodium chloride, 4.7 mM potassium chloride, 2.2 mM calcium chloride, 1.18 mM magnesium sulfate, 11 mM glucose, 25 mM sodium phosphate at pH 7.0. One-tenth ml of incubation medium containing 50x concentrated drug, biogenic amine, or amino acid, or a combination of these, was added and the samples were incubated at 37°C for 20 min. for uptake experiments and 10 min. for Km determinations. At the end of the incubation, the samples were centrifuged at 17,000 g and the pellets resuspended in 250 μl of 0.4N perchloric acid prepared in 50% ethyl alcohol. After centrifugation at 1500 g, a 200 μl aliquot was then transferred to counting vials containing 12 ml phosphor ethanol counting mixture and the radioactivity was measured by liquid scintillation spectrometry. Km and Ki values were calculated using Lineweaver-Burk curves (Mahler and Cordes, 1971). The radioactive compounds of 2, ^{3}H Dopamine (3.48 ci/mM), 1,2, ^{3}H 5-Hydroxytryptamine (1.3 Ci/mM), 2,3, ^{3}Hγ-aminobutyric acid (3.1 Ci/mM), 5, ^{3}H tyrosine (30.8 Ci/mM), ^{3}H(G) Tryptophan (2.3 Ci/mM), and methyl-^{14}C Choline (23.8 mCi/mM) were obtained from New England Nuclear Corporation, Boston, Massachusetts, and the N-methyl^{14}C Morphine (58 mCi/mM) was obtained from Amersham/Searle Corporation, Arlington Heights, Illinois.

RESULTS

Studies were carried out to examine the effect of different concentrations of morphine (10^{-7} to 10^{-3}M) on the uptake of the following putative neurotransmitters or their precursors: ^{3}H-NE, ^{3}H-DA, ^{3}H-5HT, ^{3}H-GABA, ^{3}H-tyrosine, ^{3}H-tryptophan, and ^{14}C-Choline. Morphine at a concentration of 10^{-3}M had an inhibitory effect on the uptake of ^{3}H-DA ($\downarrow$58%), ^{3}H-5HT ($\downarrow$34%), and ^{14}C-Choline ($\downarrow$44%), whereas there was no significant alteration in the uptake of ^{3}H-GABA, ^{3}H-tyrosine, or ^{3}H-tryptophan. The dose-response relationship of morphine on the uptake of ^{3}H-NE uptake, and the concentration of morphine required to inhibit 50% of ^{3}HNE uptake, or I_{50}, was 7.5 x 10^{-4}M (see Figure 1.) In order to establish whether this inhibitory effect of morphine on the uptake of ^{3}H-NE by synaptosomes was competitve or noncompetitive, kinetic experiments were carried out. The apparent Km for ^{3}H-NE uptake was found to be 2.27 x 10^{-7}M, with a Ki of 5.3 x 10^{-4}M for morphine against norepinephrine uptake. The reciprocal plot of initial uptake vs. the reciprocal of ^{3}H-NE concentrations show a simple Lineweaver-Burk type of kinetics (see Figure 2), with a competitive type of inhibition for morphine. Naloxone, a specific antagonist of morphine, also showed a weak competitive, inhibitory effect on ^{3}H-NE uptake at a concentration of 10^{-4}M, with a Ki value of 3.05 x 10^{-4}M. The combined inhibitory effects of naloxone and morphine on ^{3}H-NE uptake appeared to be additive (see Figure 3). However, naloxone alone at lower concentrations (10^{-5}M–10^{-7}M) had no significant inhibitory effects on the uptake of ^{3}H-NE.

The uptake of ^{14}C-morphine by synaptosomes was also studied. Kinetic data showed the uptake of morphine to be a temperature-dependent, saturable process. The apparent Km value of ^{14}C-morphine uptake was calculated as 2.0 x 10^{-6}M. Naloxone, at a significantly higher concentration (5 x 10^{-4}M), inhibited competitively the active uptake of ^{14}C-morphine with a calculated Ki value of 9.8 x 10^{-6}M. However,

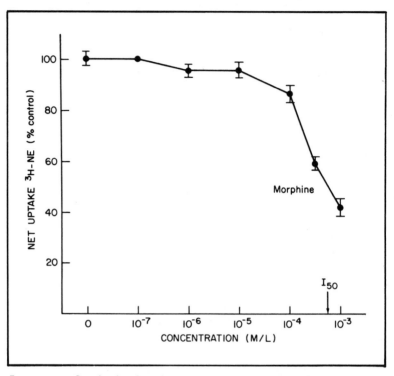

1 Graph showing the dose-response relationship of morphine on the active uptake of ^{3}H-NE into synaptosomal fractions. The synaptosomal fractions were incubated with ^{3}H-NE and various concentrations of morphine at 37°C for 20 minutes. Control uptake of ^{3}H-NE was 1.42 x 10^{6}dpm and expressed as 100%. The mean and S.E.M. are indicated.

NE, DA, and 5-HT at a similar concentration showed only weak inhibitory effects on ^{14}C-morphine uptake. The effects of all three monoamines appeared to be similar, and the Ki values obtained were of the order of 10^{-3}M (see Figure 4).

Studies of combined effects of morphine and reserpine on the uptake of ^{3}H-NE showed that morphine, at a concentration of 3 x 10^{-4}M or greater, was additive to the inhibitory effect of reserpine (5 x 10^{-9}M) on ^{3}H-NE uptake. However, addition of morphine at concentrations from 10^{-4} and higher failed to cause any displacement of the reserpine response curve to the left (see Figure 5).

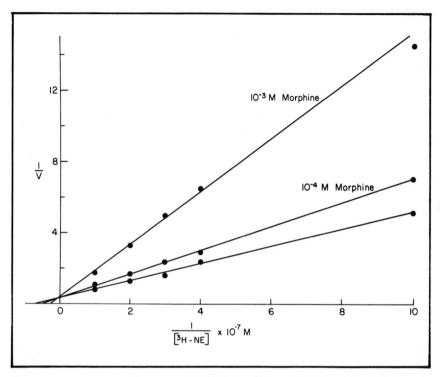

2

Lineweaver-Burk plot of the reciprocals of the initial active uptake of ^{3}H-NE into the synaptosomal fractions in the presence and absence of morphine. Morphine concentrations are indicated. The synaptosomal fractions were incubated at 37°C for 10 minutes with ^{3}H-NE at varying concentrations.

DISCUSSION

It would seem from these studies that morphine accumulates at nerve terminals and may produce some of its effect at these sites. Since synaptosomes are also the storage sites of various putative neurotransmitters and their respective enzyme systems, interaction between morphine and these neurotransmitters at these sites may account for some of the central effects of morphine. The fact that morphine at relatively high concentrations (10^{-4}M–10^{-3}M) produced inhibition of uptake of NE, DA, 5-HT, and choline—but not GABA, tyrosine, or tryptophan—

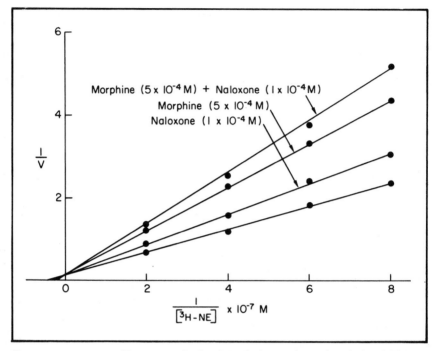

3 Lineweaver-Burk plot of the reciprocals of the initial active uptake of ³H-NE into the synaptosomal fractions in the presence of morphine and naloxone either alone or in combination. The concentrations of each compound are indicated and the control curve contains no drug. The incubations were carried out at 37°C for 10 minutes with ³H-NE at varying concentrations.

would suggest some degree of specificity for putative transmitters. These findings also suggest that one of the sites of action of morphine may be the synaptosomal and/or vesicular membranes.

Kinetic studies indicate that morphine at relatively high concentrations competitively inhibits the uptake of ³H-NE, and naloxone potentiated this inhibitory effect. Therefore, it would appear unlikely that the antagonistic action of naloxone on morphine involves their effects on ³H-NE uptake. It would appear more likely that naloxone acts competitively with morphine for binding sites since naloxone was found to inhibit the uptake of labeled morphine by synaptosomes. The monoamines also showed a weak competitive inhibition on the uptake of labeled morphine. Since the concentrations used were high, the inhibitory effect might be on the nonspecific binding sites of morphine.

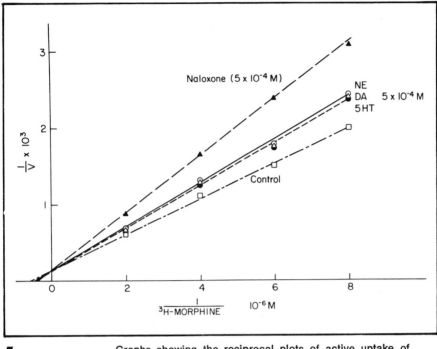

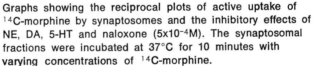

4   Graphs showing the reciprocal plots of active uptake of ^{14}C-morphine by synaptosomes and the inhibitory effects of NE, DA, 5-HT and naloxone (5x10^{-4}M). The synaptosomal fractions were incubated at 37°C for 10 minutes with varying concentrations of ^{14}C-morphine.

Recently, Goldstein et al. (1971) and Pert and Snyder (1973) showed that morphine has a high affinity for opiate receptor sites which are associated with nerve terminals, and our results appear to be consistent with these findings. The possibility that a higher concentration of morphine may be localized in specific subcellular sites in certain parts of the brain (Kuhar et al., 1973) would be consistent with our observations that a relatively high concentration of morphine was required to produce inhibitory effects on the uptake of catecholamines. On the other hand, morphine may produce some of its effect on the transmitter systems, by mechanisms other than active uptake processes. It has been shown that morphine inhibits the release of ACh from brain *in situ* and from cortical slices (Beleslin and Polak, 1965; and Sharkawi and Schulman, 1969).

The inhibitory action of morphine on ^{3}H-NE uptake appears to be additive to that of reserpine, a well-established inhibitor of ^{3}H-NE uptake and binding at nerve terminal sites (Colburn and Kopin, 1968).

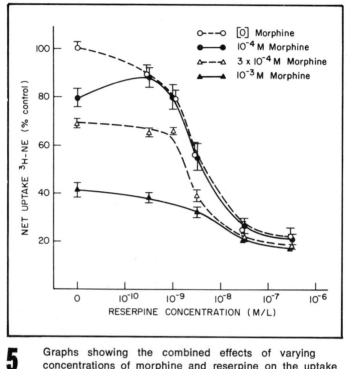

5 Graphs showing the combined effects of varying concentrations of morphine and reserpine on the uptake of ^{3}H-NE into synaptosomal fractions. Control uptake of ^{3}H-NE in the absence of either drug was 1.24 x 10^{6}dpm and expressed as 100%. The mean values and S.E.M. are indicated.

However, the dose-response curve of reserpine on ^{3}H-NE uptake was not displaced significantly in either direction in the presence of morphine, and these findings may imply different sites of action for these two drugs. The mechanism of action of reserpine on morphine analgesia is obscure. Reserpine has been reported to antagonize (Medakovic and Banic, 1964; and Verri et al., 1968), to potentiate (Garcia-Leme and Rochaeme-Silva, 1961; Dandiya and Menon, 1963; and Ross and Ashford, 1967), or to have no effect (Johannesson and Woods, 1964) on morphine analgesia. Furthermore, inhibition of catecholamine uptake by cocaine or DMI has been shown to potentiate the analgesic action of morphine (Heller et al., 1968). These observations suggest that catecholamines at synaptic sites may play an important role in the phenomenon of analgesia. Our studies provide evidence for morphine interaction with catecholamines at these subcellular sites.

SUMMARY

In basic studies of interactions between morphine and their uptake by synaptosomes, kinetic parameters found were: Ki of 5.3 x 10^{-4}M for morphine against norepinephrine, Ki of 3.0 x 10^{-4}M for naloxone against norepinephrine, Km of 2.0 x 10^{-6}M for morphine uptake, and a Ki of 5 x 10^{-4}M for naloxone against morphine. Morphine at concentrations of 3 x 10^{-4}M or greater was additive to the inhibitory effects of reserpine at 5 x 10^{-9}M or norepinephrine uptake.

REFERENCES

Beleslin, D., and R. L. Polak. 1965. Depression by morphine and chloralose of acetylcholine release from the cat's brain. *J. Physiol.* (Lond.) 177: 411–419.

Clouet, D. G., and M. Ratner. 1970. Catecholamine biosynthesis in brains of rats treated with morphine. *Science* 168: 854–855.

Colburn, R. W., and I. J. Kopin. 1968. Effects of reserpine and tyramine on release of norepinephrine from the synaptosomes. *Biochem. Pharmac.* 21: 733.

Dandiya, P. C., and M. K. Menon. 1963. Studies on central nervous system depressants (III). Influence of some tranquilizing agents on morphine analgesia. *Arch Int. Pharmacodyn.* 141: 223–232.

Garcia-Leme, J., and M. Rochaeme-Silva. 1961. Analgesic action of chlorpromazine and reserpine in relation to that of morphine. *J. Pharm. Pharmacol.* 13: 734–742.

Goldstein, A., L. I. Lowney, and B. K. Pal. 1971. Stereospecific and non-specific interactions of the morphine congener levorphanol in subcellular fractions of mouse brain. *Proc. Natl. Acad. Sci.* 68: 1742–1747.

Gunne, L. M. 1963. Catecholamines and 5-hydroxytryptamine in morphine tolerance and withdrawal. *Acta Physiol. Scand.* 58 (Suppl): 204.

Heller, B., T. M. Saavedra, and E. Fisher. 1968. Influence of adrenergic blocking agents upon morphine and catecholamine analgesic effects. *Experientia* 24: 804.

Johannesson, T., and L. A. Woods. 1964. Analgesic action and brain and plasma levels of morphine and codeine in morphine tolerant, codeine tolerant and non-tolerant rats. *Acta Pharmacol.* 21: 381–396.

Kuhar, M. J., C. B. Pert, and S. H. Snyder. 1973. Regional distribution of opiate receptor binding in monkey and human brain. *Nature* (Lond.) 245: 447–450.

Lee, J. R., Jr., and M. R. Fennessy. The relationship between morphine analgesia and the levels of biogenic amines in the mouse brain. *Eur J. Pharmacol.* 12: 65–70.

Mahler, H. R., and E. H. Cordes. 1971. *Biological Chemistry.* Harper & Row, New York.

Medakovic, M., and Banic. 1964. The action of reserpine and α-methyl-m-tyrosine on the analgesic effect of morphine in rats and mice. *J. Pharm. Pharmacol.* 16: 198–206.

Pert, C. B., and S. H. Snyder. 1973. Opiate receptor: Demonstration in nervous tissue. *Science* 179: 1011–1014.

Reis, D. J., M. Rifkin, and A. Corvelli. 1969. Effects of morphine on cat brain norepinephrine in regions with daily monoamine rhythms. *Eur. J. Pharmacol.* 8: 149.

Ross, J. W., and A. Ashford. 1967. The effect of reserpine and α-methyldopa on the analgesic action of morphine in the mouse. *J. Pharm. Pharmacol.* 19: 709–713.

Schneider, J. A. 1954. Reserpine antagonism of morphine analgesia in mice. *Proc. Soc. Exp. Biol.* (N. Y.) 87: 614–615.

Sharkawi, M., and M. P. Schulman. 1969. Inhibition by morphine of the release of (^{14}C) acetylcholine from rat brain cortex slices. *J. Pharm. Pharmacol.* 21: 546–547.

Sigg, E. G., G. Caprio, and J. A. Schneider. 1958. Synergism of amines and antagonism of reserpine to morphine analgesia. *Proc. Soc. Exp. Biol.* (N.Y.) 97: 97–100.

Smith, C. B., M. I. Sheldon, J. H. Bedarczyk, and J. E. Villarreal. 1972. Morphine-induced increases in the incorporation of ^{14}C-tyrosine into ^{14}C-dopamine and ^{14}C-norepinephrine in the mouse brain: Antagonism by naloxone and tolerance. *J. Pharmacol. Exptl. Ther.* 180: 547–557.

Tagaki, H., and M. Nakama. 1968. Studies on the mechanism of action of tetrabenazine as a morphine antagonist. II. A participation of catecholamine in the antagonism. *Jap. J. Pharmacol.* 18: 54–58.

Teller, D. N., T. DeGuzman, and L. Lajtha. 1971. Effects of morphine and phenobarbital on uptake of some amino acids into mouse cortex slices. *Trans. Amer. Soc. Neurochem.*, 114.

Verri, R. A., F. G. Graeff, and A. P. Corrado. 1968. Effect of reserpine and alpha-mythyltyrosine on morphine analgesia. *Int. J. Neuropharmacol.* 7: 283–292.

Vogt, M. 1954. The concentration of sympathin in different parts of the central nervous system under normal conditions and after the administration of drugs. *J. Physiol.* (Lond.) 123: 451, 1954.

Whittaker, V. P., I. A. Michaelson, and R. J. A. Kirkland. 1964. The separation of synaptic vesicles from nerve-ending particles ('synaptosomes'). *Biochem. J.* 90: 293–303.

Tissue Responses to Addictive Drugs
© 1976, Spectrum Publications, Inc.

Biphasic Actions of Selected Narcotics on Rat Locomotor Activity and Brain Acetylcholine Utilization

EDWARD F. DOMINO
MICHAEL R. VASKO
ANN E. WILSON

Department of Pharmacology
University of Michigan
Ann Arbor, Michigan

Narcotics have long been known to have depressant as well as stimulant effects, which are both dose and species dependent (Krueger et al., 1941). For example, in the mouse and cat, administration of narcotics causes psychomotor stimulation (Rethy et al., 1971; Cools et al., 1974). In the monkey and man, narcotics usually cause sedation and depression of behavior (Martin, 1967). The rat, however, is one species that exhibits both depressant and stimulant effects. These actions are observed on motor activity (Babbini and Davis, 1972; Buxbaum et al., 1973; Kuschinsky, 1974; Martin et al., 1963), and many other physiologic and behavioral parameters. Recently, we reviewed the literature on the effects of morphine on rat locomotor activity, body temperature, electroencephalographic activity, self-stimulation and operant behavior and related it to our own data on rat brain acetylcholine (ACh) (Domino et al., 1976).

Morphine and other narcotics have been shown to depress ACh function in the brain as measured by total levels, release, and direct or indirect turnover (see reviews by Weinstock, 1971); Smith, 1972; and Domino, 1975). Recently investigators have demonstrated that narcotics have "biphasic effects" on brain ACh as well (Mullin et al., 1973; Mullin, 1974; Vasko and Domino, 1974). In addition to antirelease, morphine causes the release of ACh from the neocortex of unanesthetized cats and rabbits (Mullin et al., 1973; Mullin, 1974). We have also demonstrated that morphine causes enhanced utilization of rat brain ACh (Vasko and Domino, 1974). The present chapter is an update of our more recent research on the locomotor depressant and stimulant effects of morphine, (−)−5α,9α diethyl−2′−hydroxy−2−methylene, cyclopropylmethyl 6,7 benzomorphan hydrochloride (L604 930, UM 747), and cyclazocine and their relationship to rat brain ACh utilization. The biphasic effects of narcotics were also studied as a function of dose, time and degree of tolerance development.

METHODS AND MATERIALS

All animals used in this study were male albino Holtzman rats 28–32 days old. They were housed 4–6 per cage and kept on a circadian rhythm of 12 hr dark (7:00 p.m. to 7:00 a.m.) and 12 hr light (7:00 a.m. to 7:00 p.m.) with food and water *ad lib.* Motor activity sessions were started one hr into the light cycle. Animals used for the ACh studies were sacrificed by decapitation 1½ to 2½ hr into the light cycle after various pretreatments of morphine sulfate (dosage calculated as base), 0.9% sodium chloride or sodium sulfate in isomolar concentrations. Unless otherwise specified, all drugs were administered s.c. Animals used in the tolerance studies were placed on the following schedule of morphine (mg/kg/24 hr):

Day 1 - 12 mg/kg	Day 9 - 140 mg/kg
Day 2 - 20 " "	Day 10 - 170 " "
Day 3 - 30 " "	Day 11 - 200 " "
Day 4 - 50 " "	Day 12 - 230 " "
Day 5 - 60 " "	Day 13 - 260 " "
Day 6 - 80 " "	Day 14 - 300 " "
Day 7 - 100 " "	Day 15 - experiment concluded
Day 8 - 110 " "	

Injections were given t.i.d. in all tolerance studies except in the initial motor activity experiment. In that series, rats were always given 10 mg/kg i.p. morphine at 8:00 a.m., run in the activity chambers and given divided doses at 4:00 p.m. and midnight to the total amount per day as shown above. All data was analyzed for statistical significance using the Student "t" for group comparison.

Locomotor Activity

Rats were removed from their home cages, given either morphine sulfate or sodium sulfate and run individually in motor activity chambers. These consisted of circular activity cages 30.5 cm in diameter, each equipped with two light beams perpendicular to each other, crossing in the center of the chamber. Each time an animal broke a light beam, one count was recorded. Six activity units were placed in one large soundproof wood chamber and two in another. Circulating fans kept the inside of the chamber at room temperature while the animals were in a session. Sessions lasted 6 to 8 hr.

Acetylcholine Assay

Brain ACh was assayed via a modification of the method of Szilagyi et al. (1972). Rats were decapitated and each brain, minus the cerebellum, was dissected out, weighed, and placed in a separate homogenizing tube containing a mixture of 9.0 ml acetonitrile (reagent grade) 3.0 ml deionized, distilled H_2O (pH 4.0-5.0) and 25 nmoles propionylcholine iodide (1 nmole/μl solution, internal standard). The time from decapitation to homogenization was always less than one min. The brain was homogenized, shaken on ice in a Dubnoff shaker for 15 min, then centrifuged for 5 min at 4000 RPM. The supernatant was decanted and the pellet washed with 1 ml of acetonitrile. Twice the volume diethyl ether was added to the supernatant to extract the aqueous phase. This solution was shaken for 5 min, centrifuged at low speed, and the ether decanted off. The ether extraction was then repeated. Ether was removed by a nitrogen stream from the final aqueous solution. One half ml of this solution was mixed with 0.5 ml water (pH 4.0-5.0), 50 μg tetramethylammonium iodide, and 0.2 ml potassium iodide-iodine solution (2 grams of potassium iodide and 1.6 grams of iodine in 10 ml of water). This mixture was chilled on ice for 30 min to precipitate the choline esters, then centrifuged for 20 min at 4800 RPM. The supernatant was decanted and the precipitate was dried. The solid was redissolved in approximately 50 μl of acetonitrile and assayed by pyrolysis gas liquid chromatography. The 8 ft stainless steel columns were packed with Chromasorb W (HMDS) coated with 20% Carbowax 6000. GC conditions were: nitrogen flow 40 ml/min; air 1.5 l/min, and hydrogen to give best peaks. The temperature of the columns was 140°C, detector 210°C, and the injection port 160°C.

Acetylcholine Utilization

ACh utilization was measured by a method involving inhibition of ACh synthesis by a hemicholinium derivative, acetylsecohemicholinium-3 (ASHC-3) (Domino et al., 1973, Domino and Wilson, 1972). The ASHC-3 was injected intraventricularly one half hr prior to sacrifice by the following procedure. Animals were anesthetized with diethyl ether-air and their bregma exposed surgically as a reference point. A puncture point was made on one side, approximately 1.5 mm posterior and 1.5 mm lateral from bregma, and 0.32 μg ASHC-3 injected into the area of the lateral ventricle in a volume of 20 μl. A microliter syringe and a needle with a stop were used to inject to a depth of 4-4.5 mm. Rats recovered from anesthesia 3-4 min later. After the ASHC-3, ACh synthesis was partially inhibited and ACh levels decreased. Any further change in levels from this new "control" reflected a drug effect on ACh utilization. Increased levels indicated a decrease in utilization of ACh. Decreased levels reflected the opposite.

RESULTS

Effects of Morphine on Locomotor Activity in Nontolerant Rats

Groups of eight rats each were given 1.0, 3.2, 10.0, 32 mg/kg of morphine sulfate or equimolar amounts of sodium sulfate. Mean locomotor activity $\pm$ S.E. was determined for each hr in the 8 hr session. (The data obtained are summarized in Figure 1). It can be noted that the control animals showed a mean $\pm$ S.E. of 240 $\pm$ 46 counts for the first hr. In each subsequent hr their activity decreased to about 100 and below. In contrast, 1.0 mg/kg of morphine caused an enhancement of activity to 420 $\pm$ 61 counts at the end of the first hr (Figure 4). This increase was significant when compared to control (P < .05). The motor activity gradually declined over the next few hours to control levels. Larger doses of morphine produced biphasic effects on locomotor activity. Initially, motor activity was depressed and subsequently enhanced over controls (see Figure 1). The larger doses produced

1

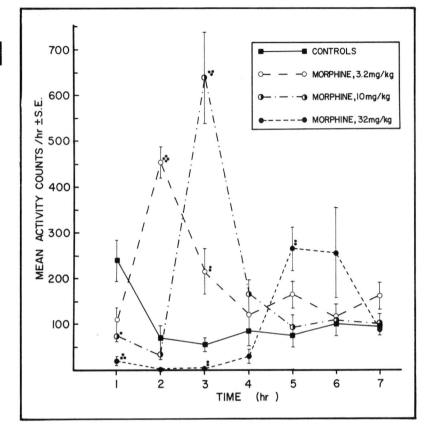

Biphasic effects of morphine on locomotor activity in nontolerant young rats.
Each point represents the mean ± S.E. activity in counts per hr on the y-axis
for groups of 8 rats. Rats were run individually and the mean data calculated.
The control animals were given equimolar sodium sulfate. Group comparison
Student "t" tests comparing the treated groups to control were run. In this and
subsequent figures the asterisks indicate: *P< .05, **P< .01, ***P< .001,
****P< .0001.

greater and more prolonged depression with the stimulant phase
delayed.

Effects of Morphine on Locomotor Activity in Tolerant Rats

Inasmuch as 10 mg/kg of morphine produced marked initial depression and subsequent stimulation of motor activity, this dose was given

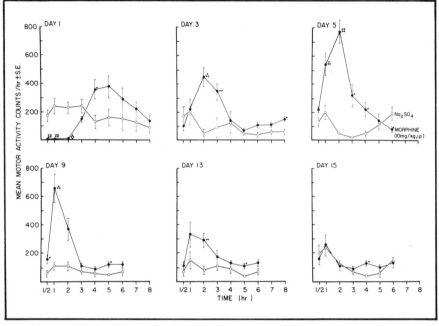

2

Differential tolerance development to the biphasic effects of morphine on locomotor activity in young rats.
    The mean motor activity ± S.E. for 10 mg/kg of morphine given i.p. and equimolar sodium sulfate are given for days 1, 3, 5, 9, 13, and 15. Additional doses of morphine were given at 4:00 p.m. and 12:00 a.m. in a rapidly incremental fashion to induce tolerance. Note that complete tolerance to locomotor depression occurs much sooner in contrast to tolerance to the stimulant effects.

each day at 8:00 a.m. The rats were observed for the next 8 hr. (The mean motor activity ± S.E. as counts per hr are plotted in Figure 2). On day 1, in contrast to the effects of an equimolar amount of sodium sulfate, morphine produced a typical biphasic effect on motor activity. These animals were given morphine on a t.i.d. incrementing dosage schedule (see Methods). The 8:00 a.m. dose was held constant at 10 mg/kg for the next 14 days and each day motor activity was recorded. The mean data for days 3, 5, 9, 13 and 15 are given in Figure 2, in comparison with the control animals. Note that tolerance to the depressant effects of morphine occurred rapidly so that by day 3 (30 mg/kg/day) only stimulant effects were observed. Stimulation was maximal by day 5 (60 mg/kg/day). Subsequently, gradual tolerance

3

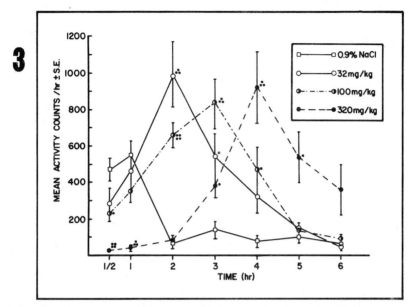

Biphasic effects of morphine on locomotor activity in tolerant young rats.
    The data obtained are similar to those of Figure 1 with a tenfold shift in the
dose-effect curve to the right. Each group of animals began the same morphine
tid tolerance schedule at 18 days of age and were injected daily for 15 days
prior to the doses given in the figure. In this case, a 0.9% NaCl control of
1.0 ml/kg was used.

to the stimulant effects of morphine was seen. By day 15 tolerance was
complete (300 mg/kg/day).

    A second group of animals were made tolerant to morphine by
equally divided t.i.d. doses (see Methods). They were given larger
doses of morphine on day 15 (32.0, 100, and 320 mg/kg) to determine
if there was a shift to the right in the dose-effect curve of motor activity,
as would be expected. (The mean motor activity ± S.E. for each hr
after morphine is summarized in Figure 3). In general, the data in
tolerant rats indicate that 32, 100, and 320 mg/kg of morphine produce
effects similar to 3.2, 10 and 32 mg/kg in the nontolerant animals.
Hence, a tenfold shift to the right in the dose-effect curve was obtained.

Relation of Biphasic Effects of Morphine on Locomotor
Activity and Acetylcholine Utilization in Non-Tolerant Rats

    Groups of 8 young rats were given 1.0, 3.2, 10 and 32 mg/kg of
morphine and sacrificed at different times, in relation to their peak

locomotor depressant or stimulant effects (see Figures 4a and b). In general, when locomotor activity was reduced by morphine, brain ACh utilization also was reduced. When locomotor activity was greatly enhanced by morphine (such as 1 hr after 1.0 and 3 hr after 10 mg/kg), brain ACh utilization also was enhanced. Following 3.2 mg/kg of morphine locomotor depressant and stimulant effects were observed, but there also was no significant change in ACh utilization. When locomotor stimulation was less marked, but still significant compared to control, brain ACh utilization was normal (5 hr after 32 mg/kg).

Relation of Biphasic Effects of Morphine on Locomotor Activity and Acetylcholine Utilization in Tolerant Rats

Groups of 8 rats each, given morphine t.i.d. for 14 days as per the dosage schedule in the Methods, were given 10, 32, 100, and 320 mg/kg morphine on day 15. Both locomotor activity and brain ACh utilization were measured at different times (see Figures 5a and b). Following 10 mg/kg, no effects were observed on either measure, indicating complete tolerance to this dose. After 32 mg/kg of morphine, a marked stimulant effect ($P < .001$) was observed at 2 hr with a slight enhancement ($P < .05$) of brain ACh utilization. In the tolerant animals, a dose of 100 mg/kg of morphine showed effects similar to 10 mg/kg in the nontolerant animals (compare Figure 5b with Figure 4b). Similarly, 320 mg/kg of morphine showed the expected depressant-stimulant effects on both locomotor activity and brain ACh utilization.

Effects of Naloxone on the Depressant-Stimulant Actions of Morphine on Locomotor Activity and Brain Acetylcholine Utilization

Naloxone, in a dose of 1.0 mg/kg i.p., was given simultaneously with morphine, 10 mg/kg, to one group of animals and 2 hr after morphine to another. Naloxone, given at the same time as morphine, antagonized the initial depression of locomotor activity and the reduced brain ACh observed with morphine alone (see Figure 6). It did not antagonize the subsequent stimulant actions 2 hr later, presumably because of its shorter duration of action.

When morphine was given first and naloxone 2 hr later, prior to the maximal morphine stimulant effect, naloxone antagonized the enhanced ACh utilization and reduced the locomotor stimulant effects (compare Figure 8 to 4b).

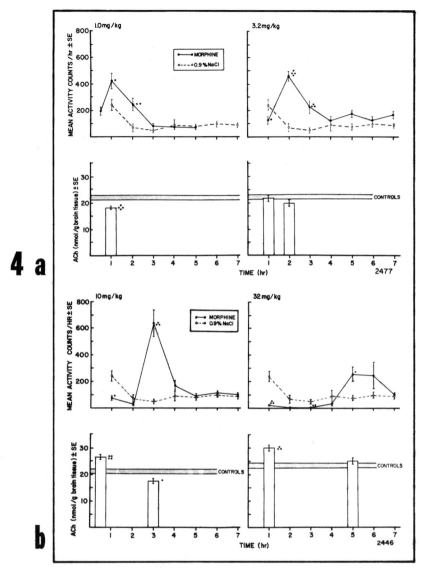

4 a

b

*Biphasic effect of morphine on locomotor activity and brain
acetylcholine utilization in nontolerant rats.*

(a) The effects of 1.0 and 3.2 mg/kg of morphine are shown. The upper line
graphs illustrate the effect on motor activity and the lower bar graphs brain ACh
in which 0.32 μg of ASHC-3 was given i.v. 30 min prior to guillotine.
The mean control level of ACh is that observed after ASHC-3. Note that
when locomotor activity was enhanced at 1.0 mg/kg brain ACh utilization was
increased. Although the locomotor effects of 3.2 mg/kg morphine were biphasic,
no significant change in ACh utilization was observed. (b) The effects of 10 and
32 mg/kg of morphine are shown. Note that at 10 mg/kg brain ACh utilization was
significantly depressed (higher level, P< .0001) at 30 min, and was enhanced
(lower level, P< .05) at 3 hr. Following 32 mg/kg of morphine, brain ACh
utilization was reduced at 1 hr (P< .001) but not altered at 5 hr. when motor
activity was significantly enhanced (P< .05) over 0.9% NaCl injection.

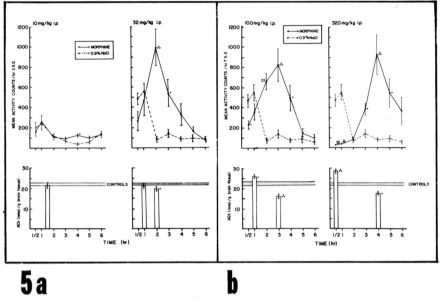

5a   b

Biphasic effects of morphine on locomotor activity and brain acetylcholine utilization in tolerant rats.

(a) The effects of 10 and 32 mg/kg of morphine i.p. are shown. The animals were almost completely tolerant to 10, but still showed a stimulant effect to 32 mg/kg in both locomotor activity (P< .001) and brain ACh utilization (P<.05). (b) The effects of 100 and 320 mg/kg of morphine i.p. are shown. With 100 mg/kg a short lasting initial depression and longer stimulation was observed. With 320 mg/kg the typical depressant-stimulant actions were observed with both endpoints.

Dissociation of Locomotor Activity and Brain Acetylcholine Utilization with UM 747 and Cyclazocine

Two synthetic narcotics have been reported to dissociate locomotor activity and catecholamine depletion in the mouse (Smith and Sheldon, 1972). Hence, it seemed of value to attempt a similar study in the rat using locomotor activity and brain ACh utilization as endpoints.

The data for UM 747 are given in Figure 7. In doses of 3.2 and 10 mg/kg i.p., this narcotic showed typical initial depressant and subsequent stimulant effects on rat locomotor activity, in contrast to its reported lack of stimulant effects in the mouse. During the maximal depressant effects at 30 min, following 10 mg/kg, brain ACh utilization was significantly reduced (P < .001), but not following 3.2 mg/kg. When maximal motor stimulation was observed for both doses 4 and 5 hr

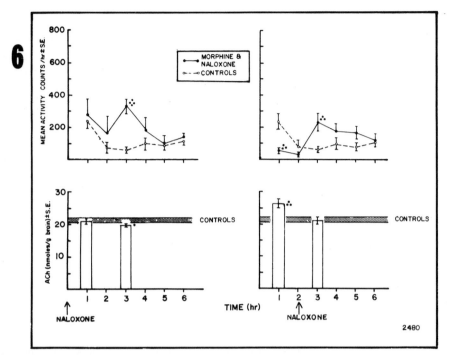

Effects of naloxone on the actions of morphine on locomotor activity and brain acetylcholine utilization in nontolerant young rats.
   Naloxone in a dose of 1.0 mg/kg i.p. was given with 10 mg/kg morphine to the first group and 2 hr after morphine to the second group. When administered with morphine, naloxone antagonized the depressant but not the stimulant effects on both endpoints. When given 2 hr postmorphine, naloxone reduced the locomotor stimulant effects and antagonized the enhanced ACh utilization.

later, brain ACh utilization was not altered, indicating a dissociation between these two phenomena.

   In contrast to UM 747, 10 mg/kg of cyclazocine produced a marked motor stimulant effect, especially 1 hr after i.p. administration (Figure 8). Brain ACh tended to be enhanced (lower levels after ASHC-3) but this was not statistically significant. Again, dissociation between these two endpoints was observed. Four hr later no significant effects of cyclazocine were seen.

DISCUSSION

   Many investigators have shown that morphine and other narcotics have biphasic effects on locomotor activity. The most extensive work,

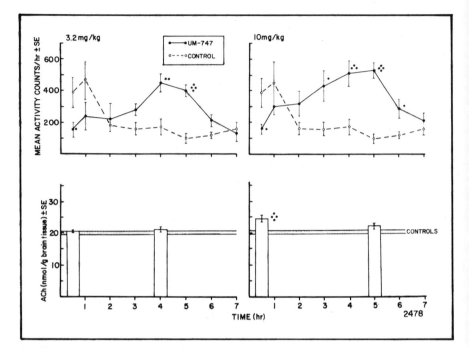

7

Biphasic effects of UM 747 on locomotor activity and brain acetylcholine utilization in nontolerant young rats. The effects of 3.2 and 10 mg/kg of UM 747 given i.p. differ from those of morphine. After 3.2 mg/kg of UM 747, when the animals showed locomotor depression, brain ACh utilization was not significantly reduced but was after 10 mg/kg. During the stimulant phase, brain ACh utilization was not enhanced.

however, was recently reported by Babbini and Davis (1972) and Buxbaum et al. (1973). Both groups of investigators were able to demonstrate stimulant effects with low doses of morphine (i.e., 4 mg/kg) and biphasic effects with higher doses (i.e., 16 mg/kg). We were able to confirm these findings with 1.0 and 10 mg/kg (see Figures 1 and 4). In addition, Babbini and Davis demonstrated rapid tolerance to the locomotor depressant effects in the rat. They could not, however, show tolerance to the stimulant effects on locomotor activity. On the contrary, they reported an enhancement of the stimulant effects after initial tolerance to the depressant actions. We also observed rapid tolerance to the depressant effect and the subsequent increase in stimulation. Following a modified tolerance schedule of Akera and Brodie (1967),

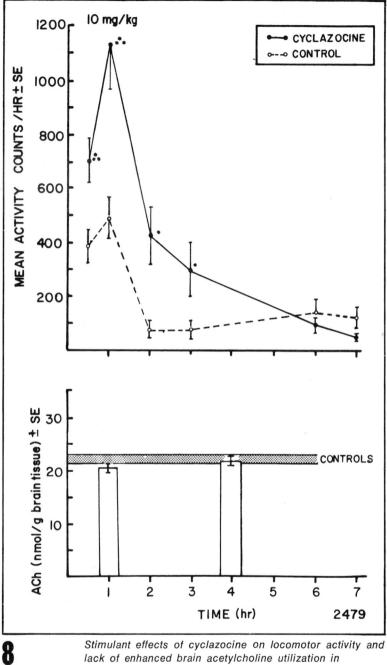

8

Stimulant effects of cyclazocine on locomotor activity and lack of enhanced brain acetylcholine utilization in nontolerant young rats.

Although there was a tendency for brain ACh utilization to be enhanced during the marked locomotor stimulation by i.p. cyclazocine the data was not significant.

we were able to demonstrate tolerance development to the stimulant effects of morphine on locomotor activity. This schedule involves large amounts of drug administered three times a day. The lack of tolerance to stimulant effects reported by Babbini and Davis and others was most likely due to conservative schedules of chronic morphine treatment. Since the tolerance we demonstrated (see Figure 2) could be an adaptive effect instead of true narcotic tolerance, we repeated the study in animals made tolerant to increasing doses of morphine, without exposure to the activity chambers. After a final dose of 300 mg/kg/day, these animals were given various doses of morphine and run in the locomotor activity cages. Tolerance did develop to both depressant and stimulant actions of morphine with an approximate tenfold shift in doses necessary to observe the biphasic effects (see Figure 3).

As an index of central cholinergic function, we used the ACh synthesis inhibitor, acetylseco-hemicholinium, as a tool for measuring indirect turnover. This method involves partial inhibition of ACh synthesis. This inhibition is not instantaneous so we do not feel our method is a quantitative measure of turnover. Rather, we use the method as an indication of utilization of ACh. Since synthesis cannot keep up with demand, increases in cholinergic activity or ACh release are reflected in lowered ACh levels.

We reported a year ago that morphine was not only a depressant of brain ACh utilization but also a stimulant in the rat (Vasko and Domino, 1974). Depending on the dose and time, morphine can have opposite effects on brain ACh (see Figures 4a and b). A small dose (1.0 mg/kg) is stimulant and a larger dose depressant one hr after administration. As mentioned above, other investigators have also found that morphine's effects on brain ACh are not totally depressant. Mullin et al. (1973) reported increases in ACh release after various doses of morphine in unanesthetized cats. This is in contrast to work with anesthetized or brainstem-transected cats and rats where morphine depressed release (Labrecque and Domino, 1974; Matthews et al., 1973; Jhamandas and Sutak, 1974).

As shown with locomotor activity, tolerance developed to both the stimulant and depressant effects on ACh utilization. Again a tenfold shift in the dose-effect curve was seen. A dose of 100 mg/kg was needed to cause the biphasic action on locomotor activity in tolerant rats, whereas 10 mg/kg was needed in the nontolerant. The lowest dose (10 mg/kg) had no effect in the tolerant rats (see Figure 5). Although not shown in the Results section, differential tolerance development to biphasic ACh utilization was also observed. As seen with locomotor activity, tolerance to decreased utilization was noted with low doses of chronic morphine, while large amounts were necessary for enhanced utilization.

In addition to tolerance development, the biphasic effects of morphine can further be shown to be specific narcotic effects since they are antagonized by naloxone. The depressant effects of 10 mg/kg morphine on locomotor activity and ACh utilization were antagonized by 1.0 mg/kg naloxone given simultaneously. This confirms previous findings (Domino and Wilson, 1973). The stimulant effects of morphine, however, were still seen presumably because of naloxone's short half-life in the body (Martin, 1967). When given just prior to the stimulant phase of morphine's actions, naloxone antagonized the enhanced ACh utilization. There was still a significant locomotor stimulant component. This may be due to the handling of the rats at 2 hr into the activity session and then returning them to the cages. The level of activity at 3 hr in the naloxone treated rats is about the same as the level of initial exploratory activity in control animals.

There seemed to be some correlation between morphine's effects on locomotor activity and ACh utilization. In general, if motor activity was enhanced, ACh utilization was enhanced and vice versa. Tolerance development also seemed to be related between the two endpoints. The correlation was not complete, however. The intermediate and large doses of morphine show differences in locomotor activity and ACh utilization, even though the trends are similar. Since a similar correlation between locomotor activity and catecholamines in the brain after narcotics was resolved using benzomorphans, we decided to use the same compounds. Smith and Sheldon (1972) showed no enhanced locomotor activity with UM 747, but increased incorporation of ^{14}C tyrosine into ^{14}C norepinephrine, and the opposite with cyclazocine. The present research with the benzomorphans also dissociated the locomotor effects of morphine from its action on brain ACh. Increases in locomotor activity after UM 747 and cyclazocine were observed but no changes in ACh utilization were noted. This dissociation was opposite to that found in the mouse since UM 747 was a motor stimulant in the rat with no significant effects on ACh unless larger depressant doses were used.

Our present report extends further the complex pharmacological actions of narcotics on the cholinergic system. An overly simple anti-release hypothesis of morphine action does not account for the biphasic effects of morphine which have been observed. It is important that future investigators take into account these biphasic effects when working with the narcotics. In addition, the stimulant effects of morphine on ACh add new dimensions to cholinergic involvement with morphine tolerance and physical dependence.

SUMMARY

Morphine has been shown to have biphasic effects on locomotor activity and ACh utilization in the rat. A dose of 1.0 mg/kg s.c. enhances locomotor activity and ACh utilization. A dose of 10 mg/kg causes an iniital depression and subsequent stimulation of both measures.

Tolerance develops to both the depressant and stimulant effects of morphine with a tenfold shift in the dose-effect curve to the right. Larger amounts of narcotic are required for tolerance to the stimulant actions.

Naloxone (1.0 mg/kg) antagonized both the depressant and stimulant effects of morphine in the rat.

Dissociation was observed between the locomotor activity and the effects on brain ACh especially with the benzomorphans. UM 747 and cyclazocine both increased locomotor activity with no change in brain ACh utilization. One half hr after 10 mg/kg of UM 747, when locomotor activity was depressed, brain ACh utilization was reduced.

ACKNOWLEDGMENTS

This study was supported in part by Grant DA–00830, USPHS. Michael Vasko was aided by Predoctoral Fellowship 5–PO1–GM–00198–16, USPHS.

REFERENCES

Akera, T., and T. B. Brodie. 1967. The addiction cycle to narcotics in the rat and its relation to catecholamines. *Biochem. Pharmacol.* 17: 675–688.

Babbini, M., and W. M. Davis. 1972. Time-dose relationships for locomotor activity effects of morphine after acute or repeated treatment. *Brit. J. Pharmacol.* 46: 213–224.

Buxbaum, D. M., G. G. Yarbrough, and M. E. Carter. 1973. Biogenic amines and narcotic effects. I. Modification of morphine-induced analgesia and motor activity after alteration of cerebral amine levels. *J. Pharmacol. Exp. Ther.* 185: 317–327.

Cools, A. R., C. Broekkamp, and H. Janssen. 1974. On the relation of neostriated and linear nuclei to morphine-induced behavior in cats. *J. de Pharmacologie* 5: 20–35.

Domino, E. F. 1975. Role of central cholinergic mechanisms in the specific actions of narcotic agonists. In P. G. Waser, Ed. *Cholinergic Mechanisms.* Raven Press, New York, pp. 433–453.

Domino. E. F., M. E. Mohrman, A. E. Wilson, and V. B. Haarstad. 1973. Acetylsecohemicholinium-3, a new choline acetyltransferase inhibitor useful in neuropharmacological studies. *Neuropharmacology* 12: 549–561.

Domino, E. F., M. Vasko, and A. E. Wilson. 1976. Mixed depressant and
    stimulant actions of morphine and their relationship to brain acetyl-
    choline. *Minireview. Life Sci.* 18: 361–376.
Domino, E. F., and A. E. Wilson. 1972. Psychotropic drug influences on
    acetylcholine utilization. *Psychopharmacologia* (Berlin) 25: 291–298.
Domino, E. F., and A. E. Wilson. 1973. Effects of narcotic analgesic agonists
    and antagonists on rat brain acetylcholine. *J. Pharmacol. Exp. Ther.*
    184: 18–32.
Jhamandas, K., and M. Sutak. 1974. Modification of brain acetylcholine re-
    lease by morphine and its antagonists in normal and morphine-dependent
    rats. *Brit. J. Pharmacol.* 50: 57–62.
Krueger, H., N. B. Eddy, and M. Sumwalt. 1941. *The pharmacology of the
    opium alkaloids.* Suppl. 165, Public Health Reports, U. S. Govt. Printing
    Office, Washington, D.C.
Kuschinsky, K. 1974. Are cholinergic mechanisms involved in morphine ef-
    fects on motility? *Naunyn-Schmiedeberg's Arch. Pharmakol.* 281: 167–173.
Labrecque, G., and E. F. Domino. 1974. Neocortical acetylcholine antirelease
    of various narcotic agonists and antagonists. *J. Pharmacol. Exp. Ther.* 191:
    189–200.
Matthews, J. D., G. Labrecque, and E. F. Domino. 1973. Effects of morphine,
    nalorphine and naloxone on neocortical release of acetylcholine in the
    rat. *Psychopharmacologia* (Berlin) 25: 113–120.
Martin, W. R. 1967. Opioid antagonists. *Pharmacol. Rev.* 19: 463–521.
Martin, W. R., A. Wikler, C. G. Eades, and F. T. Pescor. 1963. Tolerance to
    and physical dependence on morphine in rats. *Psychopharmacologia*
    (Berlin) 4: 247–260.
Mullin, W. J. 1974. Central release of acetylcholine following administration
    of morphine to unanesthetized rabbits. *Canad. J. Physiol. Pharmacol.* 52:
    369–374.
Mullin, W. J., J. W. Phillis, and C. Pinsky. 1973. Morphine enhancement of
    acetylcholine release from the brain in unanesthetized cats. *Europ. J.
    Pharmacol.* 22: 117–119.
Rethy, C. R., C. B. Smith, and J. E. Villarreal. 1971. Effects of narcotic
    analgesics upon the locomotor activity and brain catecholamine content
    of the mouse. *J. Pharmacol. Exp. Ther.* 176: 472–479.
Smith, C. B., 1972. Neurotransmitter and narcotic analgesics. In S. J. Mulé,
    and H. Brill, Eds. *Chemical and Biological Aspects of Drugs of De-
    pendence.* The Chemical Rubber Company, Cleveland, pp. 495–504.
Smith, C. B., and M. I. Sheldon. 1972. Effects of narcotic analgesic drugs
    on brain noradrenergic mechanisms. In H. W. Kosterlitz, J. E. Villarreal,
    and H. O. J. Collier, Eds. *The Pharmacology of Morphine Agonists and
    Antagonists.* McMillan Co., London. 164–175.
Szilagyi, P. I. A., J. P. Green, O. M. Brown, and S. Margolis. 1972. The
    measurement of nanogram amounts of acetylcholine in tissues by pyroly-

sis gas chromatography. *J. Neurochem.* 19: 2555–2566.

Vasko, M. R., and E. F. Domino. 1974. Biphasic effects of morphine on locomotor activity and ACh utilization in non-tolerant and tolerant rats. *Pharmacologist* 16: 204.

Weinstock, M. 1971. Acetylcholine and cholinesterase. In D. H. Clouet, Ed. *Narcotic Drugs, Biochemical Pharmacology.* Plenum Press, New York, pp. 254–260.

Tissue Responses to Addictive Drugs
© 1976, Spectrum Publications, Inc.

Assessment of the Role of Acetylcholine in Morphine Analgesia, Tolerance and Physical Dependence

E. LEONG WAY
HEMENDRA N. BHARGAVA

Department of Pharmacology
School of Medicine
University of California
San Francisco, California

and

Department of Pharmacognosy and Pharmacology
College of Pharmacy
University of Illinois at the Medical Center
Chicago, Illinois

There is considerable evidence suggesting that acetylcholine may be involved in some of the acute effects of morphine and in the expression of certain withdrawal signs. However, the findings are not always in agreement and the conflicting conclusions of various investigators have been cited in earlier publications from this laboratory (Bhargava and Way, 1975b) as well as by others (Frederickson and Pinsky, 1975). The sum of our own work indicates that although some of the acute actions of morphine and certain manifestations of abstinence might be mediated in part by acetylcholine, an alteration in cholinergic activity does not appear to influence materially the process by which the morphine tolerant-dependent state develops. These conclusions are based largely on studies assessing the analgetic response to morphine in the nontolerant and tolerant states and certain withdrawal signs in the physical dependent state after using various cholinergic agonists and antagonists to modify acetylcholine levels or actions in the central nervous system. These findings are summarized below.

ASSESSMENT OF NARCOTIC TOLERANCE AND PHYSICAL DEPENDENCE

The quantitative assessment of narcotic tolerance and physical dependence poses problems because in any given animal species, each syndrome is represented by a constellation of signs with different onset, duration and intensity. In the assessment procedure, therefore, some degree of arbitrariness needs to be imposed not only in selecting the number of signs that are to be included but also in ranking the relative importance of each sign. Practicalities limit the number of signs of tolerance and dependence that can be used for making measurements. To obtain a quantitative index of the degree of tolerance and dependence development we select a representative sign of each syndrome that is sensitive, reproducible, and can be easily measured. In using only one sign for assessing tolerance dependence, consideration must always be given to the possibility that any experimental manipulation of the tolerant-dependent state might selectively affect only the particular nervous pathway or biochemical process being measured and not the total syndrome. Any affirmative findings, therefore, need to be validated by assessing other parameters quantitatively as well as by subjective evaluation of the total syndrome. In evaluating maneuvers that might affect physical dependence development in particular, it is important to distinguish between masking and suppressing the state. An adequate dose of an agent which suppresses abstinence should inhibit all the withdrawal signs and if this be the case, then measurement of any one sign that is easily reproducible should provide an accurate indication of the degree of dependence. However, when attempts are made to apply pharmacologic manipulations to modify dependence, one must be aware that the particular sign being measured might be altered rather than the withdrawal state. This should hold true irrespective of whether one or many signs are assessed. In the latter case, a point scoring system is often used and in instances when several signs might be masked and a lower total abstinence score results, this could be misinterpreted to be inhibition of dependence development. Furthermore, since the number and kinds of withdrawal signs may vary with varying degrees of dependence (Bläsig et al., 1973) it is important also to standardize the procedures for establishing a reproducible dependent state.

In our laboratory we use the mouse and rat as models and the details appear in two published papers (Way et al., 1968; Wei et al., 1972). The rodent model appears to have validity since the classic effects of morphine such as analgesia (antinociception), tolerance and physical dependence can easily be demonstrated in both species. Our studies have been greatly facilitated by the subcutaneous morphine pellet-implantation procedure first reported by Huidobro and Maggiolo (1961). By using a modified pellet, however, we have been able to produce a much greater degree of tolerance and physical dependence within a very brief period (Way et al., 1968). It is possible to detect tolerance and dependence development within a few hours and the effect usually is maximal after three days. To produce a more protracted state of tolerance a second pellet can be implanted.

Tolerance to morphine is measured by noting the increase in the amount of the drug to produce analgesia. The classic tail-flick procedure is used to determine the median analgetic dose of morphine (AD_{50}).

Physical dependence on morphine can be assessed after abrupt withdrawal by removing the pellet or by precipitating withdrawal with the narcotic antagonist, naloxone. The withdrawal signs after abrupt withdrawal in both the mouse and rat are similar to those after precipitated withdrawal. However, they are much slower in onset, of lesser intensity and persist longer. In the mouse, the most characteristic signs of precipitated withdrawal is stereotyped jumping. The degree of dependence on morphine can be quantified with or without removal of the pellet by estimating the amount of naloxone (ED_{50}) needed to precipitate the response. An inverse relationship exists between the two parameters; the higher the degree of dependence, the lower the naloxone ED_{50}. In the rat, escape attempts and wet shakes are especially characteristic and can be used as the endpoint for estimating the naloxone ED_{50} (Wei et al., 1973a). A convenient procedure to assess the degree of dependence after abrupt withdrawal is to follow the body weight after pellet removal. Dependent animals lose considerable weight during abstinence (Hosoya, 1959; Shuster et al., 1963).

ROLE OF ACETYLCHOLINE IN MORPHINE ANALGESIA

Maneuvers to elevate and lower acetylcholine levels in the brain tended to produce modest effects on morphine antinociception as measured by the tail-flick procedure. Moreover, the alterations produced were not always consistent with respect to the changes induced in cholinergic function. Elevation of brain acetylcholine by choline-esterase inhibition with either physostigmine or diisopropyl-fluoro-phosphate (DFP) results in a modest enhancement of analgetic activity as evidenced by a 30-50% decrease in the morphine AD_{50} by the tail-flick method (Bhargava and Way, 1972). Although reducing cholinergic activity by decreasing acetylcholine synthesis with hemicholinium (HC-3) effected a slight decrease in morphine analgesia (Bhargava et al., 1974) blockade with atropine or scopolamine increased slightly morphine analgesia (Bhargava and Way, 1975a). When mice were rendered tolerant to morphine by pellet implantation, similar but perhaps slightly greater changes were obtained with the cholinergic agonist and antagonists. Occasionally a more pronounced response was obtained with tolerant animals but the effects were not particularly striking.

Thirty minutes after a single subcutaneous dose of morphine sulfate (40 mg/kg) in mice, a significant increase in the cerebral content of ACh was observed but does of 10 and 20 mg/kg were ineffective in this respect (Bhargava and Way, 1975b). These findings are consistent with those of Hano et al. (1954). Choline levels were not significantly affected by any of the three doses of morphine. In the rat morphine sulfate at a dose of 40 mg/kg did not alter the steady-state levels of ACh or choline in the brain. Giarman and Pepeu (1962), and Domino and Wilson (1973) reported that doses greater than 32 mg/kg (morphine base) are required to raise the cerebral ACh level. Since in our laboratory the s.c. tail-flick AD_{50} of morphine in mice and rats is usually about 8 mg/kg and ranges between 2.5 and 15 mg/kg, it is apparent that the doses of morphine needed to elevate total brain ACh are much higher than those necessary to produce significant analgesia.

The above studies indicate that it is possible to produce analgesia without necessarily altering the whole brain ACh content and that a dose of morphine much higher than that needed to produce analgesia is required to increase brain ACh significantly. The data are consistent with those of Howes et al. (1969) who found no correlation between the tail-flick analgesia and the brain levels of ACh in mice. These authors also found that the cholinomimetic, oxotremorine, raised the brain ACh levels and inhibited the tail-flick response in mice; however, naloxone also raised the brain ACh content without having any effect on the tail-flick reflex. Similarly in the rat, a dose of morphine sulfate as high as 40 mg/kg had no effect on the ACh contents of rat brain. This finding is in accordance with those of Giarman and Pepeu (1962) and Domino and Wilson (1973). Thus, unless highly localized changes occur in specific brain regions, it would appear that brain ACh does not play a prominent role in morphine antinociception, and any role that it may assume during morphine analgesia is secondary.

Our results also suggest that the processes involved in the augmentation of morphine analgesia after cholinesterase inhibition are still functional to the same degree in animals rendered tolerant to morphine. Despite the fact that there was a several fold elevation of the morphine AD_{50} after pellet implantation, administration of either physostigmine or DFP to the tolerant animals resulted in a relative lowering of the morphine AD_{50} to about the same degree as that in nontolerant mice. However, although the tolerant state was modified, development of the process was not. The studies leading to these conclusions will be described towards the end of this presentation.

ROLE OF ACETYLCHOLINE IN PHYSICAL DEPENDENCE

Cholinergic mechanisms appear to be involved in morphine abstinence but their precise role is not clear. Several studies have shown that morphine impairs the release of ACh in the brain (Beleslin and Polak, 1965; Sharkawi and Shulman, 1969; Jhamandas et al., 1970). The latter group suggested that the morphine withdrawal syndrome may be related to the release of ACh from the central cholinergic nerve terminals and further that the abstinence could be modified by drugs affecting the cholinergic system (Jhamandas and Dickinson, 1973). A role for ACh in withdrawal was suggested by several investigators (Paton, 1957; Collier, 1968; Pinsky et al., 1973) who proposed that excessive release of ACh from the brain occurred after abrupt discontinuance of morphine or after precipitation of abstinence with a narcotic antagonist. The lowered ACh occurring upon abrupt withdrawal after repeated long administration of morphine (Domino and Wilson, 1973) is compatible with such a hypothesis. Additionally, there are at least three studies which can be cited indicating that brain ACh utilization is enhanced by morphine withdrawal in rats made dependent on morphine by injection for many weeks (Large and Milton, 1970; Large, 1972; Domino and Wilson, 1973). In the cat, however, the situation may be more complex during naloxone precipitated withdrawal. An initial inhibition of ACh release and a subsequent return to control release levels with a possible enhanced release was observed (Labrecque and Domino, 1974). Also, attempts at modifying withdrawal with cholinergic and anticholinergic drugs have not always produced results consistent with the hypothesis that acetylcholine may be involved with withdrawal. To delve into this matter further, we have made measurements on brain acetylcholine during abrupt and antagonist withdrawal and have assessed the possible effects of cholinergic agonists and antagonists on naloxone precipitated withdrawal jumping. In general our studies support that ACh is involved in the expression of abstinence but not all our findings are in agreement with the reported literature.

BRAIN ACh LEVELS AFTER ABRUPT MORPHINE WITHDRAWAL

The experiments yielded data that was difficult to interpret. In mice rendered dependent on morphine by pellet implantation, abrupt withdrawal, induced by removal of the pellet, resulted in an elevation of brain ACh after 6 hours but after 12 and 24 hours the ACh levels had returned to normal. Brain Ch levels were not altered significantly at any of the time intervals. In rats implanted with 2 morphine pellets and withdrawn from morphine for 6 hours or with 4 morphine pellets and withdrawn from morphine for 18 hours, brain ACh of Ch levels were not materially affected (Bhargava and Way, 1975b). The increase in the ACh seen after abrupt withdrawal in mice is in agreement with the finding in the rat that an increase occurs 7 hours after discontinuance of morphine in dependent rats maintained on twice daily injections of morphine for 6 to 10 weeks. (Large and Milton, 1970; and Large, 1972). However, we failed to find a difference in the brain ACh levels between morphine and placebo withdrawn mice at 12 and 24 hours after pellet removal nor in dependent rats after 6 or 18 hours. On the other hand, Domino and Wilson (1973) reported a decrease in brain ACh after 48 hours in rats made morphine dependent by daily multiple injections. Thus, it appears that total brain level of ACh does not provide an accurate index for making meaningful conclusions and more detailed studies on regional ACh turnover are in order.

BRAIN LEVELS OF ACh and Ch DURING NALOXONE-PRECIPITATED WITHDRAWAL

Naloxone caused a rapid and significant decrease in brain ACh in mice rendered dependent on morphine by pellet implantation (Bhargava and Way, 1975b). Brain acetylcholine was lowered 21–33% during peak withdrawal ($\sim$ 5 minutes) while choline levels were unaltered (see Table I). Also, in morphine dependent rats implanted with 4 morphine pellets for 3 days naloxone effected a significant decrease (18%) in brain ACh levels 10 minutes after an injection of an ED_{50} dose of

Table I. Brain ACh and Ch Levels in Morphine Dependent Nonjumping and Jumping Mice and Rats following Naloxone Challenge

Treatment	No. Responding No. Tested	$\mu g/g \pm$ S.E. (N = 4)	
		ACh	Ch
Mice			
Saline	Non-jumping 0/10	3.95 ± 0.22	5.84 ± 0.50
Naloxone 0.025 mg/kg	Non-jumping 6/12	3.65 ± 0.18	5.50 ± 0.49
	Jumping 6/12	3.11 ± 0.07*	5.60 ± 0.50
Naloxone 0.05 mg/kg	Jumping 11/12	2.54 ± 0.05[†]	4.77 ± 0.11
Rats			
Saline	Non-jumping 0/10	2.31 ± 0.06	4.49 ± 0.29
Naloxone 20 mg/kg	Non-jumping 6/10	2.10 ± 0.09	4.43 ± 0.19
	Jumping 4/10	1.55 ± 0.18[†]	3.91 ± 0.45

Mice were rendered dependent by a s.c. implantation of a morphine pellet for 72 hours and rats by implantation of 4 pellets for 72 hours. Six hours after pellet removal, saline or naloxone, s.c., was injected to precipitate jumping and animals were separated into jumpers and nonjumpers over a 10 minute observation period. Four animals from each group were selected at random and were sacrificed for the analysis of brain ACh and Ch.

*$p < 0.05$; [†]$p < 0.001$ vs nonjumpers receiving either saline or naloxone.
(From Bhargava and Way 1975b)

naloxone. Choline levels again remained unchanged. On comparing brain ACh levels in the jumping and nonjumping animals after an ED_{50} dose of naloxone, brain ACh was found to decrease in the jumpers but not in the nonjumpers. This decrease in brain ACh in jumping mice was dependent on the dose of naloxone injected. Doubling the naloxone ED_{50} caused a decrease in brain ACh greater than 40%. On the other hand, there was no difference in the specific activity of brain AChE in jumping and nonjumping mice after naloxone or saline. A similar response was noted in the morphine-dependent rat. The rats that jumped after naloxone administration had over 30% lower brain ACh levels.

The above results indicate that naloxone-precipitated withdrawal jumping in morphine dependent mice and rats can be correlated with a decrease in brain levels of ACh. This decrease in ACh was dependent on the dose of naloxone and occurred only in mice and rats that jumped after a naloxone challenge, but not in those that failed to jump. Consistent with these findings Jhamandas and Sutak (1974) reported that antagonists produced an increase in release of brain ACh in the dependent rat and the time course corresponded closely with that of the abstinence syndrome. On the other hand Cheney and Hanin (1973) did not note a decrease in brain ACh after naloxone administration to morphine dependent mice, but their observation time was at 15 minutes. Likewise, Domino and Wilson (1975) reported negative data 30 minutes after naloxone. In our experiments we found 5 minutes to be the peak time for the jumping response in mice. The decrease in brain ACh in morphine dependent jumping mice after a naloxone challenge was not related to the specific activity of brain AChE. Since the decrease in ACh was not related to an increased rate of hydrolysis, this suggests that the release of ACh from the central neurons may be enhanced during naloxone-precipitated withdrawal jumping.

Previous studies from our laboratory also support a role for ACh in naloxone precipitated withdrawal jumping. We noted that elevation of brain ACh by cholinesterase inhibition with physostigmine or DFP greatly inhibited naloxone-precipitated withdrawal jumping. (Bhargava and Way, 1972; Iwamoto et al., 1973; Brase et al., 1974). Our data with the compound 1-phenyl-3-(2-thiazolyl)-2-thiourea (PTT) are also compatible with these findings. Although PTT has been reported to be a dopamine-β-hydroxylase inhibitor (Johnson et al., 1969), we found that independent of this action, PTT also elevated brain ACh and markedly inhibited naloxone-precipitated withdrawal jumping (Bhargava and Way, 1974). Conversely, when hemicholinium-3 was injected intracerebrally to inhibit brain ACh synthesis, naloxone-precipitated withdrawal jumping was enhanced. A dose of hemicholinium-3 which reduced brain ACh by 40% reduced the naloxone ED_{50} in the morphine-dependent mouse by 50% (Bhargava et al., 1974). We now also find that the inhibitory effect of physostigmine on jumping can be largely reversed by the anticholinergics, atropine or scopolamine and the elevation in brain ACh effected by physostigmine was also blocked (Bhargava and Way, 1975a).

CHOLINERGIC AND ANTICHOLINERGIC DRUGS ON PRECIPITATED WITHDRAWAL

Cholinergic agonists, such as the cholinesterase inhibitors eserine and diisopropylfluorophosphate (DFP) inhibited naloxone-induced jumping markedly, as evidenced by a naloxone ED_{50} 30- to 35-fold higher than that of saline controls (Bhargava and Way, 1972; Iwamoto et al., 1973; Brase et al., 1974). The centrally acting cholinergic oxotremorine was also highly effective, increasing the naloxone ED_{50} by more than 100-fold (Brase et al., 1974; Bhargava and Way, 1975a) (see Table II). On the other hand, echothiophate, a quarternary organic phosphate acetylcholinesterase inhibitor which penetrates the brain with difficulty, did not alter the naloxone jumping response (Brase et al., 1974; Bhargava and Way, 1975a).

The cholinergic antagonists elicited both an inhibition and an enhancement of naloxone precipitated withdrawal jumping and the response exhibited was time dependent. An inhibition of naloxone precipitated withdrawal jumping occurred when the anticholinergics were administered 30 minutes prior to naloxone challenge. Both atropine and scopolamine under these conditions elevated significantly the naloxone ED_{50}. However, the degree of inhibition noted was much less than that observed with the cholinergic agonists, and despite the fact that atropine and scopolamine inhibited withdrawal jumping, both compounds markedly reduced the inhibitory effects of physostigmine on withdrawal jumping. Although atropine and scopolamine each increased the naloxone ED_{50} 3- to 4-fold, the more than 30-fold increase in the naloxone ED_{50} effected by physostigmine was only about 3-fold after atropine or scopolamine pretreatment (Bhargava and Way, 1975a) (see Table II). In contrast, when atropine was given 10 minutes before challenge with naloxone, slight enhancement of withdrawal jumping was observed (Brase et al., 1974; Bhargava and Way, 1975a).

The effects elicited by the cholinergic antagonists on precipitated withdrawal are conflicting in the relevant literature. Our data indicate that atropine has a biphasic effect on the response and both an enhancement and an inhibition of naloxone precipitated withdrawal jumping can occur. The critical factor in whether a stimulatory or inhibiting response is to be elicited by atropine appear to be the time of atropine administration and the level of brain ACh. When the challenge with naloxone is initiated 10 minutes after atropine, the usual response is an enhancement of the jumping (Brase et al., 1974; Bhargava and Way, 1975a) but, 30 minutes after its administration, the response to atropine is inhibitory (Collier et al., 1972; Jhamandas and Dickinson, 1973; Jhamandas et al., 1973; Bhargava and Way, 1975a) and after 2 hours the effects of atropine are not apparent (Iwamoto et al., 1973). During peak naloxone-precipitated-withdrawal jumping, a lowering of brain ACh occurs (Bhargava and Way, 1975b) and likewise during the time when atropine produces an enhancement of naloxone-precipitated-withdrawal jumping at 10 minutes brain ACh levels are also decreased

Table II. Effect of Cholinergic Agonist and Antagonists on Naloxone Precipitated Withdrawal Jumping in Morphine Dependent Mice

Experiment	Treatment	Dose mg/kg	Route	Naloxone ED$_{50}$(mg/kg)	Potency Ratio
A	Saline	—	—	1.25 (0.89- 1.75)	—
	Eserine	0.4	s.c.	43.00 (29.70-62.26)	34.40 (20.98-56.42)[†]
	Scopolamine	50	i.p.	3.90 (2.65- 5.74)	3.12 (1.88- 5.18)[†]
	S + E	50, 0.4	i.p., s.c.	3.30 (2.23- 4.88)	2.64 (1.57- 4.44)[†]
B	Saline	—	—	1.15 (0.76- 1.74)	—
	Eserine	0.4	s.c.	35.00 (25.34-48.34)	30.44 (18.12-51.14)[†]
	Atropine	50	i.p.	4.90 (3.31- 7.26)	4.26 (2.43- 7.46)[†]
	A + E	50, 0.4	i.p., s.c.	4.45 (3.02- 6.56)	3.87 (2.21- 6.77)[†]
	Oxotremorine	0.2	i.p.	120.00 (81.69-176.28)	104.35 (59.63-182.61)[†]

*Drugs were administered 30 minutes before naloxone. In combination experiments, atropine (A) or scopolamine (S) was administered just prior to eserine (E) injection. Numbers in parentheses indicate 95% confidence limits.
[†]Significantly different controls at the 5% level or less.
(From Bhargava and Way, 1975a)

However, when at 30 minutes the potentiating action of atropine is absent, brain ACh levels are at normal levels. Several laboratories have reported previously on the biphasic effects of atropine during withdrawal (Frederickson and Pinsky, 1971; Collier et al., 1972; Pinsky et al., 1973).

In addition to ACh, dopamine also appears to be important for the manifestation of jumping in the morphine-dependent animal. Maruyama and Takemori (1973) suggested that the full expression of morphine-abstinence syndrome in morphine-dependent mice appears to require the integrity of the central stores of norepinephrine and dopamine, especially the later. It was found in studies from this laboratory that in mice rendered dependent on morphine by pellet implantation, naloxone-precipitated-withdrawal jumping was accompanied by a sudden elevation of dopamine. On the other hand, brain levels of norepinephrine and serotonin were not altered by naloxone at any of the test times. The increase in dopamine was noted to occur within 2 minutes and to reach a maximum between 5 and 10 minutes when the incidence of jumping was at its peak. The increase in dopamine was found in dependent mice that jumped after a naloxone challenge but not in those that failed to jump. The response was not caused by the act of jumping, since in dependent mice given tubocurarine to prevent jumping, naloxone still elicited a sudden rise in brain dopamine. The increase in brain dopamine occurred primarily in the corpus striatum and hardly at all in the other brain areas (Iwamoto et al., 1973). Elevation of brain ACh by cholinesterase inhibition in the morphine-dependent mouse, blocked not only naloxone-precipitated-withdrawal jumping but also the sudden elevation of brain dopamine which occurred (Iwamoto et al., 1973). Thus, both cholinergic and dopaminergic neurons participate in the manifestation of morphine withdrawal, and indeed, the two substances appear to be interrelated. The findings are compatible with the well-established relationship between cholinergic and dopaminergic function in the extrapyramidal system in which both cholinergic antagonists and dopaminergic agonists have been used to treat parkinsonism. Studies on the brain sites of morphine for initiating antagonist-precipitated withdrawal, however, indicate that the sensitive sites reside in the medial mesodiencephalic area, rather than in the extrapyramidal system (Wei et al., 1973b; Herz et al., 1972). Although the relationships of these sites to dopaminergic activity has not been clearly defined, it is of interest to note that high levels of acetylcholinesterase and cholinesterase have been found in medial thalamic nuclei (Shute and Lewis, 1967; Oliver et al., 1970), and, behaviorally, stimulation of medial thalamic and hypothalamic regions in the brain elicits avoidance behavior. (Olds and Olds, 1963; Kaelber and Mitchell, 1967; Stein, 1968).

However, it should not be excluded that morphine may act more directly on another endogenous substance which could influence cholinergic-dopaminergic relationships. While current evidence suggests that the initiating sites for some morphine effects are cholinergic, gabaminergic sites have not been eliminated from consideration. Also, the recent reports that a morphinelike factor exists in the central nervous system (Terenius and Wahlstrom, 1974) needs to be considered.

ROLE OF ACh IN TOLERANCE AND DEPENDENCE DEVELOPMENT

Although inhibitors of cholinesterase were found to enhance morphine antinociception and markedly suppress naloxone-precipitated-withdrawal jumping, these modifications in morphine action are achieved without necessarily affecting the processes which might be involved in the development of tolerance to and physical dependence on morphine. It appears that the target site(s) for tolerance and for dependence development are not those that are directly concerned with the immediate effector responses to morphine. Several experiments clearly established that acetylcholine could not play a major role in tolerance development. The administration of DFP prior to morphine pellet implantation resulted in a lowering of the morphine AD_{50} comparable to that obtained in mice that had been previously rendered maximally tolerant by implantation. The ratio of the morphine AD_{50} of tolerant over nontolerant animals receiving DFP was found to be nearly identical with the ratio in tolerant and nontolerant animals without DFP treatmet. This was interpreted to mean that cholinesterase inhibition does not affect the development of tolerance to morphine (Bhargava and Way, 1972). Additionally, pretreatment with HC-3 intracerebrally to lower brain acetylcholine prior to morphine pellet implantation did not affect the development of tolerance to morphine, although an elevation in the morphine AD_{50} was found, it was no more than that obtained in mice implanted with a placebo pellet. The negative finding was obtained with a near lethal dose of HC-3 which could not be repeated within 72 hours without causing a high mortality incidence (Bhargava et al., 1974).

Finally, daily administration of high doses of atropine had no effect on morphine tolerance development. An intraperitoneal dose of 100 mg/kg given before and repeated twice while the morphine pellet was implanted did not alter the analgetic response to morphine. Following morphine pellet implantation for 3 days the morphine AD_{50} increased from 3.9 to 44.0 mg/kg in the saline controls (11-fold tolerance), while in the atropine treated group, the AD_{50} for morphine increased from 4.8 to 48 mg/kg (10-fold tolerance).

There is considerable evidence also indicating that ACh is not primarily involved in the development of physical dependence on morphine. Pronounced inhibition of naloxone-precipitated withdrawal-jumping by cholinesterase inhibition was evidenced by a manyfold elevation of the naloxone ED_{50} after physostigmine or DFP treatment. Despite the striking response elicited, the treatment did not appear to have a significant effect on physical dependence development. Although the elevation in the naloxone ED_{50} was greater when DFP was injected before than after pellet implantation and this could be interpreted to mean that physical dependence development was inhibited by DFP, it failed to affect body weight loss after abrupt withdrawal. Had DFP produced a generalized inhibitory effect on morphine dependence development, it should have prevented, at least in part, the loss in weight which occurred upon pellet removal. In another experiment it was found that when physostigmine was injected repeatedly and its effects on naloxone-precipitated-withdrawal jumping were assessed after an interval of 24 hours, the results were negative. Decreased brain ACh by intracerebral administration of HC-3 also failed to alter physical dependence. Although naloxone-precipitated-withdrawal jumping was facilitated in morphine pellet implanted animals and enhanced by HC-3, the loss in body weight occurring after pellet removal was not altered. This, again supports the supposition that ACh is involved in the expression of abstinence jumping but not in the development of dependence (Bhargava et al., 1974).

Finally, high doses of atropine (100 mg/kg i.p. daily for 3 days) failed to alter dependence development. The naloxone ED_{50} for precipitated withdrawal jumping after morphine pellet implantation in the treated animals was identical to that of the saline controls.

SUMMARY AND CONCLUSION

The results indicate that alteration in brain ACh levels by pharmacologic manipulation influences morphine effects in different manners. Only modest effects were obtained on morphine analgesia as assessed by the tail-flick procedure: elevating brain ACh enhancing, and lowering brain ACh decreasing morphine analgesia. On the other hand, marked changes in naloxone-precipitated-withdrawal jumping was observed by manipulating brain ACh. Increasing brain ACh produced pronounced inhibition of the response and the reverse was noted upon decreasing brain ACh. Despite the occurrence of these acute changes, none of the maneuvers appear to affect the development of either tolerance or physical dependence. Thus, it would seem that the receptors concerned with mediating central acetylcholine responses of morphine are not the ones primarily concerned with the genesis of tolerance and physical dependence even though they might be indirectly involved.

ACKNOWLEDGMENT

This work was supported by Grants from The National Institute of Drug Abuse (DA–00037) and The Graduate College of the University of Illinois at the Medical Center, Chicago, Illinois.

REFERENCES

Beleslin, D., and L. Polak. 1965. Depression by morphine and chloralose of acetylcholine release from the cat's brain. *J. Physiol.* (London) 177: 411–419.

Bhargava, H. N., S. L. Chan, and E. L. Way. 1974. Influence of hemicholinium-3 on morphine tolerance and physical dependence and on brain acetylcholine. *Europ. J. Pharmacol.* 29: 253–261.

Bhargava, H. N., and E. L. Way. 1972. Acetylcholinesterase inhibition and morphine effects in morphine tolerant and dependent mice. *J. Pharmacol. Exp. Ther.* 183: 31–40.

Bhargava, H. N., and E. L. Way. 1974. Effect of 1-phenyl-3-(2-thiazolyl)-2-thiourea (PTT), a dopamine β-hydroxylase (DBH) inhibitor, on morphine analgesia, tolerance and physical dependence. *J. Pharmacol. Exp. Ther.* 190: 165-175.

Bhargava, H. N., and E. L. Way. 1975a. Morphine tolerance and physical dependence: Influence of cholinergic agonists and antagonists. *Europ. J. Pharmacol.* (In press)

Bhargava, H. N., and E. L. Way. 1975b. Brain acetylcholine and choline following acute and chronic morphinization and during withdrawal. *J. Pharmacol. Exp. Ther.* 195: 65–73.

Bläsig, J., H. Herz, K. Reinhold, and S. Zieglgänsberger. 1973. Development of physical dependence on morphine in respect to time and dosage and quantification of the precipitated withdrawal syndrome in rats. *Psychopharmacologia* (Berlin) 33: 19–38.

Brase, D. A., L. F. Tseng, H. H. Loh, and E. L. Way. 1974. Cholinergic modification of naloxone induced jumping in mice. *Europ. J. Pharmacol.* 26: 1–8.

Cheney, D. L., and I. Hanin. 1973. Effect of acute and chronic morphine on specific radioactivity of choline and acetylcholine in mouse brain. *Fed. Proc.* 32: 757.

Collier, H. O. J. 1968. Supersensitivity and dependence. *Nature* (London) 220: 228–231.

Collier, H. O. J., D. L. Francis, and C. Schneider. 1972. Modification of morphine withdrawal by drugs interacting with humoral mechanisms: some contradictions and their interpretation. *Nature* (London) 237: 220–223.

Domino, E. F., and A. Wilson. 1973. Effect of narcotic analgesic agonists and antagonists on rat brain acetylcholine. *J. Pharmacol. Exp. Ther.* 184: 18–32.

Domino, E. F., and A. E. Wilson. 1975. Brain acetylcholine in morphine pellet implanted rats given naloxone. *Psychopharmacologia* 41: 19–22.

Frederickson, R. C. A., and C. Pinsky. 1971. Morphine impairs acetylcholine release but facilitates acetylcholine actions at a skeletal neuromuscular junction. *Nature New Biol.* 231: 93–94.

Frederickson, R. C. A., and C. Pinsky. 1975. Effects of cholinergic and anticholinergic drugs and a partial cholinergic agonist on the development and expression of physical dependence on morphine in rats. *J. Pharmacol. Exp. Ther.* 193: 44–55.

Giarman, N. J., and G. Pepeu. 1962. Drug-induced changes in brain aceytlcholine. *Brit. J. Pharmacol.* 19: 226–234.

Hano, K., H. Kaneto, T. Kakunaga, and N. Moribayashi. 1964. Pharmacological studies of analgesics. VI: The administration of morphine and changes in acetylcholine metabolism in mouse brain. *Biochem. Pharmacol.* 10: 441–447.

Herz, A., Hj. Teschemacher, K. Albus, and S. Zieglgänsberger. 1972. Morphine abstinence syndrome in rabbits precipitated by injection of morphine antagonists into the ventricular system and restricted parts of it. *Psychopharmacologia* (Berlin) 26: 219–235.

Hosoya, E. 1959. Some withdrawal symptoms of rats to morphine. *Pharmacologist* 1: 77.

Howes, J. F., L. S. Harris, W. L. Dewey, and C. A. Voyda. 1969. Brain acetylcholine levels and inhibition of the tail-flick reflex in mice. *J. Pharmacol. Exp. Ther.* 169: 23–28.

Huidobro, F., and C. Maggiolo. 1961. Some features of the abstinence syndrome to morphine in mice. *Acta. Physiol. Lat. Am.* 18: 201–209.

Iwamoto, E. T., I. K. Ho, and E. L. Way. 1973. Elevation of brain dopamine during naloxone-precipitated withdrawal in morphine-dependent mice and rats. *J. Pharmacol. Exp. Ther.* 187: 558–567.

Jhamandas, K., and G. Dickinson. 1973. Modification of precipitated morphine and methadone abstinence in mice by acetylcholine antagonists. *Nature New Biol.* 245: 219–221.

Jhamandas, K., C. Pinsky, and J. W. Phillis. 1970. Effect of morphine and its antagonists on release of cerebral cortical acetylcholine. *Nature* (London) 228: 176–177.

Jhamandas, K., M. Sutak, and S. Bell. 1973. Modification of precipitated morphine withdrawal syndrome by drugs affecting cholinergic mechanisms. *Europ. J. Pharmacol.* 24: 296–305.

Jhamandas, K., and M. Sutak. 1974. Modification of brain acetylcholine release by morphine and its antagonists in normal and morphine-dependent rats. *Brit. J. Pharmacol.* 50: 57–62.

Johnson, G. A., S. J. Boukma, and E. G. Kim. 1969. Inhibition of dopamine β-hydroxylase by aromatic and alkyl-thioureas. *J. Pharmacol. Exp. Ther.* 168: 229–234.

Kaelber, W. W., and C. L. Mitchell. 1967. The centrum medianum-central tegmental fasciculus complex. A stimulation, lesion and degeneration study in the cat. *Brain* 90: 83–100.

Labrecque, G., and E. F. Domino. 1974. Tolerance to and physical dependence on morphine: Relation to neocortical acetylcholine release in the cat. *J. Pharmacol. Exp. Ther.* 191: 189–200.

Large, W. A., and A. S. Milton. 1970. The effect of acute and chronic morphine antagonists on central and peripheral cholinergic systems. Doctoral dissertation, University of London.

Large, W. A., and A. S. Milton. 1970. The effect of acute and chronic morphine administration on brain acetylcholine levels in the rat. *Brit. J. Pharmacol.* 38: 451P–452P.

Maruyama, Y., and A. E. Takemori. 1973. The role of dopamine and norepinephrine in the naloxone-induced abstinence of morphine-dependent mice. *J. Pharmacol. Exp. Ther.* 185: 602–608.

Olds, M. E., and J. Olds. 1963. Approach avoidance analysis of rat diencephalon. *J. Comp. Neurol.* 120: 259–295.

Olivier, A., A. Parent, and L. J. Poirier. 1970. Identification of the thalamic nuclei on the basis of their cholinesterase content in the monkey. *J. Anat.* 106: 37–50.

Paton, W. D. M. 1957. The action of morphine and related substances on contraction and on acetylcholine output of coaxially stimulated guinea pig ileum. *Brit. J. Pharmacol.* 12: 119–127.

Pinsky, C., R. C. Frederickson, and A. J. Vazquez. 1973. Morphine withdrawal syndrome responses to cholinergic antagonists and to a partial cholinergic agonist. *Nature* 242: 59–61.

Sharkawi, M., and M. P. Shulman. 1969. Inhibition by morphine of the release of ^{14}C-acetylcholine from the rat brain cortex slices. *J. Pharm. Pharmacol.* 21: 546–547.

Shuster, L., R. V. Hannam, and W. E. Boyle, Jr. 1963. A simple method for producing tolerance to dihydromorphinone in mice. *J. Pharmacol. Exp. Ther.* 140: 149–154.

Shute, C. C. D., and P. R. Lewis. 1967. The ascending cholinergic reticular system: Neocortical, olfactory and subcortical projections. *Brain* 90: 497–519.

Stein, L. 1968. Chemistry of reward and punishment. In D. H. Ephron, Ed. *Psychopharmacology, A Review of Progress 1957–1967*. Public Health Publication No. 1836, Washington, D. C., pp. 105–124.

Terenius, L., and A. Wahlstrom. 1974. Inhibitor(s) of narcotic receptor-binding in brain extracts and cerebrospinal-fluid. *Acta Pharmacol Toxicol.* 35: 35.

Wei, E. T., H. H. Loh, and F. H. Shen. 1968. Morphine tolerance, physical dependence and synthesis of brain 5-hydroxy-tryptamine. *Science* 162: 1290–1292.

Wei, E. T., H. H. Loh, and E. L. Way. 1972. Neuroanatomical correlates of morphine dependence. *Science* 177: 616–617.

Wei, E. T., H. H. Loh, and E. L. Way. 1973a. Quantitative aspects of precipitated abstinence in morphine-dependent rats. *J. Pharmacol. Exp. Ther.* 184: 398–403.

Wei, E. T., H. H. Loh, and E. L. Way. 1973b. Brain sites of precipitated abstinence in morphine-dependent rats. *J. Pharmacol. Exp. Ther.* 185: 108–115.

Tissue Responses to Addictive Drugs
© 1976, Spectrum Publications, Inc.

Antinociceptive Activity of Acetylcholine and its Involvement in the Actions of Morphine and Other Analgesics

WILLIAM L. DEWEY
NORMAN PEDIGO
MICHAEL KARBOWSKI
JAMES FORBES
LOUIS S. HARRIS

Department of Pharmacology
Medical College of Virginia
Richmond, Virginia

It has been hypothesized, with considerable supporting data, that most drugs, including narcotic analgesics, produce their effect on the central nervous system by either a direct or indirect action on one or another of the neurotransmitters. The data supporting acetylcholine as a neurotransmitter in the central nervous system is impressive. It is logical, therefore, to investigate the involvement of morphine as a prototype narcotic on brain cholinergic mechanisms.

Many papers have appeared which describe the effect of narcotics on one or another neurotransmitter system in the brain. Harris (1970) has pointed out that the effect of the narcotic might be due to an alteration in the balance of neurotransmitters rather than an effect on a particular biogenic amine. We have previously reviewed the role of brain cholinergic systems in the actions of narcotics and their antagonists (Harris and Dewey, 1972). We will restrict the majority of our remarks in this chapter to those studies which have been published since 1972 and will concentrate on data reported from our laboratory in the past year concerning the interaction of cholinergic systems with narcotics and their antagonists. Specifically, we will describe our results on the antinociceptive activity of intraventricularly administered acetylcholine, the effects of narcotics on brain acetylcholine levels and turnover rates, and the effects of narcotic analgesics and their antagonists on the release of acetylcholine at ganglionic sites.

Considerable evidence exists which implicates the involvement of cholinergic mechanisms in the actions of narcotic analgesics. Domino and Wilson (1973) have suggested a number of criteria which should be met before concluding a certain effect is specific as that of a narcotic agonist. The effects of morphine on central cholinergic mechanisms of the rat fulfilled most of these criteria. Cholinergic agents such as oxotremorine and physostigmine are active in many antinociceptive tests in animals (Howes, et al., 1969). Tolerance and cross tolerance with morphine develops to these effects and they are antagonized by naloxone. The prior injection of inactive doses of physostigmine causes the normally inactive narcotic-antagonist analgesics to be active in the mouse tail-flick test, suggesting cholinergic involvement in the analgesic actions of this interesting class of drugs (Harris et al., 1969). Recently, we have found that the intraventricular injection of acetylcholine resembles parenterally administered morphine in that it is active in a number of antinociceptive screening procedures including the tail-flick and phenylquinone induced writing tests. Tolerance develops to its effects on the tail-flick procedure and acetylcholine induced antinociception is antagonized by a number of the narcotic antagonists with an identical order of potency to that found for these drugs versus morphine.

When one injects acetylcholine intraventricularly into mice, there is a significant increase in tail-flick latency and an inhibition of phenylquinone induced writhing (Pedigo et al., 1975). This inhibition of the tail-flick response has been shown to be mediated by central muscarinic systems. (The data presented in Figure 1 show the dose-response curves for acetylcholine alone, and following the injection of atropine, atropine methylnitrate, neostigmine, or mecamylamine.) The muscarinic blocker, atropine, inhibited the effects of intraventricularly administered acetylcholine in the tail-flick test. However, atropine methylnitrate, which does not cross the blood-brain barrier, and mecamylamine, which is specific for blocking nicotinic sites, did not alter the response to acetylcholine. Recently, we have published additional evidence which suggests that the active site is muscarinic in nature (Dewey et al., 1975). Various isomers of alpha- and beta-methylcholine were injected into the

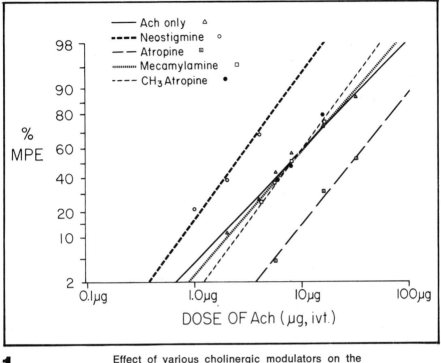

1 Effect of various cholinergic modulators on the antinociceptive activity of intraventricularly administered acetylcholine as measured by the mouse tail-flick technique. (MPE=Maximum possible effect).

lateral ventricle. The alpha- substituted methylcholines, which are active at peripheral nicotinic but not muscarinic sites, were without effect in the phenylquinone induced writing test when injected intraventricularly. Beta- substituted methylcholines, which stimulate peripheral muscarinic receptors, were quite active when given by intraventricular administration. Further, the isomer of beta-methylcholine which most closely resembles the preferred conformation of acetylcholine was the most active isomer (Dewey et al., 1975).

The effect of intraventricularly administered acetylcholine was significantly potentiated by a prior intraventricular injection of an inactive dose of neostigmine. The effect of acetylcholine also was potentiated by a prior injection of morphine. Many similarities between the antinociceptive effects of an intraventricular injection of acetylcholine and morphine given by parenteral administration have emerged. The nar-

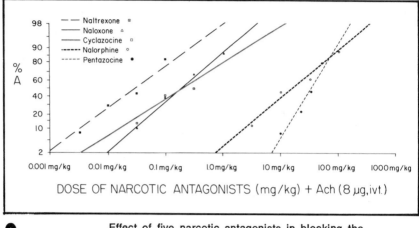

2

Effect of five narcotic antagonists in blocking the
antinociceptive activity of intraventricularly administered
acetylcholine as measured by the mouse tail-flick technique.
(A=antagonism.)

cotic antagonists pentazocine, cyclazocine, nalorphine, naloxone, and
naltrexone all blocked the activity of acetylcholine in the tail-flick test
(see Figure 2).

As has been reported previously, the *l*-isomers of pentazocine and
cyclazocine are active as antagonists of opiates in laboratory animals
and in man, also possessing analgesic activity in man. The *d-isomer*
has been found to be inactive in antagonizing opiate induced analgesia.
However, the *l*-isomers of cyclazocine and pentazocine were inactive
in blocking the antinociception-induced by acetylcholine, while the
d-isomers were active (see Table I). The *d*-isomer of cyclazocine was
equipotent with the racemic mixture and was more potent than the
d-isomer of pentazocine. In other words, the antagonistic potency of the
d-isomers of these two compounds versus acetylcholine-induced antinociception was the same order of potency as the *l*-isomers versus morphine-induced antinociception.

These observations reconfirm our hypothesis that central cholinergic mechanisms might well be involved in the analgesic action of
morphine and other narcotic analgesics. A number of other observations have also indicated an involvement of cholinergic mechanisms in
the actions of the opiates. We have performed preliminary experiments
in an attempt to confirm and extend two of these observations: morphine
and other opiates block the release of acetylcholine from neurons; and

morphine and other narcotics alter levels or turnover rates of brain acetylcholine.

Working independently, Paton (1957) and Schauman (1957) showed that morphine blocked the release of acetylcholine from electrically stimulated guinea pig ileum. This effect has been shown to be dose-related and antagonized by narcotic antagonists. In addition, a rapid tolerance and cross tolerance among narcotics have also been demonstrated. These observations have been extended and many of these studies were discussed in our previous review (Harris and Dewey, 1972). It has been suggested that the effects of narcotic analgesics on the release of acetylcholine in the stimulated ileum may serve as an experimental model and the results may be extrapolated to suggest possible effects of these drugs on central mechanisms. Reports have appeared which show that morphine causes an inhibition of the release of acetylcholine in the brain (Yaksh and Yamamura, 1975). Most of the studies have measured the release of acetylcholine into cups placed on the cortex and, for the most part, have been concerned with effects of morphine on acetylcholine in a rather large portion of the CNS.

Our approach to study the effect of morphine on acetylcholine release has utilized the superior cervical ganglion of the rat as the experimental model. The initial studies by Paton (1957) showed that the morphine effect on the guinea pig ileum was at the neuro-smooth muscular junction and not at the ganglia. Soteropoulus and Standaert (1973) have shown that morphine has a nonspecific inhibitory effect on acetylcholine release at the neuro-skeletal muscular junction in cats. To the best of our knowledge, specific inhibitory effects of morphine on acetylcholine release has not been demonstrated at nerve-nerve synapses in mammalian systems. It has been demonstrated that morphine blocks release of acetylcholine in the abdominal ganglia of *Aplysia,* but this effect was not blocked by naloxone, which in itself caused an inhibition of the release of acetylcholine in this preparation. Kosterlitz et al (1968) and Trendelenberg (1957) have shown that morphine has inhibitory effects on the contraction of the nictitating membrane induced by pre-, but not postganglionic electrical stimulation. This effect was not antagonized by narcotic antagonists and was concluded to be a nonspecific effect of the opiate. The purpose of the experiments was to investigate the effects of morphine on acetylcholine release at the rat superior cervical ganglia. We attempted to decrease the possible number of sites that morphine could be affecting, by measuring the effects of morphine on action potentials recorded from postganglionic neurons induced by electrical stimulation of preganglionic neurons. If warranted, future experiments will involve single cell recordings and measurements of the

Table I. Effect of d- and l- Isomers of Pentazocine and Cyclazocine on Morphine (10 mg/kg, i.p.) and Acetylcholine (8 µg, ivt.) Induced Antinociception

Dose (mg/kg)	Isomer	Pentazocine Percent MPE		Percent Antagonism	
		Morphine	Acetylcholine	Morphine	Acetylcholine
Control	–	79.2 ± 7.1*	56.6 ± 7.4	–	–
15	l	N.T.†	69.0 ± 7.7	N.T.	0
30	l	28.5 ± 3.5	71.2 ± 8.2	64.0	0
60	l	N.T.	77.1 ± 8.4	N.T.	0
15	d	N.T.	41.9 ± 6.3	N.T.	26.0
30	d	82.4 ± 6.7	19.7 ± 3.2	0	65.2
60	d	N.T.	13.3 ± 3.7	N.T.	76.5

AD50 of d-isomer versus acetylcholine = 25.0 (16.1 – 38.8), slope = 2.7 (1.7 – 6.5)

quantity of acetylcholine released per stimulation prior to and after the administration of morphine.

In the present experiments, large rats were anesthetized with pentobarbital and the superior cervical ganglia and adjoining nerves were isolated. The drugs were administered in a maximum volume of 0.05 ml through a 27-gauge needle inserted into the common carotid artery. Injections of saline were given prior to drug treatment as a control. The saline did not alter the postganglionic potentials as they were displayed on a Tektronix oscilloscope. The potentials were evoked with a biphasic stimulus of 0.5 msec. duration from a Grass S-4 stimulator connected to a stimulus isolation unit. The viability of the preparation was demonstrated by the ganglionic blocking agent, hexamethonium, which blocked the postganglionic action potentials induced by either the injection of acetylcholine or preganglionic electrical stimulation.

There was no specificity for the action of the narcotics, narcotic-antagonist analgesics or the narcotic antagonists in inhibiting the postganglionic potentials induced by preganglionic stimulation. Morphine, meperidine, and methadone all inhibited the postganglionic potentials; however, levorphanol, another narcotic analgesic, had no effect in this preparation. Pentazocine, a narcotic-antagonist analgesic, blocked this response; whereas cyclazocine and nalorphine, which are also narcotic-antagonist analgesics, were both without effect in this preparation (see Table II). The lack of specificity of this effect was also apparent in the completely opposite effects of the two pure narcotic antagonists that were studied. Naltrexone inhibited the preganglionic induced action potential, whereas naloxone was inactive. None of the analgesics nor antagonists blocked the action potentials induced by the injection of acetylcholine. Therefore, it may be suggested that those compounds which blocked the action potential, although nonspecifically and at very high doses, inhibited the release of acetylcholine from the preganglionic neuron. Proof for this hypothesis is still lacking. Tolerance did not develop to this effect of morphine and it was not reversed by a subsequent injection or prevented by a prior injection of a pure narcotic antagonist.

These data support previous investigations which showed that the action of morphine on inhibiting preganglionic stimulation which resulted in contraction of the nictitating membranes was a nonspecific effect. Our results indicate that the effects observed in the prior studies were effects of the opiates at the ganglionic sites rather than at the postganglionic neuro-effector junction or a direct musculatropic effect of the opiates on the nictitating membrane. These observations also agree with the conclusions of Soteropoulus and Standaert (1973) and Sokoll et al (1975), who showed that morphine and naloxone both block

**Table II. Effects of Narcotic Analgesics, Narcotic-Antagonist
Analgesics and Narcotic Antagonists on Transmission
in the Superior Cervical Ganglion of the Rat *In Vivo***

Drug	Dose Ratio	Effect on Transmission
Morphine	2.5 mg/kg, 1	inhibition
Meperidine	1 − 2	inhibition
Methadone	1/2 − 1	inhibition
Levorphanol	1/3 − 1	no effect
Pentazocine	3/5	inhibition
Cyclazocine	.1 − .2	no effect
Nalorphine	1	no effect
Naloxone	1	no effect
Naltrexone	1/2 − 1	inhibition

the neuromuscular junction in cats and frogs, and the work of Tremblay et al. (1974), who have shown that the blockade of excitatory postsynaptic potentials by morphine in the abdominal ganglia of the *Aplysia* is nonspecific.

The data appears to be convincing that morphine and other narcotic analgesics decrease or inhibit the release of acetylcholine at cholinergic presynaptic neurons. This phenomenon has been demonstrated in guinea pig ileum at the neuromuscular junction, and at ganglia of both invertebrates and vertebrates. As mentioned above, evidence also exists to suggest that narcotics block the release of acetylcholine in vertebrate central nervous systems. It is intriguing that the blockade of the release of acetylcholine induced by narcotics in the guinea pig ileum should be a specific effect of the narcotic analgesics. Certainly the action of these agents in the central nervous system is also quite specific; i.e., tolerance develops to both of these effects and the effects are reversed by narcotic antagonists. It has been known for a long time that the two organs which are most sensitive to the effects of the opiates are the brain and the gastrointestinal tract. The postganglionic fibers in the gastrointestinal tract and the cholinergic neurons in the central nervous system might differ from the others that have been shown to be sensitive to morphine-induced inhibition of acetylcholine release in that they are the only ones which are impinging upon muscarinic receptor sites. The neurons that release acetylcholine at neuromuscular junctions or ganglia are innervating receptors which are predominately nicotinic in nature. As mentioned previously, recent observations in our laboratory suggest that certain actions of acetylcholine injected into the brain resemble those of the opiates and are involved with central muscarinic sites. Obviously, additional work is needed to confirm or refute this hypothesis and to elucidate the possible importance of morphine's ability to block acetylcholine release and its actions as an analgesic or the phenomena of tolerance and physical dependence.

A number of investigators have reported an increase in rodent whole brain acetylcholine levels following an acute injection of morphine or another narcotic analgesic (Giarman and Pepeu, 1962; Crossland and Slater, 1968; Richter and Goldstein, 1970). The majority of these investigators gave doses of morphine which were considerably higher than those needed to produce complete antinociception in the species being studied. Possibly, lower doses of morphine did not produce a change in brain acetylcholine and these results were not included in the papers. Howes et al. (1969) administered 8 mg/kg morphine to mice, a dose which produced 84% antinociception, and observed a 72% increase in whole brain acetylcholine level. However, Hano et al. (1964) administered 20 mg/kg morphine subcutaneously, and Richter and Goldstein (1970) administered 36 mg/kg morphine by the intraperitonial route and observed no change in mouse brain acetylcholine levels.

The literature is not quite as contradictory on the effects of an acute injection of morphine on rat brain levels of acetylcholine. Three different papers have appeared which report that a dose of 10 mg/kg morphine did not alter rat brain acetylcholine levels. Each group gave the morphine by a different route of administration. Herken et al. (1957) used the intravenous route, Domino and Wilson (1972) confirmed their previous finding using the subcutaneous route. Few studies have shown a significant increase in rat brain acetylcholine levels at doses of less than 50 mg/kg morphine. In addition, the majority of investigations into the effects of doses of 50 mg/kg or higher on whole rat brain acetylcholine levels have shown an increase of less than 20%.

We could not find reports in the literature of a dose-response relationship between acute injections of morphine and increased levels of brain acetylcholine. In the majority of studies that have shown an increase in brain acetylcholine levels the dose was so high that it produced almost 100% analgesia with a barely significant change in brain acetylcholine which precludes an investigation into a possible correlation between the amount of antinociceptive activity and increased brain acetylcholine levels. Recent reports by Schubert et al. (1970), and confirmed in our laboratory (Karbowski et al., 1975) indicate that the turnover rate of acetylcholine in rodent brain is approximately 15 nM/g/min., and the entire pool could be replaced within 1 minute. The turnover rate recently found by Cheney et al. (1975) was a little slower. A neurotransmitter system with such rapid kinetics would probably compensate for drug-induced alterations in basal levels so fast that they would not be detected by our measurements. The conclusion of the majority of the reports that narcotics do not cause a significant dose-related effect on brain acetylcholine levels does not rule out the possibility that the narcotics affect central cholinergic mechanisms and more importantly, the possibility that central cholinergic mechanisms are involved in the mechanism of action of narcotic analgesics in relieving pain.

Obviously one would expect an alteration in brain acetylcholine level or turnover following the intraventricular administration of acetylcholine. Similarities between the effects of intraventricular acetylcholine and systemically administered morphine adds support to previous work which suggested that morphine might alter levels or turnover rates of brain acetylcholine. We investigated the effects of morphine on mouse brain levels of acetylcholine by using the radioenzymatic technique of Goldberg and McCamman (1973). As mentioned above, the data in the literature on the effects of morphine on brain acetylcholine levels are often contradictory. Many of the more recent investigations have shown that the level of brain acetylcholine does not change following acute administration of morphine. We have performed a number of preliminary experiments in which we have looked at whole mouse brain acetylcholine levels after an acute injection of morphine. There is approximately a 16% increase in the acetylcholine level 15 minutes after the injection of morphine which returned to normal within 1 hour and remained that way throughout the rest of the test period (see Figure 3). As a matter of fact, the peak increase was not significantly different from control. In another set of experiments we investigated the effects of logarithmically spaced doses of morphine from 0.3 up to 300 mg/kg on brain acetylcholine levels. There were no significant changes in the acetylcholine level at any of these doses of morphine when given 30 minutes prior to sacrifice (see Figure 4). This is the time of peak brain level of morphine and its maximal analgesic effect (Patrick et al., 1975).

These data confirm recent reports that there are no significant alterations of brain acetylcholine following the injection of morphine. Recently, Sparf and his colleagues and Costa and his colleagues have shown that they have been able to measure the turnover rate of acetyl-

MORPHINE TIME COURSE

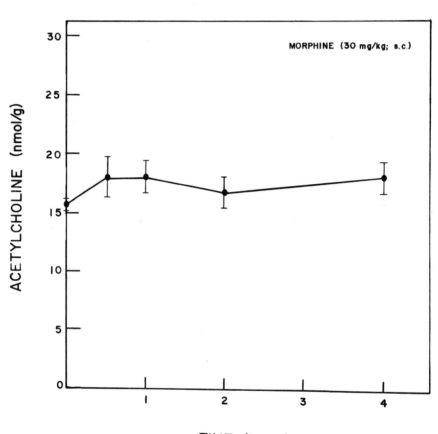

3 Whole mouse brain levels of acetylcholine 30 minutes after the subcutaneous injection of logarithmically spaced doses of morphine.

choline in the brain. We have also measured turnover rates of acetylcholine and have reported that the turnover rate is approximately 1 minute.

We reported previously (Howes et al., 1969) that there was a significant increase of brain acetylcholine level following the injection of the narcotic-antagonist analgesics, nalorphine and pentazocine. We in-

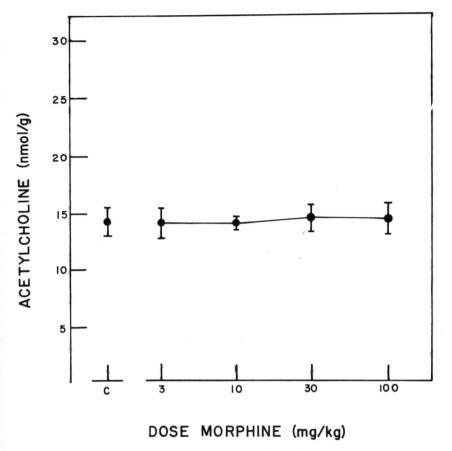

DOSE MORPHINE (mg/kg)

4 Effect of 30 mg/kg morphine sulfate given subcutaneously on whole mouse brain acetylcholine levels at various times after injection.

vestigated the effects of these agents on the brain level of acetylcholine as a portion of our present experiments. There was no significant change in acetylcholine level following the injection of either nalorphine or pentazocine (see Table III). Again, a wide range of doses was used to investigate the effects of each of these drugs on brain acetylcholine.

Finally, we investigated the possibility that although there was no alteration in brain acetylcholine levels following the acute injection of morphine, chronic medication with morphine might increase brain levels of this amine. We have rendered rats dependent on morphine by the constant intraperitoneal infusion technique as first reported by Tieger

**Table III. Lack of Effect of Narcotic Agonist-Antagonists
on Mouse Brain Acetylcholine Levels**

mg/kg	Nalorphine	Pentazocine
Control	17.4 ± 1.6	16.6 ± 1.9
0.1	–	16.8 ± 1.2
1.0	16.3 ± 1.2	17.0 ± 0.8
3.0	20.1 ± 0.6	–
10	17.8 ± 0.8	16.1 ± 0.5
30	18.3 ± 1.0	–
100	19.0 ± 2.4	17.0 ± 0.7

(1974). In this technique, animals are infused intraperitoneally 24 hrs/day, receiving 50 mg/kg the first day, 100 mg/kg the second day, and 200 mg/kg the third through sixth days. When rats are removed from this treatment schedule they lose approximately 20% of their body weight during the first 24 hours. Wet dog shakes, diarrhea, hyperexcitability and other signs of opiate withdrawal are also often seen in these rats. In this particular experiment, the rats were sacrificed at the conclusion of the infusion period. The animals were sacrificed by guillotine, brains rapidly removed and analyzed for acetylcholine content. There was no change in the acetylcholine level in the brains of rats treated chronically with morphine (see Table IV). We are in the process of carrying out experiments designed to study the effects of morphine on brain acetylcholine turnover rate in specific areas of the mouse and rat brain. The technique for measuring turnover is sensitive enough so that the study can be carried out on approximately 2 mg of tissue. We will then be able to make determinations of the effects of various drug treatments on brain acetylcholine turnover in very small areas of the brain.

The studies, which we have described, support the hypothesis that morphine and other opiates affect cholinergic mechanisms in the brain and that central cholinergic mechanisms might well be involved either directly or indirectly in the analgesic action of the opiates. Considerable work is needed in an effort to determine the relevance of the effects of opiates on blocking the release of acetylcholine and their analgesic actions. Similarly, few, if any, conclusions can be made concerning a possible effect of opiates on brain acetylcholine levels or kinetics and their analgesic activity.

Table IV. Lack of Effect of Morphine Infusion on Rat Brain Acetylcholine Levels

Control	Morphine Infused
16.2 nmol/g	14.1 nmol/g
15.8 nmol/g	14.8 nmol/g
	17.3 nmol/g
	18.9 nmol/g
	16.1 nmol/g
	11.6 nmol/g

Average	
16.0 nmol/g	15.5 ± 1.0 nmol/g

Morphine Infusion Schedule:	50 mg/kg/day (Day 1)
	100 mg/kg/day (Day 2)
	200 mg/kg/day (Days 3, 4, 5, 6)

ACKNOWLEDGMENTS

This work was supported by USPHS grant numbers DA-00326 and DA-00490.

REFERENCES

Cheney, D. L., E. Costa, I. Hanin, M. Trabacchi, and C. T. Wang. 1975. Application of principles of steady-state kinetics to the *in vivo* estimation of acetylcholine turnover rate in mouse brain. *J. Pharmacol. Exp. Ther.* 192: 288–296.

Crossland, J., and P. Slater. 1968. The effect of some drugs on the "free" and "bound" acetylcholine content of rat brain. *Brit. J. Pharmac.* 33: 42–47.

Dewey, W. L., G. Cocolas, E. Daves. and L. S. Harris. 1975. Stereospecificity of intraventricularly administered acetylmethylcholine antinociception. *Life Sciences* 17: 9–10.

Domino, A. E., and A. E. Wilson. 1972. Psychotropic drug influences on acetylcholine utilization. *Psychopharmacologia* (Berlin) 25: 291–298.

Domino, E. F., and A. E. Wilson. 1973. Effects of narcotic analgesic agonists and antagonists on rat brain acetylcholine. *J. Pharmacol. Exp. Ther.* 184: 18–32.

Giarman, N. J., and G. Pepeu. 1962. Drug induced changes in brain acetylcholine. *Brit. J. Pharmac.* 19: 226–234.

Goldberg, A. M., and R. E. McCaman. 1973. The determination of picomole amounts of acetylcholine in mammalian brain. *J. Neurochem.* 20: 1–8.

Hano, K., H. Kaneto, T. Kakunga, and N. Moribayashi. 1964. The administration of morphine and changes in acetylcholine metabolism by mouse brain. *Biochem. Pharmacol.* 13: 441–447.

Harris, L. S. 1970. Central neurohumoral systems involved with narcotic agonists and antagonists. *Fed. Proc.* 29: 28–31.

Harris, L. S., and W. L. Dewey. 1972. Role of cholinergic systems in the central action of narcotic agonists and antagonists. In H. W. Kosterlitz, H. O. J. Collier, and J. E. Villarreal, Eds. *Agonists and Antagonist Actions of Narcotic Analgesic Drugs.* McMillan Press Ltd., London, pp. 198–206.

Harris, L. S., W. L. Dewey, J. F. Howes, J. S. Kennedy, and H. Pars. 1969. Narcotic antagonist analgesics: Interactions with cholinergic systems. *J. Pharmacol. Exp. Ther.* 169: 17–22.

Herken, H., D. Mailbauer, and S. Muller. 1957. Acetylcholingehalt des Gehirns und Analgesie nach Einwirkung von Morphin und einigen 3-Oxymorphinanen. *Arch. Expt. Path. Pharmakol.* 230: 313-324.

Howes, J. F., L. S. Harris, W. L. Dewey, and C. A. Voyda. 1969. Brain acetylcholine levels and inhibition of the tail-flick reflex in mice. *J. Pharmacol. Exp. Ther.* 169: 23–28.

Karbowski, M., A. Jagoda, W. L. Dewey, and L. S. Harris. 1975. Effect of delta-9-THC on the level and turnover of acetylcholine in mouse brain. *Pharmacologist* 17: 254.

Kosterlitz, H. W., G. M. Lees, D. I. Wallis, and A. J. Watt. 1968. Nonspecific inhibitory effects of morphine-like drugs on transmission in the superior cervical ganglion and guinea pig isolated ileum. *Brit. J. Pharmac.* 34: 691–692.

Paton, W. D. M. 1957. The action of morphine and related substances on contraction and on acetylcholine output of coaxially stimulated guinea pig ileum. *Brit. J. Pharmac.* 12: 119–127.

Patrick, G. A., W. L. Dewey, T. C. Spaulding, and L. S. Harris. 1975. Relationship of brain morphine levels to analgesic activity in acutely treated mice and rats and in pellet-implanted mice. *J. Pharmacol. Exp. Ther.* 193: 876–883.

Pedigo, N. W., W. L. Dewey, and L. S. Harris. 1975. Determination and characterization of the antinociceptive activity of intraventricularly administered acetylcholine in mice. *J. Pharmacol. Exp. Ther.* 193: 845–852.

Richter, J. A., and A. Goldstein. 1970. Effects of morphine and lavorphanol on brain acetylcholine content in mice. *J. Pharmacol. Exp. Ther.* 175: 685–691.

Schauman, W. 1957. Inhibition by morphine of the release of acetylcholine from the intestine of the guinea pig. *Brit. J. Pharmac.* 12: 115–118.

Schubert, J., B. Sparf, and A. Sundwall. 1970. On the turnover of acetylcholine in nerve endings of mouse brain *in vivo. J. Neurochem.* 17: 461–468.

Sokol, M. D., E. L. Post, S. D. Gergis, and R. Cronnelly. 1975. Effects of morphine and narcotic antagonists on neuromuscular transmission in the frog. *Fed. Proc.* 311: 3014.

Soteropoulos, G. C., and F. G. Standaert. 1973. Neuromuscular effects of morphine and naloxone. *J. Pharmacol. Exp. Ther.* 184: 136–142.

Tieger, D. 1974. Induction of physical dependence on morphine, codeine and meperidine in the rat by continuous infusion. *J. Pharmacol. Exp. Ther.* 190: 408–415.

Tremblay, J. P., W. T. Schlapfer, P. B. J. Woodson, and S. H. Barodnes. 1974. Morphine and related compounds: Evidence that they decrease available neurotransmitters in *Aplysia* california. *Brain Res.* 81: 107–118.

Trendelenburg, U. 1957. The action of morphine on the superior cervical ganglion and in the nictitating membrane of the cat. *Brit. J. Pharmac.* 12: 79–85.

Yaksh, T. L., and H. I. Yamamura. 1975. Blockade by morphine of acetylcholine release from the caudate nucleus in the mid-pontine pretrigeminal cat. *Brain Res.* 83: 520–524.

Evidence for a Role of Prostaglandin in the Synaptic Effects of Opiates and Other Analgesics on Guinea Pig Ileum

S. EHRENPREIS
J. GREENBERG
J. COMATY

*New York State Research Institute
for Neurochemistry and Drug Addiction
Ward's Island, New York*

It is well known that inhibition of transmission in the guinea pig ileum by morphine and other opiates results from block of release of acetylcholine (ACh) from cholinergic nerve terminals within Auerbach's plexus (Paton, 1957; Schaumann, 1957). A neural receptor for opiates has been demonstrated by the technique of stereospecific binding, using homogenates of the tissue (Pert and Snyder, 1973). We have recently presented evidence that the naturally occurring substrate for the opiate receptor is a prostaglandin (PG) of the E series (Ehrenpreis et al., 1973; Ehrenpreis and Greenberg, 1975) and have suggested that the receptor for opiates is actually a PG receptor. In this scheme, PG acts as a modulator for ACh release. This function is blocked when an opiate combines with the PG receptor with concommitant inhibition of ACh release upon nerve stimulation. In accordance with the hypothesis, analgesics such as indomethacin and aspirin, known to inhibit synthesis of PG (Vane, 1971; Smith and Lands, 1971; Ku et al., 1975) also produced

273

morphine-like actions on the ileum. In the present paper, we review some of the earlier evidence on which this hypothesis was based and present considerable additional supportive findings.

MATERIALS AND METHODS

The isolated longitudinal muscle-nerve plexus

This preparation was set up for electrical stimulation as previously described (Ehrenpreis et al., 1972; Ehrenpreis et al., 1973; Ehrenpreis, 1975a,b). Guinea pigs weighing between 250 and 350 grams were used. Tyrode's solution was the buffer, the bath temperature was 37°C and 95% O_2, 5% CO_2 was bubbled into the organ bath. The usual stimulus parameters were 0.4–0.8 msec current duration, 60 volts, 0.1 Hz, giving about 80% maximum contraction. Current duration-response curves were determined as previously described by Ehrenpreis (1975a). After sufficient equilibration period, generally 1 hour, the current duration was reduced to the subthreshold level and gradually increased by small increments until maximum contraction was obtained. The tissue was stimulated for a period of 1–2 min. at each current duration. The same procedure was repeated in the presence and after washout of indomethacin (IM) or 5,8,11,14-eicosatetraynoic acid (ETA). Data are plotted as % maximum contraction height at a given current duration. The advantages of this procedure in the study of drug effects on electrically-induced contractions are discussed in detail by Ehrenpreis (1975a).

PG effects on drugs blocking contractions

Many types of drugs block electrically-induced contractions of the ileum. The efficacy of various PGs in reversing block of the following drugs was determined: morphine and a number of other opiates, PG receptor inhibitors, e.g., SC19220 (Sanner, 1971; Bennett and Posner, 1971), 7-oxaprostynoic acid (Fried et al., 1969), PG synthetase inhibitors including IM, phenylbutazone, aspirin and ETA (Ku et al., 1975; Ku and Wasvary, 1975), and a variety of other drugs (barbiturates, atropine, chlorpromazine, norepinephrine (NE), GABA, cyclic AMP). Following block (75% or greater) by any one of these drugs, progressively increasing concentrations of PG were added to the bath. Standard parameters of stimulation were use in these experiments with the exception of those involving IM and ETA for which complete current duration-response curves were determined in the presence and absence of PG as described above.

In some instances, particularly with IM and ETA, it was noted that block of contractions could be irreversible or semireversible. Effectiveness of PG's in restoring contractions was determined following washout of these drugs.

PG action was also examined on longitudinal muscles removed from guinea pigs administered IM, 25 mg/kg twice daily for several days either by mouth or ip.

Physostigmine effects on block by morphine, IM and chlorpromazine

Following block of contractions by these drugs, physostigmine was added to the bath in increasing concentrations; the concentration was increased at 2 min. intervals up to 80ng/ml.

Arachidonic acid (AA) effect on the longitudinal muscle preparation

AA, a precursor for PG synthesis, causes a pronounced contraction of the preparation. This effect is due to its conversion to PG and hence can be used as an assay for synthetase activity of the tissue. Contracture can be quantitated by tracing the polygraph record on weighing paper and weighing a cut-out of the trace.

We have found that AA contraction shows marked tachyphylaxis; accordingly, many precautions had to be taken in order to utilize this compound to determine drug effects on synthetase activity. To avoid tachyphylaxis the tissue was exposed only once to AA: either in the presence of IM or after washout of IM. In each case the tissue was exposed to the IM for 30 minutes.

Interaction between PG and naloxone: In vitro

This interaction was studied on the ileum preparation as follows: A high concentration of morphine (or other opiate) was applied to two strips to produce complete block of contractions. PG was added to one of these at a concentration which failed to cause reversal of the block. Next, naloxone was added in increasing concentration to both strips until reversal of the block was complete.

Interaction between PG and naloxone: In vivo

The parameter studied was morphine-induced respiratory depression in several species. A large dose of morphine was administered to

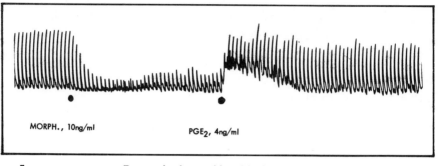

1 Reversal of morphine block of electrically-induced contractions of longitudinal muscle by PGE$_2$. The morphine, 10ng/ml, was applied for 5 minutes followed by the PG. Recovery is approximately 80%. (From Ehrenpreis et al., 1973.)

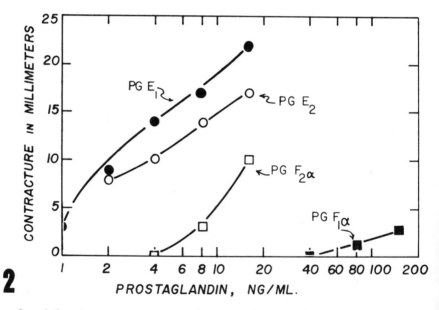

2 Cumulative dose-response curves for reversal of morphine block by various prostaglandins. Note that in the case of PGF$_1\alpha$ and F$_2\alpha$ the concentration of morphine was half that with PGE$_1$ and E$_2$. In each experiment, the tissue was exposed to the morphine for 5 minutes prior to adding the particular PG. (From Ehrenpreis et al., 1973.)

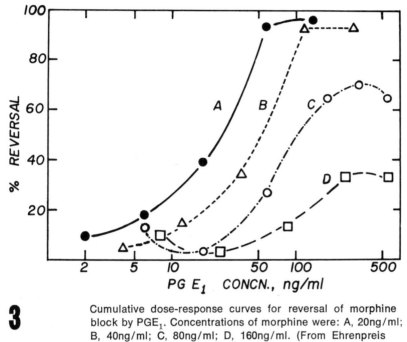

3 Cumulative dose-response curves for reversal of morphine block by PGE_1. Concentrations of morphine were: A, 20ng/ml; B, 40ng/ml; C, 80ng/ml; D, 160ng/ml. (From Ehrenpreis et al., 1973.)

rabbits (100-150 mg/kg, ip), mice (100 mg/kg, ip), and rats (20 mg/kg, i.v.). The duration and intensity of naloxone reversal of respiratory depression was determined in animals given PG (1 mg/kg, ip in rabbits and mice, 5–20μg/kg, i.v. in rats) just prior to the naloxone and compared with suitable controls not given the PG.

RESULTS AND DISCUSSION

PG reversal of morphine block of contractions

Block of contractions by morphine is readily reversed by very low concentrations of PGE_2 (see Figure 1) and PGE_1. Other PGs are much less effective in this regard (see Figure 2); in fact, PGA_1 and A_2, PGB_1 and B_2, PGF_1, α, and β are completely inactive. At least in a certain range of morphine concentrations reversal of block by PGE_1 is competitive (see Figure 3); at higher morphine concentrations, the block becomes

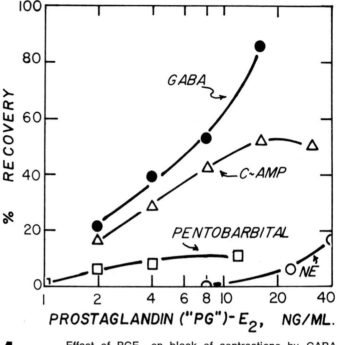

4

Effect of PGE$_2$ on block of contractions by GABA
(50μg/ml), cyclic AMP (2μg/ml), pentobarbital
(66μg/ml) and norepinephrine (8μg/ml).

noncompetitive and insurmountable. A similar series of curves is obtained for naloxone reversal of morphine block.

PGE$_1$ and E$_2$ reverse other opiates including methadone, meperidine, levorphanol, and codeine. On the other hand, PGE failed to reverse· block by nonopiates such as pentobarbital, norepinephrine[1] (see Figure 4), chlorpromazine, isoproterenol, and gave a partial reversal of block by GABA and cyclic AMP.

These results suggest that morphine and other opiates block cholinergic transmission in the ileum by interfering with the endogenous actions of PG. We have suggested that PG functions as a modulator for ACh release; inhibition of PG action results in inhibition of such release (Ehrenpreis et al., 1973; Ehrenpreis and Greenberg, 1975) with resultant

[1]PGE at very high concentrations (1 μg/ml) can reverse block of contractions by NE. This may result from an acceleration of NE oxidation by PG (S. Ehrenpreis and S. Krugyr, unpublished experiments).

block of contractions. Thus a PG, most likely of the E series, is considered to be the naturally occurring substance with which opiates compete in producing their effect on transmission. PG may have a similar modulatory role in other tissues with predominantly cholinergic transmission, e.g., salivary glands (Taira and Satoh, 1974; Hahn and Patil, 1972, 1974).

It is further suggested that the receptor with which opiates combine in the ileum is a PG receptor. Evidence in support of the presence of such a receptor was obtained through the use of compounds known to act as PG receptor inhibitors in other tissues. SC192220 and 7-oxaprostynoic acid block electrically-induced contractions, both being reversed by low concentration of PGE_1 or E_2. These compounds have been reported to be highly specific PG receptor inhibitors (Fried et al., 1969; Sanner, 1971; Bennett and Posner, 1971) and such findings provide strong support for the involvement of a PG receptor system in transmission.

Despite the considerable data to support a direct antagonism between PG and opiates on the same receptor, other interpretations are possible particularly since PG's are smooth muscle stimulants and apparently can sensitize the ileum to effects of ACh (Harry, 1968). Thus, reversal of opiate action by PGE could result from a postsynaptic mechanism totally unrelated to the proposed presynaptic site of action involving ACh release. However, other evidence seems to rule out such a site of action. Although PGE_1 or E_2 does increase the height of contraction produced by electrical stimulation, thereby suggesting a postsynaptic sensitization, this effect is quite minimal, compared with the reversal of morphine block (see Figure 5). Furthermore, PGE_1 or E_2 failed to alter the midpoint of the duration-response curve or to enhance the potency of egogenous ACh, thereby ruling out an action which involves sensitization of the tissue to ACh. Finally, PCE_1 fails to reverse the block of contractions produced by atropine (see Figure 6). Thus, the site of action of PG in reversing morphine block is considered to be presynaptic as expected from the presynaptic site of action of morphine itself on this tissue.

Another interpretation for the PG–opiate antagonism is possible on the basis of recent work by Ho et al. (1973), and by Collier and Roy (1974) who apparently showed an involvement of the adenylate cyclase system in analgesic and other actions of opiates. In particular, Collier and Roy presented evidence for the specific inhibition by opiates of PG activation of adenylate cyclase and consider that this constitutes the molecular basis for opiate action. Although PGE antagonism of opiate effects on the ileum are consistent with this hypothesis, other evidence

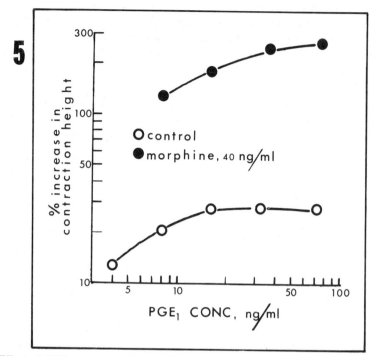

Effect of PGE₁ on contractions elicited by electrical stimulation on untreated ileum (control) and one blocked by morphine, 40ng/ml. Note that although the PG does cause an increase in contraction height of the control tissue, this reaches a maximum of less than 30% at about 15ng/ml and levels off. The dose-dependent increase in contraction height in the presence of morphine is apparent and is far greater than the control at all concentrations of PG.

rules out involvement of the adenylate cyclase system either in transmission itself in the ileum or opiate effects on synaptic events. Thus norepinephrine, isoproterenol and dopamine, all of which are known to activate adenylate cyclase, *block* transmission. Inhibitors of phosphodiesterase, such as theophylline or papaverine, fail to reverse morphine block of electrically-induced contractions. Indeed, these drugs mimic morphine action on transmission. The above facts, as well as others discussed elsewhere (Ehrenpreis, Comaty, and Greenberg, in preparation) are inconsistent with the proposed adenylate cyclase hypothesis of opiate drug action.

Actions of PG synthetase inhibitors

The pioneering studies of Vane and co-workers on the mechanism of analgesic action for various synthetase inhibitors (Vane, 1971; Ferreira,

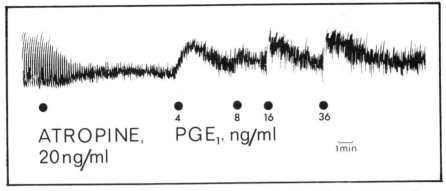

ATROPINE,   PGE₁, ng/ml

20 ng/ml

6 Lack of effect of PGE₁ in reversing block of electrically-induced contractions caused by atropine.

Moncada, and Vane, 1973) stimulated a great amount of research of a biochemical nature with these compounds. Surprisingly little has been done on their effects on synaptic transmission, and most of this has been concerned with the adrenergic system (Samuelsson and Wennmalm, 1971; Ambache et al., 1972; Stjarne, 1973). With the longitudinal muscle preparation, all of the agents of this type studied caused a block of transmission; this was reversed by PGE_1 or E_2 at very low concentrations. Figure 7 shows block of electrically induced contractions by IM and its reversal by PGE_2 at only 2 ng/ml. Following washout of PG, the block is reinstated but contractions could be restored by PGE_2. The potency of a series of PGs in reversing IM block is indicated in Table I; once again, PGs of the E series are most potent. Other PGs examined (of the A, B and F_1 series) were essentially inactive.

The finding that IM causes irreversible block of contractions is consistent with reports that this drug is an irreversible inhibitor of the synthetase (Smith and Lands, 1971; Ku et al., 1975a,b). However, complete irreversibility was not always observed; washout of IM following essentially complete block by the drug almost invariably resulted in partial recovery. In about 100 experiments involving concentrations of IM between 10 and 40 μg/ml applied for 30 minutes, most tissues showed 50–60% irreversible effect of the drug although in some instances 100% block was observed. This lack of complete irreversibility of IM effect is explained in part by recent reports (Ku et al., 1975a; Ku and Wasvary, 1975) that the synthetase may be very resistant to inhibitors; in fact, beyond a certain concentration, additional inhibition greater than 50–60% was not attained. This finding explains why IM at 0.1 mM does not at all times produce an irreversible block of contractions even

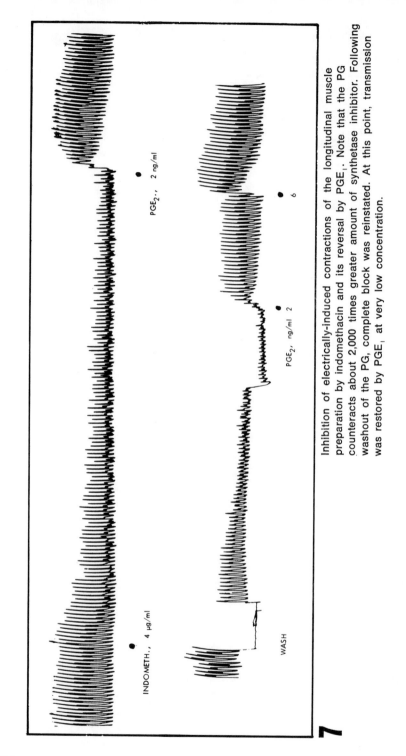

Inhibition of electrically-induced contractions of the longitudinal muscle preparation by indomethacin and its reversal by PGE_1. Note that the PG counteracts about 2,000 times greater amount of synthetase inhibitor. Following washout of the PG, complete block was reinstated. At this point, transmission was restored by PGE_1 at very low concentration.

INDOMETH., 4 μg/ml

WASH

PGE_2, ng/ml 2

PGE_2, ng/ml 6

PGE_2, 2 ng/ml

7

Table I. Potency of Various Prostaglandins in Reversing Indomethacin Block of Electrically Induced Contractions of Guinea Pig Ileum

Prostaglandin	ED_{50} for complete reversal* ng/ml
A_1	340
B_1	70
E_1, E_2	2
$F_{2\alpha}$	270

*These values refer to reversal of block following washing out the indomethacin (see text for explanation).

though this concentration is about 50 times greater than the Ki for the enzyme. In the presence of such a high concentration of IM, however, 100% block is almost always noted (see Figure 8). This may be explained on the basis of some nonspecific actions of IM, or other synthetase inhibitors, as shown by block of contractions of exogenous ACh (see Figure 9) when the concentration of IM exceeds about $5 \times 10^{-5}M$ ($16\mu g/ml$). If the drug is washed out this nonspecific effect is reversed while the enzyme remains partially inhibited. Another factor may be that even a small fraction of the enzyme which is not blocked is sufficient to synthesize enough PG to maintain partial transmission. It is evident that very small amounts of PG are required for this purpose as shown by the experiment (see Figure 7) where only 2ng/ml in the bath can restore transmission following almost complete block by IM. Finally, Ku et al. (1975a) indicate that a spectrum of synthetases may be present in tissues with very different affinities for a given inhibitor. If true, then the degree of block by such a compound may well be expected to be quite variable. On the whole, the finding of even partial irreversibility of effects on the ileum by IM as well as ETA, fits in very well with the known effects of these drugs on synthetase activity.

Further support for the involvement of the synthetase in transmission is indicated (see Table II) by data showing ED_{50} blocking electrically-induced contractions as well as the corresponding Ki for a number of synthetase inhibitors. It is apparent that the correlation between both parameters is almost perfect over a very wide spread of potencies. It may be noted that PGE_1 at 2ng/ml gave complete reversal of all of these synthetic inhibitors when applied at the ED_{50} concentrations.

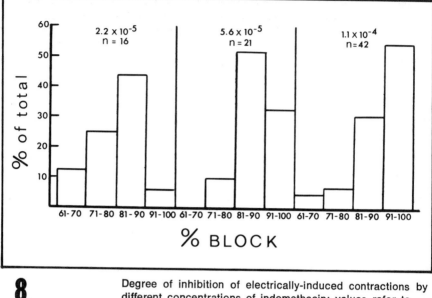

8

Degree of inhibition of electrically-induced contractions by different concentrations of indomethacin; values refer to effect produced in the presence of the drug. Note variability of extent of block at all concentrations. n refers to number of tissues used.

Figures 10 and 11 show complete duration-response curves obtained in the presence and following washout of IM and ETA. The partial irreversible nature of the block of contractions is noted, and that PGE_1 shifts the entire curve almost to control values, indicating that this PG can "repair the biochemical lesion" produced by the synthetase inhibitors.

Administration of IM, 25mg/kg, i.p. or orally to guinea pigs resulted in an ileum which at times (3 out of 6) failed to respond adequately to electrical stimulation (see Figure 12). This apparently reflects the irreversible inactivation of the synthetase since transmission was restored fully by very small concentrations of PGE_1. Washout of the PG resulted once again in greatly diminished response to electrical stimulation. Thus the *in vivo* administration of IM exactly parallels what is observed *in vitro*.

Site of action of synthetase inhibitors

Many different types of drugs can block electrically-induced contractions in the ileum; some of the mechanisms of blockade are discussed

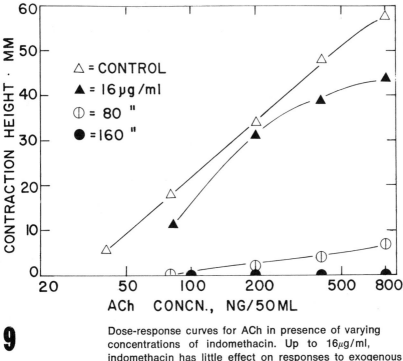

9 Dose-response curves for ACh in presence of varying concentrations of indomethacin. Up to 16μg/ml, indomethacin has little effect on responses to exogenous ACh while causing 80-100% block in most tissues (see Figure 8, middle panel).

Table II. Relationship Between Potency of Various PG Synthetase Inhibitors in Blocking Electrically-Induced Contractions and Inhibition of the Enzyme

Drug	ED_{50} Block of contractions	Ki, PG Synthetase*
Indomethacin	1.3×10^{-6}M	6.5×10^{-6}
ETA	4.0×10^{-6}M	4.9×10^{-6}
Phenylbutazone	70×10^{-6}M	98×10^{-6}
Aspirin	700×10^{-6}M	$5,800 \times 10^{-6}$

*Values from Ku and Wasvary (1975).

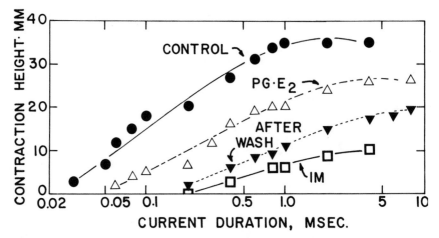

10 Duration-response curves obtained in the presence and after washout of indomethacin (15μg/ml). Also shown is that PGE₁ (4ng/ml) antagonizes the irreversible effect of indomethacin at all current durations.

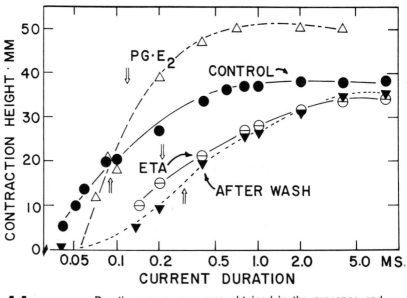

11 Duration-response curves obtained in the presence and after washout of ETA (8μg/ml). The irreversible action of the drug is to be noted as in the case of indomethacin. PGE₁ (4ng/ml) reverses the entire duration-response curve back to control. The double arrow (↑↑) shows the midpoint of the curves.

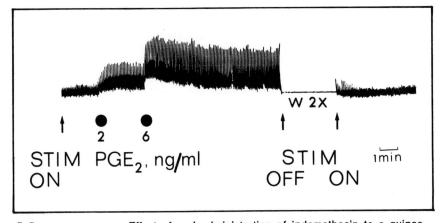

12
Effect of oral administration of indomethacin to a guinea
pig on response of longitudinal muscle to electrical
stimulation and to PGE$_2$. Note that initially the tissue gives
almost no response to electrical stimulation and that
PGE$_2$ causes a rapid increase in contraction height.
Following washout of the PG, electrical stimulation is again
ineffectual in eliciting a contraction.

in detail elsewhere (Ehrenpreis, 1975a,b). The most prominent mechanisms are: a) inhibition of ACh release; b) block of axonal conduction; c) inhibition of ACh receptors; d) extrajunctional membrane stabilization; and e) other extrajunctional effects, e.g., at the level of the sarcoplasmic reticulum. Considerable evidence has been obtained that both IM and ETA have a presynaptic mode of action which most likely involves inhibition of ACh release.

Block of electrically-induced contractions by IM can occur without any marked effect on contractions of the tissue by ACh. This is also true for ETA (see Figure 9). Furthermore, the block could not be reversed by very large concentrations of ACh. Thus these drugs do not exhibit atropinic-type action. However, as indicated above, if the IM concentration is increased much beyond 15μg/ml then ACh responses may also be blocked. This effect is considered to occur by mechanisms d and/or e, and possibly involves inhibition of Ca binding as noted by Northover (1973) to occur when smooth muscle is exposed to IM at concentrations of 10^{-4}M and above.

Block of contractions by IM is reversed by physostigmine (see Figure 13). Interestingly, the effectiveness of physostigmine in reversing

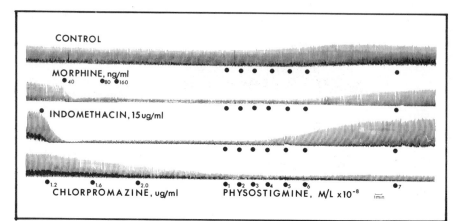

13   Effect of physostigmine on block of electrically-induced contractions by morphine, indomethacin, and chlorpromazine. The parallel reversal of morphine and IM is apparent. Absence of effect of physostigmine on chlorpromazine block or on contractions of untreated tissues is noted.

IM is identical to that of morphine when the block of contractions was the same for both drugs. It has been established (Paton, 1957; Schaumann, 1957) that morphine block results from inhibition of ACh release. This experiment shows that at equivalent degree of blockade, IM and morphine cause essentially the same reduction in ACh output and that reversal by physostigmine represents potentiation of the same small amount of ACh released under the influence of both drugs. It may be noted that physostigmine fails to reverse block by chlorpromazine which evidently acts in a much more nonspecific manner than IM or morphine.

Effect on ACh release. The ultimate proof for the site and mechanism of action of the PG synthetase inhibitors is the demonstration that they diminish the output of ACh from the tissue, either at rest or during stimulation. Botting and Salzman (1974) reported that IM reduces ACh output at rest but only occasionally during stimulation. However, they reported that IM at $10 \mu g/ml$ failed to cause a significant block of electrically-induced contractions, whereas in our hands this concentration of IM almost invariably gave about 80% block. One possible explanation for this discrepancy is that Botting and Salzmann used whole ileum whereas we used longitudinal muscle for most experiments. Using gas chromatography to estimate ACh, we have shown that indeed IM at a concentration which blocks contractions by 80% or more reduces ACh output by greater than 75% (S. Ehrenpreis, E. Maruyama, I. Sawa, and E. Hosoya, unpublished findings). Recent confirmation of this finding has come from the work of Masek and Kadlec (1975) who reported that IM inhibited ACh release in the ileum and that this was reversed by PGE_2. Thus, under appropriate conditions of concentration and time of exposure of the tissue, it is readily demonstrated that IM does reduce output of ACh from the ileum. One possible explanation for the lack of agreement may be the improper use of physostigmine to inhibit cholinesterases during the collection of ACh. The very high concentrations of this drug frequently used (e.g., $2\mu g/ml$ by Botting and Salzmann) may cause a large release of ACh which can counteract that diminished by the IM.

Arachidonic acid experiments

Arachidonic acid has been used as an index for synthetase activity in rat stomach fundal strip (Splawinski et al., 1973) and guinea pig tracheal muscle (Lambley and Smith, 1975). It is necessary to carry out these experiments with proper controls since, unlike the stomach or trachea, AA effect on the ileum shows a very pronounced tachyphylaxis. Thus successive application of AA alone results in progressively diminished contractions of the tissue; eventually no response is noted. The contraction evidently reflects conversion to PG since it is blocked by SC19220. In view of the tachyphylaxis, we resorted to the single dose technique to assess whether IM inhibits the synthetase when it blocks transmission. In other words, the tissue was exposed only once to the AA. Since responses to AA do vary considerably, and no control was possible, the results can only be semiquantitative. Nevertheless, it is apparent that when irreversible block of transmission by IM was almost complete, AA failed to cause significant contraction (see Figure 14). If recovery following IM was partial, a large AA-induced contraction was noted.

Interaction between PGE_1 or E_2 with naloxone

That PGE can combine with the opiate receptor was indicated by reversal of block of contractions produced by morphine and other narcotics. Evidence of a different nature was obtained in terms of the ability of PG to potentiate naloxone reversal of morphine action *in vitro* and *in vivo*. The presence of PGE_1 or E_2 greatly enhances the effectiveness of naloxone in reversing morphine block of electrically-induced contractions. A plot of dose-response curves (see Figure 15) shows that this potentiation is about 6-fold under the conditions indicated. Similar

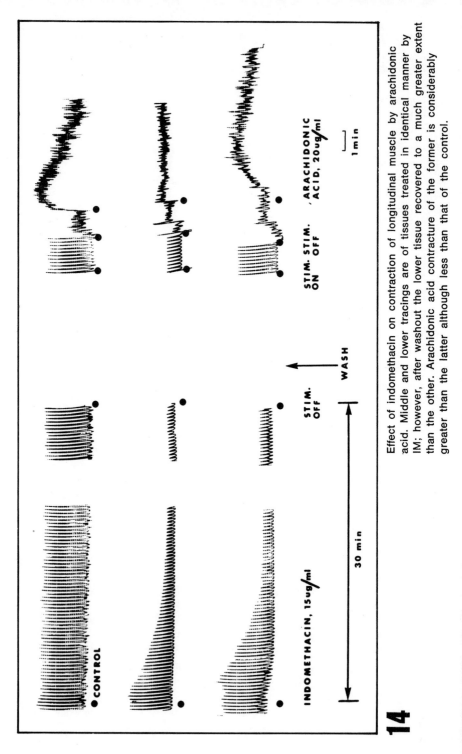

Effect of indomethacin on contraction of longitudinal muscle by arachidonic acid. Middle and lower tracings are of tissues treated in identical manner by IM; however, after washout the lower tissue recovered to a much greater extent than the other. Arachidonic acid contracture of the former is considerably greater than the latter although less than that of the control.

14

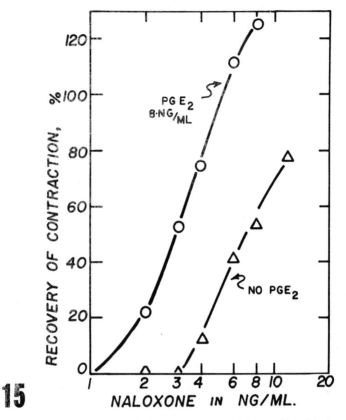

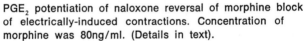

15

PGE$_2$ potentiation of naloxone reversal of morphine block of electrically-induced contractions. Concentration of morphine was 80ng/ml. (Details in text).

potentiation was noted with methadone and meperidine. Prompted by this observation, we found that PGE$_1$ or E$_2$ could also greatly potentiate naloxone reversal of morphine respiratory depression in rabbit (see Figure 16), mouse, and rat. Both intensity and duration of action of naloxone were augmented by doses of PGE which by themselves failed to influence respiration. At the present time we are investigating whether the PG also potentiates naloxone antagonism of opiate analgesia.

CONCLUSIONS

The present results provide considerable evidence that a number of diverse types of drugs affect cholinergic transmission in the guinea pig

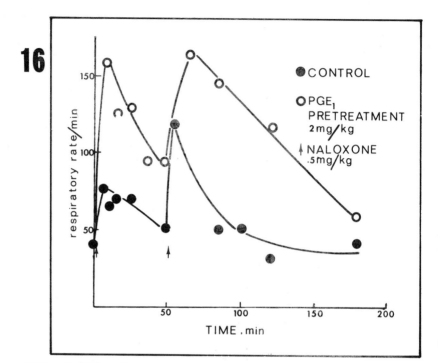

PGE₁ potentiation of naloxone reversal of respiratory depression produced by morphine in the rabbit. Zero time refers to respiratory rate after morphine. At this time one rabbit (0) was given PGE₁ plus naloxone while the other rabbit (●) was given naloxone only. Note potentiation of naloxone effect by the PG. At 50 minutes both rabbits were subjected to the same drug administration as at zero time.

ileum by altering the activity of a PG system. Opiates, inhibitors of PG synthesis, and PG receptor inhibitors all have a similar action: they block electrically-induced contractions of the tissue. Furthermore, this effect can be reversed by PG's, particularly of the E series, unlike other drugs which block transmission by mechanisms not associated with the PG system. The findings presented extend our original hypothesis that the PG system plays an essential role in transmission in this tissue. This hypothesis provides a unified synaptic mechanism of analgesia which is considered to be a resultant of inhibition of some key cholinergic pathways in the CNS that are controlled by the PG system. Such inhibition can be brought about either by PG receptor inhibitors or by inhibitors of PG synthesis and indeed drugs of both types exhibit analgesic activity. It is of considerable interest in this connection that Ferri et al

(1974) have shown that, as predicted from the ileum results, PGE_1 administered intraventricularly antagonized morphine analgesia in rats.

SUMMARY

Opiates, prostaglandin (PG) receptor inhibitors, and inhibitors of PG synthetase block electrically-induced contractions of the longitudinal muscle of the guinea pig ileum. This blockade is selectively reversed by some PGs, particularly those of the E series. Many other types of drugs which block transmission are not reversed by PGs. There is a very close parallel between the potency with which a series of synthetase inhibitors block transmission and inhibit the enzyme. The mechanism of inhibition of transmission by indomethacin involves block of acetylcholine (ACh) release as shown by assay for ACh and by the fact that physostigmine can readily reverse the block. Other evidence for a presynaptic site of action for the synthetase inhibitors is suggested by the lack of effect of blocking concentrations on response of the tissue to exogenous ACh. PGE_1 and E_2 greatly potentiate naloxone reversal of opiate block of transmission in the ileum and also potentiate naloxone antagonism of morphine depression of respiration in rat, mouse, and rabbit. These results are compatible with the postulate that (a) a prostaglandin system is directly involved with the release of acetylcholine in the ileum; (b) opiates act as PG receptor inhibitors; and (c) such receptor inhibition results in blockade of PG modulatory function and reduced ACh output. The adenylate cyclase system most likely is not involved in the mechanism of ACh release or with the effects of opiates or PG as postulated by Collier (1974).

ACKNOWLEDGMENTS

We wish to thank Dr. J. Pike of the Upjohn Co. for generous samples of prostaglandins, Dr. J. Sanner for SC19220, and Dr. J. Fried for 7-oxaprostynoic acid. We thank Mrs. L. Mussolini for expert secretarial assistance.

This work was supported in part by USPHS grant DA 00496.

REFERENCES

Ambache, N., L. P. Dunk, J. Verney, and M. Aboo Zar. 1972. Inhibitory nature of the adrenergic innervation in the guinea-pig vas deferens. *Brit. J. Pharmacol.* 44: 359–360P.

Bennett, A., and J. Posner. 1971. Studies on prostaglandin antagonists. *Brit. J. Pharmacol.* 42: 584–594.

Botting, J. H., and R. Salzmann. 1974. The effect of indomethacin on the release of prostaglandin E_2 and acetylcholine from guinea pig isolated ileum at rest and during field stimulation. *Brit. J. Pharmacol.* 50: 119–124.

Collier, H. O. J., and A. C. Roy. 1974. Morphine-like drugs inhibit the stimulation by E prostaglandins of cyclic AMP formation by rat brain homogenate. *Nature* (London) 248: 24–27.

Ehrenpreis, S. 1975a. Determination of action of narcotic analgesics and their antagonists on electrically stimulated guinea pig ileum. In S. Ehrenpreis and A. Neidle, Eds. *Methods in Narcotics Research.* Marcel Dekker, New York. pp. 67–82.

Ehrenpreis, S. 1975b. Actions of opiates and their antagonists on cholinergic transmission in the guinea pig ileum. In T. Narahashi and P. Bianchi, Eds. *Advances in General and Cellular Pharmacology.* Plenum Pub. Co., N. Y. pp. 111–125.

Ehrenpreis, S., and J. Greenberg. 1975. Mechanism of the synaptic effects of morphine, indomethacin and prostaglandins. In E. M. Sellers, Ed. *Clinical Pharmacology of Psychoactive Drugs.* Alcoholism and Drug Addiction Foundation, Toronto, pp. 171–182.

Ehrenpreis, S., J. Greenberg, and S. Bellman. 1973. Prostaglandins reverse inhibition of electrically-induced contractions of guinea pig ileum by morphine, indomethacin, and acetylsalicylic acid. *Nature New Biol.* 245: 280–282.

Ehrenpreis, S., I. Light, and G. Schonbuch. 1972. Use of the electrically stimulated guinea pig ileum to study potent analgesics. In J. M. Singh, L. H. Miller, and H. Lal, Eds. *Drug Addiction: Experimental Pharmacology.* Futura Publishing Co., Mt. Kisco, N.Y. pp. 319–342.

Ferreira, S. H., S. Moncada, and J. R. Vane. 1973. Prostaglandins and the mechanism of analgesia produced by aspirin-like drugs. *Brit. J. Pharmacol.* 49: 86–97.

Ferri, S., A. Santagostino, P. C. Braga, and I. Galatuas. 1974. Decreased antinociceptive effect of morphine in rats treated intraventricularly with prostaglandin E_1. *Psychopharmacologia* (Berlin) 89: 231–235.

Fried, J., T. S. Santhanakrishnan, J. Himizu, C. H. Lin, S. H. Ford, B. Rubin, and E. O. Grigas. 1969. Prostaglandin antagonists: Synthesis and smooth muscle activity. *Nature* (London) 233: 298–300.

Hahn, R. A., and P. N. Patil. 1972. Salivation induced by prostaglandin $F_{2\alpha}$ and modification of the response by atropine and physostigmine. *Brit. J. Pharmacol.* 44: 527–533.

Hahn, R. A., and P. N. Patil. 1974. Further observations on the interaction of prostaglandin $F_{2\alpha}$ with cholinergic mechanisms in canine salivary glands. *Eur. J. Pharmacol.* 25: 279–286.

Harry, J. D. 1968. The action of prostaglandin E_1 on the guinea-pig isolated intestine. *Brit. J. Pharmacol.* 33: 213–214P.

Ho, I. K., H. H. Loh, and E. Leong Way. 1973. Cyclic adenosine monophosphate antagonism of morphine analgesia. *J. Pharmacol. Exp. Therap.* 185: 336–346.

Ku, E. C., and J. M. Wasvary. 1975. Inhibition of prostaglandin synthase by pirprofen. Studies with sheep seminal vesicle enzyme. *Biochim. Biophys. Acta* 384: 360–368.

Ku, E. C., J. M. Wasvary, and W. D. Cash. 1975. Diclofenac sodium (GP 45840, Voltaren), a potent inhibitor of prostaglandin synthetase. *Biochem. Pharmacol.* 24: 641–643.

Lambley, J. E., and A. P. Smith. 1975. The effects of arachidonic acid, indomethacin and SC–19220 on guinea-pig tracheal muscle tone. *Eur. J. Pharmacol.* 30: 148–153.

Masek, K., and O. Kadlec. 1975. The effect of prostaglandins of the E type on peripheral and central release of neurotransmitters. *Abstracts, International Conference on Prostaglandins,* Florence, May, 1975, p. 17.

Northover, B. J. 1973. Effect of antiinflammatory drugs on the binding of calcium to cellular membranes in various human and guinea-pig tissues. *Brit. J. Pharmacol.* 48: 496–504.

Paton, W. D. M. 1957. The action of morphine and related substances on contraction and on acetylcholine output of coaxially stimulated guinea pig ileum. *Brit. J. Pharmacol.* 12: 119–127.

Pert, C. B., and S. W. Snyder. 1973. Opiate Receptor: Demonstration in nervous tissue. *Science* 179: 1011–1014.

Samuelsson, B., and A. Wennmalm. 1971. Increased nerve stimulation induced release of noradrenaline from the rabbit heart after inhibition of prostaglandin synthesis. *Acta Physiol. Scand.* 83–92.

Sanner, J. 1971. Prostaglandin inhibition with a dibenzoxazepine hydrazide derivative and morphine. *Ann. N.Y. Acad. Sci.* 180: 396–409.

Schaumann, W. 1957. Inhibition by morphine of the release of acetylcholine from the intestine of the guinea pig. *Brit. J. Pharmacol.* 12: 115–118.

Smith, W. L., and W. E. M. Lands. 1971. Stimulation and blockade of prostaglandin biosynthesis. *J. Biol. Chem.* 246: 6700–6704.

Splawinski, J. A., A. S. Nies, B. Sweetman, and J. A. Oates. 1973. The effects of arachidonic acid, prostaglandin E_2 and prostaglandin $F_{2\alpha}$ on the longitudinal stomach strip of the rat. *J. Pharmacol. Exp. Therap.* 187: 501–510.

Stjarne, L. 1973. Prostaglandin-verses α-adrenoceptor-mediated control of sympathetic neurotransmitter secretion in guinea-pig isolated vas deferens. *Eur. J. Pharmacol.* 22: 233–238.

Taira, N., and S. Satoh. 1974. Differential effects on the sialogenous and vasodilator actions of prostaglandin E_2 in the dog salivary gland. *Life Sci.* 15: 987–993.

Vane, J. R. 1971. Inhibition of prostaglandin synthesis as a mechanism of action of aspirin-like drugs. *Nature New Biol.* 231: 232–235.

Tissue Responses to Addictive Drugs
© 1976, Spectrum Publications, Inc.

Opiates and the Brain Adenylate Cyclase System

DORIS H. CLOUET

New York State Drug Abuse Control Commission
Testing and Research Laboratory
Brooklyn, New York

KATSUYA IWATSUBO

The University of Osaka Dental School
Osaka, Japan

A synapse consists of three elements: a presynaptic neuron with axons terminating in nerve-endings; an extracellular cleft; and a postsynaptic neuron with membrane receptors, adjoining the cleft. The nerve impulse, characterized in its simplest form, is a transfer of charge (a change in membrane potential) from the presynaptic neuron to the postsynaptic neuron across the cleft by the secretion of neurotransmitters which interact with postsynaptic receptors. Each element of the synapse contains many regulatory and effector mechanisms. In the presynaptic nerve-ending: ions are transferred across the cell membrane to effect a change in membrane potential; cellular components are synthesized in the perikaryon of the neuron and transported along the axons to the nerve-endings; enzyme activities in the nerve-endings are activated or inhibited; neurotransmitters and ions are transported across the synaptic membrane, and transynaptic regulation of neurotransmitter biosynthesis and release occurs either through presynaptic receptors or

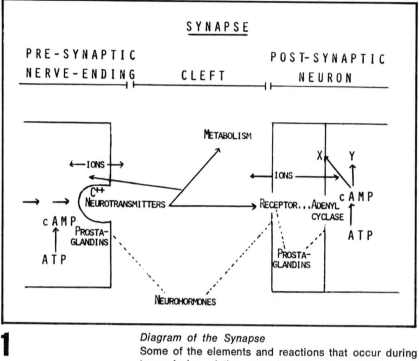

1

Diagram of the Synapse
Some of the elements and reactions that occur during
transmission of the nerve impulse are depicted
diagramatically. C++ = cations; X and Y represent
proteins phosphorylated by protein kinase.

along other nerve pathways. In addition to accommodating the transfer
of ions and transmitters, the synaptic cleft is the route of entry to the
postsynaptic membrane of regulators which are not released from the
presynaptic nerve-ending, and is one site of catabolism of neurotransmitters. In the postsynaptic neuron the synaptic membrane contains
receptors for a variety of neurotransmitters and other neurohormones,
ion pore systems, and an elaborate 'second messenger' system to effect
the many actions which modulate nerve impulse flow, and direct cell
metabolism (see Figure 1).

The relationships at the synapse of polypeptide hormones, neurotransmitters, the cAMP-adenylate cyclase system and opiates will be
reviewed, both because the synapse has been indicated as the site of
action of opiates (Clouet, 1972), and because brain poplpeptides have
been suggested as the natural ligands of the 'opiate receptor' in nervous
tissue (Wahlstrom and Terenius, 1974; Hughes, 1975).

Table I. Peptide Hormones that have been Shown to Alter Adenylate Cyclase Activity in the Anterior Pituitary

Releasing Factor	Activity	Reference
LH-RH*	Release of LH and FSH	Borgeat et al., 1972; Kaneko et al., 1973; Lipmann, 1975
CRH	Release of ACTH	Fleisher et al., 1969
GH-RH	Release of GH	Steiner et al., 1970
TRH	Release of TSH	Bowers, 1971
PRH	Release of Prolactin	Lemay and Labrie, 1972
Somatostatin	Inhibition of release of GH and TSH	Brazeau et al., 1973
PR-IH	Inhibition of release of Prolactin	Lemay and Labrie, 1972

*RH = releasing hormone; LH = luteinizing hormone; FSH = follicle-stimulating hormone; ACTH = adrenocorticotropin; GH = growth hormone; TSH = thyrotropin; PR = prolactin; MSH = melanocyte-stimulating hormone.

In addition, the results of some experiments performed in our laboratory which have a bearing on the site of opiate action at the synapse will be described.

POLYPEPTIDE HORMONES

In endocrine glands and in other tissue, polypeptide hormones have been shown to act by binding to specific sites in cell membranes and thereby activating an adenylate cyclase system in the membrane, changing the levels of cyclic nucleotide in the locus and effecting secondary responses in cyclic nucleotide-sensitive systems. FSH and LH (see legend to Table I for list of abbreviations) act directly on Sertoli cells and interstitial cells of the testis, respectively, to produce an increase in cAMP levels followed by an increased biosynthesis of androgens in the interstitial cells (Heindel et al., 1975). Similarly, vasopressin acts on the kidney plasma membrane to increase cAMP levels and renal transport (Anderson and Brown, 1963; Walter et al., 1972), and ACTH acts in the adrenal to increase cAMP levels and corticosteroid activity (Lefkowitz et al., 1970).

In the anterior pituitary gland, the hypothalamic polypeptide releasing-factors alter adenylate cyclase activity to effect or inhibit the

Table II. Neuronal Activity of Polypeptide Hormones

Polypeptide	Tissue-Effect	Reference
ACTH*	Increase in spontaneous firing in spinal cord	Sawyer et al., 1968
Substance P	Increase in firing rate in: spinal cord cerebral cortex cuneate nucleus	Takahashi et al., 1974; Phillis and Limacher, 1974; Krnjevic et al., 1974
Angiotensin	Increase in spiking frequency in superoptic nucleus	Marks et al., 1974
Bradykinin	Increase in firing in spinal cord	Krivoy et al., 1963
β - MSH	Increase in firing in spinal cord	Krivoy et al., 1974
Physalemin	Increase in firing rate in frog spinal motorneurons	Konishi and Otsuka, 1974
TRH	Decrease in neuronal firing in: cuneate nucleus cerebellar cortex cerebral cortex; hypothalamus	Renaud et al., 1975

*Abbreviations listed in legend to Table I.

release of trophic hormones (see Table I). The involvement of cGMP as well as cAMP in the mechanism of peptide hormone action has been indicated in a study in which somatostatin added to rat pituitaries *in vitro* increased the levels of cGMP and decreased the levels of cAMP while inhibiting GH release (Oka et al., 1975).

Many of the peptide hormones have, in addition to action at specific endocrine receptors, a direct effect on nerve impulse transmission (see Table II). Some peptides (ACTH, substance P, angiotensin, and bradykinin) have been shown to increase the frequency or amplitude of firing in the spinal cord or brain, while other peptides, (TRH, LH-RH, somatostatin, and vasopressin) have been shown to decrease neuronal firing as do some peptides isolated from nonmammalian sources (di Caro et al., 1974).

A possible role for cyclic nucleotides in the direct effects of peptides on neuronal firing has not been investigated as yet.

The administration of opiates has important effects on hypothalamic-pituitary peptides, and on nerve transmission. (Both of these subjects are discussed elsewhere in this volume.)

OPIATES AND ADENYLATE CYCLASE IN BRAIN

The relationship between opiates and the cAMP-adenylate cyclase system has been examined in a number of ways. When cAMP was administered to animals by peripheral injection, the analgesia induced by acute morphine administration was antagonized, and withdrawal signs in morphine-tolerant animals were increased (Ho et al., 1972; 1973). The injection of cAMP into the lateral ventricles of rats also increased withdrawal signs in tolerant animals (Collier and Francis, 1975). In addition to cAMP, adenine, adenosine and ATP pretreatment has been shown to decrease the acute effect of morphine (Gourley and Beckner, 1973), suggesting that the effects of cAMP and related compounds were due to the adenine or adenosine moiety.

In two experiments, the addition of morphine sulfate to brain homogenates increased basal adenylate cyclase activity (Chou et al., 1971; 1975). A PGE₁-stimulated adenylate cyclase in rat brain homogenates was inhibited by morphine sulfate (Collier and Roy, 1974).

There are several reports of the effects of opiate administration on the levels of cAMP in brain, or on adenylate cyclase activity (see Table III). There is no agreement or discernible pattern in the responses reported. As discussed later in regard to our experiments, cAMP is both ubiquitous and ephemeral, so that its levels in whole tissue might be expected to fluctuate widely. When nervous tissue is grown in tissue culture, adenylate cyclase in the cells are sensitive to prostaglandins and catecholamines. Cells derived from a neuroblastoma, or hybrid cells of a neuroblastoma x glioma, contain a PGE-sensitive adenylate cyclase which is inhibited by morphine (Traber et al., 1974; Sharma et al., 1975). Cells derived from a glioma, and from a glioma x fibroblast hybrid, also contain a PGE-stimulated adenylate cyclase, which, however, is not inhibited by morphine (see Table IV). Also seen in neuroblastoma x glioma hybrid cells was an increase in cGMP levels which was induced by active narcotics but not by an inactive isomer or a narcotic antagonist (Traber et al., 1974). Several of the glial lines had norepinephrine-sensitive adenylate cyclase which was also unaffected by morphine. It is interesting that, in mice glial cells grow in culture, the clones with highly-inducible norepinephrine-sensitive adenylate cyclase were found to have the lowest amounts of cell surface antigens (Sundarraj et al., 1975).

Two other aspects of the regulation of adenylate cyclase activity should be considered in relation to opiates: the role of ionic calcium; and changes in the sensitivity of adenylate cyclase to neurohormones. An

Table III. Opiates and Brain Adenylate Cyclase Activity

Tissue	Effect	Reference
A. *Opiates Administered to Animals*		
Rat striatal homogenate	Basal AC* increased 1 hr after morphine in dose-dependent way	Puri et al., 1975
Rat cortex, cerebellar, thalamic homogenates	AC unaltered after acute administration of morphine, but decreased in withdrawal	Singhal et al., 1973
Rat cortex homogenate	AC increased 1 hr after morphine	Chou et al., 1971
Rat brainstem homogenate	AC decreased morphine	Chou et al., 1971
Rat striatal cAMP levels	Increased after morphine	Costa et al., 1973
Rat mid-brain thalamus cAMP levels	Increased 20 min after morphine	Brammer and Paul, 1974
B. *Opiates Added 'In Vitro'*		
Mouse cortex homogenate	Basal AC activated at 10^{-3}M morphine.SO_4	Chou et al., 1971
Rat brain homogenate	PGE-stimulated AC inhibited by 10^{-4}M morphine.SO_4	Collier and Roy, 1974
Rat striatal homogenate	Basal AC activated by 10^{-4}M morphine.SO_4	Puri et al., 1975

*AC = adenylate cyclase activity

increase in calcium ion concentration inhibits adenylate cyclase activity in many tissues, probably by increasing the activity of the cAMP-catabolizing enzyme, phosphodiesterase. A Ca^{++}-protein activator complex increases phosphodiesterase activity (Teshima and Kakiuchi, 1974) and, thus, decreases cAMP (and cGMP) levels. The acute administration of morphine has been shown to decrease Ca^{++} levels in mouse brain (Kaneto, 1971), an effect that might be expected to result in local increases in cAMP levels.

The regulation of adenylate cyclase activity by changes in hormonal sensitivity of the enzyme requires a longer time than does regulation by concentration of cAMP, ATP, ADP, ions, etc., or neurohormonal stimulation. A supersensitivity to norepinephrine was found

Table IV. Opiates and Adenylate Cyclase Activity in Cultures of Nervous Tissue

Line	Adenylate Cyclase		Opiate	Reference
	Basal	+ PGE		
Mouse neuro-blastoma		Stimulated		
N4TG3	NC*	Antagonized by	Morphine, 10^{-6}M	Traber et al., 1974
Rat glioma		Stimulated		
C6-BU-1	NC	NC		
Hybrid: Glioma x fibroblast		Stimulated		
54SCC11	NC	NC		
Hybrid: Glioma x neuroblastoma		Stimulated		
	NC	Antagonized by	Morphine, 10^{-5}M	
Mouse neuro-blastoma		Stimulated		Sharma et al., 1975
N18TG2	NC	Sl. antagonized by	Morphine, 10^{-5}M	
Rat glioma		Stimulated		
C6-BU-1	NC	NC		
Hybrid: Glioma x neuroblastoma		Stimulated		
NG108-15	Sl. Inhibited	Antagonized by	Morphine, 10^{-5}M (Reversed by naloxone)	
NG108-15-morphine-tolerant		Stimulated Large stimulation by	Naloxone	

*NC = no change

in adenylate cyclase in cortex slices isolated from young rats treated with a denervation agent, 6-OH dopamine; and a subsensitivity to norepinephrine was found in the adenylate cyclase of an astrocytoma grown in culture containing norepinephrine (Perkins et al., 1975). Pineal glands grown in culture have a light-sensitive adenylate cyclase that increases in norepinephrine-sensitivity in light or after denervation and decreases in dark, or with isoproterenol (Romero and Axelrod, 1975). The temporally longer mode of control seems to require protein synthesis, since cycloheximide blocks the change in adenylate cyclase sensitivity.

In neurons, adenylate cyclase is localized in postsynaptic membranes, in neuronal perikarya, and in presynaptic nerve-endings. Adenylate cyclase is one of the particulate enzymes that is transported by fast migration through the axons into the nerve-endings (Bray et al., 1971). The particulate enzymes have been shown to travel in dopaminergic pathway from cells in the substantia nigra to the caudate nucleus of the rat in a few hours (Fibiger et al., 1973). In the experiments described below, an hypo-osmotically shocked synaptosomal preparation was used as a source of adenylate cyclase activity in order to include both pre- and post-synaptic enzymes and exclude glial enzymes. The experiments have been reported in detail in appropriate journals (Iwatsubo and Clouet, 1975; Clouet et al., 1975).

EXPERIMENTAL RESULTS

The Effect of Opiates on Adenylate Cyclase 'in vitro'

Basal adenylate cyclase in shocked nerve-ending particles prepared from rat brain areas was inhibited by the addition of 1 mM morphine, l-methadone or levorphanol (see Table V). The addition of the same concentrations of inactive isomers (d-methadone, dextrorphan) or a narcotic antagonist (naloxone) inhibited basal cyclase activity to the same extent, indicating that the inhibition was not specific. The addition of PGE_1 or PGE_2 to the assay had no effect on adenylate cyclase activity in the shocked nerve-ending preparations.

The addition of dopamine to shocked striatal nerve-ending particles *in vitro* increased the activity of adenylate cyclase (Table VI), as found previously in striatal homogenate (Kebabian, et al., 1973). Dopamine-stimulated adenylate cyclase was completely inhibited in this tissue preparation by haloperidol at 3 μM concentration, but was not affected by the addition of morphine in concentrations as high as 3 X 10^{-4}M (see Figure 2). Other opiates also had no effect on dopamine-sensitive adenylate cyclase of shocked striatal synaptosomes in concentrations as high as 10^{-4}M. At higher drug concentrations both basal and dopamine-sensitive adenylate cyclase were inhibited (Iwatsubo and Clouet, 1975).

Table V. Adenylate Cyclase Activity in Nerve-Ending Preparations from Rat Brain Assayed in the Presence of Opiates

Brain Area	Control Levels (pmol cAMP/min/ mg protein)	Adenylate Cyclase Activity % Control Activity					
		Morphine 10^{-4}	10^{-3}	Levorphanol 10^{-4}	10^{-3}	Dextrorphan 10^{-4}	10^{-3}M
Midbrain	218 ± 87*	99	98	81	37	84	37
Striatum	430 ± 49	96	90	101	49	106	57
Medulla	193 ± 22	102	99	91	47	87	39
Cortex	392 ± 47	91	70	90	56	98	48
Hypothalamus	380 ± 36	105	89	72	42	82	49
Cerebellum	617 ± 75	115	108	104	59	100	50

* = standard deviation.

Rats were killed by decapitation, the brains removed and dissected into six areas. The tissues were homogenized in 0.32M sucrose and a crude mitochondrial-synaptosomal fraction was isolated by centrifugation (Chakrin and Whittaker, 1969). The assay in which ATP^{32} is converted to cAMP^{32} is described in detail in Clouet et al., 1975. The underlined values were significantly different from control values.

Table VI. Dopamine-Sensitive Adenylate Cyclase of Striatal Nerve-Ending Preparations

	Adenylate Cyclase Activity (pmol cAMP/min/mg protein)	
	Basal Activity	Dopamine-sensitive
Acute Morphine		
0 (Control)	355 ± 35	505 ± 25
15 minutes	*440 ± 20	605 ± 45
30 minutes	*450 ± 40	*630 ± 25
60 minutes	*580 ± 45	*815 ± 35
120 minutes	445 ± 60	*700 ± 35
240 minutes	345 ± 20	505 ± 15
Morphine Pellets		
0 (Control)	355 ± 35	505 ± 25
1 day	340 ± 40	520 ± 30
2 day	380 ± 45	*605 ± 10
3 day	360 ± 50	*960 ± 25

*Indicates significantly different values.
Morphine was injected acutely at a dose of 60 mg/kg sc. Morphine pellets were implanted s.c. Dopamine was added to adenylate cyclase assays at a concentration of 100 μM.

The Effect of Morphine Treatment on the cAMP-adenylate Cyclase System

The levels of cAMP were measured in homogenates of rat brain areas after the animals were sacrificed by microwave irradiation. An acute injection of morphine (60 mg/kg) produced significant increases in cAMP levels in midbrain, cerebellum, striatum and cortex 15 to 30 minutes after the injection. In three areas (hypothalamus, medulla and cerebellum) the levels of cAMP were significantly lower than control values two hours after the injection of morphine (Clouet, et al., 1975). The two hour values were lower than the levels 15 to 30 minutes after morphine injection in all areas. In morphine-tolerant rats killed two hours after the last of twice daily injections for 10 days, the levels of cAMP were at control levels or higher, indicating that tolerance to decreased cAMP levels had developed (Clouet et al., 1975).

Adenylate cyclase activity was increased in midbrain and striatum one hour after the injection of 60 mg/kg morphine or 15 mg/kg levorphanol, but not after 15 mg/kg dextrorphan. The enzyme activity was decreased only in cerebellum by active narcotic agonists (see Table VII). In tolerant animals, cerebellar adenylate cyclase activity was

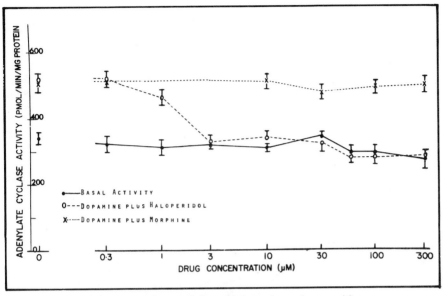

2

Effect of adding morphine or haloperidol on dopamine-sensitive adenylate cyclase of rat striatal synaptosomes
    In the absence of added dopamine, the addition of morphine or haloperidol had little effect on basal adenylate cyclase activity (● - - - - - - - ●). In the presence of 100 μM dopamine, adenylate cyclase activity was measured in the presence of various amounts of morphine (X - - - - - - -X) or haloperidol (O - - - - - - - O).

increased by a morphine challenge, as it was in midbrain and cortex again indicating a tolerance in cerebellar cyclase (Clouet, et al., 1975).

Dopamine-sensitive Adenylate Cyclase in Striatal Nerve-endings

Dopamine-sensitive adenylate cyclase activity in shocked preparations of striatal synaptosomes was increased by acute morphine treatment above control dopamine-stimulation (see Table VI). Even though basal cyclase activity was also increased above control levels from 15 to 60 minutes after morphine injection, the absolute stimulation by 100 μM dopamine was significantly higher at 30 minutes to 2 hours after the injection of the opiate than stimulation by dopamine in preparations from untreated rats. The percent stimulation by dopamine,

**Table VII. Effect of Morphine Treatment on Adenylate Cyclase Activity
in Shocked Nerve-Ending Preparations from
Rat Brain Regions**

| Brain Area | Adenylate Cyclase Activity Naive Rats | | (% Control Activity) Morphine-tolerant Rats |
	Morphine	Levorphanol	Morphine Challenge
Midbrain	*149 ± 8	130 ± 11	*167 ± 10
Striatum	*148 ± 9	*152 ± 8	103 ± 7
Medulla	129 ± 12	92 ± 8	115 ± 11
Cortex	100 ± 10	95 ± 12	*143 ± 8
Hypothalamus	101 ± 11	105 ± 10	87 ± 4
Cerebellum	* 79 ± 8	* 61 ± 5	*148 ± 13

*Indicates a significant difference.

Naive rats were injected with 60 mg/kg morphine or 15 mg/kg levorphanol and killed two hours later. The tolerant rats were injected twice daily with increasing doses of morphine for 10 days. A challenge dose of 100 mg/kg morphine was injected and the rats killed two hours later. Adenylate cyclase activity was measured as described by Clouet et al. (1975).

however, was similar at each time point after acute morphine treatment (Iwatsubo and Clouet, 1975).

Morphine pellets were implanted subcutaneously into groups of rats that were killed at daily intervals thereafter. The basal adenylate cyclase activity in striatal nerve-endings was unchanged for three days after pellet implantation (Table VI). However, on days 2 and 3 after implantation, there was an increased sensitivity of the enzyme to dopamine.

DISCUSSION OF EXPERIMENTAL RESULTS

After the acute administration of morphine, the levels of cAMP in rat brain regions had a general tendency to fall well below control levels by two hours after drug treatment. A transient but significant rise in cAMP levels preceded the fall in some brain areas. Because cAMP levels in a whole tissue represent the sum total of cAMP in various compartments which may or may not be reacting to the presence of the drug, one would not expect a necessary relationship beween cAMP levels in whole tissue and adenylate cyclase activity in shocked nerve-ending preparations from the same tissue. Such a relationship was not found in any brain area except cerebellum, where both the levels and the rates of biosynthesis of cAMP were substantially decreased. The transient fluctuations in cAMP levels and adenylate cyclase activity may explain the seemingly contradictory results found in the literature.

Three significant conclusions may be drawn from the results of these experiments:

1 Opiates do not act directly on the postsynaptic dopamine receptor, as neuroleptics do.

2 Opiates do not inhibit basal adenylate cyclase activity in shocked nerve-ending preparations when the drugs are added to the assay.

3 Dopamine supersensitivity in striatal synaptosomes develops with chronic morphine treatment.

The third conclusion may be related to the pharmacological supersensitivity to dopaminergic agonists such as apomorphine seen in morphine-tolerant animals (Gianutsos et al., 1974).

GENERAL DISCUSSION

The molecular site of opiate action in the central nervous system lies, at least in part, in the general area of the synaptic plasma membrane. The distinction between pre- and postsynaptic membranes, so obvious in simple axonal:receptor cell systems (as depicted in Figure 1) becomes blurred in the brain. Although the principal neuronal connections in brain, as in the periphery, are axonal:dendrite or axonal:cell soma, other synaptic interactions (dendro:dendrite, axonal:axon spine, etc.) are numerous in the central nervous system (Haycock, 1975). Cells may be coupled by serial and reciprocal synapses, so that the same cell membrane may have areas of synaptic vesicles (= output) and areas of "postsynaptic fuzz" (= input) in adjacent segments. Thus, it is possible for opiates to act on an "input region" of the synaptic plasma membrane on either the pre- or postsynaptic cell.

Information on the molecular relationship between membrane receptors in the brain and the regulation of cyclic nucleotide systems by polypeptide hormones, neurotransmitters and prostaglandins is far from complete. Little is known of the molecular architecture of the catalytic, GTP-binding and receptor units of adenylate cyclase in the membranes and its molecular transitions in response to ligand binding. In other tissues, the possibility of both positive and negative cooperativity has been recognized (Rodbell et al., 1975). The competition between membrane stabilizing anesthetics and opiates for stereospecific opiate binding sites (described in this volume by Musacchio et al.) suggests that opiates may bind generally on external membranes surfaces, while other evidence (discussed by Pasternack and Snyder in this volume) suggests a more specific site such as the ion pore. Further experimentation should shed light on this question, as well as on the nature of the biochemical consequences of the initial opiate:membrane interaction.

ACKNOWLEDGMENT

The experimental work described in this paper was supported in part by HEW-NIDA Grant DA-00087.

REFERENCES

Anderson, W. A., and E. Brown. 1963. The influence of arginine-vasopressin upon the production of cAMP by adenyl cyclase from the kidney. *Biochem. Biophys. Acta* 67: 674–676.

Borgeat, P., G. Chavancy, A. Dupont, F. Labrie, A. Arimura, and A. V. Schally. 1972. Stimulation of adenosine 3′, 5′ cyclic monophosphate accumulation in the anterior pituitary gland *in vitro* by synthetic LHRH-FSHRH. *Proc. Nat. Acad. Sci.* 69: 2677–2681.

Bowers, C. Y. 1971. Studies on the role of cyclic AMP in the release of anterior pituitary hormones. In G. A. Robison, G. Nahas, and L. Triner, Eds. *Cyclic AMP and Cell Function*. Ann. New York Acad. Sci. 185, pp 263–291.

Brammer, G. L., and M. I. Paul. 1974. Cyclic AMP and morphine analgesia. *Lancet* Nov. 2, 1084–1085.

Brazeau, P., W. Vale, R. Burgus, N. Line, M. Butcher, J. Rivier, and R. Guillemin. 1973. Hypothalamic polypeptide that inhibits the secretion of immunoreactive pituitary growth hormone. *Science* 179: 77–79.

Bray, J. J., C. M. Kon, and B. M. Breckenridge. 1971. Adenylate cyclase, cyclic nucleotide diesterase and axoplasmic flow. *Brain Res.* 26: 385–394.

Chakrin, L. W., and V. P. Whittaker. 1969. The subcellular distribution of (N-Me-H³) acetylcholine synthesized by brain *in vivo*. *Biochem. J.* 113: 97–107.

Chou, W. S., A. S. K. Ho, and H. H. Loh. 1971. Effect of acute and chronic morphine and norepinephrine on brain adenyl cyclase activity. *Proc. West. Pharmacol. Soc.* 14: 42–46.

Clouet, D. H. 1972. Theoretical biochemical mechanisms for drug dependence. In S. J. Mulé and H. Brill, Eds. *Chemical and Biological Aspects of Drug Dependence.* Chemical Rubber Company Press, Cleveland, Ohio pp. 545–561.

Clouet, D. H., G. J. Gold, and K. Iwatsubo. 1975. Effects of narcotic analgesics on the cyclic AMP-adenylate cyclase system in rat brain. *Brit. J. Pharmacol.* 54: 541–548.

Collier, H. O. J., and D. L. Francis. 1975. Morphine abstinence is associated with increased brain cyclic AMP. *Nature* (London) 255: 159–162.

Collier, H. O. J., and A. C. Roy. 1974. Morphine-like drugs inhibit the stimulation by E prostaglandins of cAMP formation by rat brain homogenates. *Nature* (London) 248: 24–27.

Costa, E., A. Carenzi, A. Guidotti, and A. Revuelta. 1973. Narcotic analgesics and the regulation of neuronal catecholamine stores. In E. Usdin and S. Snyder, Eds. *Frontiers in Catecholamine Research.* Pergamon Press, New York, pp. 1003–1010.

diCaro, G., L. G. Micossi, and F. Venturi. 1974. Behavioral and electrocortical modifications induced in the rat by intraventricular injection of physalaemin and eledoism. *Psychopharmacol.* (Berlin) 38: 211–218.

Fibiger, H. C., E. G. McGeer, and S. Atmadja. 1973. Axoplasmic transport of dopamine in nigro-striatal neurons. *J. Neurochem.* 21: 373–385.

Fleischer, H., R. A. Donald, and R. W. Butcher. 1969. Involvement of adenosine 3' 5' monophosphate in the release of ACTH. *Am. J. Physiol.* 5: 1287–1291.

Gianutsos, G., M. D. Hynes, S. K. Puri, R. B. Drawbaugh, and H. Lal. 1974. Effect of apomorphine and nigrostriatal lesions on aggression and striatal dopamine turnover during morphine withdrawal: Evidence for dopamine supersensitivity in protracted abstinence. *Psychopharmacolog.* (Berlin) 34: 37–44.

Gourley, D. R. J., and S. K. Beckner. 1973. Antagonism of morphine analgesia by adenine, adenosine and adenine nucleotides. *Proc. Soc. Exp. Biol. Med.* 144: 774–778.

Haycock, J. 1975. New varieties of synaptic interactions. In *Soc. Neurosci. Symp.* (IV Ann. Meeting, Brain Information Service) U. Calif. Los Angeles, Calif. pp. 41–47.

Heindel, J. J., R. Rothenberg, G. A. Robison, and A. Steinberger. 1975. LH and FSH stimulation of cyclic AMP in specific cell types isolated from the testis. *J. Cyclic Nucleotide Res.* 1: 69–70.

Ho, I. K., H. H. Loh, and E. L. Way. 1972. Effect of cAMP on morphine analgesia, tolerance and dependence. *Nature* (London) 238: 397–398.

Ho, I. K., H. H. Loh, and E. L. Way. 1973. Cyclic adenosine monophosphate antagonism of morphine analgesia. *J. Pharmacol. Exp. Therap.* 185: 336–346.

Hughes, J. 1975. Isolation of an endogenous compound from the brain with pharmacological properties similar to morphine. *Brain Res.* 88: 295–308.

Iwatsubo, K., and D. H. Clouet. 1975. Dopamine-sensitive adenylate cyclase of the caudate nucleus of rats treated with morphine or haloperidol. *Biochem. Pharmacol.* 24: 1499–1503.

Kaneko, T., S. Saito, H. Oka, T. Oda, and N. Yanaihara. 1973. Effects of synthetic LH-RH and its analogs on rat anterior pituitary cAMP and LH and FSH release. *Metabolism* 22: 77–78.

Kaneto, H. 1971. The role of calcium on the action of narcotic analgesic drugs. In D. H. Clouet, Ed. *Narcotic Drugs: Biochemical Pharmacology.* Plenum Press, New York, pp. 300–309.

Konishi, S., and M. Otsuka. 1974. Excitatory action of hypothalamic substance P on spinal motor neurons of newborn rats. *Nature* (London) 252: 734–735.

Krebabian, J. W., G. L. Petzold, and P. Greengard. 1973. Dopamine-sensitive adenylate cyclase in the caudate nucleus of rat brain and its similarity to the 'dopamine receptor'. *Proc. Nat. Acad. Sci.* 69: 2145–2149.

Krivoy, W., M. Bodansky, and S. Lande. 1963. Neurological and oxytocic actions of some nonapeptides related to bradykinin. *Biochem. Pharmacol.* 12: 179–180.

Krivoy, W., D. Kroeger, A. N. Taylor, and E. Zimmerman. 1974. Antagonism of morphine by β-melanocyte-stimulating hormone and by tetracosactin. *Eur. J. Pharmacol.* 27: 339–345.

Krnjevic, K., and M. E. Morris. 1974. An excitatory action of substance P on cuneate neurons. *Canad. J. Physiol. Pharmacol.* 52: 736–744.

Lefkowitz, R. J., J. Roth, W. Pricer, and I. Pastan. 1970. ACTH receptors in the adrenal: Specific binding of ACTH-[125] and its relation to adenyl cyclase. *Proc. Nat. Acad. Sci.* 65: 745–752.

Lemay, A., and F. Labrie. 1972. Calcium-dependent stimulation of prolactin release in rat anterior pituitary *in vitro* by N[6]-monbutyryl adenosine 3' 5' monophosphate. *FEBS Letters* 20: 7–10.

Lipmann, W. 1975. Stimulation of cAMP accumulation in rat anterior pituitary *in vitro* by analogs of LH-RH. *Experientia* 31: 403–404.

Marks, B. H., K. K. Satai, J. M. George, and A. Koestner. 1974. A new technique for studying neuroendocrine systems. In E. Zimmerman and R. George, Eds. *Narcotics and the Hypothalamus.* Raven Press, New York, pp. 96–106.

Oka, H., T. Kaneko, M. Munemura, T. Oda, and N. Yanaihara. 1975. *In vitro* effects of synthetic somatostatin on cyclic nucleotide levels and GH release in rat anterior pituitary gland. In G. I. Drummond, P. Greengard and G. A. Robinson, Eds. *Adv. Cyclic Nucleotide Res.* Vol. 5. Raven Pres, New York, pp. 804–814.

Perkins, J. P. M., M. M. Moore, A. Kalisher, and Y-F Su. 1975. Regulation of cAMP content in normal and malignant brain cells. In Drummond et al., Eds. *Adv. Cyclic Nucleotide Res.,* Vol 5. Raven Press, New York, pp. 641–660.

Phillis, J. W., and J. J. Limacher. 1974. Substance P excitation of cerebral cortical beta cells. *Brain Res.* 69: 158–163.

Puri, S. K., J. Cochin, and L. Volicer. 1975. Effect of morphine sulfate on adenylate cyclase and phosphodiesterase activities in rat corpus striatum. *Life Sci.* 16: 759–768.

Renaud, L. P., J. B. Martin, and P. Brazeau. 1975. Depressant action of TRH, LH-RH and somatostatin on activity of central neurons. *Nature* (London) 255: 233–235.

Rodbell, M., M. C. Lin, Y. Salomon, C. Londos, J. P. Harwood, B. R. Martin, M. Rendell, and M. Berman. 1975. Role of adenine and guanine nucleotides in the activity and response of adenylate cyclase systems to hormones. In Drummond et al., Eds. *Adv. Cyclic Nucleotide Res.*, Vol. 5. Raven Press, New York, pp. 3–30.

Romero, J. A., and J. Axelrod. 1975. Regulation of sensitivity to β-adrenergic stimulation in induction of pineal N-acetyltransferase. *Proc. Nat. Acad. Sci.* 72: 1661–1665.

Sawyer, C. H., M. Kakakami, B. Meyerson, D. I. Whitmeyer, and J. J. Lilley. 1968. Effects of ACTH, dexamethasone and asphyxia on electrical activity of the rat hypothalamus. *Brain Res.* 10: 213–226.

Sharma, S. K., M. Nirenberg, and W. A. Klee. 1975. Morphine receptors as regulators of adenylate cyclase activity. *Proc. Nat. Acad. Sci.* 72: 590–594.

Singhal, R. L., S. Kacew, and R. Lafreniere. 1973. Brain adenyl cyclase in methadone treatment of morphine dependency. *J. Pharm. Pharmacol.* 25: 1022–1024.

Steiner, A. L., G. T. Peake, R. D. Utiger, I. E. Karl, and LDM Kipnis. 1970. Hypothalamic stimulation of growth hormone and thyrotropin release *in vitro* and pituitary 3″ 5″ adenosine cyclic monophosphate. *Endocrinol.* 86: 1354–1364.

Sundarraj, N., M. Schactner, and S. E. Pfeiffer. 1975. Biochemically different mouse glial cell lines carrying a nervous system-specific cell surface antigen. *Proc. Nat. Acad. Sci.* 72: 1927–1931.

Takahashi, T., S. Konishi, D. Powell, S. E. Leeman, and M. Otsuka. 1974. Identification of the motor neuron-depolarizing peptide in bovine dorsal root as hypothalamic substance P. *Brain Res.* 73: 59–69.

Terenius, L., and A. Wåhlstrom. 1974. Inhibition of narcotic receptor binding in brain extracts and cerebrospinal fluid. *Acta Pharmacol. Toxicol.* 34: 55.

Teshima, Y., and S. Kakiuchi. 1974. Mechanism of stimulation of Ca^{++} plus Mg^{++}-dependent phosphodiesterase from rat cerebral cortex by the modulator protein and Ca^{++}. *Biochem. Biophys. Res. Comm.* 56: 489–495.

Traber, J., K. Fischer, S. Latzin, and B. Hamprecht. 1974. Morphine antagonizes the action of prostaglandin in neuroblastoma cells but not of PGE or norepinephrine in glioma and glioma X fibroblast hybrid cells. *FEBS Letters* 49: 260–263.

Walter, R., M. A. Kirchberger, and V. J. Hruby. 1972. Competitive inhibitors of neurohypophyseal hormones on adenylate cyclase from toad urinary bladder. *Experientia* 28: 959–960.

Tissue Responses to Addictive Drugs
© 1976, Spectrum Publications, Inc.

The Opiate Receptor: Relevance of Binding to Pharmacological Activity

IAN CREESE
SOLOMON H. SNYDER

*Departments of Pharmacology and Experimental Therapeutics
and
Psychiatry and the Behavioral Sciences
Johns Hopkins University School of Medicine
Baltimore, Maryland*

A major reason for concluding that stereospecific opiate receptor binding in the brain involves the pharmacologically relevant opiate receptors is that the affinities of a large number of opiate agonists and antagonists for the opiate receptor parallel, in general, their analgesic potency or their ability to antagonize the actions of opiate agonists in intact animals and man (Pert and Snyder, 1973a; Simon et al., 1973; Pert et al., 1973; Pert and Snyder, 1974; and Terenius, 1974). However, it is inherently difficult to establish vigorous correlations between *in vivo* pharmacological effects and *in vitro* binding affinities, because *in vivo* potencies are determined in part by the differential metabolism of the drugs as well as variations in the ability of drugs to penetrate from the circulation into the brain. In order to relate, with precision, features of opiate receptor binding to pharmacological activity, it is important that both pharmacological activity and binding be measured in a functional tissue where these problems can be minimized.

315

The guinea pig intestine is a valuable *in vitro* model system for studying the actions of opiates. The ability of opiate agonists to inhibit the electrically induced contractions of the longitudinal muscle of the ileum, or the ability of opiate antagonists to reverse this inhibition, closely parallels their *in vivo* pharmacological potency (Paton, 1957; and Kosterlitz et al., 1973). The site of opiate action is neuronal, within the myenteric plexus, and is mediated by a decrease in the release of acetylcholine following the electrical stimulation (Paton, 1957; Cox and Weinstock, 1966; and Lees et al., 1973). Stereospecific opiate receptor binding has been identified in the ileum preparation (Terenius, 1972). It is restricted to the myenteric plexus and is not present on the longitudinal muscle itself (Pert and Snyder, 1973a).

The guinea pig intestine thus affords an excellent system in which to determine the pharmacological potency of opiates *in vitro* in functioning tissue and correlate it directly with receptor binding.

CHARACTERISTICS OF OPIATE RECEPTOR BINDING IN THE GUINEA PIG INTESTINE

Stereospecific opiate receptor binding of the tritiated antagonist, naloxone, was measured by a modification of the rapid filtration method of Pert and Snyder (1973a). Since it was the intention to directly investigate the relationship between drug receptor occupation at equilibrium and the pharmacological response of the tissue to the drug, it was, of necessity, imperative that both opiate receptor binding and the pharmacological response to the opiate be measured under identical conditions. It has been previously demonstrated that opiate receptor binding is extremely sensitive to the ionic environment; for example whereas sodium selectively decreases the binding of opiate agonists while increasing antagonist binding (Pert et al., 1973; Pert and Snyder, 1974; and Simon et al., 1975), low concentrations of manganese and other divalent cations can selectively enhance opiate agonist binding without affecting that of opiate antagonists (Pasternak et al., 1975b). Thus, in the studies reported here, both the opiate receptor binding and the *in vitro* pharmacological response to opiates were investigated in a full, physiological, ion complement, Krebs buffer. It is also important to note that in the binding studies incubations were conducted at the physiological temperature, 37°C, to equilibrium and the samples then filtered immediately—without the cooling on ice as performed by many investigators. This is an important methodological and theoretical

**Table I. Stereospecificity of Opiate Binding to
Homogenates of Guinea Pig Intestine**

Opiate	IC_{50} for Inhibition of Stereospecific ^{3}H-Naloxone Binding (nM)
(−)-3-Hydroxy-N-allyl-morphinan (Levallorphan)	2.9
(+)-3-Hydroxy-N-allyl-morphinan (Dextrallorphan)	2800
Levorphanol	30
Dextrorphan	8500
(−)-Methadone	180
(+)-Methadone	2200

consideration as the brief cooling on ice before filtration is sufficient only to disturb the equilibrium reached at 37°C and, moreover, temperature itself can have profound influences on opiate agonist and antagonist receptor binding (Creese et al., 1975). The binding of unlabeled opiates was investigated by determining the concentrations required to inhibit the binding of ^{3}H-naloxone by 50% (IC_{50}). The complete details of these methods have been published elsewhere (Creese and Snyder, 1975).

The properties of ^{3}H-naloxone binding in homogenates of the guinea pig intestine were very similar to those previously described in rat brain homogenates (Pert and Snyder, 1973a; and Pert and Snyder, 1973b). Since the pharmacological experiments in this study employed strips of the longitudinal muscle and myenteric plexus, we compared the binding of ^{3}H-naloxone to minces of such strips which contain intact pieces of tissue, with its binding to homogenates of the strips. ^{3}H-Naloxone binding was saturable in both homogenates and minces with the same K_D value of about 4 nM for both preparations.

Binding was highly stereospecific (see Table I); levorotatory isomers were much more potent inhibitors of ^{3}H-naloxone binding than dextrorotatory isomers. The lesser stereospecificity of the methadone isomers, similar to previous findings with brain homogenates (Pert and Snyder, 1973b), may be related to the greater comformational mobility of methadone as compared to levorphanol.

COMPARISON OF OPIATE RECEPTOR BINDING IN HOMOGENATES OF THE GUINEA PIG INTESTINE AND RAT BRAIN

There was a highly significant correlation between the relative potencies of an extensive series of opiate agonists, mixed agonist-antagonists, and antagonists in their ability to inhibit ^{3}H-naloxone binding to homogenates of guinea pig intestine and to homogenates of rat brain when assayed in the presence of sodium (see Figure 1). A linear regression analysis of the relative potencies of opiates (morphine = 1 in each case) in the intestine and brain receptor binding assays yielded a slope of 1.10 which was not significantly different from 1.0 ($p < 0.05$). The correlation coefficient between the relative potencies of the opiates in the brain and intestine was highly significant ($r = 0.96$, $p < 0.001$). Since intestinal assays were performed in physiological buffer which contained sodium, the IC_{50} values, especially for agonists, were much more similar to those for the brain assayed with, rather than without, sodium (see Table II). This close agreement in absolute IC_{50} values is even more impressive in light of the fact that the assay conditions were somewhat different for brain and intestine.

COMPARISON OF THE EFFECTS OF OPIATES ON RECEPTOR BINDING AND ELECTRICALLY INDUCED CONTRACTIONS OF THE GUINEA PIG INTESTINE

The detailed methods for the investigation of opiate effects on the electrically induced contractions of the longitudinal muscle and myenteric plexus strips have been published elsewhere (Creese and Snyder, 1975). In brief, the strip is suspended in an organ bath in oxygenated buffer at 37°C and stimulated by supramaximal electrical field stimulation once every 10 seconds. The contractions of the strip are measured by an attached force-displacement transducer and recorded on an oscillograph. Opiates are added in small volumes to the bath and are allowed to remain in contact until a maximal pharmacological response is achieved. The differences in the time taken to reach a maximal response for different opiates (see Figure 2) are related to their lipid solubility (Kosterlitz, personal communication).

Normorphine is a useful drug for evaluating opiate effects on electrically induced contractions of the guinea pig intestinal strips because of its quick onset of action and the rapid recovery of contractions when normorphine is washed out (Kosterlitz et al., 1973) (see Figure 2). The potency of normorphine in inhibiting the electrically

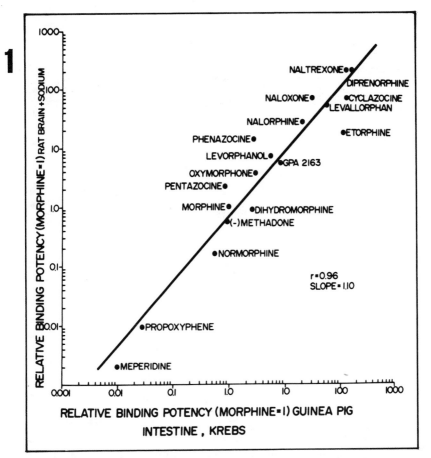

Correlation between the relative potencies of opiates to inhibit ^{3}H-naloxone binding in the guinea pig intestine and rat brain homogenates. The relative potencies of opiates were calculated from IC_{50} determinations for each drug to inhibit stereospecific ^{3}H-naloxone binding in either homogenates of the guinea pig intestine longitudinal muscle and myenteric plexus preparation (assayed in Krebs-Tris, 37°C, pH 7.4) or homogenates of rat brain (assayed in 50 mM Tris + 100 mM NaCl, 25°C, pH 7.7). The IC_{50} for morphine was taken as the standard in each system and given the value of 1. (The rat brain data is taken from Pert and Snyder (1974.)

induced contractions of the intestinal strips correlated closely with its potency in inhibiting ^{3}H-naloxone binding (see Figure 3). Indeed, at all concentrations of normorphine examined the extent of the inhibition of ^{3}H-naloxone binding and of the electrically induced contractions was essentially the same. The slopes of the dose response curves generated

Table II. IC_{50} Values for the Inhibition of ^{3}H-Naloxone Binding by
Opiates in Homogenates of the Guinea Pig Intestine and Rat Brain

Opiate	IC_{50} for Inhibition of Stereospecific ^{3}H-Naloxone Binding (nM)		
	Guinea Pig Intestine	Rat Brain	Rat Brain
	(Krebs-Tris)	(Tris + 100 mM NaCl)	(Tris No NaCl)
Diprenorphine	0.97	0.5	0.5
Cyclazocine	1.25	1.5	0.9
Naltrexone	1.25	0.5	0.5
Etorphine	1.4	6.0	0.5
Levallorphan	2.9	2.0	1.0
Naloxone	5.3	1.5	1.5
Nalorphine	8.0	4.0	1.5
GPA 2163	23	20	100
Levorphanol	30	15	1.0
Oxymorphone	57	30	1.0
Phenazocine	60	8.0	0.6
Dihydromorphine	65	140	3.0
Morphine	170	110	3.0
(−) Methadone	180	200	7.0
Pentazocine	200	50	15
Normorphine	300	700	15
Propoxyphene	6,000	12,000	200
Meperidine	17,500	50,000	3,000

Guinea pig intestine was homogenized in Krebs-Tris solution and assayed at 37°C (pH 7.4). Rat brain was homogenized in 0.05 M Tris and assayed at 25°C (pH 7.7) ± 100 mM NaCl. [The rat brain data is taken from Pert and Snyder (1974).]

for normorphine in the binding assay and in the pharmacological assay were closely similar and the IC_{50} for both processes was the same, about 250 nM.

To compare in greater detail the correlation between potency for receptor binding and for pharmacological actions, we evaluated a wide range of opiate agonists and antagonists, determining ID_{50} values for agonist activity corresponding to the molar concentration for a 50% maximal pharmacological response and K_e values for antagonist activity. The IC_{50} values for opiate receptor binding were transformed into apparent K_D values by correcting for the small fraction of opiate sites occupied by the ^{3}H-naloxone in the assay system (Colquhoun, 1973). The resultant K_D values presumably represent the concentrations of the various drugs required to occupy 50% of receptor binding sites and were compared with the ID_{50} concentrations of these drugs to inhibit the

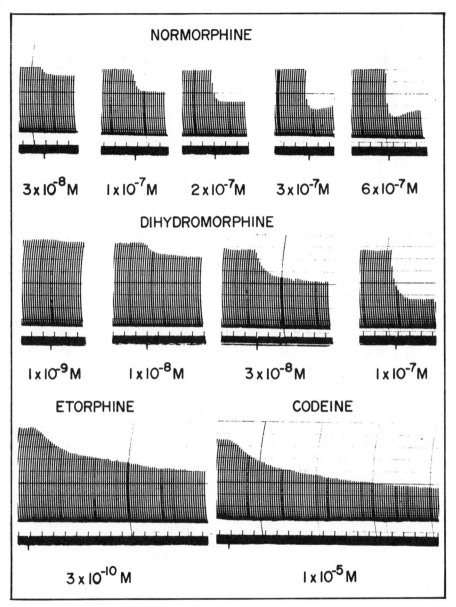

NORMORPHINE

3×10^{-8} M 1×10^{-7} M 2×10^{-7} M 3×10^{-7} M 6×10^{-7} M

DIHYDROMORPHINE

1×10^{-9} M 1×10^{-8} M 3×10^{-8} M 1×10^{-7} M

ETORPHINE   CODEINE

3×10^{-10} M 1×10^{-5} M

2 Inhibition of the electrically induced contractions of the guinea pig intestine by opiate agonists. The upper trace represents the degree of contraction of the myenteric plexus and longitudinal muscle strip which was supramaximally stimulated every 10 sec for 1.5 msec. The lower trace is a time scale, deflections upwards indicating 1 min intervals and deflections downwards the addition of drug.

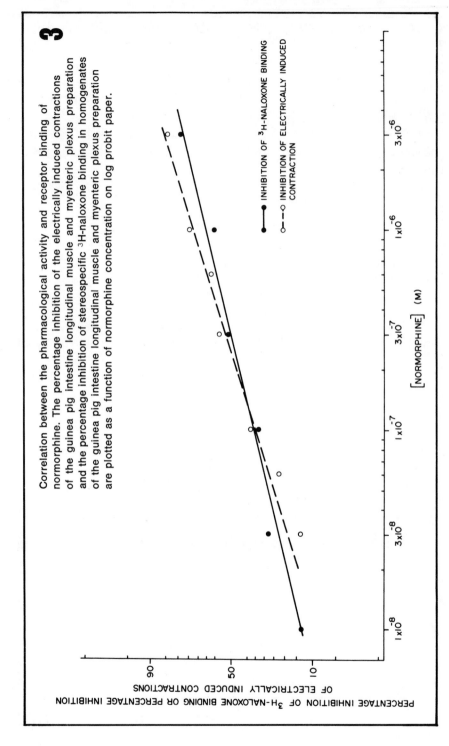

3

Correlation between the pharmacological activity and receptor binding of normorphine. The percentage inhibition of the electrically induced contractions of the guinea pig intestine longitudinal muscle and myenteric plexus preparation and the percentage inhibition of stereospecific ^{3}H-naloxone binding in homogenates of the guinea pig intestine longitudinal muscle and myenteric plexus preparation are plotted as a function of normorphine concentration on log probit paper.

INHIBITION OF ^{3}H-NALOXONE BINDING

INHIBITION OF ELECTRICALLY INDUCED CONTRACTION

[NORMORPHINE] (M)

PERCENTAGE INHIBITION OF ^{3}H-NALOXONE BINDING OR PERCENTAGE INHIBITION OF ELECTRICALLY INDUCED CONTRACTIONS

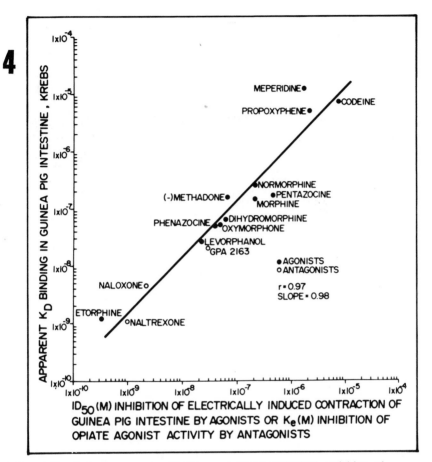

Correlation between receptor binding and pharmacological activities of opiates in the guinea pig intestine. The K_D values (determined by the inhibition of stereospecific ^{3}H-naloxone binding in homogenates of the guinea pig intestine longitudinal muscle and myenteric plexus preparation) for a series of opiate agonists and antagonists are plotted against the ID_{50} concentration, for agonists, required to inhibit the electrically induced contractions of the guinea pig intestine longitudinal muscle and myenteric plexus preparation by 50%, or the K_e value for antagonist inhibition of agonist activity in the same preparation.

electrically induced contractions of the guinea pig intestinal strip by 50% or with the K_e concentration for antagonists (see Figure 4).

There was an extremely close correlation between the effects of drugs on ^{3}H-naloxone binding and on electrically induced contractions. The extent of the correlation between opiate effects on binding and on contraction appeared to be the same for pure agonists, mixed agonist-antagonists and for relatively pure antagonists. The linear regression analysis for these values for all drugs described a line with a slope of 0.98 which did not differ significantly from 1.0, representing a perfect correlation. The extent of the correlation was statistically impressive ($r = 0.97$, $p < 0.001$) (see Figure 4).

In our initial studies of opiate receptor binding in the rat brain we found evidence for only one saturable component of opiate binding (Pert and Snyder, 1973b). More recently, using opiates of much higher specific activity it has been possible to demonstrate a novel higher affinity binding in addition to the initially described sites of somewhat lower affinity (Pasternak and Snyder, 1975a). In guinea pig intestine homogenates as well as in rat brain homogenates assayed in Krebs-Tris solution at 37°C there was evidence for two saturable components of ^{3}H-dihydromorphine binding (see Figure 5). The high affinity site determined by Scatchard analysis in both tissues had a K_D of about 0.9 nM, while the K_D for the low affinity sites was 25 nM in rat brain and 65 nM in intestinal homogenates. The significance of this apparent 2.6-fold difference in K_D values for guinea pig intestine and rat brain is unclear. Since the concentration of dihydromorphine which inhibited electrically induced contractions of the intestine by 50% was 62 nM, the low affinity binding sites for dihydromorphine in the intestine may be the ones which are pharmacologically relevant. Similar experiments were performed for ^{3}H-levorphanol binding. High affinity and low affinity binding components for ^{3}H-levorphanol had respective K_D values of about 1 nM and about 20 nM. The concentration of levorphanol which inhibited electrically induced contractions of the intestinal strips was 30 nM, corresponding to the K_D value for the low affinity binding site. However, if high and low affinity binding represents opiate interactions with two interconvertible receptor conformations (Pasternak and Snyder, 1975a), other interpretations may be appropriate (see Discussion section below). Interestingly, in the guinea pig intestinal homogenates, we did not detect evidence for multiple binding sites for ^{3}H-naloxone as observed in the brain (Pasternak and Snyder, 1975a). The significance of this result is unclear and could merely be a technical artifact related to the greater difficulty of receptor assay in intestine than brain. For the brain, with numerous tritium labeled ligands, the total number of receptors is a constant value (Pert and Snyder, 1973b; Simon et al., 1973; and Pert and Snyder, 1974).

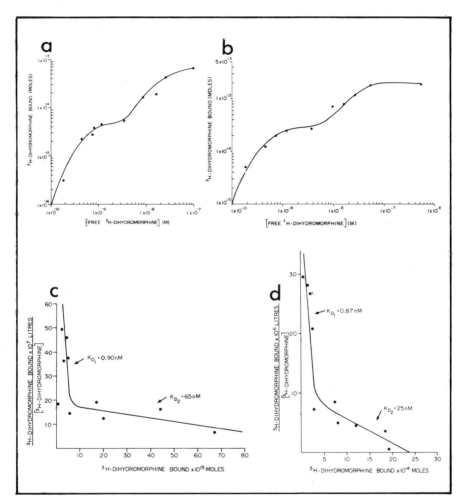

5 Binding of ³H-dihydromorphine in homogenates of guinea pig intestine and rat brain assayed in Krebs-Tris at 37°C. a) Saturation of stereospecific ³H-dihydromorphine binding in homogenates of the guinea pig intestine longitudinal muscle and myenteric plexus preparation. b) saturation of stereospecific ³H-dihydromorphine binding in homogenates of rat brain. c) Scatchard plot of ³H-dihydromorphine binding in homogenates of the guinea pig intestine longitudinal muscle and myenteric plexus preparation. d) Scatchard plot of ³H-dihydromorphine binding in homogenates of rat brain.

RELATIONSHIP BETWEEN OPIATE AND SEROTONINERGIC MECHANISMS IN THE INTESTINE

Gaddum and Picarelli (1957) and Gintzler and Musacchio (1974) have demonstrated complex interactions between serotonin, LSD, and morphine in the guinea pig intestine. Moreover, Schulz and Goldstein (1973) demonstrated an apparent supersensitivity to the spasmogenic action of serotonin in this preparation following opiate addiction. We investigated this interaction by studying the binding of d-^{3}H-LSD, a potent peripheral serotonin antagonist, to the myenteric plexus and longitudinal muscle preparation. d-^{3}H-LSD binding showed a high degree of stereospecificity (see Figure 6). Scatchard analysis (see Figure 7) demonstrated that the stereospecific binding of LSD was of a high affinity, 12 nM, similar to that found in the brain (Snyder and Bennett, 1975). ^{3}H-LSD binding was displaced by serotonin with an IC_{50} of about 1 μM corresponding to the ID_{50} concentration for the spasmogenic action of serotonin. Other LSD and tryptamine analogs displaced ^{3}H-LSD binding with similar affinities in the intestine to those found in the brain (see Table III). Investigation of the stereospecific binding of ^{3}H-LSD and ^{3}H-naloxone to innervated and denervated sections of the longitudinal muscle indicated that whereas naloxone binding was neuronal, LSD binding took place to both the muscle and the myenteric plexus (see Table IV). Moreover, the recent intracellular recording of responses of myenteric neurones to serotonin by North (personal communication) has demonstrated two distinct serotonin sensitive neurones as well as the serotonin receptor on the longitudinal muscle itself. The presence of three distinct receptor sites for serotonin (which also have distinct pharmacological properties) makes valid comparisons between binding and pharmacological data difficult. However, we can state that, in collaboration with Dr. J. P. Bennett, Jr., we were unable to show any interaction between pharmacologically active concentrations of opiates and ^{3}H-LSD binding in the intestine or brain, nor could we find any evidence for an increase in the number of LSD receptors in the intestine or brain, and serotonin receptors in the brain, in the opiate addicted guinea pig or rat.

DISCUSSION

The major finding of the present study is the extraordinarily close correlation between the affinity for opiate receptor binding sites and the ability of opiate agonists and antagonists to influence the electrically induced contractions of the guinea pig intestine. These data provide

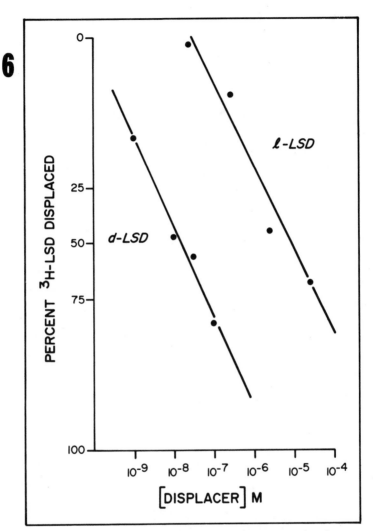

Stereospecificity of d-³H-LSD binding in guinea pig intestine myenteric plexus and longitudinal muscle preparation. Homogenates of myenteric plexus and longitudinal muscle were assayed at 37° in Tris buffer (pH 7.2) + 0.1% ascorbic acid with d-³H-LSD and varying concentrations of d- and l-LSD.

strong evidence that the receptor binding sites investigated here and in our previous studies are those which are "pharmacologically relevant."

The detailed comparison of binding and pharmacological potencies in the present study may have bearing on certain questions regarding the mechanisms of drug-receptor interaction. Some receptor theories,

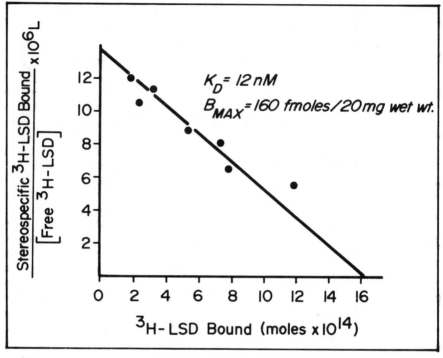

$K_D = 12\,nM$

$B_{MAX} = 160\,fmoles/20\,mg\ wet\ wt.$

7   Scatchard plot of d-^{3}H-LSD binding in guinea pig myenteric plexus and longitudinal muscle preparation.

Table III. Comparison of the Displacement of Stereospecific ^{3}H-LSD Binding from Guinea Pig Longitudinal Muscle-Myenteric Plexus Intestinal Preparations and Rat Brain Cerebral Cortex Membranes

	Guinea Pig Intestine IC_{50} nM	Rat Brain* IC_{50} nM
d-LSD	17	9.5
l-LSD	10,000	20,000
2-Bromo LSD	3.5	7.5
Methysergide	60	100
Serotonin	1,000	3,000
Bufotenine	780	2,000

*Rat brain data from Snyder and Bennett (1975).

**Table IV. The Effect of Denervation of the Longitudinal
Muscle-Myenteric Plexus Preparation of the Guinea Pig
Intestine on Receptor Binding**

	Innervated	Denervated	% Decrease
	(fmoles/mg protein)		
Stereospecific ^{3}H-LSD	62.6	25.3	60
Stereospecific ^{3}H-Naloxone	43.3	7.6	82

based on studies of drug effects on guinea pig intestinal contractions, posit that for many agonist drugs, a maximal pharmacological response can be elicited when only a small fraction of the pharmacologically active receptors are occupied (Stephenson, 1956; Nickerson, 1956; and Ariens et al., 1960). However, in these previous studies receptor occupation was never measured directly with a radioactively labeled ligand, but inferred from the pharmacological response. If a substantial proportion of opiate receptors are "spare receptors," then there should be major differences between the concentration of drugs which occupy 50% of receptor sites, as measured in binding studies, and the concentrations which produce 50% of the maximal pharmacological response. For four ^{3}H-opiate agonists and antagonists the K_D value, representing the concentration of drug for 50% receptor occupation, was determined directly from the binding of the drug to receptor sites. For a large number of nonradioactive opiate agonists and antagonists the K_D value was determined from the concentration of the drug which inhibited ^{3}H-naloxone binding by 50%. In all cases the K_D value for receptor binding corresponded closely to the ID_{50} or K_e value for the pharmacological response. There was no evidence for major, systematic discrepancies. There was also an excellent agreement between the complete dose response curves for normorphine in the binding and pharmacological studies. Thus, our data suggest that pharmacological responses to opiates in the guinea pig intestine can be explained without evoking the concept of spare receptors. It is possible that some of the binding demonstrated may correspond to "silent receptors" (Goldstein, 1949) which bind opiates but do not provide a biological effect.

It has been suggested that the many variations in pharmacological potency among drugs are determined by the relative contribution of affinity for receptor sites and "intrinsic activity" (Ariens, 1954; and Ariens et al., 1957) or "efficacy" (Stephenson, 1956). According to these

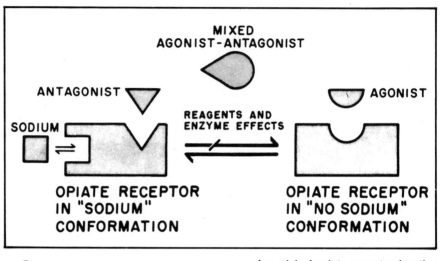

8

A model of opiate receptor function

theories a series of drugs may all have the same affinity for the receptor but differ in their capability to initiate the biological response, that is, intrinsic activity, and accordingly have different pharmacological potencies. However, the fact that for almost all opiate agonists examined, the concentration required to occupy 50% of the receptor binding sites corresponded to the concentration required to produce 50% of the maximal pharmacological response indicates that receptor affinity alone would suffice to account for the pharmacological potency of opiate agonist drugs.

One major rationale for invoking the concept of intrinsic activity is the need to explain the actions of pharmacological antagonists. It is usually postulated that an antagonist occupies the agonist receptor site but has no intrinsic activity. While the precise mechanism of action of opiate antagonists is unclear, data from our laboratory on the differential influence of sodium on receptor binding of opiate agonists and antagonists may provide a molecular mechanism accounting for the different "intrinsic activity" of opiate agonists and antagonists. Sodium enhances the binding of antagonists and diminishes the binding of agonists (Pert et al., 1973), suggesting that the opiate receptor exists as a reversible equilibrium between two interconvertible conformations (see Figure 8) (Pert and Snyder, 1974). We have hypothesized that sodium acts as an allosteric effector, driving the equilibrium in the direction favoring the binding of antagonists while concurrently decreasing the binding of agonists (Pert and Snyder, 1975). Whereas antagonists have a high affinity for the "sodium" form of the receptor, agonists have a very low affinity. However, agonists have a substantial affinity for the "nonsodium" form of the receptor. Mixed agonist-antagonists have intermediate affinities for the two forms (Pert, et al., 1976). The high and low affinity binding of the agonist dihydromorphine seen in these experiments, and in the brain (Pasternak and Snyder, 1975a), may thus involve "nonsodium" and "sodium" receptor states of the receptor respectively.

This model provides a simple molecular mechanism to explain opiate agonist and antagonist activity (Snyder, 1975). If the pharmacological effects of opiate agonists are mediated by the "nonsodium" receptors, then by binding to the "sodium" form of the receptor, opiate antagonists would lower the available number of "nonsodium" receptors by moving the receptor conformation equilibrium to the left, thereby hindering the pharmacological actions of opiate agonists. With normal body sodium levels the receptor would exist predominantly in the antagonist form. While agonists can half saturate the few "nonsodium" receptors at low K_D concentrations, the shifting of the equilibrium between the two receptor conformations, to obtain sufficient numbers of "nonsodium" receptors to mediate pharmacological agonist responses, would require 10-100 times greater agonist concentrations. This may explain why relatively high concentrations of agonists, corresponding to the agonist affinity for the "sodium" receptor state, are required to elicit pharmacological responses. The concept of interconversion of the receptor between two different conformations, which would involve modifications in the protein-lipid structure of the receptor, has been supported by studies with protein-modifying reagents and enzymes (Pasternak and Snyder, 1974 and 1975b; and Wilson et al., 1975).

The postulated interconversion of agonist and antagonist conformations of the opiate receptor resembles models for the behavior of the nicotinic cholinergic receptor (Changeux, 1966; Karlin, 1967; Changeux and Podleski, 1968; and Colquhoun, 1973). In these models, it is postulated that the binding of acetylcholine to the receptor, in addition to causing a transition between two conformations of the receptor, opens the ionophone, transforming acetylcholine recognition into an excitatory postsynaptic potential. If the endogenous morphine-like substance (Hughes, 1975; Terenius, 1975; and Pasternak et al., 1975a) is a neurotransmitter, one might speculate that the influence of sodium on the opiate receptor indicates that sodium is the ion whose conductance is changed by the synaptic activity of this new putative neurotransmitter.

ACKNOWLEDGMENTS

This research was supported by USPHS Drug Abuse Research Center grant DA–00266, RSDA Award MH–33128 to S.H.S. and DA–05328 to I.C. We thank Adele Snowman for her inspired technical assistance.

REFERENCES

Ariens, E. J. 1954. Affinity and intrinsic activity in the theory of competitive inhibition. *Arch. Int. Pharmacodyn. Therap.* 99: 32–49.

Ariens, E. J., J. M. Van Rossum, and A. M. Simonis. 1957. Affinity, intrinsic activity and drug interactions. *Pharmacol. Rev.* 9: 218–236.

Ariens, E. J., J. M. Van Rossum, and P. C. Koopman. 1960. Receptor reserve and threshold phenomena. I. Theory and experiments with autonomic drugs tested on isolated organs. *Arch. Int. Pharmacodyn.* 127: 459–477.

Changeux, J. P. 1966. Responses of acetylcholinesterase from Torpedo marmorate to salts and curarizing drugs. *Mol. Pharmacol.* 2: 369–392.

Changeux, J. P., and T. R. Podleski. 1968. On the excitability and cooperativity of the electroplax membrane. *Proc. Nat. Acad. Sci., USA* 59: 944–950.

Colquhoun, D. 1973. The relation between classical and cooperative models for drug action. In H. P. Rang, Ed. *Drug Receptors.* Macmillan Press, London, pp. 149–181.

Cox, B. M., and M. Weinstock. 1966. The effect of analgesic drugs on the release of acetylcholine from electrically stimulated guinea-pig ileum. *Br. J. Pharmacol. Chemother.* 27: 81–82.

Creese, I., and S. H. Snyder. 1975. Receptor binding and pharmacological activity of opiates in the guinea pig intestine. *J. Pharm. Exp. Ther.* 194: 205–219.

Cresse, I., G. W. Pasternak, C. B. Pert, and S. H. Snyder. 1975. Discrimination by temperature of opiate agonist and antagonist receptor binding. *Life Sci.* 16: 1837–1842.

Gaddum, J. H., and Z. P. Picarelli. 1957. Two kinds of tryptamine receptor. *Brit. J. Pharmacol.* 12: 323–328.

Gintzler, A. R., and J. M. Musacchio. 1974. Interaction between serotonin and morphine in the guinea pig ileum. *J. Pharm. Exp. Ther.* 189: 484–492.

Goldstein, A. 1949. Interactions of drugs and plasma proteins. *Pharmacol. Rev.* 1: 102–165.

Hughes, J. 1975. Isolation of endogenous compound from the brain with pharmacological properties similar to morphine. *Brain Res.* 88: 285–308.

Karlin, A. 1967. On the application of a "plausible model" of allosteric proteins to the receptor for acetylcholine. *J. Theor. Biol.* 16: 306–320.

Kosterlitz, H. W., J. A. H. Lord, and A. X. J. Watt. 1973. Morphine receptor in the myenteric plexus of the guinea-pig ileum. In H. W. Kosterlitz, H. O. S. Collier and J. E. Villarreal, Eds. *Agonist & Antagonist Actions of Narcotic Analgesic Drugs.* University Park Press, Baltimore, pp. 45–61.

Lees, G. W., H. W. Kosterlitz, and A. A. Waterfield. 1973. Characteristics of morphine-sensitive release of neurotransmitter substances. In H. W. Kosterlitz et al., Eds. *Agonist & Antagonist Actions of Narcotic Analgesic Drugs.* University Park Press, Baltimore, pp. 142–152.

Nickerson, M. 1956. Receptor occupancy and tissue response. *Nature* (London) 178: 697–698.

Pasternak, G. W., R. Goodman, and S. H. Snyder. 1975a. An endogenous morphine-like factor in mammalian brain. *Life Sci.* 16: 1765–1769.

Pasternak, G. W., A. M. Snowman, and S. H. Snyder. 1975b. Selective enhancement of ^{3}H-opiate agonist binding by divalent cations. *Mol. Pharmacol.* 11: 735–744.

Pasternak, G. W., and S. H. Snyder. 1974. Opiate receptor binding: Effects of enzymatic treatments. *Mol. Pharmacol.* 10: 183–193.

Pasternak, G. W., and S. H. Snyder, 1975a. Identification of novel high affinity opiate receptor binding in rat brain. *Nature* (London) 253: 536–565.

Pasternak, G. W., and S. H. Snyder. 1975b. Opiate receptor binding: Enzymatic treatments discriminate between agonist and antagonist interactions. *Mol. Pharmacol.* 11: 478–484.

Paton, W. D. M. 1957. The action of morphine and related substances on contraction and on acetylcholine output of coaxially stimulated guinea-pig ileum. *Br. J. Pharmacol.* 12: 119–127.

Pert, C. B., G. W. Pasternak, and S. H. Snyder. 1973. Opiate agonists and antagonists discriminated by receptor binding in brain. *Science* 182: 1359–1361.

Pert, C. B., and S. H. Snyder. 1973a. Opiate receptor; demonstration in nervous tisse. *Science* 179: 1011–1014.

Pert, C. B., and S. H. Snyder. 1973b. Properties of opiate receptor binding in rat brain. *Proc. Nat. Acad. Sci., USA* 70: 2243–2247.

Pert, C. B., and S. H. Snyder. 1975. Opiate receptor binding of agonists and antagonists affected differentially by sodium. *Mol. Pharmacol.* 10: 868–879.

Pert, C. B., and S. H. Snyder. 1975. Differential interactions of agonists and antagonists with the opiate receptor. *Neurosciences Res. Prog. Bull.* 13: 73–79.

Pert, C. B., S. H. Snyder, and E. L. May. 1976. Opiate receptor interactions of benzomorphans in rat brain homogenates. *J. Pharm. Exp. Ther.* (In press)

Schulz, R., and A. Goldstein. 1973. Morphine tolerance and supersensitivity to 5-hydroxytryptamine in the myenteric plexus of the guinea pig. *Nature* (London) 244: 168–170.

Simon, E. J., J. M. Hiller, and I. Edelman. 1973. Stereospecific binding of the potent narcotic analgesic [^{3}H]etorphine to rat brain homogenate. *Proc. Nat. Acad. Sci., USA* 70: 1947–1949.

Simon, E. J., J. Hiller, J. Groth, and I. Edelman. 1975. Further properties of stereospecific opiate binding sites in rat brain: On the sodium effect. *J. Pharm. Exp. Ther.* 192: 531–537.

Snyder, S. H. 1975. A model of opiate receptor function with implications for a theory of addiction. *Neurosciencees Res. Prog. Bull.* 13: 137–141.

Snyder, S. H., and J. P. Bennett, Jr. 1975. Biochemical identification of the postsynaptic serotonin receptor in mammalian brain. In E. Usdin and W. E. Bunney, Eds. *Pre- and Postsynaptic Receptors.* Marcel Dekker, Inc., New York, pp. 191–205.

Stephenson, R. P. 1956. A modification of receptor theory. *Brit. J. Pharmacol.* 11: 379–393.

Terenius, L. 1972. Specific uptake of narcotic analgesics by subcellular fraction of the guinea-pig ileum. *Acta Pharmacol. et Toxicol.* Suppl. 1, 31: 50.

Terenius, L. 1974. Contribution of "receptor" affinity to analgesic potency. *J. Pharmacy & Pharmacology* 26: 146–148.

Terenius, L. 1975. Narcotic receptors in guinea pig ileum and rat brain. *Neurosciences Res. Prog. Bull.* 13: 39–42.

Wilson, H. A., G. W. Pasternak, and S. H. Snyder. 1975. Differentiation of opiate agonist and antagonist receptor binding by protein modifying reagents. *Nature* (London) 253: 448–450.

Tissue Responses to Addictive Drugs
© 1976, Spectrum Publications, Inc.

Studies on Opiate Receptors in Animal and Human Brain

J. M. HILLER
E. J. SIMON

Department of Medicine
New York University School of Medicine
New York, N.Y.

Stereospecific binding of opiates and their antagonists to homogenates of animal and human brain was originally demonstrated in three laboratories (Pert and Snyder, 1973; Simon et al., 1973; Terenius, 1973), based on an assay suggested by Goldstein et al. (1971). The level of binding, its saturability, its restriction to nervous tissue, and the correlation between binding affinity and pharmacological efficacy of a variety of agonist and antagonist drugs are all consistent with the hypothesis that these bindings sites represent pharmacological opiate receptors.

This chapter will discuss the results from three avenues of research which are being employed in our laboratory to characterize further the properties of the opiate receptor: differences in receptor distribution in the brains of various species; further evidence of receptor conformational changes; and solubilization of an opiate-macromolecular complex.

DIFFERENCES IN OPIATE RECEPTOR DISTRIBUTION IN THE BRAINS OF VARIOUS MAMMALIAN SPECIES

Early effects in mammals after acute morphine administration include changes in behavior. While depressive behavior is observable in dog, monkey and man, excitatory behavior is elicited in cat, sheep and cow among others. In an effort to ascertain if the species difference in behavioral change caused by morphine is reflected in the distribution pattern of opiate binding sites in the brain, we undertook a survey of the binding of tritiated etorphine in selected areas of the brains of various species.

The methods used for the binding assay are the same as those described by us for mapping the distribution of opiate binding sites in human brain tissue obtained at autopsy (Hiller et al., 1973). Table I shows the stereospecific binding of ^{3}H-etorphine in various areas of the brain of six species. Except for the amygdala and the frontal cortex areas, the same anatomical area from different species showed rather good reproducibility. Table II shows the ratios of binding levels of the amygdala and frontal cortex compared to an arbitrarily chosen baseline, the caudate—an area of consistently high and reproducible binding from species to species. In both the amygdala and frontal cortex, the ratios for the "depressed" species are at least twofold greater than the ratios seen in the "excited" species. While the motor cortex seems to fall into this category of differential opiate binding, incomplete data prevent its definitive inclusion in this group.

The interpretation of these findings is difficult. Both the amygdala and frontal cortex are part of the limbic system wherein most of the regions with high opiate binding in man (Hiller et al., 1973) and monkey (Kuhar et al., 1973) are located. It has been reported that bilaterally amygdalectomized monkeys were rendered placid (Mark and Sweet, 1974), while the same procedure performed on cats produced a sustained ferocity (Bard and Mountcastle, 1948). Thus, amygdalectomy mimics the effects seen in acute morphine administration to these species. The removal of the frontal cortex in man may leave the perception of pain unaffected while the anxiety associated with pain is markedly diminished (Jacobson, 1972). This observation has also been made in patients in pain who are receiving morphine.

CONFORMATIONAL CHANGES IN THE OPIATE RECEPTOR

Sodium effect

Since the presence of salt in the incubation medium was reported to decrease the binding of etorphine (Simon et al., 1973) and increase the binding of naloxone (Pert et al., 1973), we suggested that this differential effect may reflect a general difference in the manner in

Table I. Distribution of Stereospecific Binding of ³H-Etorphine in Brain Regions of Mammalian Species

Anatomical Area	Stereospecific ³H-Etorphine Binding pMoles/mg Protein					
	Cow (6)	Cat (5)	Sheep (3)	Dog (2)	Monkey (1)	Man (8)*
Caudate	0.080 ± 0.020	0.126 ± 0.063	0.089 ± 0.006	0.094	0.085	0.103 ± 0.029
Hypothalamus	0.054 ± 0.008	0.075 ± 0.024	0.025	0.089	0.151	0.101 ± 0.033
Putamen	0.053 ± 0.015	0.152 ± 0.125	0.058 ± 0.010	0.158	—	0.085 ± 0.033
Amygdala	0.050 ± 0.020	0.056 ± 0.016	0.059 ± 0.002	0.121	0.142	0.195 ± 0.074
Thalamus	0.035 ± 0.025	0.052 ± 0.014	0.042 ± 0.010	0.050	0.074	0.106 ± 0.022
Motor Cortex	0.030 ± 0.005	—	0.041 ± 0.015	0.067	0.068	0.106 ± 0.051
Cerebellum	0.028 ± 0.012	0.030	—	0.023	0.033	0.040 ± 0.003
Occipital Cortex	0.027 ± 0.004	0.033 ± 0.008	0.031 ± 0.010	0.064	0.021	0.052 ± 0.022
Hippocampus	0.027 ± 0.004	0.047 ± 0.016	0.047 ± 0.006	0.079	0.052	0.042 ± 0.018
Frontal Cortex	0.024 ± 0.007	0.036 ± 0.007	0.042 ± 0.005	0.082	0.075	0.110 ± 0.053
Medulla	0.017 ± 0.009	—	0.013 ± 0.004	0.026	—	0.023
Pons	0.009 ± 0.009	—	0.013 ± 0.005	0.023	0.044	0.016
Cerebral White	0.008	0.019	—	0.007	0.011	0.023 ± 0.012

Figures in parentheses represent the numbers of brains assayed.
*Data from Hiller et al., 1973.

Table II. Comparison of Stereospecific Binding of ^{3}H-Etorphine in Selected Anatomical Areas of Brain from Various Species

Anatomical Area	Stereospecific ^{3}H-Etorphine Binding pMoles/mg Protein					
	Cow	Cat	Sheep	Dog	Monkey	Man
Amygdala	0.050	0.056	0.059	0.121	0.142	0.195
Frontal Cortex	0.024	0.036	0.042	0.082	0.075	0.110
Caudate	0.080	0.126	0.089	0.094	0.085	0.103
Amygdala/Caudate	0.6	0.4	0.7	1.3	1.7	1.9
Frontal Cortex/Caudate	0.3	0.3	0.5	0.9	0.9	1.1

which agonists and antagonists bind to the receptor (Simon et al., 1973). It was shown that discrimination between agonists and antagonists is in fact a specific property of sodium salts (Pert et al., 1973). Our recent studies on the mechanism of the sodium effect (Simon et al., 1975b) suggest that sodium acts as an allosteric effector causing a conformational change in the receptor molecule. The resulting "sodium-dependent" form has a higher affinity for antagonists and a lower affinity for agonists than the "sodium-free" form, but the total number of receptor sites does not change. In order to understand better the role of the SH-group in the opiate receptor, we embarked on a study of the kinetics of receptor inactivation by sulfhydryl reagents. In the course of this study we came upon unexpected, independent evidence of receptor conformational change caused by sodium (Simon and Groth, 1975).

Kinetics of NEM inactivation

The inactivation of stereospecific etorphine binding in rat brain homogenate by sulfhydryl reagents was reported earlier by us (Simon et al., 1973). We now present kinetic studies of the inactivation of receptor binding by the SH-alkylating agent, N-ethylmaleimide (NEM). Results to be presented will show that an SH group essential for binding is present and can be protected from inactivation by opiates. Independent evidence for the conformational change in receptor sites caused by sodium ions is also provided.

Rat brain mitochondrial-synaptosomal fraction (P_2) was prepared as described previously (Simon et al., 1975b) from brains of Sprague-Dawley rats after removal of the cerebellum. For inactivation studies, 2 ml of P_2 fraction (about 1 mg protein/ml) were incubated in 0.05 M Tris-Hcl, pH 7.4, with NEM and appropriate additions. (Concentrations of salts and reagents, temperature and length of incubation are indicated in the legend to the table and figures.)

When rat brain P_2 membranes are incubated with NEM, there is a progressive decrease in their capacity to bind ^3H-naltrexone stereospecifically. The rate of inactivation follows pseudo-first order kinetics, as would be expected at high NEM concentration (NEM concentration being essentially constant) if reaction occurs with a single SH-group on the receptor (see Figure 1). Strong temperature dependence is exhibited, the half time of inactivation being increased from 9 minutes at 37°C to 35 minutes at 26°C. When residual binding of ^3H-etorphine is assayed, both the rate and extent of inactivation by NEM are the same as for naltrexone. Inactivation by p-hydroxymercuribenzoate or iodoacetamide follow similar first order kinetics.

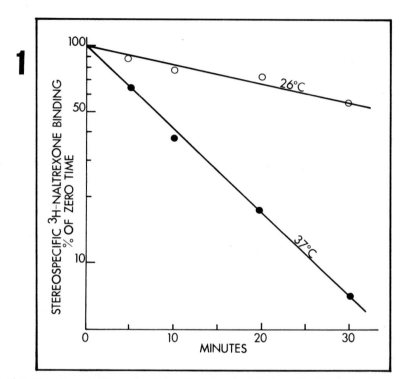

Effect of temperature on the rate of inactivation of stereospecific binding of ^{3}H-naltrexone by rat brain P_2 fraction. Rat brain P_2 fraction was preincubated with 0.5 mM NEM for various intervals at 26°C and 37°C. The reaction was stopped by addition of tris-(2-carboxyethyl)-phosphine (2.5mM). Stereospecific binding of ^{3}H-naltrexone (sp. act. 15.3 C/mmole, concentration 1×10^{-9}M) was assayed. Results are expressed as percent of activity remaining as compared to a sample treated with NEM and phosphine immediately (zero time).

Protection against NEM inactivation by opiates

When preincubation of membranes with NEM is performed in the presence of an opiate or opiate antagonist there is considerable protection of the receptor. Figure 2 shows the rate of inactivation by NEM in the presence and absence of naltrexone. The half time of inactivation is increased from 9 to 25 minutes. Similar protection is observed with levorphanol. This indicates that binding of opiates to the receptor makes the SH-group less accessible for inactivation, and suggests a close proximity of the SH-group to the opiate binding site. However, a con-

2

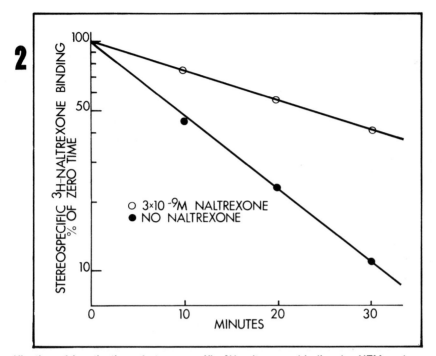

Kinetics of inactivation of stereospecific ^{3}H-naltrexone binding by NEM and protection by pretreatment with naltrexone. Inactivation was carried out as in legend to Figure 1 at 37°C. P$_2$ fraction was preincubated for 5 min with or without unlabeled naltrexone (3x10^{-9}M before addition of NEM. For the binding assay ^{3}H-naltrexone was added to the final concentration of 2x10^{-9}M (total concentration of naltrexone 5x10^{-9}M).

formational change resulting in masking of an SH-group at some distance from the binding site cannot be ruled out.

Protection against NEM inactivation by sodium ions

When preincubation of P$_2$ membranes with NEM is carried out in 100 mM NaCl, the half time of inactivation is increased from 9 minutes to 30 min (see Figure 3). Protection by sodium is observed whether residual binding is measured with ^{3}H-naltrexone or ^{3}H-etorphine. The possibility that NaCl retards the alkylation of SH-compounds was investigated. The reaction of NEM with glutathione in the presence

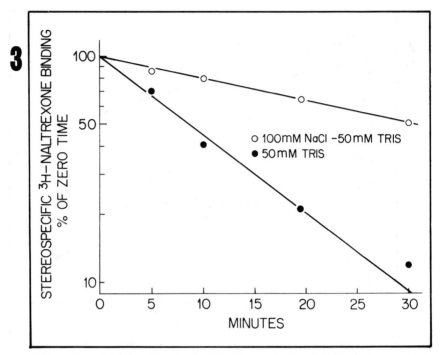

Kinetics of inactivation of stereospecific binding by NEM in the presence and absence of NaCl. Preincubation with NEM was carried out in the presence and absence of 100 mM NaCl. Reaction was stopped and assay for stereospecific naltrexone binding was done as described in legend to Figure 1.

and absence of 100 mM NaCl was monitored spectrophotometrically. No change in the rate of alkylation was observed. We therefore postulate that the effect of sodium is the result of a conformational change in the receptor which renders the SH-group less accessible to alkylation by NEM.

Specificity of protection by sodium ions

Our evidence suggests, further, that the alteration reflected in the protection of SH group by Na$^+$ may be identical to that which results in enhanced antagonist and decreased agonist binding. Table III shows the effect of different alkali metal salts on the rate of inactivation. In addition to sodium only lithium has a slight protective effect, whereas potassium, rubidium and cesium are totally inactive. The cation specificity is the same as that previously demonstrated for enhancement of

Table III. Effect of Alkali Metal Cations on Inactivation of Receptor Binding Capacity by NEM

Time of Preincubation (min)	Tris only	KCl	RbCl	CsCl	LiCl	NaCl
			Binding of ^{3}H-Naltrexone (% of Zero Time)			
5	73	72	75	—	81	85
10	45	51	51	50	65	78
20	22	24	27	24	42	65
30	12	11	17	12	32	48

All preincubations were carried out in the presence of 0.5 mM NEM in 50 mM Tris with the appropriate salt added to final concentration of 100 mM. The reaction was stopped after the appropriate interval and stereospecific binding of ^{3}H-naltrexone was measured. Results are expressed as percent of zero time preincubation in the appropriate salt. All results are means of three closely similar experiments.

antagonist binding (Pert et al., 1973). The protective effect of various concentrations of sodium are presented in Figure 4. Protection increases with the concentration of NaCl from essentially none at 1 mM to maximal protection at 100 mM. This concentration response is identical to that which we reported for the enhancement of antagonist binding (Simon et al., 1975b).

Evidence for inactivation of alkylated binding sites and binding characteristics of residual receptors

Saturation experiments with and without sodium were carried out with P_2 fraction in which binding capacity had been reduced 80% by treatment with NEM. We find that the degree of inactivation remains constant throughout the concentration range of naltrexone studied (10^{-10}-10^{-8} M) providing evidence that alkylated binding sites do not simply have reduced affinity but are totally inactivated over this concentration range and under these experimental conditions. The remaining active binding sites are found to be identical to those in untreated membranes with respect to the affinity of naltrexone in the absence (K_D = 1.1 mM) and presence (K_D = 0.5 mM) of NaCl, indicating that they retain their original properties. Pasternak and Snyder (1975) reported recently that treatment with SH-reagents causes the receptors to "freeze" in the sodium-dependent form ("antagonist conformation"

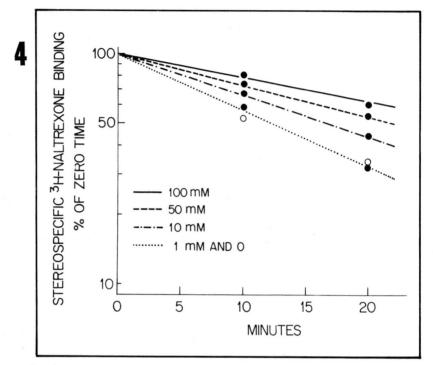

Kinetics of inactivation of stereospecific binding of ^{3}H-naltrexone by NEM in the presence of various concentrations of NaCl. Incubation with NEM was carried out in the concentrations of NaCl shown.

in the authors' language). The findings presented above are at variance with their conclusions.

Model for conformational changes caused by sodium ions

Based on the evidence cited, we have previously postulated the following model (Simon, 1975) (see Figure 5). The reason for postulating a dimer is our observation (Simon et al., 1975a) that binding of opiates to the receptor exhibits positive cooperativity, implying an oligomeric structure. It is suggested that the binding of sodium to allosteric sites results in a conformational change in the receptor that alters the shape of the binding site. This altered binding site exhibits greater affinity towards antagonists and lower affinity towards agonists than the conformation characteristics of sodium-free media. However, both conformational states can bind both types of ligand. Moreover, the results

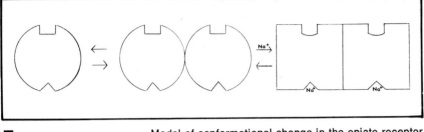

Model of conformational change in the opiate receptor in the presence of sodium.

on the protection of receptors by sodium against inactivation by NEM suggest that the same conformational change also causes an alteration in the position of the SH-group essential for binding, rendering it less accessible to inactivation by NEM.

Our evidence (Simon et al., 1975a) also suggests that the dimer can dissociate into monomers which cannot be readily converted to the sodium-dependent state. These monomers are thought to account for the residual sodium-free form found to persist even in 100 mM NaCl (Simon et al., 1975b).

The significance of this conformational change in the presence of sodium is not clear. The sodium-dependent form is thought to be the physiologically important one. However, the binding of opiate agonists may result in release of sodium ions, a phenomenon that may be involved in the mode of action of these drugs.

Conformational change produced by lowering of temperature and its interaction with the change due to sodium

At the International Narcotics Research Club Meeting at Airlie, Va., in May 1975, Dr. Ian Creese reported that the sodium effect on the binding of agonists and antagonists is observable most strikingly when the temperature of the 25°C or 37°C incubation is dropped to 0°C for a period of time prior to filtration. We have confirmed this observation and have performed experiments directed at understanding the basis of this phenomenon.

Table IV shows the binding of ^{3}H-naltrexone and ^{3}H-etorphine at 37°C, in the presence or absence of 100 mM NaCl, filtered immediately or after cooling in ice for 15 min. It can be seen that increased binding of antagonist and decreased binding of agonist in the presence of salt is considerably increased when incubates are filtered following the

Table IV. Effect of Incubation Conditions on the Stereospecific Binding of Labeled Antagonist and Agonist

Incubation Conditions	Stereospecific Binding cpm/sample					
	37°C–15 min		37°C–15 min 0°C–30 min		37°C–15 min 0°C–30 min 37°C–15 min	
	–NaCl	+NaCl	–NaCl	+NaCl	–NaCl	+NaCl
^{3}H-Naltrexone	3448	2883	3732	5835	2646	2488
^{3}H-Etorphine	5223	4023	4583	1621	5317	3258

The concentration of ^{3}H-naltrexone (sp. act. 15.3 C/mmole) used was 1×10^{-9}M.
The concentration of ^{3}H-etorphine (20.7 C/mmole) used was 5×10^{-10}M.

downshift in temperature to 0°C. A small shift in binding can also be seen when Tris-immediate and Tris-0° binding values are compared, i.e., agonist binding is slightly decreased, antagonist binding is slightly increased. Table IV also shows that returning the incubation mixture to 37°C reversed the low temperature effect almost completely. We have also determined that the changes seen at low temperature are completed for the antagonist in less than five minutes and for the agonist in about 30 minutes.

The first question we raised was whether the conformational change caused by sodium is real or a laboratory artifact caused entirely by a shift to low temperature. Evidence that a conformational change does occur at 37°C is provided by the following. Sodium greatly decreased the rate of inactivation of the opiate receptor by NEM at 37°C with no requirement for low temperature. When competition experiments are carried out between a labeled antagonist and an unlabeled agonist there is a large increase (10-60-fold) in the ED$_{50}$ of the agonist in 100 mM NaCl, as first shown by Pert et al. (1973). We performed experiments in which five different agonists (etorphine, bezitramide, piritramide, fentanyl, phenoperidine) were allowed to compete against labeled naltrexone at 37°C, in Tris and in salt, followed by immediate filtration or by filtration after 15 minutes at 0°C. Figure 6 shows the competition between etorphine and labeled naltrexone plotted on log-probit paper. A twofold increase in ED$_{50}$ in the presence of NaCl is seen even when samples were filtered immediately. However, when samples were cooled to 0°C prior to filtration, the samples in NaCl showed a 10-fold increase

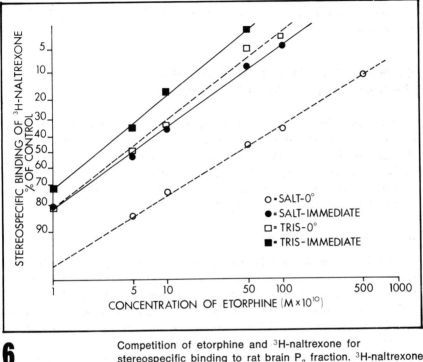

6

Competition of etorphine and ^{3}H-naltrexone for stereospecific binding to rat brain P_2 fraction. ^{3}H-naltrexone (sp. act. 15.3 C/mmole) at a concentration of 1×10^{-9}M was used. Data are presented as probit-log plots.

in the ED_{50} of etorphine. Similar results were obtained for all five agonists used. It was therefore concluded that a conformational change in the receptor does occur at 37°C in the presence of salt but that the effect is amplified at 0°C.

We, therefore, wish to propose the following addition to our previously stated model. In the sodium-free state, low temperature causes a small conformational change similar, by our criteria, to that caused by sodium. However, in the sodium dependent state a further conformational change is induced by low temperature which is greater in magnitude than the conformational change induced by low temperature in the sodium-free state. Thus, what we are observing is a synergistic effect between sodium and low temperature resulting in a larger than additive conformational change in the receptor.

The fact that changes in temperature can cause alterations in the conformation of macromolecules is not surprising. What is somewhat unexpected is that the conformational change induced by low temperature is so similar to that induced by sodium, at least by the criteria of increased affinity of the receptor for antagonists and decreased affinity for agonists.

SOLUBILIZATION OF A STEREOSPECIFIC OPIATE-MACROMOLECULAR COMPLEX

The exact chemical structure of the opiate receptor and many aspects of receptor-drug interaction can only be learned when receptor molecules are available in soluble and highly purified form. As a first step towards this end we report here the solubilization of etorphine bound stereospecifically to a macromolecular moiety and present data suggesting that this moiety may be the opiate receptor.

Solubilization procedures

The brains of Sprague-Dawley rats were used to prepare mitochondrial-synaptosomal (P_2) fraction as described earlier in this chapter. Prior to extraction, the P_2 membranes are incubated with ^{3}H-etorphine at 37°C for 20 minutes. As described in our earlier reports (Simon et al., 1973; Simon et al., 1975b), incubations are carried out in the presence of the active narcotic analgesic, levorpanol (10^{-6}M), or an equal concentration of its inactive enantiomorph, dextrorphan, in order to establish stereospecificity of etorphine binding (Goldstein et al., 1971). The membrane fraction is then centrifuged at 20,000 x g for 15 minutes at 4°C. The resulting pellet is resuspended in 1/10 the original volume of an ice cold 1% solution of the nonionic detergent Brij 36T in 0.01 M Tris buffer containing 0.2 mM dithiothreitol and 1 mM EDTA (Pollock et al., 1974). This suspension is mixed briefly on a Vortex vibrator and immediately centrifuged in a Beckman preparative ultracentrifuge at 100,000 x g for 90 minutes. Free and bound etorphine in the supernatant are separated by passage through a column of XAD-4 amberlite and elution with cold 0.05 M Tris buffer, pH 7.4. Effluent fractions of 1 ml are collected and radioactivity and protein content are determined.

Detection of solubilized bound ^{3}H-etorphine

Free ^{3}H-etorphine binds firmly and quantitatively ($> 99\%$) to an XAD column and can only be eluted with methanol or ethanol. Figure 7 shows another control in which ^{3}H-etorphine is added to a Brij extract of P_2 membranes (no binding of drug occurs in the presence of 1% Brij 36T). When the supernatant from ultracentrifugation of the extract

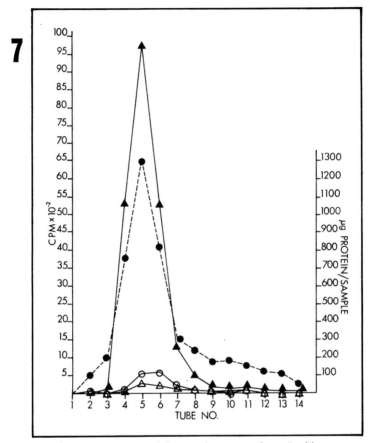

Elution profile on XAD-4 of Brij extract of P_2 membranes prebound with
³H-etorphine. P_2 membranes (2 mg protein/ml) were incubated with ³H-etorphine
((1 x 10⁻⁹ M, 20.7 Ci/mmole) and subsequently extracted with 1% Brij 36T
as described in the text. A 1 ml aliquot of the supernatant following ultracentrifugation was placed on a 2 x 10 cm column of XAD-4 (Rohm and Haas)
and eluted with cold 0.05 M Tris buffer. △ ³H-etorphine prebound in the
presence of 10⁻⁶ M dextrorphan (cpm/ml). O ³H-etorphine prebound in the
presence of 10⁻⁶ M levorphanol (cpm/ml). △ ³H-etorphine added to Brij
extract of P_2 membranes subsequent to extraction and ultracentrifugation
(cpm/ml). ● Protein concentration (µg/ml).

is passed through the XAD-4 column more than 85% of the protein is
recovered, while less than 1% of the radioactivity is eluted.

Figure 7 also shows the results of a typical solubilization experiment.
When ³H-etorphine was prebound to P₂ membranes in the presence
of a 1000-fold excess of dextrorphan followed by solubilization, as de-

scribed above, chromatography of the resultant extract on XAD-4 yields a peak of radioactivity coincident with the eluted protein peak. In contrast, when the identical extraction procedure is performed on membranes prebound with ³H-etorphine in the presence of 1000-fold excess of levorphanol, the amount of radioactivity eluted is negligible. This experiment clearly demonstrates the stereospecificity of the etorphine-bound complex solubilized by Brij 36T.

Characterization of the solubilized ³H-etorphine-bound moiety

The solubilized material is quite stable at 0°C and can be dialyzed in the cold overnight with only minimal loss of radioactivity. At 37°C the solubilized bound material has a half life of dissociation of about 10 minutes, considerably faster than the dissociation rate for intact etorphine-bound membranes, which is about 45 minutes.

The etorphine-bound moiety is sensitive to an SH reagent, proteolytic enzymes and heat, suggesting involvement of a protein. Thus, incubation at 37°C for 30 min with 1×10^{-3}M NEM reduces bound radioactivity by 90% while trypsin (1 mg/ml) or pronase (60 μg/ml) reduces bound ligand by 60% in 10 min at 25°C as compared to control samples incubated for the same length of time. Heating at 50°C for 10 min results in 84% loss of bound radioactivity.

Molecular weight determination of the bound complex

When the bound extract is chromatographed on a column of Sepharose 6B, 25–30% of the radioactivity emerges in a peak at an elution volume consistent with the binding of ³H-etorphine to a macromolecule. The remaining radioactivity is eluted at the same volume as free etorphine. Chromatography of the extract on a Sepharose 6B column calibrated with proteins of known molecular weight (see Figure 8) yields an estimate of about 370,000 daltons for the molecular weight of the ³H-etorphine-bound macromolecular complex.

Attempts at binding drug to unbound solubilized macromolecular material

We are encountering a difficulty faced by other investigators in their early attempts to solubilize receptors, i.e., inability to demonstrate binding of drug to unbound or dissociated solubilized macromolecular material. This may be due to the presence of an inhibitory concentration of detergent. A large portion of the detergent seems to be

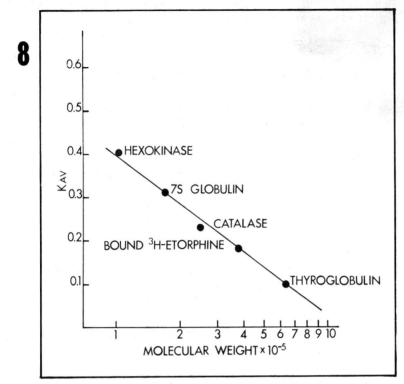

Estimation of the molecular weight of solubilized ^{3}H-etorphine-bound complex on Sepharose 6B. Gel filtration was carried out on a column measuring 1 x 52 cm. Eluting solution was 0.05 M Tris buffer, pH 7.4. Data are expressed in terms of K_{av} as defined by Laurent and Killander (1964),

$$K_{av} = (V_e - V_o)/(V_t - V_o),$$

where V_e is the elution volume corresponding to the peak concentration of solute (marker proteins monitored by absorbance at 280 nm, ^{3}H-etorphine-bound complex monitored by radioactivity determination), V_o is the void volume as determined by the appearance of dextran blue and V_t is the total liquid volume as determined with free ^{3}H-etorphine. V_o and V_t values were 20 and 65 ml, respectively. The relationship between logarithm of the molecular weight and K_{av} was used to obtain the molecular weight of the ^{3}H-etorphine-bound complex.

removed by the XAD-4 column, but we have no quantitative assay for Brij and therefore do not know its residual level in the eluate. The reduced affinity for etorphine binding may point to some distortion of the binding site. This may result in good retention of already bound drug, but inability to rebind. Efforts to obtain this solubilized macro-

352   HILLER, SIMON

molecular material in a form able to bind opiates and purification of the ³H-etorphine-bound macromolecular complex are in progress.

CONCLUSIONS

Much progress has been made in the study of opiate receptors in the two years since their discovery. The evidence that these binding sites are, in fact, pharmacological receptors is accumulating at an ever increasing rate. The recent discovery of what appears to be the endogenous ligand for this receptor (Hughes, 1975) adds further excitement to this very active field of investigation.

This chapter demonstrates some of the major directions in which our laboratory is moving. The finding that it is possible to detect reproducible differences in opiate receptor distribution between the brains of animal species whose primary reaction to opiates is depression and those whose primary response is excitement is of interest and may ultimately provide explanations for these differences. The conformational change in receptor structure produced in a highly specific manner by Na⁺ ions may shed light on the molecular mode of opiate action. Meanwhile, it serves as a useful assay for the relative agonist and antagonist potencies of new drugs.

An important goal in these studies is the solubilization and purification of active opiate receptors. We have not yet attained this difficult objective but we feel that our ability to solubilize an ³H-etorphine-macromolecular complex with properties consistent with those of an ³H-etorphine-receptor complex is a first step in this direction.

A thorough understanding of the nature of opiate receptors and their interactions with endogenous and exogenous ligands should aid greatly in our comprehension of the mechanisms of opiate action and of tolerance and physical dependence.

REFERENCES

Bard, P., and V. B. Mountcastle. 1948. Some forebrain mechanisms involved in expression of rage with special reference to suppression of angry behavior. *Res. Publ. Ass. Nerv. Ment. Dis.* 27: 362.

Goldstein, A., L. I. Lowney, and B. K. Pal. 1971. Stereospecific and nonspecific interactions of the morphine congener levorphanol in subcellular fractions of mouse brain. *Proc. Nat. Acad. Sci. USA* 68: 1742–1747.

Hiller, J. M., J. Pearson, and E. J. Simon. 1973. Distribution of stereospecific binding of the potent narcotic analgesic etorphine in the human brain: Predominance in the limbic system. *Res. Commun. Chem. Pathol. Pharmacol.* 6: 1052–1062.

Hughes, J. 1975. Isolation of an endogenous compound from the brain with properties similar to morphine. *Brain Res.* 88: 295–308.

Jacobson, S. 1972. Taste olfaction and the emotional brain. In: B. A. Curtis, S. Jacobson and E. M. Marcus, Eds. *An Introduction to the Neurosciences.* Saunders, New York, pp. 425–436.

Kuhar, M. J., C. B. Pert, and S. H. Snyder. 1973. Regional distribution of opiate receptor binding in monkey and human brain. *Nature* (London) 245: 447–450.

Laurent, T. C., and J. J. Killander. 1964. A theory of gel filtration and its experimental verification. *J. Chromat.* 14: 317–330.

Mark, V. H., and W. H. Sweet. 1974. The role of limbic brain dysfunction in aggression. *Res. Publ. Ass. Nerv. Ment. Dis.* 52: 186–200.

Pasternak, G. W., and S. H. Snyder. 1975. Identification of novel high affinity opiate binding in rat brain. *Nature* (London) 253: 563–565.

Pert, C. B., G. Pasternak, and S. H. Snyder. 1973. Opiate agonists and antagonists discriminated by receptor binding in the brain. *Science* 182: 1359–1361.

Pert, C. B., and S. H. Snyder. 1973. Opiate receptor: Demonstration in nervous tissue. *Science* 179: 1011–1014.

Pollock, J. J., M. Nguyen-Disteche, J. Ghysen, J. Coyette, R. Linder, M. R. Salton, K. S. Kim, H. R. Perkins, and P. Reynolds. 1974. Fractionation of the DD-carboxypeptidase-transpeptidase activities solubilized from membranes of *Escherichia coli* K12, strain 44. *Eur. J. Biochem.* 41: 439–446.

Simon, E. J. 1975. Opiate receptor binding with ^{3}H-etorphine. *Neurosciences Res. Prog. Bull.* 13: 43–50.

Simon, E. J., and J. Groth. 1975. Kinetics of opiate receptor inactivation by sulfhydryl reagents: Evidence for a conformational change in the presence of sodium ions. *Proc. Nat. Acad. Sci. USA* 72: 2404–2407.

Simon, E. J., J. M. Hiller, and I. Edelman. 1973. Stereospecific binding of the potent narcotic analgesic ^{3}H-etorphine to rat brain homogenate. *Proc. Nat. Acad. Sci. USA* 70: 1947–1949.

Simon, E. J., J. M. Hiller, I. Edelman, J. Groth, and K. D. Stahl. 1975a. Opiate receptors and their interactions with agonists and antagonists. International Narcotics Research Club Meeting, Airlie, Virginia, May, 1975.) *Life Sciences* 16: 1795–1800.

Simon, E. J., J. M. Hiller, J. Groth, and I. Edelman. 1975b. Further properties of stereospecific opiate binding sites in rat brain: On the nature of the sodium effect. *J. Pharmacol. Exp. Ther.* 192: 531–537.

Terenius, L. 1973. Stereospecific interaction between narcotic analgesics and a synaptic membrane fraction of rat cerebral cortex. *Acta Pharmacol. Toxicol.* 32: 317–320.

Tissue Responses to Addictive Drugs
© 1976, Spectrum Publications, Inc.

A Model System for Opiate-Receptor Interaction

HORACE H. LOH
T. M. CHO

Langley Porter Neuropsychiatric Institute
and
Department of Pharmacology
University of California
San Francisco, California

It is widely recognized that opiates exert their pharmacological effects by interacting with specific receptors located at nerve membranes. However, the exact mechanism of interaction between the opiate and its receptor is unknown. According to classical receptor theory, (Ariens and Simonis, 1964; Clark, 1937) and its modification (Stephenson, 1956), two major factors are involved, i.e., affinity between opiate and its receptor, and the efficacy (i.e., how drug-receptor complex elicits its pharmacological effect). Other problems needing resolution are: the relationship between affinity and efficacy; and whether binding is necessary and sufficient to give pharmacological effect. It has been suggested that the nerve transition between resting and excited states is related to the conformational change between two macromolecular states in the nerve membrane (Tasaki, 1968) and that opiates work by blocking the transition of these states. Even though some information is available to support this theory, the exact mechanism is still not clear.

Such information may be obtained by isolating the receptor and characterizing the physicochemical properties of the drug-receptor complex which can then be compared with the pharmacological activity. However, the purification and isolation of opiate receptors has not been achieved. In order to resolve this difficulty, we have selected an *in vitro* receptor model which appears to fulfill most of the criteria for the opiate receptor and used this model to examine the physicochemical properties of the opiate-receptor complexes.

In this chapter we will describe our reasons for using cerebroside sulfate, a membrane acidic lipid as an opiate receptor model; present some data to determine the validity of this model; and discuss a possible role of acidic lipids in opiate action.

In order to understand opiate actions at the molecular level, it is essential to have a pure receptor which permits the study of its interaction with drugs *in vitro*. Since the purification of these receptors from nerve membrane has not been achieved, we have been looking for a model system for this purpose.

Several lines of evidence have shown that the prime mode of opiate receptor interaction is the formation of an electrostatic bond between the protonated nitrogen of opiate and an anionic site of the receptor molecule. Beckett (1958) has shown that the analgesic activity of various opiates decreased with an increase in the "effective width" of the basic group. Based on the structure-activity relationships, Portoghese (1965) has concluded that the nitrogen atom plays a pivotal role in the association of analgesics with their receptors and that the receptors should have either some degree of flexibility or there should be more than one receptor. Additionally, Harris et al. (1975) have shown that lanthanum, an inorganic cation, when administered intraventricularly, exhibited analgesic activity which was antagonized by naloxone, a pure opiate antagonist. It is very likely, therefore, that the anionic group of some macromolecules are involved in opiate receptor interactions.

The anionic site that seems to be an essential feature of opiate receptors can be found in three types of anionic derivatives in the nerve membrane: carbohydrates, phosphates, or sulfates, which are present in macromolecular species in the CNS. Anionic derivatives of protein and carbohydrates have not been purified from nerve membranes. However, acidic lipids such as cerebroside sulfate (CS), gangliosides and acidic phospholipids can be obtained in a pure state (Radin, 1969).

When we examined the molecular model of CS, an acidic lipid membrane component, we recognized the similarity between it and the opiate receptor postulated by Beckett and Casy (1954). If we fixed

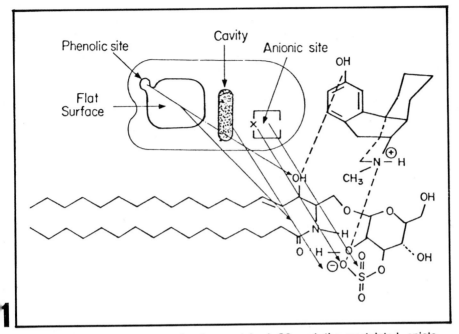

A comparison between the molecular model of CS and the postulated opiate receptor and sites of interaction between CS and a narcotic drug.

the ceramide moiety of the cerebroside sulfate in the antiplanar structure (which is believed to be most stable) (see Figure 1) the freedom of motion of the cerebroside sulfate would be much more restricted and the galactose moiety could only move around the axis which is the bond connecting the ceramide and the galactose moiety.

When an opiate with a rigid ring structure, such as morphine, approaches cerebroside sulfate, the opiate molecule could induce the flexible cerebroside sulfate molecule to fit the rigid structure of the opiate. Thus, the phenyl group with high polarizability would interact with the complementary part of the ceramide moiety which also has a high polarizability (due to the π-bonding) by Van der Waals bonding which is proportional to the polarizability. The phenolic hydroxy group could bind with the hydroxyl group in ceramide moiety through hydrogen bonding. The piperidine ring of levorphanol which is located under the molecular plane of levorphanol would fit the space between the ceramide moiety and galactose group of cerebroside sulfate by hydrophobic bonding. The protonated nitrogen of levorphanol interacts with anionic sulfate group of cerebroside sulfate by electrostatic bond. This seems to fulfill all the requirements of the receptor postulated by Beckett and Casy (1954). Moreover, Eddy et al. (1952) found that in compounds structurally related to methadone, the alteration of the ketonic carbonyl group causes a profound change in the enantiomeric potency ratio. For example, comparing the analgesic potency of the enantiomeric pairs of methadone, α-methadol and α-methadol acetate, the more active enantiomers are the 6R($-$)methadone, 6S($+$) α-methadol, and 6R($-$) α-methadol acetate. This could be explained using cerebroside sulfate as a model receptor. Assuming that the keto group of methadone would interact with 2-hydroxyl group on galactose by hydrogen bond (see Figure 1), the reduction of the keto group to α-hydroxyl group may preferentially bind with the carbonyl group of the ceramide moiety of cerebroside sulfate by hydrogen bond and the acetylation of the hydroxyl group preferentially interacts with 2-hydroxyl group of the galactose moiety of cerebroside sulfate like methadone. Thus, the carbonyl group of the cerebroside sulfate may play a role as a hydrogen acceptor, while the 2-hydroxyl group on the galactose ring may act as a hydrogen donor. Furthermore, Bently and Lewis (1973) found that a compound prepared by ozonolysis of etorphine is as potent as morphine despite the absence of aromatic ring. This could also be due to the interaction of the carbonyl group in a newly formed esteric moiety of the compound with the hydroxyl group of ceramide moiety in CS by a hydrogen bond. Thus, CS not only fits the Beckett and Casy model receptor, but also provides an explanation for the results of methadone series and etorphine derivative as reported by Eddy et al. (1952) and Bently and Lewis (1973), respectively.

BINDING OF OPIATE TO CEREBROSIDE SULFATES

In our early studies, the binding of opiates to liposomes prepared from commercial cerebrosides was studied according to a modification of the method of Goldstein et al. (1971). Using this system, substantial amounts of ^{3}H-naloxone and ^{3}H-etorphine were shown to be bound (Loh et al., 1974), with about 20–30% of the total binding stereospecific. However, the commercial source of cerebroside consists of four different compounds: cerebroside, hydroxycerebroside, cerebroside sulfate, and hydroxycerebroside sulfate. The latter two sulfated derivatives comprise about 10–15% of the total material (our unpublished data). Thus, when concentration binding curves were made four plateaus were observed indicating multiple binding affinities. With ^{3}H-etorphine, the highest affinity binding appeared to reach saturation at about 10 nM and this was attributed to binding to hydroxycerebroside sulfate; another binding plateau at 40 nM was found to be due to the binding to cerebroside sulfate. The other two sites of lesser affinity but higher capacity might be related to ^{3}H-etorphine binding to hydroxy and nonhydroxycerebroside. The binding affinities of other opiates to cerebrosides liposome were also determined (Loh et al., 1974). Within the small series of those drugs we examined, binding affinities seemed to correlate with their pharmacological potency. The liposome as a model lipid membrane for studying binding presents some experimental difficulties; low yield of binding (only 5–10% of the total radioactivity were found in the liposomes); lack of control of the particle size; and differentiation of binding of the drug from solubility of the drug in liposomes. Therefore, in subsequent studies, we have used cerebroside sulfates and have measured binding in an organic solvent/water partition system as described by Weber et al. (1971) and by Lowney et al. (1974). For a typical experiment, a 1 ml aqueous solution containing 5×10^{-8} M ^{3}H-levorphanol and varying concentrations of an unlabeled narcotic was adjusted to pH 6.0 and vortexed with 1 ml of organic solvent containing 4 μg of CS. The organic solvent consisted of heptane, chloroform, and methanol in the proportion of 1500:2:1.

In our hands, 80% of the ^{3}H-levorphanol was bound to CS at a 5×10^{-8} M concentration. The saturable component of the binding was distributed with 96% at the interface and 4% in heptane phase. Based on the drug concentration added to the partition system, dissociation constants of 9.1×10^{-8} M (capacity 0.45 nmole) and 1×10^{-6} M (capacity 1.4 nmole) were obtained. The former is for hydroxycerebroside sulfate while the latter is for nonhydroxycerebroside sulfate. The concentration of nonradioactive drug required to displace 50% of the ^{3}H-levorphanol from CS (ID50) was determined for over 20 narcotics including the complete series of ten N-alkylnorketobemidones. The results (see Figures 2 and 3) indicate that the ID50 of each of these drugs for binding to CS closely correlates with their pharmacologic potencies in both humans and other animals (Loh et al., 1975).

The ID50 based on the concentration of drugs added to the total partition system closely parallels their analgetic activity when the drugs were given by intravenous or subcutaneous administration, while the ID50 based on the concentration of drugs in heptane phase is more closely related to the potency by intraventricular administation of these drugs (Kutter et al., 1970). For example, a drug such as l-methadone with a high partition in heptane ($P_{H/w} = 45$) was about three times more potent than morphine with a low solubility ($P_{H/w} = 5 \times 10^{-4}$) based on the drug concentration added in water. However, based

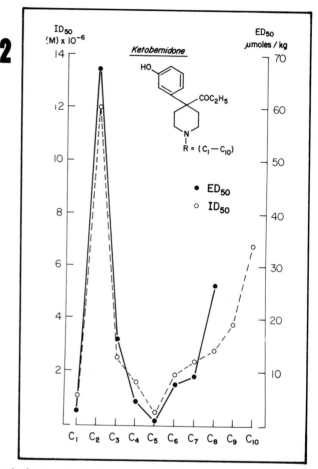

2

Comparison of ID50 and pharmacological potency (ED50) of N-alkylnorketobemidones. The inhibition of 1 μM ^{3}H-levorphanol (26 mCi/mMole) binding to 10 μg cerebroside sulfate by N-alkylnorketobemidones was determined with increasing concentrations of the homologs by the heptane:water partition method. The ID50 is defined as the concentration of the homologs required to inhibit ^{3}H-levorphanol binding to cerebroside sulfate by 50%.

on the drug concentration in the heptane phase, morphine was 628 times more potent than *l*-methadone. This is consistent with the report that *l*-methadone was about five times more potent than morphine by intravenous administration, while given by intraventricular administration, morphine is 30 times more potent than *l*-methadone (Kutter et al., 1970). However, there is an apparent discrepancy between the relative potency of morphine (30 $\times$ methadone) by intraventricular administration and

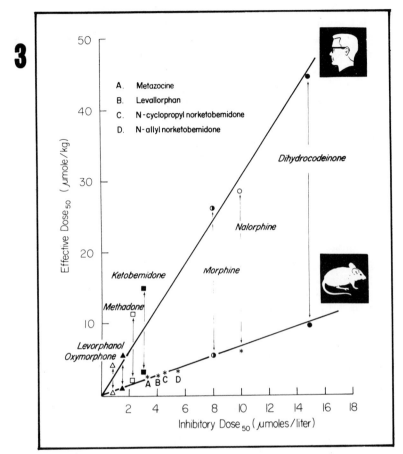

Correlation between the ID50 and analgetic activity (ED50). The ID50 is the concentration of the narcotic analgetics required to inhibit the binding of 5 x 10⁻⁸ M, ³H-levorphanol (3 Ci/mMole) with 4 μg of cerebroside sulfate by 50%. (The analgetic activities (ED50's) of the drug were taken from E. L. May et al. (1965) and converted into μmoles/kg.)

its relative ID50 (628 × methadone) in heptane. This is probably due to the fluid/membrane partition

POSSIBLE ROLE OF MEMBRANE ACIDIC LIPIDS IN THE PHARMACOLOGIC EFFECT OF OPIATES

While the identification of opiate receptor(s) in the CNS have been reported by several laboratories (Snyder, 1975), only Lowney et al.

(1974) have described attempts to purify the receptor. In 1974, they isolated a partially purified opiate receptor, from a mouse brain, which they reported to be a proteolipid. The receptor binds the opiate in a stereospecific manner. In examining different regions of the brain, they found that the greatest binding resided in areas of white matter where the proteolipids are more concentrated. However, by careful chemical, chromatographic analysis, as well as by its narcotic binding properties, we have provided evidence that the opiate receptor isolated by Lowney et al (1974) is virtually identical to cerebroside sulfate. Further attempts to determine the extent to which cerebroside sulfate could mimic the behavior of the purified opiate receptor involved comparison of the elution pattern of cerebroside sulfate and its levorphanol complex with that of the opiate receptor and its levorphanol complex on a Sephadex LH-20 column as described by Soto et al. (1969) and by Lowney et al. (1974). Our results shows that a mixture of hydroxy and nonhydroxy CS is eluted in the same fractions as the Lowney receptor. Moreover, when CS is complexed with levorphanol, the complex also migrates on the column to a more lipophilic region. Various chemical determinations of these purified fractions were also used to further establish the similarity between CS and the purified opiate receptors. Thus, CS appears to be at least the major, if not entire, constituent of the opiate receptor reported by Lowney et al. (1974).

In addition to the *in vitro* experiment discussed above, we have carried out several *in vivo* experiments in which we have attempted to alter the availability of brain CS and to determine the effects of this alteration on the antinociceptive effects of morphine. In the first experiment, we evaluated the effects of morphine on Jimpy mutant B6CBA mice and their normal littermates. These mutants were used since they are known to have low levels of brain cerebrosides but normal levels of brain phospholipids and gangliosides in comparison to their normal littermates (Bauman et al., 1968; Sidman et al., 1964).

The jimpy mice were found to be quite resistant to morphine as the median analgesic dose (AD50) was 11-fold higher in the jimpy mutants than in the normal controls. In another experiment, we reduced the availability of CS in normal mice by injecting agents which have been found to bind strongly to CS. These agents, Azure A and cetylpyridinium chloride (CPC), were found to antagonize the effects of morphine as they increased the AD50 by three and eight times, respectively (Loh et al., 1975). CPC was found to be quite toxic when injected intracerebrally (i.c.) but this toxicity was reduced by complexing CPC with chondroitin sulfate and injecting this mixture. Thus, three different conditions which reduced the availability of brain CS also reduced the

**Table I. Comparison of ^{3}H-Morphine and ^{3}H-Naloxone Binding
by Octanol-Water Partition and Equilibrium Dialysis**

	^{3}H-Morphine Bound (M)	^{3}H-Naloxone Bound (N)	M/N
Octanol-water partition	14.95	2.48	6.00
Equilibrium dialysis	24.10	38.60	0.65

The data were taken from Cho et al., (1975).

effectiveness of morphine. Although these experiments cannot be considered conclusive, they do suggest that the interaction of narcotic drugs with CS may be an important step in the production of the pharmacological effects of these drugs.

PHYSICOCHEMICAL PROPERTIES OF OPIATE-CS COMPLEX

Results presented above seem to indicate that CS fulfilled most of the criteria used to identify opiate receptor *in vitro*. We feel, therefore, that CS may be used as an opiate receptor model to study the opiate-CS interactions that may aid in understanding opiate actions at the molecular level. Below we will describe some preliminary results obtained with the model system.

It has been concluded that one of the prime modes of opiate-receptor interaction is the formation of an electrostatic bond between the protonated nitrogen of opiate and an anionic locus on the receptor. This interaction should be dependent on the physicochemical properties of the cationic center of the opiate such as the size, hydration, polarizability of the anionic center on the receptor. The nature of the interaction determines the physiochemical properties of the drug-receptor complex and the physiochemical properties of agonist-cerebroside sulfate complex may differ from those of the antagonist complex. Consequently, the differences in these properties may influence the affinity of the drug to the receptor and may even be drug "efficacy," as postulated by Stephenson (1956). In this chapter evidence will be presented to show that the narcotic agonist-cerebroside sulfate complex is more hydrophobic while that of the narcotic antagonist is more hydrophilic in nature.

The binding of ^{3}H-morphine and ^{3}H-naloxone in an organic solvent and in water was determined by octanol-water partition and equilibrium dialysis, respectively. As shown in Table I, the ^{3}H-morphine binding to

Table II. Comparison of ID50 of Narcotic Agonist to Its Respective Antagonist

Drugs	ID50[1] Water (M x 10^6)	Heptane (M x 10^9)[2]	$P_{H/W}$[3]
Morphine	5.0	2.5	5×10^{-4}
Nalorphine	6.0	20.9	3.5×10^{-3}
Oxymorphone	5.0	10.0	2×10^{-3}
Naloxone	14.0	112.0	8×10^{-3}
Levorphanol	1.5	15.0	1×10^{-2}
Levallorphan	1.8	69.0	4×10^{-2}
GPA-1657	0.75	190.0	3.4×10^{-1}
GPA-2163	2.0	2016.0	1.1×10

[1] ID50 is defined as the concentration of the drug required to inhibit the binding of 5×10^{-8} M, ^{3}H-levorphanol to 4 μg of cerebroside sulfate by 50%.

[2] The ID50's of the drugs in heptane were obtained by multiplying those of the drugs in water by their respective partition coefficient between heptane and water.

[3] Partition coefficients of the drugs between heptane and water (pH 7.4) were determined in our laboratory.

CS was six times higher than that of ^{3}H-naloxone at equimolar concentration in octanol, while in water, ^{3}H-naloxone significantly bound more with CS than ^{3}H-morphine (Cho et al., 1975).

The concentration of various labelled narcotic agonists and antagonists required to inhibit the binding of 5×10^{-8} M ^{3}H-levorphanol with 4 μg of CS by 50% (ID50) was estimated by log-probit analysis (Cho et al., 1976). When the ID50's and the heptane solubility of the narcotic agonists were compared with those of their corresponding antagonists (see Table II), it was observed that agonists were generally more potent than their corresponding antagonists by this method. However, antagonists were more soluble in heptane than their corresponding agonists.

Chromatographic analysis of the individual CS-drug complexes on Sephadex LH-20, as described above, revealed distinct differences in their solubility behavior. Three to four elution peaks were obtained in order of increasing polarity. Free CS was eluted last in the most polar fraction (67–72). The drug-CS complexes were eluted mainly in two less polar fractions (19–26 and 42–46) and the yields for each fraction was

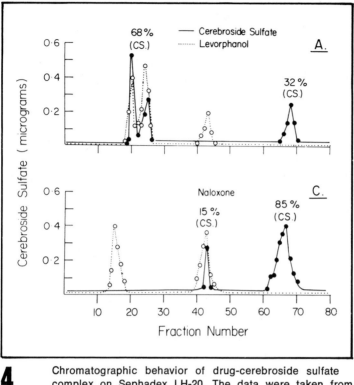

4 Chromatographic behavior of drug-cerebroside sulfate complex on Sephadex LH-20. The data were taken from Cho *et al.* (1975).

dependent on the drug (see Figure 4). Levorphanol exhibited the most binding (68%) of the levorphanol-CS complex was eluted in the most hydrophobic fraction (19–26) but not in fraction 42–46. In contrast, the naloxone complex appeared in more polar fraction (42–46) than in the fraction in which the levorphanol-CS complex was eluted but not in fraction (19–26). Recently, using four pairs of agonists and antagonists, we have confirmed that the yields of agonist-CS complexes are higher than the complexes formed with the corresponding antagonists. Gray and Robinson (1974) have prepared a number of salts of methadone, cyclazocine, and naloxone with various mono- and polybasic organic acids in order to obtain a long acting antagonist preparation. From this study, they found that salts of methadone (an agonist) were more insoluble than cyclazocine (a partial agonist) which were more insoluble than naloxone (a pure antagonist). This is consistent with our result that opiate agonist-CS complex is more hydrophobic than the corresponding antagonist-CS complex.

The higher binding of agonist to CS and the hydrophobic nature of agonist-CS complex in organic solvent may be attributed to the solubility of the drug, the affinity of the drug to CS and the solubility of the complex. Since the solubility of antagonists in an organic solvent is higher than that of corresponding agonists, it is surprising that the agonist binding in an organic solvent is higher than that of the antagonist.

The affinity and the solubility of the drug-CS complex may be dependent on the types of electrostatic bond between the protonated nitrogen of the drug and the anionic sulfate group of CS. It has been shown that there are two types of electrosatic bond: intimate ion pairs and solvent separated (dissociated) ion pairs (Winstein and Robinson 1958). Polyatomic organic cations, unlike uniatomic inorganic cations, can still associate with CS by hydrogen bonding and hydrophobic bonding even if the electrostatic bonds are partially dissociated. The extent of formation of intimate ion pairs for a given ionic concentration is greater, the smaller the size of the ions, and the lower the dielectric constants of the solvent as described by the following equation (Bockris and Reedy, 1970; Conway, 1970):

$$E = \frac{1}{e} \frac{q^+}{(r^+} \times \frac{q^-}{r^-)}$$

where E = electrostatic bond between cation (drug) and anion (receptor); e = dielectric constant; q^+ and q^- are the charges of drug and receptor, respectively; and r^+ and r^- are the radius of the cationic drug and anionic receptor.

The effective size of the ion in solution includes water bound to the ion. This may differ considerably from the size of the dehydrated ion. It follows, therefore, that hydration in aqueous solution is an important factor in intimate ion pair formation. Antagonists can form more hydrated ion pairs with the CS than their corresponding agonists because they possess a larger N-alkyl group, an unsaturated alkyl group, and a $14-\beta-OH$ group (e.g., naloxone). All three structural modifications tend to increase reactivity with water to form hydrated ion pairs. In a solvent of low dielectric constant such as octanol or heptane, where the force of attraction between ions of opposite sign is great, there is an increased tendency for the occurrence of intimate ion pairs. On the other hand, in a solvent of high dielectric constant such as water, solvent separated (hydrated) ion pairs would be increased. Therefore, we may conclude that an agonist interacts with CS to form more intimate ion pairs while an antagonist would yield more hydrated ion pairs. A solvent of low dielectric constant increases the ratio of the intimate pairs to dehydrated ion pairs while a solvent of high dielectric constant decreases the ratio. Thus, the affinity and solubility of the drug-CS complex are dependent on the types of electrostatic bonds formed between the protonated nitrogen of the drug and the anionic sulfate group of CS. The ratio of the intimate ion pairs to hydrated ion pairs discriminates between agonist and antagonist; a high ratio would indicate agonistic properties and a low ratio antagonistic properties.

SUMMARY

Recent studies of Snyder (1975), Simon et al. (1973) and Terenius (1973) have established unequivocally the existence of opiate binding sites in the CNS. This work has been confirmed by many other investigators (Snyder, 1975). Further studies on the anatomical localization, subcellular distribution and biochemical characterization have also been reported. It is generally assumed, based on these studies, that the opiate binding sites are protein in nature. In 1974, Lowney et al. reported the isolation and partial purification of opiate receptors from the mouse brain which they reported to be a proteolipid. Simon and Hiller, at this volume, reported the solubilization and isolation of a protein-etorphine complex which they suggested might be the opiate receptor.

Despite the fact that opiates have a profound effect on lipid metabolism (Mulé, 1970), the question of whether lipid plays a role in opiate-receptor interaction is as yet unanswered. Recent publications from our laboratory employing the same criteria used by other investigators to demonstrate opiate-receptor interaction have shown that CS, an acidic lipid membrane component, exhibits high affinity and stereoselective binding to a number of narcotic drugs. The binding also can be correlated with the analgesic potency of these drugs in both man and rodents indicating that CS demonstrates many of the properties that are thought to be necessary, if not sufficient, for the identification of an "opiate receptor." Cerebroside sulfate appears to fulfill many of the structural requirements of a hypothetical opiate receptor. It is an endogenous component of nerve tissue and, in fact, a partially purified opiate receptor from mouse brain has now been shown to be CS. Other animal experiments indicate, at least indirectly, that reduced availability of brain CS decreases the analgesic effects of morphine, suggesting that the interaction of opiates with CS observed *in vitro* may also have importance *in vivo*.

Recently, Abood and Hoss (1975) have investigated various membranous components for morphine binding. They found that morphine binds to phosphatidylserine (the major acidic lipid in biological membranes) stereospecifically with high affinity. Even the relation between binding affinity and biological potency was not consistent. They suggested that phospatidylserine "may play an important role in regulating the association of the opiates and many cationic drugs with their biological receptors." The exact role of acidic lipids in opiate action cannot be established at the present time, but the possible involvement of these natural membrane components as "prosthetic groups" of the opiate receptor has been suggested (Snyder, 1975). In the case of enzymology, a substrate first binds with the prosthetic group and then the catalytic sites of apoenzyme (proteins) convert the substrate into a product. If this is the case, the receptor protein with acidic lipid as a prosthetic group should have a function such as eliciting the analgesic activity, and that the binding of opiates to a pure acidic lipid (e.g., CS) should neither correlate with the *in vivo* potency nor can it distinguish agonists from antagonisis. However, this is contradictory to our findings.

As we have shown above, the binding of opiate agonists to CS correlates well with their *in vivo* potency and that agonists are stronger than their corresponding antagonists in forming an electrostatic bond between protonated nitrogen of the drugs and the anioic sulfate group of CS. This electrostatic bond not only enhances the affinity of the drug for CS but also distinguishes the agonist from its antagonist, suggesting the affinity of the drug to the receptor cannot be separated from its efficacy (Ariens and Simonis, 1964; Stephenson, 1956).

Based on our experimental observations described above, using cerebroside sulfate as a model receptor for opiate, we have proposed that the analgesic action of opiates may be attributed to the dehydration of the surface membrane by narcotic analgesics through the formation of intimate ion pairs between the protonated nitrogen of the drug (agonist) and anionic site of the receptor. The receptors could contain protein, carbohydrate or lipid and they should have anionic sites and possess high affinity to the drug.

Our proposed mechanism provides explanations for some observations. An antagonist cannot produce analgesic effects since it forms mainly the hydrated ion pairs with the receptors but not the intimate (hydrophobic) ion pairs. In the case of partial agonists, at low concentrations of the drugs, they behave like antagonists but at higher concentrations, exhibit agonistic effects, since the ratio between intimate ion pairs and hydrated ion pairs increases with increasing concentrations of the drug (Bockris and Reedy, 1970; Conway, 1970). The analgesic action elicited by nonopiate drugs such as general anesthetics and alcohols can also be explained by this proposed mechanism. Benson and

King (1965) have reported that the reversible absorption of anesthetics to the ionic sites of surface membrane due to electrostatic bond such as dipole-ion and induced dipole-ion interaction alter the surface potentials and impede the conduction of charges across the interfaces, thereby, providing a pathway for anesthetic action. This may indicate that when the ions at the interface are hydrated, anesthetics like organic solvents could remove the hydrated water, resulting in an increased formation of intimate ion pairs (hydrophobic) to give pharmacological action, since the formation of the intimate (hydrophobic) ion pairs increases with decreasing dielectric constants of the solvent used.

If one assumes the resting state of nerve membrane is more hydrophobic than the excited state opiate, agonists could stabilize the resting state through interaction with their receptors resulting in inhibition of ion conductance. This provides an explanation for the interpretation that opiates and general anesthetics act as electrical stabilizers (Seeman, 1972).

ACKNOWLEDGMENTS

The authors wish to express their gratitude for the excellent technical assistance of Mrs. Jung Sook Cho. We also wish to acknowledge Miss Barbara Halperin for assistance in preparation of this paper.

This work was supported by U.S. Army Contract DADA–17–73–C–3006. H. H. Loh is a recipient of a NIMH Research Scientist Career Development Award, K2–DA–70554.

REFERENCES

Abood, L. G., and W. Hoss. 1975. Stereospecific morphine adsorption to phosphatidylserine and other membranous components of brain. *Europ. J. Pharmacol.* 326: 66–75.

Ariens, E. J., and A. M. Simonis. 1964. Drug-receptor interaction. In E. J. Ariens, Ed. *Molecular Pharmacology.* Vol. 1. Academic Press, New York, pp. 119–286.

Baumann, N., C. Jacque, S. Pollet, and M. L. Harplin. 1968. Fatty acid and lipid composition of the brain of a myelin deficient mutant, the quaking mouse. *Europ. J. Biochem.* 4: 340–344.

Beckett, A. H. 1958. Analgesics and their antagonists: some steric and chemical considerations. *J. Pharm. Pharmacol.* 8: 848–859.

Beckett, A. H., and A. F. Casy. 1954. Synthetic analgesics: Stereochemical considerations. *J. Pharm. Pharmac.* 6: 968–1001.

Benson, S. W., and J. W. King. 1965. Electrostatic aspects of physical adsorption: Implications for molecular sieves and gaseous anesthesia. *Science* 150: 1710–1713.

Bently, K. W., and J. W. Lewis. 1973. The relationship between structure and activity in the 6, 14-endoethenotetrahydrothebaine series of analgesics, In H. W. Kosterlitz et al., Eds. *Agonist and Antagonist Actions of Narcotic Analgesic Drugs*. University Park Press, Baltimore, pp. 7–16.

Bockris, J. O., and A. K. N. Reedy. 1970. Temporary ion association in an electrolytic solution: formation of pairs, triplets. etc. In Bockris, J. O. Eds. *Modern Electrochemistry*, Vol. I, Chapter 3, Plenum Press, New York, pp. 257–267.

Cho, T. M., J. S. Cho, and H. H. Loh. 1976. A model system for opiate-receptor interaction: mechanism of opiate-cerebroside sulfate interaction. *Life Sci.* 18: 231–244.

Cho, T. M., H. H. Loh, and E. L. Way. 1975. Physicochemical properties of opiate-cerebroside sulfate complex. *Proc. West. Pharmacol. Soc.* 18: 176–180.

Clark, A. J. 1937. Concentration-Actions I. In *Handbuch der Experimentellen Pharmakologic*, Erganzungswerk, Bd. 4, Springer-Verlag, Berlin, p. 61.

Conway, B. E. 1970. Some aspects of the thermodynamic and transport behavior of electrolytes. In H. Eyring, Ed. *Physical Chemistry, An Advanced Treatise*, Volume IXA, *Electrochemistry*, Chapter 1. Academic Press, New York, pp. 1–155.

Eddy, N. B., E. L. May, and E. Mosettig. 1952. Chemistry and pharmacology of the methadols and acetyl-methadols. *J. Org. Chem.* 17: 321–326.

Goldstein, A., W. I. Lowney, and B. K. Pal. 1971. Stereospecific and non-specific interactions of the morphine congener levorphanol in subcellular fractions of mouse brain. *Proc. Nat. Acad. Sci.* 68: 1742–1747.

Gray, A. P., and D. S. Robinson. 1973. Insoluble salts and salt complexes of cyclazocine and naloxone. In Braude, M. C., et al. Eds. *Narcotic Antagonists. Advances in Biochemical Pharmacology*, Vol. 8, Chapter IV. Raven Press, New York, pp. 555–568.

Harris, A., E. T. Iwamoto, H. H. Loh, and E. L. Way. 1975. Site-dependent analgesia after microinjection of morphine or lanthanum in rat brain. *West. Pharmacol. Soc.* 18: 275–278.

Kutter, E., A. Herz, H. S. Teschmacher, and R. Hess. 1970. Structure-activity correlations of morphine-like analgesics based on efficiencies following intravenous and intraventricular applications. *J. Med. Chem.* 13: 801–805.

Loh, H. H., T. M. Cho, Y. C. Wu, and E. L. Way. 1974. Stereospecific binding of narcotics to brain cerebrosides. *Life Sci.* 14: 2231–2245.

Loh, H. H., T. M. Cho, Y. C. Wu, R. A. Harris, and E. L. Way. 1975. Opiate binding to cerebroside sulfate: A model system for opiate-receptor interaction. *Life Sci.* 16: 1811–1818.

Lowney, L. I., K. Schultz, P. J. Lowery, and A. Goldstein. 1974. Partial purification of an opiate receptor from mouse brain. *Science* 183: 749–753.

May, E. L., and L. J. Sargent. 1965. Morphine and its modifications. In de Stevens, G. Ed. *Analgetics: Medicinal Chemistry*, Volume 5, Chapter IV, Academic Press, New York, pp. 123–174.

Mulé, S. J. 1970. Morphine and the incorporation of 32-orthophosphate *in vivo* into phospholipids of the guinea pig cerebral cortex, liver and sub-cellular fractions. *Biochem. Pharmacol.* 19: 581–593.

Portoghese, P. S. 1965. A new concept on the mode of interaction of nar-cotic analgesics with receptors. *J. Med. Chem.* 8: 609–616.

Radin, N. S. 1969. Preparation of lipid extracts, In J. M. Lowenstein Ed. *Methods in Enzymology*, Volume XIV, Lipids, Section VII, Academic Press, New York, pp. 245–255.

Seeman, P. 1972. The membrane actions of anesthetics and tranquilizers. *Pharmacol. Rev.* 24: 583–655.

Sidman, R. L., M. M. Dickie, and S. H. Appel. 1964. Mutant mice (quaking and jimpy) with deficient myelination in the central nervous system. *Science* 144: 309–311.

Simon, E. J., J. M. Hiller, and E. Edelman. 1973. Stereospecific binding of the potent narcotic analgesic [³H]-etorphine to rat brain homogenate. *Proc. Nat. Acad. Sci.* 70: 1947–1949.

Snyder, S. H. 1975. II. Biochemical identification of receptors. *Neuroscience Res. Prog. Bull*, Vol. 13, No. 1: 35–38.

Soto, E. F., J. M. Pasquini, R. Placido, and J. L. La Torre. 1969. Fractiona-tion of lipids and proteolipids from cat gray and white matter by chromatography on an organophilic dextran gel. *J. Chromat.* 41: 400–409.

Stephenson, R. P. 1956. A modification of receptor theory. *Brit. J. Pharmacol.* 11: 379–393.

Tasaki, I. 1968. Macromolecular state of axon membrane. In I. Tasaki, Ed. *Nerve Excitation*. Charles Thomas Co. Springfield. pp. 87–129.

Terenius, L. 1973. Stereospecific interaction between narcotic analgesics and a synaptic plasma membrane fraction of rat cerebral cortex. *Acta Pharmacol. Toxicol.* 32: 317–320.

Weber, G., D. P. Borris, E. De Robertis, F. J. Barrantes, J. L. LaTorre, and M. De Carlin. 1971. The use of cholinergic fluorescent probe for the study of receptor proteolipid. *Mol. Pharmacol.* 7: 530–537.

Winstein, S. S., and G. C. Robinson. 1958. Salt effects and ion pairs in solvolysis and related action. *J. Am. Chem. Soc.* 80: 169–181.

Tissue Responses to Addictive Drugs
© 1976, Spectrum Publications, Inc.

Photoaffinity Labeling
of Opiate Receptors

B. M. COX
K. E. OPHEIM
AVRAM GOLDSTEIN

*Stanford University
and Addiction Research Foundation
Palo Alto, California*

The analysis of receptor structure and function has been facilitated by the complementary use of both reversible and irreversible ligands (Furchgott, 1954; Gill and Rang, 1966; Karlin et al., 1973). We have explored the possibility that synthetic opiate analogues might be induced to form covalent complexes with opiate receptors. The technique of photoaffinity labeling (Knowles, 1972) offered the theoretical advantage that reversible drug-receptor interactions could be studied in the absence of photolytic activation of reactive substituents, but that at any desired point in an experiment the photosensitive ligand could be activated by UV irradiation to form a highly reactive intermediate which would react in a nonselective manner with surrounding molecules.

Initial attempts to attach a photoreactive ligand to opiate receptors were made by Winter and Goldstein (1972), who described the synthesis and pharmacologic properties of N-β-(p-azidophenyl) [α-^{3}H]-ethylnorlevorphanol (^{3}H-APL). Arylazides undergo photolytic convertion to aryl nitrenes (Fleet et al., 1969), which are capable of direct insertion into carbon-hydrogen bonds, or cyclo-addition and may be attacked by nucleophiles.

APL has potent opiate-like pharmacological activity in whole mice and the isolated guinea pig ileum preparation. Exposure to UV radiation resulted in significant incorporation of the drug into tissue proteins or into bovine serum albumen (Winter and Goldstein, 1972). However at the concentrations used in their binding experiments (10^{-6} – 10^{-5}M) it was not possible to demonstrate a component of binding attributable to opiate receptors, as defined by inhibition of binding by levorphanol but not by dextrorphan (Goldstein, Lowney and Pal, 1971). The synthesis of ^{3}H-APL at higher specific activity (DeGraw and Engstrom, 1975) has enabled the study of the interaction of the compound with tissue constituents at lower drug concentrations which parallel the concentrations required to demonstrate opiate effects of the drug in *in vitro* preparations. Unlabeled APL, and its dextro enantiomorph (APD) synthesised from dextrorphan, have been used in some experiments. Measurement of the specific optical rotations of the hydrochloride salts of APD and APL gave values of $[\alpha]_D^{19}$ + 81.2° (c = 1.2 in methanol), and $[\alpha]_D^{19}$ −81.1°C (c = 1.1 in methanol), respectively.

We have also synthesised the quaternary nitrogen derivative of APL, N-methyl-N-β(p-azidophenyl) [α-^{3}H] ethylnorlevorphanol (MAPL) by the following procedure. A methanolic solution of ^{3}H-APL (S. A. 1.0 Ci/mmol) was treated with excess methyl iodide and a trace of sodium bicarbonate. (Here and subsequently all manipulations of APL and MAPL were conducted in the dark at 23°C unless otherwise indicated). The conversion of APL to MAPL was followed by TLC (SiO$_2$; CHCl$_3$:-CH$_3$OH, 9:1; APL R$_f$ = 0.55; MAPL R$_f$ = 0.05). Upon completion of the reaction, the methyl iodide and methanol were evaporated under nitrogen and the residue was taken up in water. The aqueous solution was purified first with ether extraction (to remove nonpolar material) and then by chromatography on Dowex 1–X8 anion exchange resin to separate MAPL, having a free phenolic group, from O-methyl MAPL, the presumed major impurity. The final product showed no trace of APL by TLC (system as above). ^{3}H-MAPL appeared as the only mobile component in two other TLC systems, (SiO$_2$; ethanol:acetic acid:water, 6:3:1; R$_f$ = 0.73, and SiO$_2$; ethanol:28% ammonia, 7:3; R$_f$ = 0.69) though a small amount of radioactivity remained at the origin. The overall yield averaged 10%. (The structure of APL, MAPL and levorphanol are shown in Figure 1.)

The demonstration of photoaffinity labeling of opiate receptors requires the differentiation of stereospecific binding (SSB), a reversible

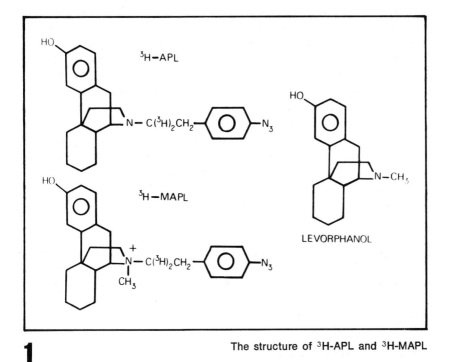

1 The structure of ³H-APL and ³H-MAPL

process occurring in the dark, from stereospecific attachment (SSA) which occurs when the photosensitive ligand is activated by light and reacts with the receptor forming a covalent bond. In all experiments stereospecificity has been determined by preincubation with either dextrorphan or levorphanol (Goldstein et al., 1971). Binding and attachment may be distinguished from each other by:

1. Prolonged washing with aqueous buffer. For drugs that can be removed from receptors by aqueous buffer in the absence of photolytic activation, this procedure offers the simplest demonstration of light induced attachment. However, APL cannot be removed from brain or ileum by repeated washing in aqueous media, and the process is slow for MAPL.

2. Extraction by organic solvents. Reversible receptor binding is usually dissociated by organic solvent extraction. APL and MAPL can be extracted from tissues by mixtures of chloroform and methanol. Thus drug remaining in tissue following solvent extraction is presumably covalently attached. It is also necessary to analyze the extract since drug receptor complexes may

be soluble in the extracting medium. This is most conveniently achieved by chromatography or gel filtration in an organic solvent. Comparison should be made between irradiated and nonirradiated samples. Autoradiography of conventionally prepared sections also allows the demonstration of covalent drug attachment since the fixation media and dehydration and clearing solvents efficiently extract free drug.

3. Analysis of receptor function may allow the distinction between reversible and irreversible drug effects. This has not so far been possible with brain homogenate, where the consequences of receptor activation are not known, but is a useful approach in the guinea pig ileum longitudinal muscle-myenteric plexus preparation where the effects of opiate receptor activation can readily be determined.

In the following discussion the term "binding" is used to refer to a) reversible binding in the absence of photolytic activation, or b) the sum of covalently attached and reversibly bound drug photolysis product, in tissues that have been irradiated with APL and MAPL but in which binding and attachment have not been distinguished by one of the procedures described above.

METHODS AND MATERIALS

Binding of APL and MAPL to brain homogenate

Mouse brain homogenate was preincubated at 23°C with dextrorphan or levorphanol, and then exposed to ^{3}H-etorphine, or ^{3}H-APL in the dark. Aliquots of the incubate were assayed for bound radioactive drug by the filtration assay technique (Pert and Snyder, 1973; Simon et al., 1973). The results (see Figure 2) show that a stereospecific saturable component of binding (SSB) was demonstrable with either drug. Quantitatively the SSB was of the same order for either drug as that previously reported for ^{3}H-etorphine binding to rat brain homogenate (Simon et al., 1973). However the nonspecific binding (NSB, i.e. binding occurring in the presence of a saturating concentration of levorphanol) was seven- to eightfold higher for ^{3}H-APL than for ^{3}H-etorphine.

Table I shows the results of a comparison of the binding of ^{3}H-APL and ^{3}H-MAPL to brain homogenate. At a concentration of 3nM the NSB of ^{3}H-MAPL was substantially lower than that of ^{3}H-APL but no SSB was observed. At a 20-fold higher concentration of ^{3}H-MAPL (approximately its ID_{50} concentration in the guinea pig ileum longitudinal muscle-myenteric plexus preparation) the ^{3}H-MAPL NSB was increased

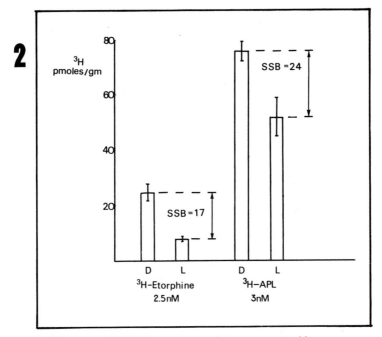

Binding of ³H-etorphine and ³H-APL to mouse brain homogenate. Mouse brains without cerebelli were homogenized in Tris-HCl buffer (0.1M, pH 7.4, 1 gm tissue/100 ml buffer). 2 ml aliquots were incubated at 23°C with dextrorphan, 1μM (D), or levorphanol, 1μM (L), for 20 min prior to the addition of ³H-etorphine (final concentration, 2.5 nM) or ³H-APL (3nM). The incubations were continued for 20 min, and the samples then filtered through Whatman GF/B filters. The filters were washed with 2 x 4 ml cold buffer (for etorphine) or 10 x 4 ml cold buffer (for APL), and radioactivity remaining in the filter determined. (Results are the means ± S.E.M. of triplicate or quadruplicate determinations.)

proportionately, and the variability between individual measurements was greater than the amount of SSB that might be expected.

Table I also demonstrates the effect of exposure to UV irradiation on ³H-APL and ³H-MAPL binding. A short exposure resulted in an increase in NSB for ³H-APL with no change in SSB. The increase in ³H-MAPL NSB was much smaller. A more prolonged irradiation of ³H-APL with brain homogenate increased NSB still further and there was some loss of SSB. Other experiments have confirmed that there is a time dependent loss of SSB of opiate drugs to brain homogenate during irradiation with UV light (H. Teschemacher, personal communication).

Table I. Binding of ^{3}H-APL and ^{3}H-MAPL to Mouse Brain Homogenate: Effects of UV Irradiation

Group	Drug	n	$h\upsilon$	pmoles bound / gm. tissue ± S.E.M.		
				+ levorphanol	+ dextrorphan	SSB
1	^{3}H-APL, 3nM,	4	–	52 ± 7	76 ± 2	24
2	^{3}H-APL, 3nM,	4	+ (2 mins.)	99 ± 3	118 ± 4	19
3	^{3}H-APL, 3nM,	6	+ (20 mins.)	143 ± 13	156 ± 17	13
4	^{3}H-MAPL, 3nM,	4	–	23 ± 1	25 ± 2	2
5	^{3}H-MAPL, 3nM,	4	+ (2 mins.)	26 ± 2	27 ± 4	2
6	^{3}H-MAPL, 60nM,	4	–	436 ± 31	405 ± 29	–31
7	^{3}H-MAPL, 60nM,	4	+ (2 mins.)	456 ± 23	459 ± 53	3

For all groups except 3, the procedures were essentially as described in Figure 2. After incubation with ^{3}H-APL or ^{3}H-MAPL some samples ($h\upsilon$,+) were exposed to UV irradiation (Hanovia 450W Hg lamp, with Kimax filter; samples were held in Kimax tubes, 8cm from the lamp, immersed in water at 23°C), for the time indicated. After filtration the filters were washed with 10 x 4 ml of cold Tris-HCl buffer. Binding to filter blanks has been subtracted. For group 3, the samples were centrifuged following irradiation, and the pellet washed four times with cold buffer by dispersion and recentrifugation prior to radioactivity determination. The SSB obtained in treatments 1, 2, and 3 was significantly different from zero ($p < 0.05$); n = number of samples.

These results establish that ³H-APL binds to opiate receptors in mouse brain homogenate but do not indicate whether UV irradiation promotes the attachment of the drug to receptors. It seems probable that the demonstration of the attachment of ³H-MAPL to receptors in brain homogenate will require extensive fractionation subsequent to irradiation.

In the following experiments the nature of the ³H-APL retained in tissue following UV irradiation has been examined in more detail. Brain homogenate was incubated with levorphanol or dextrorphan (1 μM), and exposed to ³H-APL (3 nM) for 20 min. The period of UV irradiation was extended to 20 min to ensure complete photolytic conversion of the arylazide. After buffer wash the pelleted particulate material was extracted twice with chloriform:methanol (2:1, v/v) and the extracts pooled. The chloroform:methanol insoluble pellet was dissolved in 1% sodium dodecyl sulfate (SDS). Two-thirds of the radioactivity initially retained by the brain homogenate particulate material was found in chloroform:methanol extract, and the stereospecific difference attributable to the initial incubation with either levorphanol or dextrorphan was also found in this extract. This radioactivity could not be precipitated by the addition of four volumes of ice-cold diethyl ether to the chloroform:methanol extract. On TLC it showed similar R_f values in four solvents systems to those obtained when chloroform:methanol extracts from ³H-APL previously photolysed in Tris buffer alone were chromatographed (see Table II).

In these experiments there was no stereospecific difference in the amounts of ³H bound to the CM insoluble residue. The ³H bound to brain proteins was further analyzed in another series of experiments. Following incubation with levorphanol or dextrorphan, and ³H-APL (3nM), the incubate was exposed to UV radiation for 20 min and then centrifuged. The pellet was extracted twice with diethyl ether and following buffer wash was solubilised in 3% SDS in Tris-HCl buffer (pH 7.4) containing 3M urea. Samples of this material were fractionated by polyacrylamide gel electrophoresis. Apart from a small amount of radioactivity remaining at the origin, two major peaks resulted; a relatively broad peak closely following the ion front which did not correspond to any visibly stained protein band, and a more slowly migrating discrete peak running in the leading edge of a heavily stained protein band (see Figure 3). The radioactivity in these peaks was not modified by the presence of levorphanol or dextrorphan in the incubation. In nonirradiated samples the second peak was reduced by 95% and the first by 80%. Essentially similar results were obtained when the nonradioactive ligands levorphanol and dextrorphan were replaced in the

Table II. Analysis of Chloroform:methanol Extractable Radioactivity Following Irradiation of ^{3}H-MAPL with Mouse Brain Homogenate or Tris Buffer

Solvent system		R_f values of ^{3}H spots after incubation and irradiation with:	
	^{3}H-APL + Tris	Brain + Lev. + ^{3}H-APL + Tris	Brain + Dex. + ^{3}H-APL + Tris
A	0.00	0.00	0.00
	0.45	0.45	0.45
B	0.00	0.00	0.00
	0.55	0.60	0.55
	0.80		
C	0.00	0.00	0.00
	0.95	0.95	0.95
D	0.95	0.95	0.95

The chloroform:methanol extracts were evaporated to dryness under a stream of N_2, taken up in a small volume of the same solvent, and applied to TLC plates (SiO_2). Solvents used for development were: A, chloroform:methanol 9:1; B, benzene:butanol, 3:1; C, chloroform:methanol:acetone:triethylamine, 30:4:10:20; and D, chloroform:methanol:water: 28% ammonia, 130:70:8:0.5. Plates were cut into 1 cm squares for radioactivity determination.

incubation mixture by nonradioactive APL or APD at a concentration of 100 nM.

These results suggest that the photolytic activation of ^{3}H-APL in combination with opiate receptors in mouse brain homogenate does not result in covalent attachment of the drug to the receptor, under the conditions studied here. Perhaps for steric reasons, the drug may react preferentially with solvent whilst bound to the receptor. In view of the high affinity of APL for opiate receptors it seems unlikely that the drug dissociates from the receptor, becomes photolytically activated in solution, reacts with solvent, and then returns to the receptor.

Effects of APL and MAPL on the guinea pig ileum longitudinal muscle-myenteric plexus preparation

In the absence of UV irradiation APL produces a dose dependent inhibition of the responses of the ileum preparation to electrical stimulation, a 50% inhibition of maximal contractions being produced at concentrations around 3 nM. APD is without effect at these concentra-

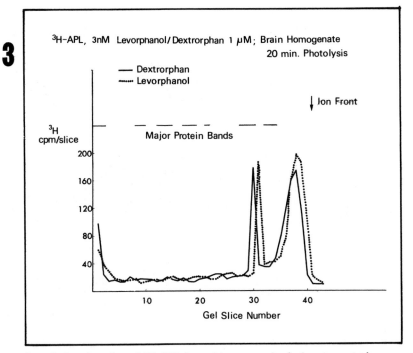

3

³H-APL, 3nM Levorphanol/Dextrorphan 1 µM; Brain Homogenate
20 min. Photolysis

—— Dextrorphan
······ Levorphanol

↓ Ion Front

Major Protein Bands

³H
cpm/slice

Gel Slice Number

Electrophoretic fractionation of ³H-APL bound to mouse brain homogenate by UV irradiation. Mouse brain homogenate was exposed to UV irradiation for 20 min. with ³H-APL (3 nM), following incubation with levorphanol or dextrorphan (1µM). The homogenate was centrifuged (10,000 g, 20 min) and extracted twice with 10 ml diethyl ether to remove unbound drug and photolysis products, washed twice with Tris-HCl buffer, and then solubilised by heating in 2 ml 3% sodium dodecyl sulfate (SDS) in Tris-HCl buffer containing 3M urea. Samples of this material were fractionated by polyacrylamide gel electrophoresis using 1 cm diameter 7.5% acrylamide gels in a Tris-Tricinate buffer giving a resolving pH of 8.1. 0.1% SDS was present in all gel and buffer solutions. A current of 1 mA/tube was applied for 18 hr. At the end of the run the gels were either frozen on solid CO_2 and cut into 2mm slices which were placed in scintillation vials for radioactivity determination, or were stained with 1% Amido Black in 7% acetic acid. The results indicate that attachment of ³H-APL to the tissue was not altered by prior incubation with levorphanol.

tions (see Figure 4). MAPL has approximately one-fifteenth (0.06 ± 0.01; APL = 1) of the activity of APL, but the rate of onset of its effect is more rapid (see Figure 4). While the effect of MAPL can be reversed by repeated washing, this has proved to be impossible with APL. The effects of both drugs can be reversed by naloxone (see Figure 4). After washing out the naloxone the inhibitory effect of APL returns to the

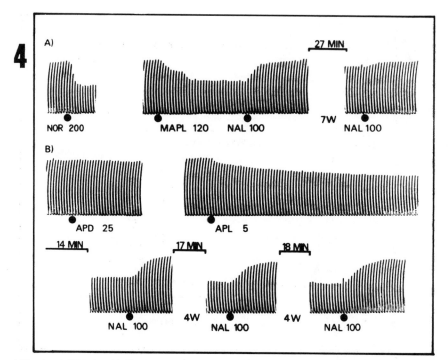

Effects of APL and MAPL on the guinea pig ileum longitudinal muscle-myenteric plexus preparation. Strips of longitudinal muscle with attached myenteric plexus from guinea pig ileum were set up as described by Paton and Vizi (1969), in a 5 ml organ bath containing Krebs-bicarbonate Ringer oxygenated with 95% O_2 plus 5% CO_2 at 37°C. The preparation was electrically stimulated at 0.1 Hz, 0.5 msec pulse duration, at maximal voltage (80 V). Responses were recorded with a Grass FT.03 strain gauge on a Grass Polygraph. The tissue was maintained under a resting tension of 1 gm, and the experiment was conducted in subdued light throughout. Panel A shows the effects and reversibility of MAPL. Panel B shows the effects of APD and APL.

NOR=normorphine; NAL=naloxone; 7W, 4W, refer ot the number of times the bathing fluid was changed during the time period indicated. Figures refer to the final bath concentration of drug (nM).

level observed prior to naloxone application. The naloxone reversal can be repeated several times with no further addition of APL to the preparation. The ability of the quarternary nitrogen derivative MAPL to produce typical opiate effects provides evidence that opiate receptors are situated on the external surface of cells. In most of the subsequent experiments MAPL has been employed rather than APL because of the reversibility of its effects in the absence of photolytic activation.

The effects of MAPL on the output of acetylcholine from the guinea pig ileum preparation have recently been described by Schulz and Goldstein (1975). They found that in the dark MAPL produced an inhibition of the electrically stimulated acetylcholine output which could be reversed by repeated washing, or blocked by the simultaneous presence of naloxone. Irradiation of the tissue with MAPL resulted in a permanent inhibition of the acetylcholine output which was not reversed on repeated washing of the tissue or by the addition of naloxone. Irradiation of the preparation in the presence of MAPL and naloxone did not result in any inhibition of acetylcholine output. Thus it appears that when the receptors are not occupied by naloxone, photolytic activation of MAPL with the tissue results in a permanent opioid effect not sensitive to a subsequent application of naloxone. These results suggest that naloxone competes with the opiates for a common receptor. Permanent occupation of that receptor by a covalently attached agonist results in a persistent opioid effect.

Binding of opioid drugs to the guinea pig ileum preparation

We initially studied the binding of a drug that had been successfully employed in studies of opiate receptors in brain, ^{3}H-etorphine (Simon et al., 1973; and above). Figure 5 shows a Scatchard plot of ^{3}H-etorphine binding to the ileum preparation. In the presence of dextrorphan a high affinity component of binding with an apparent K_D of about 4×10^{-10}M was observed. This corresponds closely to the observed concentration of 5×10^{-10}M required to give 50% inhibition of the electrically induced contractions of the ileum preparation. This high affinity component was not seen in the presence of levorphanol. Extrapolation to the abscissa suggests a maximum number of stereospecific high affinity binding sites of about 6 pmoles/gm tissue. The high affinity component of etorphine binding to the intact ileum preparation could be inhibited by APL (10 nM) but not by APD at the same concentration, and did not appear to be affected by the exposure of the tissue to UV irradiation for 20 min. (see Figure 6)

Because the pharmacologic evidence (Schulz and Goldstein, 1975) provided a clear indication of permanent opioid effects resulting from the irradiation of ileum preparations with MAPL, we have studied MAPL binding. It has proved difficult to obtain consistent SSB of ^{3}H-MAPL to the ileum preparation, although this has been observed in some experiments with low MAPL concentrations. In general the total level of MAPL binding at concentrations giving more than 50% inhibition of the electrically induced contractions of the ileum preparation has been so high as to preclude the observation of the small fraction of binding attributable to receptor occupation. Nonspecific binding of MAPL by

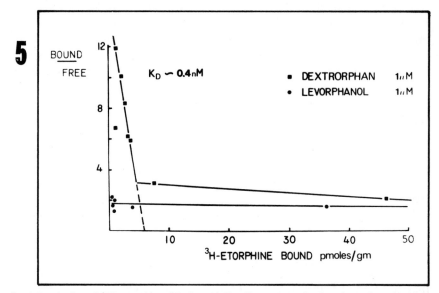

5

Scatchard plot of ³H-etorphine binding to the ileum preparation. Lengths of longitudinal muscle-myenteric plexus preparation from guinea pig ileum were spread on a plastic sheet and frozen on solid CO_2. The strips were cut longitudinally in half and each half assigned to a dextrorphan or levorphanol pretreatment group. After a preliminary wash the tissues were blotted, weighed and incubated with levorphanol or dextrorphan (1 μM, 20 min) as previously determined. ³H-etorphine was added and the incubation continued for a further 20 min. The tissues were then rinsed with three changes of 5 ml Krebs (0°C.) containing levorphanol or dextrorphan as appropriate. Finally the tissues were dissolved in 1 ml Soluene (Packard) and radioactively determined. Ordinate: Bound ³H/ Free ³H (pmoles/gm tissue : pmoles/ml incubate).

ileum preparation homogenates was substantially higher than by intact strips. Attempts to remove reversibly bound radioactivity following irradiation, by washing the preparation with organic solvents, still left very high levels of radioactivity attached to the tissue.

We have sought an indication of the localization of ³H-MAPL binding by autoradiography. Silver grain distribution over nonirradiated ³H-MAPL treated sections was little higher than background. However, following irradiation of the tissue with ³H-MAPL, many more silver grains were observed over the tissue sections. Analysis of silver grain counts over ganglia and longitudinal muscle revealed consistently higher grain density over ganglia previously treated with dextrorphan than over levorphanol treated ganglia (see Figure 7). Grain densities over

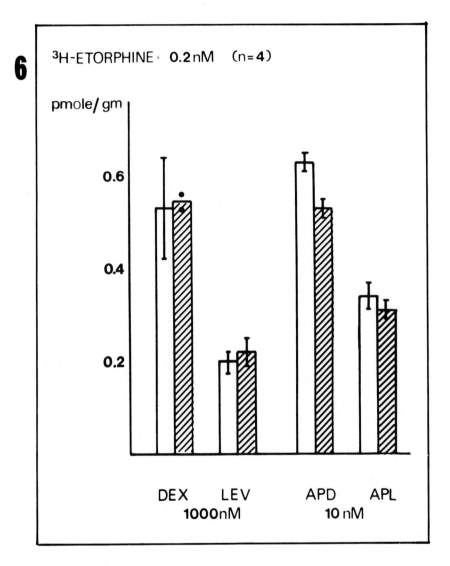

6

^{3}H-ETORPHINE · 0.2 nM   (n=4)

pmole/gm

0.6

0.4

0.2

DEX   LEV   APD   APL
1000nM   **10 nM**

Effects of APL, APD and UV irradiation on high affinity binding of ^{3}H-etorphine to the ileum preparation. The procedure was essentially as described in Figure 5, except that for some samples preincubation with levorphanol or dextrorphan was replaced by preincubation in APL or APD. Some samples (hatched columns) were irradiated (for 20 min, 23°C.) after the etorphine incubation. ^{3}H-etorphine concentration was 0.2 nM. (Results are the means ± S.E.M. from 4 determinations.) Dex=dextrorphan; Lev=levorphanol.

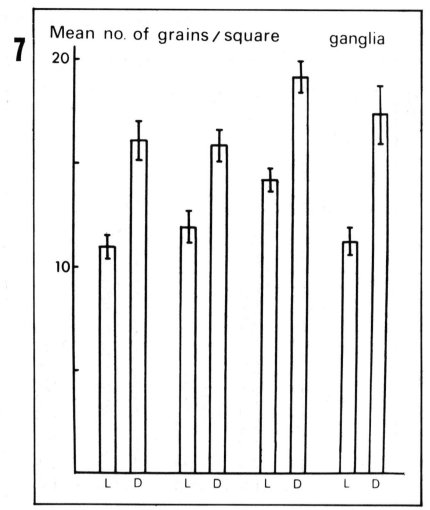

Autoradiography of ^{3}H-MAPL in the ileum preparation. Silver grain density over ganglia of the myenteric plexus. Paired lengths of longitudinal muscle-myenteric plexus preparation were mounted on strips of plastic with the ganglia side uppermost. After a preliminary wash in Krebs solution, the mounted tissues were incubated with either leverphanol (L) or dextrorphan (D), 1 μM. ^{3}H-MAPL was added to a final concentration of 60 nM and the incubation continued for 20 min. The tissues were irradiated (20 min, 23°C) with the ganglia surface facing the lamp. Following irradiation the tissues were rinsed in Krebs solution, fixed in formalin-saline, dehydrated in ethanol, cleared in xylene and blocked in paraffin wax. 5 μ sections were mounted on glass slides, dipped in Kodak NTB 2 emulsion and exposed (21 days over anhyd. CaSO$_4$ at 2°C). Following development and fixation, sections were stained with toluidine blue. The sections were examined at 640 x magnification using a Zeiss Photomicroscope I fitted with an eyepiece grid defining tissue areas of approximately 400 μ^2. Silver grains were counted over 30 areas orientated over ganglia of the myenteric plexus in each tissue. (Results are the mean ± S.E.M. (n=30) obtained from 4 pairs of tissues. Counts were made by an observer blind to the experimental conditions.)

longitudinal muscle did not differ consistently in the levorphanol or dextrorphan preparations. Thus there appeared to be a stereospecific attachment of ^{3}H-MAPL over the ganglia of the myenteric plexus.

DISCUSSION

It has been shown that APL binds to opiate receptors in brain homogenate in the dark. UV irradiation resulted in a progressive increase in the total amount of drug binding, but there was a time dependent decrease in SSB. The stereospecific component of binding could be extracted into chloroform-methanol, and chromotographic analysis of this extract suggested that covalent attachment of the drug to receptors had not occurred under the conditions employed in these experiments. It seemed probable that when APL, reversibly bound to receptors, was irradiated, the photolytically generated arylnitrene, remaining in a reversible complex with the receptor, reacted preferentially with surrounding solvent molecules. In view of the very high total binding of ^{3}H-MAPL by brain homogenate, we have not as yet demonstrated whether attachment of this drug to receptors occurs.

In the guinea pig ileum preparation, the autoradiographic data clearly show a stereospecific attachment of MAPL to the ganglia of the myenteric plexus. This interpretation is supported by the functional studies which show that a permanent opioid effect is produced by irradiation of MAPL with the tissue. The difficulty of demonstrating either SSB or SSA of MAPL in the intact preparation, despite the autoradiographic demonstration of SSA over ganglia, probably arises because the myenteric plexus is only a small fraction of the total mass of the intact preparation, and there is substantial binding and attachment of the drug by longitudinal muscle.

The very high affinity of APL for opiate receptors suggests that this drug should be a good photoaffinity label. It is therefore surprising that we have not obtained evidence of SSA with APL, but appear to have achieved opiate receptor labeling with MAPL, a drug with lower receptor affinity. The most useful results with photoaffinity labeling have been obtained under circumstances which are particularly favorable to selective labeling. Thus in the experiments of Westheimer and his colleagues (Singh et al., 1962; Shafer et al., 1966), and Fleet et al. (1969) there was clearly a close juxtaposition between the active site surfaces and the photoreactive labeling groups. Singer et al. (1973) also emphasize the importance of steric factors in discussing the difficulty they experienced in obtaining true photoaffinity labeling of acetylcholine binding sites. It is possible that the preferred orientation of the *p*-azido-phenylethyl nitrogen substituent of APL may be subtly shifted by addition of another nitrogen substituent, thus allowing the photoreactive group of MAPL to be more closely aligned with the receptor surface. This hypothesis would suggest that careful analysis of MAPL covalently attached to brain homogenate would reveal a component of binding attributable to receptor occupation.

Alternatively there may be minor differences in structure between ileum and brain receptors which facilitate covalent attachment in the former tissue but impede it in the latter. A more trivial explanation would be that homogenization of tissue results in subtle changes in membrane receptor conformation.

We have shown that under certain circumstances arylazide analogues of opiate drugs may be used to label opiate receptors of the guinea pig ileum myenteric plexus irreversibly. This approach has provided an additional tool in the pharmacological analysis of receptor function, and may subsequently allow the isolation of the drug receptor complex.

ACKNOWLEDGMENTS

This work was supported by grants DA–972 and DA–1199 from the National Institute on Drug Abuse. We thank Pat Lowery and Rekha Padhya for expert technical assistance.

REFERENCES

DeGraw, J. I., and J. S. Engstrom. 1975. The synthesis of ^{14}C and ^{3}H-labeled N-p-azidophenethylnorlevorphanol. *J. Label. Cpds.* 11: 233–239.

Fleet, G. W. J., R. R. Porter, and J. R. Knowles. 1969. Affinity labeling of antibodies with arylnitrene as reactive group. *Nature* (London) 224: 511–512.

Furchgott, R. F. 1954. Dibenamine blockade in strips of rabbit aorta and its use in differentiating receptors. *J. Pharmacol. Exp. Ther.* 111: 265–284.

Gill, E. W., and H. P. Rang. 1966. An alkylating derivative of benzilylcholine with specific and long-lasting parasympatholytic activity. *Mol. Pharmacol.* 2: 284–297.

Goldstein, A., L. I. Lowney, and B. K. Pal. 1971. Stereospecific and nonspecific interactions of the morphine congener levorphanol in subcellular fractions of mouse brain. *Proc. Nat. Acad. Sci. U.S.A.* 68: 1742–1747.

Karlin, A., D. A. Cowburn, and M. J. Reiter. 1973. Molecular properties of the acetylcholine receptor. In H. P. Rang, Ed. *Drug Receptors.* Macmillan, London, pp. 193–209.

Knowles, J. R. 1972. Photogenerated reagents for biological receptor-site labeling. *Account Chem. Res.* 5: 155–160.

Paton, W. D. M., and E. S. Vizi. 1969. The inhibitory action of noradrenaline and adrenaline on the acetylcholine output by guinea pig ileum longitudinal muscle strip. *Brit. J. Pharmacol.* 35: 10–28.

Pert, C. B., and S. H. Snyder. 1973. Opiate receptor: its demonstration in nervous tissue. *Science* 179: 1011–1014.

Schulz, R., and A. Goldstein. 1975. Irreversible alteration of opiate receptor function by a photoaffinity labeling reagent. *Life Sci.* 16: 1843–1848.

Shafer, J., P. Baronowsky, R. Laursen, F. Finn, and F. H. Westheimer. 1966. Products from the photolysis of diazoacetyl chymotrypsin. *J. Biol. Chem.* 241: 421–427.

Simon, E. J., J. M. Hiller, and I. Edelman. 1973. Stereospecific binding of the potent narcotic analgesic ^{3}H-etorphine to rat brain homogenate. *Proc. Nat. Acad. Sci. U.S.A.* 70: 1947–1949.

Singer, S. J., A. Ruoho, H. Kiefer, J. Lindstrom, and E. S. Lennox. 1973. The use of affinity labels in the identification of receptors. In H. P. Rang, Ed. *Drug Receptors.* Macmillan, London, pp. 183–190.

Singh, A., E. R. Thornton, and F. H. Westheimer. 1962. The photolysis of diazoacetylchymotrypsin. *J. Biol. Chem.* 237: PC3006–3008.

Winter, B. A., and A. Goldstein. 1972. A photochemical affinity-labelling reagent for the opiate receptor(s). *Mol. Pharmacol.* 6: 601–611.

Tissue Responses to Addictive Drugs
© 1976, Spectrum Publications, Inc.

Effect of Sodium on Specific Binding of ³H-Dihydromorphine and ³H-Naloxone to Striatal Membranes of Rat Brain

DAVID T. WONG
JONG S. HORNG

The Lilly Research Laboratories
Indianapolis, Indiana

Goldstein et al. (1971) first suggested that displacement of bound radioactive opiate drug by nonradioactive nonopiate enantiomer could be used to identify specific binding to particulate matter in the central nervous system. This displacement principle enabled three laboratories to demonstrate independently the specific binding of opiate and opiate antagonist drugs to brain fractions (Terenius, 1973; Pert and Snyder, 1973; Simon et al., 1973), and this binding has been confirmed in our laboratory (Wong and Horng, 1973).

The specific binding of both opiates (³H-etorphine and ³H-dihydromorphine) and opiate antagonist (³H-naloxone) could be displaced by pharmacologically active opiates or opiate-like drugs and by opiate antagonists (Pert and Snyder, 1973; Simon et al., 1973; Wong and Horng, 1973), the effectiveness of displacement being proportional to the pharmacological potencies of the displacing drugs. Thus binding sites may represent the pharmacologic receptor for opiates.

Simon et al. (1973) showed that sodium reduced the binding of ^{3}H-etorphine to brain homogenates. This observation was confirmed by Pert et al. (1973) who also showed that sodium increased the binding of ^{3}H-naloxone. There has been disagreement about the mechanism of action of sodium. The cation was found to exert its influence on the affinity (Simon et al., 1975) and on the number of binding sites (Pert and Snyder, 1974; Pasternak and Snyder, 1975) for both opiate and opiate antagonist. We are reporting here our own studies on the characteristics of sodium action in enhancing ^{3}H-naloxone binding and antagonizing ^{3}H-dihydromorphine binding to striatal membranes of rat brain.

MATERIALS AND METHODS

Male rats (110 g) of Wistar strain fed *ad libitum* on Purina Chow were killed by decapitation. The corpus striatum was immediately removed from the brain and kept in ice-chilled 0.32M sucrose solution. Tissue was homogenized in either 50 mM Tris-Cl, pH 7.4 or 0.32M sucrose as 1% or 10% homogenate, respectively. The sucrose homogenate was centrifuged at 1085 x g for 10 min. The supernatant fraction was spun at 100,000 x g for 60 min as a washing step. In some cases, this washing step was repeated. The determination of specific binding of ^{3}H-dihydromorphine (^{3}H-DHM, NEN, 46 Ci/mM) or ^{3}H-naloxone (^{3}H-NLX, NEN, 38 Ci/mM) was made by the filtration technique as described by Wong and Horng (1973). Specific binding was defined as the difference in amounts of ^{3}H-ligands bound in the absence and presence of 10^{-7}M levorphanol or ^{3}H-naltrexone. When the equilibrium binding was done at various concentrations of ^{3}H-ligands, the dissociation constant and density of binding sites were estimated by means of the Scatchard method (Scatchard, 1949). The intercepts were determined by means of best fit into a single or two straight lines which would have the least sum of squared deviations utilizing computer analysis. Experiments were repeated two to four times to establish their validity.

RESULTS

Among six gross brain regions (see Table I), the capacity for the binding of ^{3}H-DHM and ^{3}H-NLX was greatest in washed membranes of corpus striatum, midbrain and hypothalamus, 70-80 fmole ^{3}H-ligands/ mg protein; intermediate in pons + medulla, and cerebral cortex; and lowest in the cerebellum. NaCl at 100 mM almost doubled the binding

Table I. The Specific Binding of ^{3}H-DHM and ^{3}H-NLX to Washed Membranes from Six Rat Brain Regions

Brain Regions	Specific binding of		
	^{3}H-DHM	^{3}H-NLX	
		$-Na^+$	$+NA^+$, 100 mM
	10^{-14} mole/mg protein*		
Corpus striatum	7.96 ± 0.24	7.49 ± 0.57	11.91 ± 0.14
Midbrain	7.68 ± 0.51	8.11 ± 0.55	12.93 ± 1.10
Hypothalamus	6.58 ± 0.37	6.78 ± 0.38	11.92 ± 0.12
Pons + Medulla	4.37 ± 0.67	4.65 ± 0.95	7.64 ± 0.16
Cerebral cortex	2.17 ± 0.19	3.63 ± 0.33	5.61 ± 0.20
Cerebellum	1.30 ± 0.12	0.87 ± 0.26	0.84 ± 0.22

*Mean values ± S.E.M. were obtained from triplicate samples with either 5 x 10^{-9}M ^{3}H-DHM or 5 x 10^{-9}M ^{3}H-NLX.

of ^{3}H-NLX to the membranes of the first five regions. We chose striatal membranes throughout our studies because of their high binding capacity.

Figure 1 shows the effects of varied concentrations of NaCl on binding of ^{3}H-DHM and ^{3}H-NLX to striatal membranes. The binding of ^{3}H-DHM was reduced to about 50% at 20 mM NaCl and was gradually reduced to 10% of control binding with increasing NaCl concentration up to 100 mM. The binding of ^{3}H-NLX was increased with NaCl concentration up to 20 mM but was not further increased at 50 or 100 mM NaCl.

The binding of ^{3}H-DHM to the membranous fraction of corpus striatum homogenate is a saturable process (see Figure 2B) with concentration range of ^{3}H-DHM between 0.5 and 6 nM. The presence of 10^{-7}M dextrorphan did not change the binding of ^{3}H-DHM indicating the binding was specific (Wong and Horng, 1973). In the absence or the presence of 10^{-7}M dextrorphan, the binding of ^{3}H-DHM appeared monophasic with similar dissociation constants (Kd values) of 2.88 nM and density of binding sites (n values) of 99.9 fmole/mg protein (see Figure 2A).

After the addition of 20 mM NaCl, the binding of ^{3}H-DHM was substantially reduced. The number of binding sites was reduced to 63.4 fmole/mg with the same Kd value of 2.92 nM as in the absence of NaCl (see Figure 2A). At a higher concentration of NaCl (40 mM),

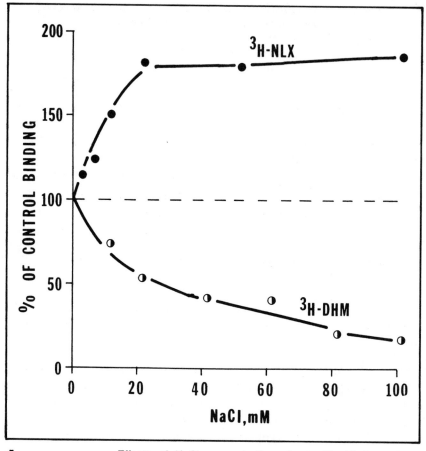

1

Effects of NaCl concentration of specific binding of
^{3}H-DHM and ^{3}H-NLX to striatal membranes.
  Aliquots of striatal membranes were incubated at 37°C
for 15 min in 50 Tris-Cl, pH 7.4 containing either 1 x 10^{-9}M
^{3}H-DHM or 2 x 10^{-9}M ^{3}H-NLX and NaCl between 1 and
100 mM.

however, the binding was further reduced due to an increase of the
Kd value (4.47 nM) without greater decrease of sites.

When the maximum concentration of ^{3}H-DHM was raised to 20
nM, two components were resolved in the Scatchard plots (see Figure 3);
a high affinity and a low affinity component having Kd values of 1.04
and 4.98 nM respectively and the corresponding n values of 68.6 and

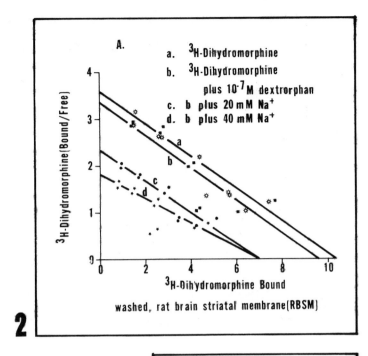

a. ^{3}H-Dihydromorphine
b. ^{3}H-Dihydromorphine plus 10^{-7}M dextrorphan
c. b plus 20 mM Na$^+$
d. b plus 40 mM Na$^+$

washed, rat brain striatal membrane(RBSM)

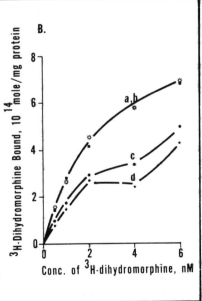

Effect of low NaCl concentrations on the specific binding of ^{3}H-DHM to striatal membranes as illustrated by Scatchard plots (A) and saturation curves (B).

The striatal membranes were prepared by repeated sedimentation at 100,000 x g and was resuspended in 50 mM Tris-Cl, pH 7.4. Aliquots of membranes were incubated at 37°C for 15 min in 50 mM Tris-Cl pH 7.4 buffer containing various concentrations of ^{3}H-DHM (a) and also with 10^{-7}M dextrorphan (b) as well as 20 mM NaCl (c) or 40 mM NaCl (d). Data from individual samples were used for the Scatchard plots when means of duplicate samples were plotted on the saturation curves.

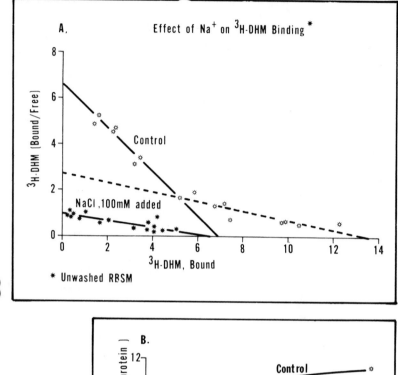

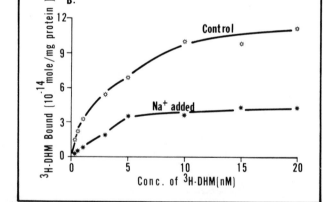

Effect of high NaCl concentration on the high and the low affinity binding of
^{3}H-DHM to striatal homogenate as illustrated by Scatchard plots (A) and
saturation curves (B).

Aliquots of striatal homogenate in 50 mM Tris-Cl, pH 7.4 were incubated
in various concentrations of ^{3}H-DHM between 8.5 to 20 nM. NaCl at 100 mM
was also included at each concentration of ^{3}H-DHM in duplicate samples.
Data were treated in identical manner as in Figure 2. The solid line and the
dotted line drawn over the open rosettes represent a high and a low affinity
binding components for ^{3}H-DHM.

136.7 fmole/mg protein. In the presence of 100 mM NaCl, only a single binding component remained having a Kd value of 6.76 nM and a n value of 67.2 fmole/mg protein. Seemingly, NaCl at 100 mM had completely abolished the sites of the high affinity component and partially the sites of the low affinity component because the computer analysis of the Scatchard plot showed unreasonably large x-intercept with data from low concentration of ^{3}H-DHM (below 5 nM) but gave reasonable x- and y- intercepts when higher concentrations of ^{3}H-DHM (up to 20 nM) were included for computations. Thus, only the low affinity component remained in the presence of 100 mM NaCl with a further decrease in affinity for ^{3}H-DHM.

The binding of the opiate antagonist, ^{3}H-naloxone (^{3}H-NLX), was increased by 100 mM NaCl and appeared to be monophasic in the absence or presence of NaCl (see Figure 4a and 4b). The increase in ^{3}H-NLX binding could not be reversed by the addition of 10^{-7}M dextrorphan. Under these three sets of conditions, the Kd values were practically identical (0 Na$^+$, 1.6 nM; 100 mM Na$^+$, 2.3 nM; 100 mM Na$^+$ and 10^{-7}M dextrorphan, 1.9 nM). However, the density of binding sites for ^{3}H-NLX was increased from 52 fmole/mg protein to 90 and 93 fmole/mg protein in the presence of 100 mM NaCl or 100 mM NaCl and 10^{-7}M dextrorphan. In this experiment, the highest concentration of ^{3}H-NLX was 10 nM (see Figure 4b). In other experiments when the maximum concentration of ^{3}H-NLX was increased to 20 nM, the binding of ^{3}H-NLX remained monophasic indicating the participation of a single binding component.

The effects of NaCl on the binding of ^{3}H-DHM was readily reversed by simply resuspending the membranes in the NaCl-free buffer (see Table II). However, the binding of ^{3}H-NLX to such membranes remained partially activated. An additional washing step by recentrifugation and resuspension to the original volume of buffer was able to return the ^{3}H-NLX binding activity to normal (see Figure 5). Like before, NaCl did not alter the dissociation constants, Kd values (control-washed, 7.4 nM; Na$^+$ treated-washed, 6.5 nM; Na$^+$ treated-washed Na$^+$ incubated, 5.5 nM). The greater Kd values here were probably caused by the extra washing of the membranes. However, the increased density of binding sites for ^{3}H-NLX was returned from 280 fmole/mg protein to 163 fmole/mg protein, as in control-washed membranes.

Besides sodium, the effects of other monovalent cations were also examined. LiCl and NaCl were most effective in reduction of ^{3}H-DHM binding to twice washed striatal membranes (see Figure 6). However, only NaCl was capable of doubling the binding of ^{3}H-NLX in the same preparation of striatal membranes. In a separate experiment, we exam-

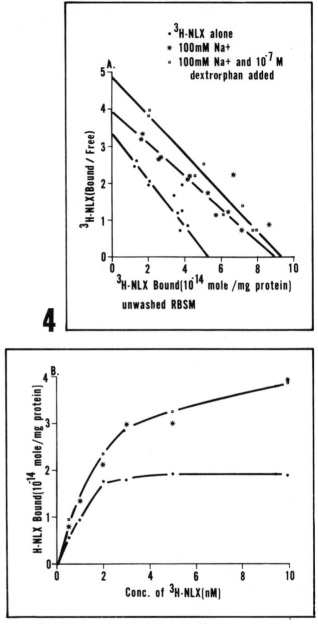

Effect of NaCl on the specific binding of ^{3}H-NLX to striatal homogenate as illustrated by Scatchard plots (A) and saturation curves (B).

Striatal homogenate was incubated with various concentrations of ^{3}H-NLX between 0.5 and 10 nM. At each concentration of ^{3}H-NLX, duplicate samples also contained either 10^{-7}M naltrexone, 10^{-7}M dextrorphan or 100 mM NaCl and samples contained only ^{3}H-NLX as control. Treatment of data was identical to Figure 2.

Table II. Reversibility of Sodium Effect on Specific Binding of
^{3}H-DHM and ^{3}H-NLX

Ligand	Control	100 mM NaCl Added	100 mM NaCl Treated and Resuspended
		10^{-14}mole/mg protein	
^{3}H-DHM	5.81 ± 0.34	1.06 ± 0.02 $P < 0.001$	5.30 ± 0.38
^{3}H-NLX	3.61 ± 0.07	7.29 ± 0.62 $P < 0.001$	5.21 ± 0.54 $P < 0.05$

A 10% striatal homogenate in 0.32M sucrose was centrifuged at 1085 x g for 10 min. The supernatant fraction was diluted to 1% homogenate with 50 mM Tris-Cl, pH 7.4 in the absence and presence of 100 mM NaCl. The suspensions stood for 30 min at 37°C and were centrifuged at 100,000 x g for 60 min at 4°C. The pellets were suspended in 50 mM Tris-Cl, pH 7.4. Striatal membranes were incubated for 15 min at 37°C with 2 x 10^{-9}M ^{3}H-DHM or ^{3}H-NLX. The difference in amount of ^{3}H-ligand bound in the absence and presence of 10^{-7}M levorphanol or 10^{-7}M naltrexone was considered as specific binding.

ined the effect of 100 mM LiCl on various concentrations of ^{3}H-NLX. Again, no increase in ^{3}H-NLX binding was found (unpublished results).

The binding of ^{3}H-DHM to the twice washed striatal membranes was increased with temperature and reached a maximum level between 36°C and 44°C (see Figure 7). The inhibitory effect of 100 mM NaCl increased as incubation temperature increased from 0°C to 44°C. The binding of ^{3}H-NLX to the control membranes had similar temperature profile as the binding of ^{3}H-DHM. However, in the presence of 100 mM NaCl, the degree of ^{3}H-NLX binding was as great at 0°C as 36°C. The effect of NaCl was more pronounced at 0°C and 24°C.

The binding of ^{3}H-DHM and ^{3}H-NLX also had different pH profiles (see Figure 8). The optimum pH for ^{3}H-DHM binding was about pH 8.4 in the absence or the presence of 100 mM NaCl. However, the optimum pH for ^{3}H-NLX binding was about pH 7.2. The addition of 100 mM NaCl changed the pH optimum toward pH 8.4 at which the increase in ^{3}H-NLX binding by NaCl was most noticeable.

DISCUSSION

The present study not only confirms our earlier finding that a high affinity binding component for ^{3}H-DHM exists in striatal membranes but also confirms our suggestion that a second binding component with a lower affinity for ^{3}H-DHM may exist in the same tissue (Wong

Reversibility of sodium effect on specific binding of ^{3}H-NLX to striatal membranes as illustrated by saturation curves (A) and Scatchard plots (B).

Striatal homogenates were incubated in 50 mM Tris-Cl, pH 7.4 buffer in the absence and presence of 100 mM NaCl. After standing at 4°C for 30 min, the homogenates were sedimented at 100,000 x g for 60 min. The pellets were suspended in Tris buffer and centrifuged again at 100,000 x g for 60 min. The final sediments were resuspended in the Tris buffer as control and sodium-treated striatal membranes. The two preparations of striatal membranes were incubated with ^{3}H-NLX between 0.5 and 6 nM. Aliquots of the sodium-treated striatal membranes also had samples containing 100 mM NaCl. Data from individual samples were used for the saturation curves (A) and Scatchard plots (B).

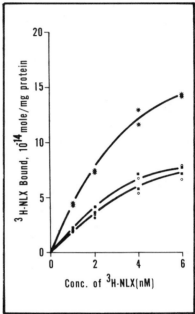

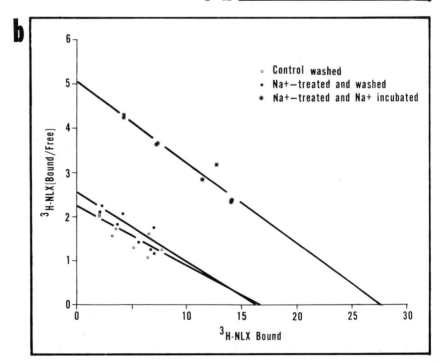

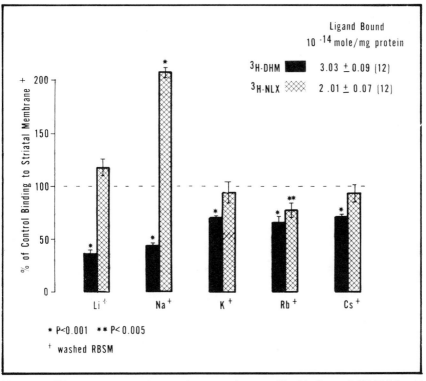

6   Effects of monovalent cations on the specific binding of ^{3}H-DHM and
^{3}H-NLX to striatal membranes of rat brain.
Aliquots in triplicate samples of striatal membranes after two
washing steps were incubated at 37°C for 15 min with 2×10^{-9}M
^{3}H-DHM or ^{3}H-NLX in the absence and the presence of 100 mM
monovalent cation chloride salt of lithium, sodium, potassium, rubidium
or cesium. Data were presented in percentage of control with p
values as indicated.

and Horng, 1973). These two components have Kd values about 1 and
5 nM for ^{3}H-DHM; much lower than the value of 20 nM for the
^{3}H-DHM binding component in homogenate of whole rat brain (Pert
and Snyder, 1974). The same laboratory recently also reported the
existence of two ^{3}H-DHM binding components with Kd values of 0.3
and 3 nM (Pasternak and Snyder, 1975).

The high affinity binding component for ^{3}H-DHM was completely
abolished by 20 mM NaCl. Snyder and associates made similar observations but they used a higher concentration of NaCl (100 mM). In the
presence of 100 mM NaCl, however, we observed that the affinity of

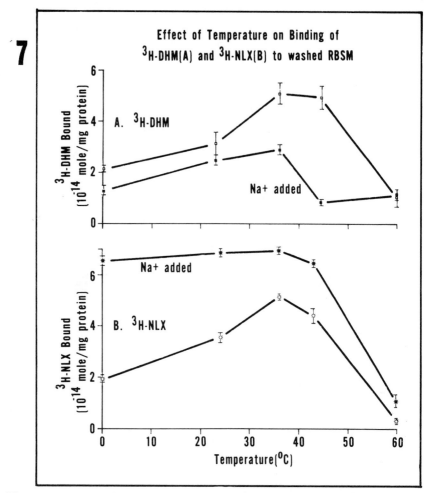

7

Effect of Temperature on Binding of
³H-DHM(A) and ³H-NLX(B) to washed RBSM

The temperature profiles on specific binding of ³H-DHM (A) and 3H-NLX (B) to striatal membranes of rat brain in the absence and presence of NaCl.

Aliquots of striatal membranes after two washing steps were incubated with 2 x 10⁻⁹M ³H-DHM or ³H-NLX at temperatures between 0°C and 60°C for 15 min. NaCl at 100 mM was included in samples at each temperature.

the low affinity binding sites for ³H-DHM was further reduced. This observation was in agreement with that reported by Simon et al. (1975) who observed a reduction in the binding affinity for ³H-etorphine by 100 mM NaCl.

We consistently observed the monophasic binding of ³H-NLX to striatal membranes of rat brain with a Kd value of 1.6-2.3 nM. The number of ³H-NLX binding sites was increased by 100 mM NaCl as reported by Pert and Snyder (1974). An additional low affinity binding

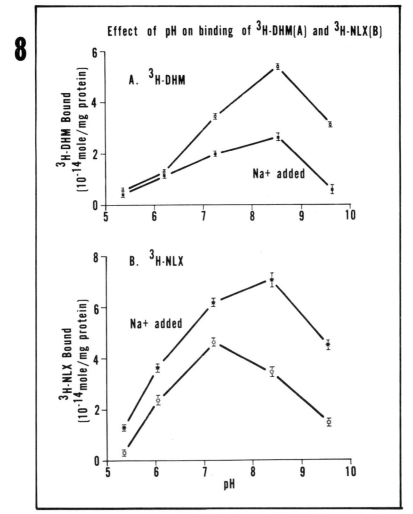

8

The pH profiles on specific binding of ^{3}H-DHM (A) and ^{3}H-NLX (B) to striatal membranes of rat brain in the absence and presence of NaCl.

Aliquots of striatal membranes after two washing steps were incubated with 2 x 10-[9]M ^{3}H-DHM or ^{3}H-NLX in 100 mM Tris-Cl buffer pH between 5.4 and 9.6 at 37°C for 15 min. NaCl at 100 mM was included in each buffer solution to examine the effects of Na+ at each pH.

component with a Kd value of 30 nM for ^{3}H-NLX was also reported but was not sensitive to 100 mM NaCl (Pasternak and Snyder, 1975). In here, we used ^{3}H-naloxone concentration up to 20 nM but we failed to observe more than a single component for the specific binding of ^{3}H-NLX.

In the presence of sodium, the specific binding of ^{3}H-DHM was temperature dependent whereas the specific binding of ^{3}H-NLX was at its maximum level between 0°C and 36°C. Sodium perhaps caused conformational changes in the two types of binding sites so differently that the opiate antagonist sites became more accessible to ^{3}H-NLX whereas the opiate agonist sites were unfolded only by an increase in temperature. Sodium also shifted the pH profile of ^{3}H-NLX binding toward higher pHs without affecting the pH profile for ^{3}H-DHM. Since all these experiments were performed with relatively low concentration (1 to 2 nM) of ^{3}H-DHM and ^{3}H-NLX, the specific binding therefore reflected the high affinity binding sites for the two ligands.

In our laboratory, among the five alkali metal cations tested, only sodium was able to increase the specific binding of ^{3}H-NLX by increasing the number of binding sites. However, Pert and Snyder (1974) also observed some stimulatory effect of lithium on ^{3}H-NLX binding. All five alkali metal cations reduced the specific binding of ^{3}H-DHM with lithium and sodium most effectively. Sodium also seemed to have different affinities for the two types of binding sites. At 20 mM NaCl, ^{3}H-NLX specific binding was increased to its maximum level when ^{3}H-DHM specific binding was reduced by half. Perhaps this difference more reflected the participation of a second component for ^{3}H-DHM binding. Despite these differences in the specific binding of ^{3}H-DHM and ^{3}H-NLX, the concomittant disappearance of ^{3}H-DHM binding sites and the appearance of ^{3}H-NLX binding sites favor the model that sodium brought about the interconversion of the two types of binding sites (Pert and Snyder, 1974; Pasternak and Snyder, 1975). However, this question rests on the isolation of pure receptors for the opiates and opiate antagonists.

On the mechanism of action of sodium, our findings and those of Snyder and associates agreed that sodium at 100 mM abolished the high affinity binding sites for ^{3}H-DHM but increased the binding sites for ^{3}H-NLX. However, Simon and associates observed that sodium reduces the affinity for ^{3}H-DHM and increased the affinity for ^{3}H-NLX. This major discrepancy was perhaps due to the fact that Simon and associates pretreated the brain homogenates with 10^{-6}M dextrorphan, a concentration sufficient to displace about 10% of specific binding of ^{3}H-DHM in our hand due to the law of mass action. On the other hand, Snyder and associates routinely used 10^{-7}M dextrorphan; at this concentration we found no effect on the specific binding of ^{3}H-DHM or ^{3}H-NLX (see Figures 2 and 4) and 10^{-7}M dextrorphan was only used in our early experiments.

We found that sodium reduced the affinity as well as the number of binding sites of the low affinity binding component for ³H-DHM but Pasternak and Snyder (1975) found no effect of sodium on this component. Snyder and associates also reported the existence of a third binding component for ³H-DHM with a Kd value of 20 nM (Pert and Snyder, 1974) and a second binding component for ³H-NLX with a Kd value of 30 nM (Pasternak and Snyder, 1975). However, we have not observed the presence of these two components by studying the binding of either ³H-ligand at concentration up to 20 nM. Perhaps the difference was due to the choice of tissue in the two laboratories. Snyder and associates consistently used whole brain homogenates of rat or mouse, and the low affinity binding they observed for ³H-DHM and ³H-NLX may therefore have been due to the heterogeneity of particulate matter in these whole brain homogenates. We chose to use striatal membranes throughout our studies, for corpus striatum was one of the few brain regions that had high binding capacities for ³H-DHM and ³H-NLX in the absence and presence of sodium. The choice of corpus striatum seems particularly appropriate since this region of the brain has recently been found to contain four times higher concentration of the endogenous opiate-like factor than other brain regions (Hughes, 1975).

SUMMARY

Among six rat brain regions, binding capacity for ³H-dihydro-morphine (³H-DHM) and ³H-naloxone (³H-NLX) was greatest in corpus striatum, midbrain and hypothalamus, intermediate in pons + medulla and cerebral cortex, and lowest in cerebellum. The addition of NaCl approximately doubled the binding of ³H-NLX in all regions except cerebellum. In striatal membranes, NaCl at 20 mM maximally stimulated the binding of ³H-NLX but reduced the binding of ³H-DHM by about 50%; the remaining portion of ³H-DHM binding was gradually reduced as the NaCl concentration was increased to 100 mM.

Two binding components for ³H-DHM were detected, a high affinity component with a Kd value of 1 nM and a lower affinity component with a Kd value of 5 nM for ³H-DHM. Only a single component of ³H-NLX binding with a Kd value of 2 nM was found in striatal membranes. NaCl at 20 mM abolished the high affinity binding sites for ³H-DHM. The number of low affinity binding sites and the binding affinity to these sites were reduced by 100 mM NaCl. NaCl at 100 mM increased the number of ³H-NLX binding sites. The effects of NaCl on ³H-DHM binding and on ³H-NLX binding were reversible, with the effects on ^{3}H-DHM binding being more readily reversed.

In the presence of NaCl, the binding of ^{3}H-NLX showed little temperature dependence between 0°C and 36°C. The binding of ^{3}H-DHM was reduced most by NaCl at 44°C. The pH optimum for ^{3}H-NLX binding was shifted by NaCl toward a more alkaline pH, whereas the pH profile for ^{3}H-DHM binding was not changed by NaCl. Of 5 alkaline metal cations tested (Li$^+$, Na$^+$, K$^+$, Rb$^+$ and Cs$^+$), only Na$^+$ stimulated ^{3}H-NLX binding but all reduced ^{3}H-DHM binding with Na$^+$ and Li$^+$ most effective.

The effects of sodium may be explained by a simple model in which sodium reversibility transforms the opiate sites into opiate antagonist sites. However, differences in the characteristics of these types of binding sites cannot be fully explained. Possible explanations are suggested for differences that have been reported from other laboratories in the mechanism of sodium action on opiate and opiate antagonist binding.

ACKNOWLEDGMENTS

The authors deeply thank Mr. L. L. Simms, Drs. W. E. Dusenberry and B. J. Cerimele for their assistance in statistical analysis. We also appreciate the assistance of Dr. R. W. Fuller in the preparation of the manuscript.

REFERENCES

Goldstein, A., L. I. Lowney, and B. K. Pal. 1971. Stereospecific and nonspecific interactions of the morphine congener: Levorphanol in subcellular fractions of mouse brain. *Proc. Nat. Acad. Sci.* 68: 1742–1747.

Hughes, J. 1975. Isolation of an endogenous compound from the brain with pharmacological properties similar to morphine. *Brain Res.* 88: 295–308.

Pasternak, G. W., and S. H. Snyder. 1975. Identification of novel high affinity opiate receptor binding in rat brain. *Nature* (London) 253: 563–565.

Pert, C. B., G. Pasternak, and S. H. Snyder. 1973. Opiate agonists and antagonists discriminated by receptor binding in brain. *Science* 182: 1359–1361.

Pert, C. B., and S. H. Snyder. 1973. Opiate receptor: Demonstration in nervous tissue. *Science* 179: 1011–1014.

Pert, C. B., and S. H. Snyder. 1974. Opiate receptor binding of agonists and antagonists affected differentially by sodium. *Mol. Pharmacol.* 10: 868–879.

Scatchard, G. 1949. The attractions of proteins for small molecules and ions. *N. Y. Acad. Sci.* 51: 660–672.

Simon, E. J., J. M. Hiller, and I. Edelman. 1973. Stereospecific binding of the potent narcotic analgesic ^{3}H-etorphine to rat brain homogenate. *Proc. Nat. Acad. Sci.* 70P 1947–1949.

Simon, E. J., J. M. Hiller, J. Groth, and I. Edelman. 1975. Further properties of stereospecific opiate binding sites in rat brain: On the nature of the sodium effect. *J. Pharmacol. Expt. Therap.* 192: 531–537.

Terenius, L. 1973. Stereospecific interaction between narcotic analgesics and a synaptic membrane fraction of rat cerebral cortex. *Acta Pharmacol. Toxicol.* 32: 317–320.

Wong, D. T., and J. S. Horng. 1973. Stereospecific interaction of opiate narcotics in binding of ^{3}H-dihydromorphine to membranes of rat brain. *Life Sci.* 13: 1543–1556.

Tissue Responses to Addictive Drugs
© 1976, Spectrum Publications, Inc.

The Specificity of Binding of
³H-Etorphine in Rat Brain in Vivo

S. J. MULE
G. CASELLA
D. H. CLOUET

New York State Office of Drug Abuse Services
Testing and Research Laboratory
Brooklyn, New York

An opiate "receptor" has two kinds of specificity in interactions with narcotic drugs: a pharmacological specificity, which is related to narcotic agonist activity and detected through experimental use of narcotic antagonists; and a stereospecificity, which distinguishes between active and inactive isomers of optically active narcotic drugs (Goldstein, et al., 1971). In *in vitro* systems, stereospecific binding of opiate agonists and antagonists has been demonstrated in whole brain homogenate and in synaptic membranes isolated from the brain (Pert and Snyder, 1973a,b; Simon et al., 1973). In these experiments, the binding of low concentrations of the radioactive drug was measured in the presence of large excesses of *d*-(inactive) or *l*-(active) isomers of another opiate, with the *d*-minus *l*-difference representing stereospecific binding of the labeled drug. A pharmacological specificity was suggested in these systems by the difference in binding characteristics between agonists and antagonists related to Na^+ concentration in the incubation medium (Simon et al., 1973; Pert, et al., 1973).

409

In *in vivo* systems, however, when opiates have been administered to experimental animals in pharmacologically effective doses, the drugs were not localized in any particulate fraction of brain. The patterns of distribution were related to the lipid solubility of each drug rather than to its pharmacological efficacy or stereoisomerism (Hertz and Tesche-macher, 1971; Mulé, 1971; Clouet and Williams, 1973). The lack of correlation between the amounts of the various narcotic drugs in brain tissue and the pharmacological responses in the drug-treated animals suggested that most of the drug found in brain was not bound to specific opiate receptors.

The potent narcotic agonist etorphine was examined because an equipotent dose was about 1/500th that of morphine or methadone, when the drugs were administered i.c. (Mulé et al., 1974). In this chapter we describe the binding of ^{3}H-etorphine in synaptic membranes of rat brain which, in part, is both pharmacologically specific and stereospecific.

METHODS

Etorphine, 15- 16-^{3}H .HCl (specific activity: 1.64 Ci/mmol) was provided by Reckitt and Coleman. The labeled drug was subjected to purification before use by counter-current distribution between 0.2M phosphate buffer, pH 7, and *n*-heptane. Diprenorphine.HCl, the cy-clorphan isomers and naloxone.HCl were gifts from NIDA, Hoffman-LaRoche and Endo Laboratories, respectively.

Male Wistar rats (180 to 220 g) were injected with ^{3}H-etorphine i.c. under light ether anesthesia and killed ten minutes later by decapi-tation. The dose of etorphine in all experiments, 0.75 µg/kg, produced analgesia within two minutes of injection and lasted for thirty minutes. The analgesia was antagonized by 25 µg/kg *l*-cyclorphan i.c., or by 1 mg/kg naloxone, 0.5 mg/kg *l*-cyclorphan or 0.5 mg/kg diprenorphine i.p. The analgesic activity of etorphine and its antagonism by narcotic antagonists was measured by the hot plate test (Eddy and Leimbach, 1953). The pharmacologically inactive *d*-isomer of cyclorphan was injected in the same dose as the active *l*-isomer and an equal volume of saline was injected instead of an antagonist solution in rats receiving etorphine alone. The time sequence and route of antagonist administra-tion are described for each experiment.

After the heads were removed by decapitation, the brains were dissected out, homogenized in 0.32 M sucrose buffered with 50 mM Tris.HCl, pH 7, and fractionated by sucrose density gradient procedures described by Rodriquez de Lores Arnaiz et al., (1967). The mito-chondrial synaptic membrane fraction (M_1), prepared by sedimenta-tion after hypo-osmotic shock of the crude mitochondrial-synaptosomal fraction, was further fractionated on a discontinuous sucrose gradient into M_1 (0.8), (0.9), (1.0), (1.2), and mitochondrial pellet fractions (DeRobertis et al., 1967). Fractions M_1 (0.9) and (1.0), and to a lesser extent (1.2) were enriched in synaptic membranes, as verified by electron micrographic examination. Each fraction was collected separately, and an aliquot was removed for the measurement of protein (Lowry, et al., 1951) and the rest of the sample examined for total radioactivity by liquid scintillation spectrometry. In some experiments, brains were dis-sected into six areas as previously described (Clouet and Williams, 1973).

The amount of ^{3}H-etorphine in each fraction has been expressed both as concentration (pg etorphine/mg protein in fraction) and as total amount (pmol etorphine/g wet weight brain). Two rat brains were pooled for each assay with at least three replications. The data were examined statistically by paired t-tests.

RESULTS

Localization of ^{3}H-etorphine in Subcellular Fractions of Brain

The levels ($\pm$ S.E.) of ^{3}H-etorphine in brain homogenates were 52 ± 2 pg/mg protein, or 14.94 ± 0.75 pmol/g wet weight brain, about 8% of the injected dose calculated on a g brain basis ten minutes after the i.c. injection of ^{3}H-etorphine (see Table I). As found in our earlier experiments also (Mulé et al., 1974) etorphine was concentrated in the M_1 (0.9) and (1.0) synaptic membrane fractions, although only 0.7% of the total drug in brain was in these fractions.

Effect of Pretreatment with Antagonists on the Binding of ^{3}H-etorphine in Synaptic Membranes

The i.p. administration of naloxone (1.0 mg/kg) or diprenorphine (0.5 mg/kg) 15 minutes prior to ^{3}H-etorphine injection, which blocked the pharmacological responses to etorphine, significantly reduced the concentration of ^{3}H-etorphine in all M_1 fractions except the mitochon-drial pellet (see Figure 1). In the M_1 (0.9) and (1.0) fractions, ^{3}H-etorphine binding was reduced by one-third to one-half following pretreatment with antagonists.

Table I. ^{3}H-etorphine in Synaptic Membrane Fractions of Rat Brain

| Fraction | ^{3}H-Etorphine | |
	Concentration pg/mg protein	Amount pmol/g wet weight brain
Homogenate	52 ± 2	14.94 ± 0.75
M$_1$ (total)	33 ± 2	0.55 ± 0.02
M$_1$ 0.8	40 ± 3	0.11 ± 0.01
M$_1$ 0.9	82 ± 7	0.06 ± 0.01
M$_1$ 1.0	72 ± 8	0.05 ± 0.00
M$_1$ 1.2	42 ± 3	0.10 ± 0.01
M$_1$ Pellet	23 ± 2	0.16 ± 0.02

The rats were killed ten minutes after 0.75 μg/kg ^{3}H-etorphine i.c. (^{3}H-etorphine levels (± S.E.) expressed as concentration and as amount, were derived from seven groups of experiments, two rats each.)

Effect of Stereoisomers of Cyclorphan on ^{3}H-etorphine Binding

Pretreatment of rats with levocyclorphan (0.5 mg/kg i.p.) 15 minutes prior to the injection of etorphine decreased significantly the concentration of ^{3}H-etorphine in the M$_1$ (0.9) and (1.0) synaptic membrane fractions (see Figure 2a). The administration of levocyclorphan (25 μg/kg i.c.) 5 minutes after the injection of ^{3}H-etorphine, which also antagonized the pharmacological responses produced by etorphine, decreased significantly the concentration of etorphine in the M$_1$ (0.9) and (1.0) fractions and in the mitochondrial pellet (see Figure 2b). The administration of d-cyclorphan in the same doses by the same routes as the l-isomer had no effect on the analgesic response to etorphine and no effect on the binding of ^{3}H-etorphine in any fraction (see Figure 2). The stereospecific binding of ^{3}H-etorphine in the M$_1$ (0.9) and (1.0) fractions was 0.040 and 0.062 pmol/g wet weight brain in the two experiments. The pharmacologically specific binding of ^{3}H-etorphine in the same two membrane fractions ranged from 0.025 to 0.056 pmol/g wet weight brain. The significant differences between ^{3}H-etorphine binding in membranes (specific and stereospecific) as determined by narcotic antagonist treatment are shown in Table II.

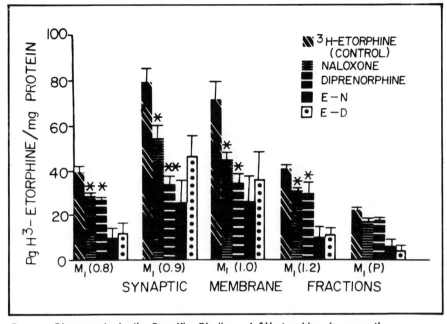

1 *Pharmacologically Specific Binding of ³H-etorphine in synaptic membrane fractions.* In all treatment groups the rats received 0.75 μg/kg ³H-etorphine i.c. ten minutes prior to sacrifice. Naloxone (1 mg/kg), diprenorphine (0.5 mg/kg) or saline (control) was injected i.p. fifteen minutes before etorphine was administered. N = three groups of two rats each for each treatment. The concentration of ³H-etorphine (E) is shown for all treatment groups, as is the decrease produced by naloxone (E-N) or by diprenorphine (E-D). $*p < 0.05$; $**p < 0.01$.

Regional Specificity of Binding of ³H-etorphine in Brain

Pharmacologically specific binding in synaptic membranes of rat brain areas was observed in the midbrain, hypothalamus and striatum (see Tables III and IV). The difference between ³H-etorphine plus saline and ³H-etorphine plus naloxone were large and approached significance in the medulla. There were no differences detected in the cerebellum or cortex. The pharmacologically specific binding in the M_1 (0.9) and (1.0) fractions was 30% to 42% of the total binding in the fractions.

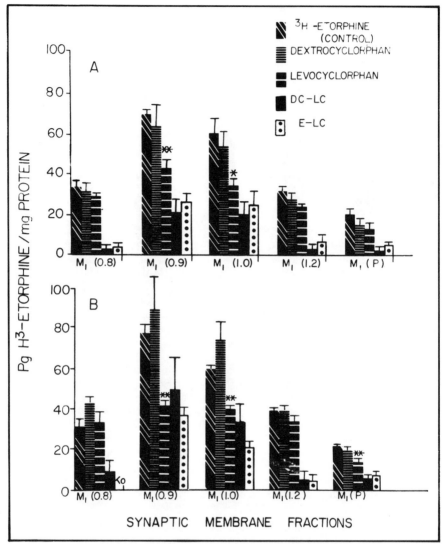

2 Stereospecific binding of ³H-etorphine in synaptic membrane fractions. In all treatment groups the rats received 0.75 μg/kg ³H-etorphine i.c. ten minutes prior to sacrifice. In (a) the rats were pretreated with saline (control), levocyclorphan (0.5 mg/kg) or dextrocyclorphan (0.5 mg/kg) i.p. fifteen minutes prior to ³H-etorphine administration. In (b) the rats received saline (control), levocyclorphan (25 μg/kg) or dextrocyclorphan (25 μg/kg) i.c. five minutes after ³H-etorphine administration. The decrease produced by levocyclorphan compared to etorphine alone (E-LC) and the dextrocyclorphan minus the levocyclorphan (DC-LC) effect on etorphine are shown. *p<0.05; **p<0.01.

Table II. Specific Binding of ^{3}H-Etorphine in Synaptic Membranes of Rat Brain

Membrane Fraction	Pharmacologically Specific Binding				Stereospecific Binding	
	E-N	E-D	D-LC$_A$	E-LC$_B$	E/DC$_A$-E/LC$_A$	E/DC$_B$-E/DC$_A$
M$_1$ (0.8)	0.037*	0.026*	—	—	—	—
M$_1$ (0.9)	0.033**	0.025*	0.014*	0.031**	0.023**	0.043**
M$_1$ (1.0)	0.023**	0.024**	0.011*	0.012*	0.017*	0.019*
M$_1$ (1.2)	0.042**	—	—	—	—	—
M$_1$ (0.9 + 1.0)	0.056	0.049	0.025	0.043	0.040	0.062

Pharmacologically specific binding is defined by the significant differences in membrane levels of ^{3}H-etorphine between rats receiving etorphine and saline (E), and those receiving etorphine and an antagonist, naloxone (N), diprenorphine (D) or levocyclorphan (LC). Stereospecific binding is defined by the significant differences in membrane levels of ^{3}H-etorphine between rats treated with etorphine and d-cyclorphan (E/DC) and those treated with etorphine and l-cyclorphan (E/LC). The differences, expressed in pmol ^{3}H-etorphine/g wet weight brain, were significant at $p < 0.05$* and $p < 0.01$** or were not significant (–). The values in each column were calculated by paired comparisons of ^{3}H-etorphine binding in each fraction between three groups of two rats each treated with ^{3}H-etorphine and saline (or ^{3}H-etorphine and d-cyclorphan) and three groups of two rats each treated with ^{3}H-etorphine and an antagonist, as described in the legend to Figures 1, 2a and 2b.

Table III. Pharmacologically Specific Binding of ^{3}H-Etorphine in Areas of the Rat Brain

FRACTIONS

(pg ^{3}H-etorphine/mg protein ± S.E.)

Brain Area	M_1 (0.8)			M_1 (0.9)			M_1 (1.0)			M_1 (1.2)		
	E	N	E-N	E	N	E-N	E	N	E-N	E	N	E-N
Midbrain	38 ± 2	22 ± 2	15** ± 3	79 ±10	41 ± 5	37** ±11	75 ±11	49 ± 6	27* ±12	40 ± 3	34 ± 4	6 ± 5
Hypothalamus	44 ±10	26 ± 5	18 ±11	60 ±10	38 ± 6	23* ±12	67 ±10	45 ±10	22* ±14	26 ± 3	24 ± 4	2 ± 5
Striatum	19 ± 1	13 ± 2	6** ± 2	35 ± 3	19 ± 2	16** ± 4	39 ± 3	26 ± 3	13** ± 4	20 ± 2	19 ± 3	1 ± 3

The control rats (E) were injected with 0.2 ml of saline intraperitoneally 15 minutes prior to 0.75 µg/kg of ^{3}H-etorphine and sacrificed 10 minutes later. The experimental rats (N) were injected with 1 mg/kg of naloxone intraperitoneally 15 minutes prior to 0.75 µg/kg of ^{3}H-etorphine and sacrificed 10 minutes later. The values were calculated as means ± S.E. from six experiments of six rats each and the differences were significant at $p < .05$* and $p < .01$**. The E-N data is the control minus the naloxone pretreated values and represents the pharmacologically specific bound etorphine in the membrane fractions of the specific brain areas.

Table IV. Pharmacologically Specific Binding of ^{3}H-Etorphine in Areas of the Rat Brain

FRACTIONS
(pg ^{3}H-etorphine/gm tissue $\pm$ S.E.)

Brain Area	M_1 (0.8)			M_1 (0.9)			M_1 (1.0)			M_1 (1.2)		
	E	N	E-N	E	N	E-N	E	N	E-N	E	N	E-N
Midbrain	371	258	113*	194	124	69*	99	74	25	162	141	21
	±16	±40	±43	±27	±10	±29	±16	±8	±18	±9	±12	±15
Hypothalamus	324	178	145	171	108	63*	102	74	27	179	149	30
	±84	±30	±89	±26	±20	±33	±13	±17	±21	±20	±25	±32
Striatum	60	43	17*	40	23	17*	30	20	10*	54	46	8
	±4	±8	±9	±6	±4	±7	±3	±4	±5	±5	±8	±10

[1]See Table III for details.

Development of Tolerance to Etorphine

Male Wistar rats (12) were made tolerant to etorphine by the administration of 3 μg/kg of the drug subcutaneously twice daily for a period of ten days. On the eleventh day, 0.75 μg/kg of ^{3}H-etorphine was injected i.c. and the rats sacrificed ten minutes later. Control rats (16) receiving saline for the same period of time were given the same concentration of ^{3}H-etorphine i.c. and sacrificed in ten minutes. There were no statistically significant differences in ^{3}H-etorphine binding between the control and etorphine-tolerant rats in either the crude subcellular or nerve ending fractions.

DISCUSSION

^{3}H-etorphine localization in the synaptic membrane fractions of rat brain in our experiments might be expected to be altered from the levels *in situ* at the time of sacrifice of the rats by two general mechanisms: a redistribution of the labeled drug during the fractionation procedures that might change the subcellular localization of the drug, and so alter drug:receptor interaction; and a dissociation of the etorphine-receptor complex during the time required to isolate the synaptic membranes. The question of the possible redistribution of ^{3}H-etorphine was answered to some extent by our earlier studies in which we showed that ^{3}H-etorphine added to the brains of untreated rats before homogenization was fairly evenly distributed and not concentrated to the same extent in the synaptic membrane fractions as that administered to animals in effective doses (Mule' et al., 1974). Because the half-life of dissociation of the etorphine-receptor binding in brain homogenates *in vitro* is one hour at 22°C (Simon et al., 1975) rather than less than a minute for naloxone-receptor binding (Pert and Snyder, 1973b) the possible loss of labeled drug by dissociation was minimized by the use of etorphine in the present experiments. Our values for ^{3}H-etorphine binding in the synaptic membranes of brain are approximate, however, because they have not been corrected for incomplete recovery of membranes or for redistribution or dissociation.

It was difficult to adapt the techniques used so successfully in *in vitro* binding studies to studies in the living animal because the potency range for narcotic agonists is relatively narrow, so that the administration of an excess of unlabeled agonist after a radiolabeled agonist tended toward lethality; because a difference in the rate of uptake of labeled drug into brain from circulating blood or CSF might be expected between narcotic-depressed and normal animals; and because rapid drug-receptor fixation is not possible when fractionation procedures are used. The use of a low effective dose of etorphine both minimized the differences in drug uptake due to the physiological state of the animal, and made it possible to administer a large excess of the unlabeled drug. In addition, the use of optical isomers of the antagonist cyclorphan eliminated the problem of lethality which would follow the administration of an active agonist in addition to etorphine.

The replacement of etorphine by an antagonist in the M_1 (0.9) plus (1.0) synaptic membrane fractions ranged from 0.025 to 0.062 pmol/g, a 2.5-fold difference. The dose about an ED_{15}, and the duration of exposure of the rats to ^{3}H-etorphine (ten minutes) were kept constant in all experiments. However, the various doses of both antagonists were only approximately equipotent because the hot plate test for analgesia and temperature measurements were not sensitive assays, and because the duration of antagonist activity varied with the antagonist or partial antagonist used. The doses of antagonists and routes of administration used did completely prevent etorphine-induced analgesia ten minutes after etorphine injection, the time of sacrifice of the rats. Because the extent of competition might be expected to vary with the ratio of agonist:antagonist at receptor sites in brain, the specific binding of ^{3}H-etorphine measured by antagonist replacement in each experiment would be a function of the level at the "receptor" sites of each antagonist at the time of sacrifice. Thus, the range of values may be an expression of antagonist levels at the opiate "receptor" site.

The stereospecific binding of ^{3}H-etorphine and ^{3}H-naloxone in rat brain homogenates *in vitro* ranged from 20 to 30 pmol/g wet weight brain (Simon et al., 1973; Pert and Snyder, 1973b). In the present experiments, the stereospecific binding of ^{3}H-etorphine in synaptic membranes of whole brain *in vivo* was considerably less that found *in vitro* in homogenates. There are a number of possible reasons for these large differences in ^{3}H-etorphine binding. Pharmacological responses may be produced when only a few strategically located receptors are occupied. Many chemical receptors for opiates in the brain may not be pharmacological receptors. Opiate receptors may be mainly located in subcellular fractions other than M_1 (0.9) and (1.0) membrane fractions. Etorphine:receptor dissociation may indeed be a major factor in reducing the apparent ^{3}H-etorphine binding in synaptic membranes in the present experiments. Homogenization may expose more receptors. However, when synaptic membranes were isolated from rat brain and incubated *in vitro* with ^{3}H-etorphine or ^{3}H-naloxone, the stereospecific binding of the labeled drugs was 0.096 pmol/mg membrane protein (Pert et al.,

1974) as compared to 0.075 pmol/mg protein *in vivo* in the present experiments, suggesting that etorphine:receptor dissociation possibility was not likely. In regard to the third possibility, we noted earlier that naloxone pretreatment tended to shift ^{3}H-etorphine administered i.c. from the nuclear to the supernatant fraction of brain (Mulé et al., 1974) indicating that etorphine may be replaced by an antagonist at receptors located in the crude nuclear fraction of brain. We have not included the reduction of ^{3}H-etorphine binding in the M_1 (0.8) and M_1 (1.2) fractions by pretreatment by naloxone or diprenorphine in the calculations of pharmacologically specific binding because similar reductions were not produced by pretreatment with levocyclorphan, suggesting that pharmacologically specific sites were not saturated by levocyclorphan. The lack of effect of treatment with dextrocyclorphan on ^{3}H-etorphine binding similarly suggests that nonspecific opiate binding sites in brain were not saturated.

Thus, evidence for pharmacologically specific or stereospecific binding of an opiate in the CNS and especially in the specific areas of the midbrain, hypothalamus and striatum, has been obtained for the first time after administration of an effective dose of the drug to experimental animals. The number of stereospecific sites for ^{3}H-etorphine in the synaptic membranes of the rat brain is very similar to the number of pharmacologically specific sites in the same membrane fractions: about 0.04 pmol/g brain or 2.5×10^{10} sites/g brain if the receptor is monovalent.

ACKNOWLEDGMENT

This study was supported in part by grants from NIDA: DA–00061 and DA–00087.

REFERENCES

Clouet, D. H., and N. Williams. 1973. Localization in brain particulate fractions of narcotic analgesic drugs administered intracisternally to rats. *Biochem. Pharmacol.* 22: 1283–1293.

DeRobertis, E., M. Alberici, G. Rodriguez de Lores Arnaiz, and J. M. Azcurra. 1966. Isolation of different types of synaptic membranes from the brain cortex. *Life Sci.* 5: 577–582.

Eddy, N. B., and D. Leimbach. 1953. Synthetic analgesic II. Dithienylbutylamines. *J. Pharmacol. Exp. Therap.* 107: 385–393.

Gollstein, A., L. I. Lowney, and B. K. Pal. 1971. Stereospecific and nonspecific interactions of the morphine cogener levorphanol in subcellular fractions of mouse brain. *Proc. Nat. Acad. Sci.* 68: 1742–1747.

Hertz, A., and H. J. Teschemacher. 1971. Activities and sites of antinociceptive action of morphine-like analgesics. In N. J. Harper and A. B. Simonds, Eds. *Advances in Drug Research.* Academic Press, New York, pp. 79–119.

Lowry, O. H., N. J. Rosebrough, A. L. Farr, and R. J. Randall. 1951. Protein measurement with the Folin phenol reagent. *J. Biol. Chem.* 193: 265–275.

Mulé, S. J. 1971. Physiological disposition of narcotic agonists and antagonists. In D. H. Clouet, Ed. *Narcotic Drugs: Biochemical.* pp. 99–121.

Mulé, S. J., G. Casella, and D. H. Clouet. 1974. Localization of levo ^{3}H-methadone in synaptic membranes of rat brain. *Res. Commun. Chem. Path. Pharmacol.* 9: 55–77.

Pert, C. B., A. M. Snowman, and S. H. Snyder. 1974. Localization of opiate receptor binding in synaptic membrane fractions of rat brain. *Brain Res.* 70: 184–188.

Pert, C. B., and S. H. Snyder. 1973a. Opiate receptor: Demonstration in nervous tissue. *Science* 179: 1011–1014.

Pert, C. B., and S. H. Snyder. 1973b. Properties of opiate receptor binding in rat brain. *Proc. Nat. Acad. Sci.* 70: 2243–2247.

Pert, C. B., G. Pasternak, and S. H. Snyder. 1973. Opiate agonists and antagonists discriminated by receptor binding in brain. *Science* 182: 1359–1361.

Rodriguez de Lores Arnaiz, G., M. Alberici, and E. DeRobertis. 1967. Ultrastructural and enzymic studies of cholinergic and non-cholinergic synaptic membranes isolated from brain cortex. *J. Neurochem.* 14: 215–225.

Simon, E. J., J. M. Hiller, and I. Edelman. 1973. Stereospecific binding of the potent narcotic analgesic ^{3}H-etorphine in rat brain homogenates. *Proc. Nat. Acad. Sci.* 70: 1947–1949.

Simon, E. J., J. M. Hiller, J. Groth, and I. Edelman. 1975. Further properties of stereospecific opiate binding sites in rat brain: On the nature of the sodium effect. *J. Pharmacol. Exp. Therap.* 192: 531–537.

Tissue Responses to Addictive Drugs
© 1976, Spectrum Publications, Inc.

Pharmacological Discrimination of Narcotic Receptor Mechanisms

ALFRED A. SMITH
MARSHA CROFFORD
FERDINAND HUI
JOHANNA HAGEDOORN

Departments of Pharmacology and Anatomy
New York Medical College
Valhalla, New York

Equianalgesic doses of opioids depress respiratory function in a corresponding way. These observations suggest a similarity or an identity of the receptor for these responses. The analgesic and cataractogenic responses to a series of opioids also show similar features (Weinstock, 1961). The lenticular effect arises from the intense sympathetic stimulation of the eye of the mouse produced by parenterally administered opioids but not by such narcotic antagonists as nalorphine. In the response to opioids, the eyelids retract, the iris dilates, and the orbit is pushed forward resulting in increased exposure of the cornea with enhanced evaporation rate of transudate from the anterior segment of the eye. Hyperosmolarity of this fluid withdraws water from the lens, thus transiently diminishing its clarity. Although much larger dosages of opioids are required to produce the transient cataracts than for antinociceptive effect, a close correspondence is obtained for the two effects. The pA_2 for analgesic and lenticular effects was found to be

423

the same for a given opioid (Cox and Weinstock, 1964). Because the concentrations of the agonist-antagonist pair at the receptor is assumed to be equal to the dosages injected into the animal, the pA_2 is considered to be only an apparent rather than absolute value.

In a study undertaken nearly a decade ago we discovered that a large single dosage of an opioid conferred acute and long-term tolerance to transient cataract formation induced by opioids. Development of long-term tolerance could be prevented by the prior administration of inhibitors of RNA or protein synthesis. A single dosage of opioid did not produce analgesic tolerance in the mouse and most studies of tolerance in this animal rely on morphine pellet implantation, or repeated injections of opioid to induce tolerance. It seemed unlikely that a single receptor for the lenticular and antinociceptice effect would employ different mechanisms for tolerance. However, the lenticular effect is enhanced by conditions of hypoxia or hypercapnia. Perhaps tolerance develops rapidly to the respiratory depression induced by opioids. The data to be presented indicates that tolerance to respiratory depression does not occur measurably after a single large dosage of levorphanol. Furthermore, the analgesic and respiratory responses to levorphanol and morphine were not equally displaced by a given dosage of the dosage of the antagonist, naloxone, further suggesting the dissimilarity of the receptor mechanisms for these responses.

It is the purpose of this chapter to present data suggesting that at least four different opiate receptors can be pharmacologically discriminated. Additional studies will show that blockade of growth in salamanders and in the growing mouse by methadone administration is correlated with a significant decrement in ^{3}H-uridine incorporation into RNA. This chapter will show that the decrement in uptake occurs in tissues dependent on neurotrophism.

METHODS AND DISCUSSION

The injection of large dosages of levorphanol tartrate (50 mg/kg) i.p. into Swiss-Webster mice increases motor activity, induces the Straub tail response and causes the development of transient cataracts of the lens (Weinstock, 1961). The cataract may appear only as a few pinpoint opacities or coalesce to reduce the clarity of the lens. As little as fifteen minutes may be required for development of the cataract and the opacity may persist for up to two hours. Data reported elsewhere (Smith et al., 1964) show that concomitant administration of norepinephrine, 10 μg injected s.c. or cocaine, 5 mg/kg shifts the dose-response curves sig-

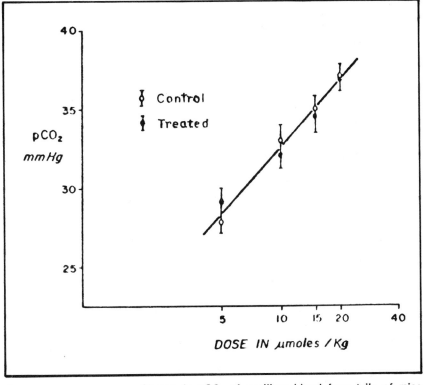

1 Change in pCO_2 of capillary blood from tails of mice injected with graded dosages of levorphanol. Closed circles indicate mean values in mice treated 24 hr earlier with levorphanol 150 μmoles/kg. (No change in dose-effect curve is noted.)

nificantly to the left, indicating that adrenergic activity is involved in the phenomenon. This was later to be shown by the elegant experiment of Weinstock and Marshall (1969), in which unilateral destruction of the superior cervical ganglion prevented cataract formation in the ipsilateral but not contralateral lens of a mouse treated with an adequate dosage of opioid.

The striking aspect of the lenticular response is the development of acute and chronic tolerance. A single large dosage of levorphanol will confer long-lasting resistance to the cataractogenic effects of a subsequent dosage of the drug. Tolerance to the respiratory depressant effect of levorphanol does not occur after a single dosage (see Figure 1). The dose-response curve is unchanged, ruling out the possibility that a change in respiratory parameters influences the long-lasting tolerance.

Takemori (1974) found that tolerance changes the pA_2 for morphine-naloxone interaction at the analgesic "receptor." These investigators conclude that the receptor participates fundamentally in tolerance development. We do not as yet know if the receptor mechanism for lenticular opacity will show a change in the pA_2 corresponding to degree of tolerance development and different from the pA_2 for the analgesic effect.

Analgetic and Respiratory Responses

More than two decades ago Schneider (1954) showed that treatment of the mouse with reserpine diminished the analgetic effect of morphine. Our studies confirmed this findings; reserpine was injected in a dosage of 2 mg/kg 24 hours before obtaining the AD_{50} for the opioid, levorphanol. Treatment with reserpine shifted the analgesic dose-response curve significantly to the right (see Figure 2); the AD_{50} rose from 5.4 mg/kg to 18 mg/kg as measured on the hot plate (55°C). However, respiratory depression, as indicated by a log-dose related rise in capillary blood pCO_2 remained virtually unchanged. To determine whether attenuation of the analgesia was caused by a serotonergic mechanism or catecholaminergic depletion, the inhibitor of tryptophan-hydroxylase, parachlorphenylalanine-methyl ester, was injected i.p. four hours before testing in a dosage of 300 mg/kg. Biogenic amines apparently play no role in the mediation or modulation of the respiratory depressant action of levorphanol. Presumably acteylcholine is the only neurotransmitter involved, although gamma amino butyric acid cannot be excluded. Specific histamine depletors were also not used, although reserpine does have an histaminolytic action on diencephalic stores of this putative transmitter.

With the finding that respiratory and analgesic responses are pharmacologically different, the possibility of separate receptor mechanisms was considered. This question arose because of the difficulty in assuming mediation of two activities by a single receptor, one on respiration and the other affecting nociception. It seemed simpler to consider that the actions of opioids on the two functions are a consequence of discrete receptor systems. In order to test this hypothesis we injected naloxone 0.3 mg. s.c. and levorphanol or morphine was administered i.p. Twenty-five minutes later the mouse was placed on the hot plate and "analgesia" determined. Those mice remaining on the plate (55°C) for more than 30 seconds were considered analgesic. The mice were then

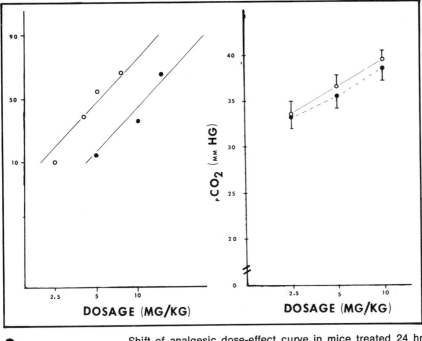

2

Shift of analgesic dose-effect curve in mice treated 24 hr earlier with reserpine, 2mg/kg (left). Lack of shift of respiratory dose-effect curve in similarly treated mice (right).

injected s.c. with 500 units of heparin and five minutes later capillary blood was drawn from a tail incision into a 100 mm. capillary tube. The pH and pCO_2 were then determined as previously described (Hayashida and Smith, 1971) using a Radiometer BMS–3 instrument.

Unlike the nearly sixfold shift of the analgesic dose-response curve that we obtained, only a twofold shift of the respiratory response curve was obtained for levorphanol, whereas the shift of the morphine dose-response curve was approximately fourfold (see Figure 3). These discepancies strongly suggest different receptor mechanisms for respiratory versus analgesic responses. As a result we determined the apparent pA_2 for these separate responses, using the method of Cox and Weinstock (1964). The apparent pA_2 for the analgetic receptor was determined and the value found to be 7.68 $\pm$ .014 whereas the respiratory receptor pA_2 was found to be 6.38 $\pm$ .09, nearly a 20-fold difference ($p < 0.01$). The pA_2's for morphine differ remarkably from levorphanol, since nearly

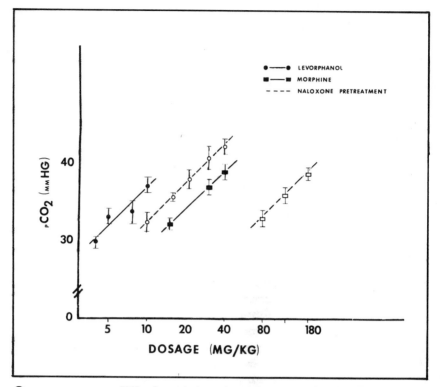

3 Shift of respiratory dose-effect curve in mice concomitantly treated with naloxone 0.3 mg/kg, s.c. The shift for levorphanol is about half that obtained for morphine.

equivalent shifts of the analgesic and respiratory curves were induced by naloxone. For analgesia the morphine-naloxone combination was found to be $7.35 \pm .07$ and for respiration 6.7 ± 0.1 ($p < .02$). These results confirm that respiratory and analgesic responses were separately mediated and the receptors may distinguish between morphine and levorphanol.

Effect of opioids or antagonists on growth

We have recently demonstrated (Smith and Hui, 1973) that the daily injection into the salamander of methadone, 2 mg/kg, or levorphanol, 10 mg/kg, effectively prevents regeneration of the amputated stump. This study arises from the earlier observation (Hui and Smith, 1970) that hemicholinium-3 (HC-3) injection, in dosages of 1 to 3 mg/kg on alternate days, also inhibits limb regeneration in the sala-mander, *Ambystoma tigrinum*. Other cholinolytic agents such as curare also blocked growth whereas atropine in the large dosage of 40 mg/kg was ineffective. The explanation for these findings probably lies in that neither a muscarinic nor nicotinic receptor is involved in regulation of trophic nerve activity. Curare has considerable activity in preventing Ach release which, we believe, is fundamental for regeneration of the limb, probably by some permissive effect on neurotrophic activation.

Singer states that "neither central connections nor reflex circuitry are required for the (trophic) effects." This statement is in accord with the fact that HC-3 blocks regeneration but does not enter the central nervous system. We therefore feel that the action of opioids on growth of the salamander limb occurs at the peripheral sensory level where it may prevent release of Ach, acting in concert with the neurotrophic factor.

Recent biochemical studies indicate that blockade by methadone is associated with a profound inhibition of ^{3}H-uridine incorporation into RNA. In untreated salamanders, the uptake of ^{3}H-uridine, 5 μc/g (i.p.) measured 24 hours later was increased more than 50% over tissues from the contralateral limb. However, the incorporation of ^{3}H-uridine by drug treated salamanders into the regenerating limb bud was the same as in the normal limb, yielding ratios equal or close to unity. Neoplasia was reduced to negligible levels (see Figure 4). That naltrexone inhibits growth is somewhat surprising since naloxone, a related antago-nist, fails to block growth at all. Obviously naltrexone in this dosage, and given on alternate days possessed some agonistic activity.

In contrast with the profound blockade of RNA synthesis by metha-done and three antagonists, the synthesis of DNA is less affected than the sythesis of RNA. Despite the lesser effect, each drug significantly reduces thymidine incorporation, as compared with control. Curiously, the incorporation of ^{3}H-leucine into protein was not altered in any significant way by methadone. Wound healing and scarring do not seem to be under trophic control, judging from the enormous epidermal cap seen covering the blastema in the treated animal. This excessive epi-dermal reaction obviously requires protein synthesis.

In the mouse treated from birth with a very large daily dosage of methadone (8 mg/kg), from birth to four weeks of age, the overall growth deficit compared with saline-treated litter mates is about 40% (Smith et al., 1974). RNA incorporation of ^{3}H-uridine is profoundly reduced in brain and in muscle of these animals but not in the heart or intestine of treated mice. The first two organs are trophically dependent on nerve for growth, whereas the latter two are more autonomous.

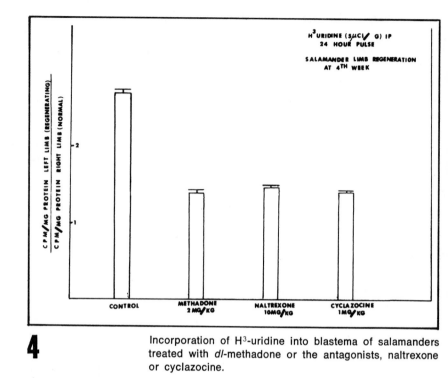

4   Incorporation of H³-uridine into blastema of salamanders treated with *dl*-methadone or the antagonists, naltrexone or cyclazocine.

We have found (Hui et al., 1975) that the greater deficit occurs in muscle. This tissue is rapidly growing throughout the first four to six weeks of life, whereas brain growth is complete at two weeks of age. Failure of muscle growth is reflected in the large weight differences between methadone-treated mice and controls. Preliminary biochemical results indicate that the findings are similar in mice treated at 2 mg/kg and at 4 mg/kg methadone.

Neuroanatomical correlates of methadone treatment

Neonatal rat pups were treated for ten days with methadone, 2 mg/kg, whereas their litter mates were injected with saline. Under ether anesthesia the chest was opened and glutaraldehyde perfused through the heart after saline exchange. The fixed tissues were separated and kept in 2% glutaraldehyde until selected portions were embedded in epoxylite. Thick sections were cut for light microscopy and ultrathin sections for electron microscopy (EM). The first tissues to be examined by EM were the sural nerves of the rat pups. The rationale for this examination arises from the findings in dysautonomia by Aguayo et al. (1971) and by Pearson et al. (1974) of reduced numbers of unmyelinated axons and increased endoneural collagen. In this heritable disease, growth is profoundly retarded, intelligence slightly but significantly diminished, taste buds are missing, and a generalized parasympathetic deficiency exists. All of these findings are thought to be due to a single gene or enzyme defect (Riley, 1974). We believe the enzyme defect is that of a relative deficiency of an isozyme of cholineacetyltransferase (CAT) whose locus of action includes sensory and parasympathetic regions. This would possibly account for the curious distribution of patho-physiology to sensory receptors and the parasympathetic system. Thus the insufficiency of CAT in the sensory nerve inhibits activity of the trophic nerve stuff by providing too little ACh. Methadone or HC-3 treatment prevents release (presumably) or synthesis of ACh, thus mimicking the dysautonomic process by blocking growth of regenerates and causing degeneration of taste bud or lateral line organs (Hui and Smith, 1972). It was therefore decided to look for neuropathology (in methadone-treated animals) where it had been observed in dysauto-nomics. We were rewarded by finding diminished numbers of unmyeli-nated and myelinated fibers as well as a pronounced increase in endoneural collagen. Strikingly similar changes are found in the dysautonomic sural nerve. Although methadone treatment does not induce "dysautonomia" in rats and mice the blockade of ACh may cause some similar and possibly persistent changes in growing animals and perhaps in man during fetal development.

SUMMARY AND CONCLUSIONS

Tolerance to the cataractogenic but not the analgesic or respiratory effects of opioids occurs after a single dose of the opioid. This finding favors the notion that the receptor mechanism for lenticular response to opioids differs from either the antinociceptive or respiratory responses. Evidence is presented that the pA_2's for levorphanol-naloxone or morphine-naloxone combinations differ significantly when comparing analgesic versus respiratory responses. It may be concluded that these central effects of opioids are mediated by separate receptors. In view of the ability of opioids and mixed agonist-antagonist drugs to inhibit growth of the salamander limb and block incorporation of ^{3}H-uridine into RNA, a peripherally mediated response, it is likely that receptors for these opioid or antagonist drugs are present in the peripheral nerv-ous system. This view is supported by the finding of changes induced in a peripheral nerve (sural) of neonatal mice treated for 10–30 days with *dl*-methadone. Blockade of the growth-inhibiting effect of methadone by naloxone indicates that the peripheral receptor is stereospecific. Thus at least four receptors can be distinguished pharmacologically by differences in tolerance development, pA_2 and by growth inhibiting action almost certainly mediated by a peripheral mechanism.

More recent evidence obtained since preparation of this chapter indicates that when narcotic analgesics are administered subcutaneously rather than intraperitoneally and the antagonist naloxone injected in an adjacent site, the pA_2 for analgesia, respiratory depression and for lenticular response is found to be approximately 7.0 for each. This finding indicates that the receptor protein mediating each response must be the same. But induction of tolerance produces no shift in the pA_2 for lenticular effect whereas the analgesic and respiratory depressive pA_2 rise to about 7.5. The analgesic dose response curve is then shifted to the right but not the respiratory dose response curve which confirms the notion that these receptor mechanisms differ. The earlier results showing marked differences in pA_2 for analgesic and for respiratory responses probably arose from early or rapid transport to the respiratory modulating center and less rapidly to the region mediating analgesic response. The hypothesis that these responses lie in different regions will require neuroanatomical location by stereotactic lesioning.

REFERENCES

Aguayo, A., C. P. V. Nair, and M. Bray. 1971. Peripheral nerve abnormalities in the Riley-Day syndrome. *Arch. Neurol.* 24: 106–116.

Cox, B. M., and M. Weinstock. 1964. Quantitative studies of the antagonism by nalorphine of some of the actions of morphine-like analgesic drugs. *Brit. J. Pharmacol.* 22: 289–300.

Hayashida, K., and A. Smith. 1971. Reversal by sotalol of the respiratory depression induced in mice by ethanol. *J. Pharm. Pharmacol.* 23: 718–719.

Hui, F., E. Krikun, and A. Smith. 1975. Selective inhibition by methadone of RNA synthesis in brain and muscle of growing mice. *The Pharmacologist* 17: 239.

Hui, F., and A. Smith. 1970. Regeneration of the amphibian limb: Retardation by hemicholinium-3. *Science* 170: 1313–1314.

Hui, F., and A. Smith. 1972. Degeneration of taste buds and lateral line organs in the salamander treated with cholinolytic drugs. *Exptl. Neurol.* 34: 331–341.

Pearson, J., F. Axelrod, and J. Dancis. 1974. Current concepts of dysautonomia: Neuropathological defects. *Ann. N. Y. Acad. Sci.* 228: 288–300.

Riley, C. 1974. Familial dysautonomia: Clinical and pathophysiological aspects. *Ann. N. Y. Acad. Sci.* 228: 283–287.

Schneider, J. A. 1954. Reserpine antagonism of morphine analgesia in mice. *Proc. Soc. Exp. Biol. Med.* 87: 614–615.

Smith, A., J. Gavitt, and M. Kaplan. 1964. Some relationships between catecholamines and morphine-like drugs. *Rec. Adv. Biol. Psychiat.* 6: 208–213.

Smith, A., and F. Hui. 1973. Inhibition of neurotrophic activity in salamanders treated with opioids. *Exptl. Neurol.* 39: 36–43.

Smith, A., F. Hui, and M. Crofford. 1974. Retardation of growth by opioids. In J. Dancis and J. C. Hwang, Eds. Raven Press, New York, pp. 195–201.

Takemori, A. E. 1974. Determination of pharmacological constants: Use of narcotic antagonists to characterize analgesic receptors. In M. C. Braude, L. S. Harris, E. L. May, J. P. Smith, and J. E. Villarreal. *Narcotic Antagonists.* Raven Press, New York, pp. 335–344.

Weinstock, M. 1961. Similarity between receptors responsible for the production of analgesia and lenticular opacity. *Brit. J. Pharmacol.* 17: 433–441.

Weinstock, M., and A. S. Marshall. 1969. Factors influencing the incidence of reversible lens opacities in solitaray and aggregated mice. *J. Pharmacol. Exp. Therap.* 170: 168–172.

Tissue Responses to Addictive Drugs
© 1976, Spectrum Publications, Inc.

Some Effects of Agonists and Antagonists on the Development of Tolerance and Dependence

BARRY E. MUSHLIN
JOSEPH COCHIN

Department of Pharmacology
Boston University School of Medicine
Boston, Massachusetts

The nature of tolerance to and dependence on the narcotic analgesics has been the subject of continuing interest and research in our laboratory for the past decade and a half. In a continuation of work begun at the National Institutes of Health in the early 1960's, Cochin and Kornetsky (1964) have described a form of tolerance that can be detected some nine to twelve months after either a single dose or after the termination of chronic administration of morphine in the rat. In further studies, we have shown that there are some aspects of tolerance to the narcotic analgesics that resemble an immune process and that are affected by agents known to modify the immune response such as cycloheximide (Feinberg and Cochin, 1972), Freund's adjuvant (Cochin and Mushlin, 1972), and total body irradiation (Mushlin and Cochin, 1974). We have also examined the role of dose interval on the development of tolerance; our research in this area has led us to believe that there are two types of tolerance that develop: "short term," which can

435

be seen after doses at intervals of less than a week apart; and "long term," which develops with dose intervals longer than one week apart (Mushlin et al., 1976).

In earlier studies of the effects of coadministration of agonists and antagonists, Orahovats et al. (1953) and Cochin and Axelrod (1959) have shown that rats injected chronically with a mixture of morphine and nalorphine exhibited significantly less tolerance to morphine than animals injected with morphine alone. Both groups used doses of nalorphine that only partially blocked the analgesic effects of morphine. Eddy et al. (1960) reported a study in humans in which morphine and levallorphan were concomitantly administered. Again, they used doses of antagonist insufficient to completely block morphine analgesia. They found that the coadministration of morphine and levallorphan caused a partial blockade of the development of tolerance to morphine. Deneau and Seevers (1960) also observed that mixtures of morphine and levallorphan were capable of reducing the extent to which tolerance and physical dependence to morphine develop in the monkey.

In this chapter we discuss a series of experiments performed in order to examine systematically the effects of concurrent morphine and naloxone administration on the development of tolerance and physical dependence to morphine. We have endeavored to approach pharmacologically the question of whether the receptor site activated by the narcotic analgesics is also the site blocked by the narcotic antagonists and whether, as a consequence, complete blockade of the agonist action would prevent the subsequent development of tolerance and physical dependence. It was our hypothesis that any occupation of the receptor site by the agonist would result in tolerance and dependence, even though one could not detect agonist activity with standard assay techniques.

MATERIALS AND METHODS

The animals used were adult male Wistar-Lewis rats, obtained from Charles River Laboratories, Wilmington, Massachusetts. The rats were housed in general animal quarters with food and water available *ad libitum*, and were removed to the testing laboratory only when experimental procedures were performed. Drugs used were morphine sulfate (15 mg/kg), naloxone hydrochloride (6 and 10 mg/kg) and saline. All injections were administered subcutaneously.

Analgesia was measured by means of the hot-plate assay (Mushlin et al., 1976); the area under the time-response curve being used as the measure of analgesia. A decrease in area as compared to control values

Table I. Partial Blockade of Morphine Tolerance by Naloxone[1]

Treatment	Day 1	Day 4	Day 9
Morphine	2318 ± 224 (21)	666 ± 84 (20)	831 ± 158 (18)
Morphine plus Naloxone	28 ± 31 (24)	−44 ± 30 (24)	1715 ± 252 (21)*
Naloxone	14 ± 25 (24)	−10 ± 22 (24)	2134 ± 210 (23)

[1]Areas under the time-response curve, in minute-seconds, are expressed as the mean ± S.E., the number of rats is indicated in parentheses.

*Different from morphine group on day 1 ($P < 0.05$, single-tailed t-test)

was taken to indicate the presence of tolerance to morphine. Physical dependence was measured by a modification of the method of Wei et al. (1973). Rats were observed for escape behavior, wet-dog shakes, diarrhea, and ptosis for 15-minute periods immediately before and after injections of saline or 10 mg/kg of naloxone. Acute 3-hour weight loss was also determined; all rats were weighed at the time of the saline or naloxone injection and again three hours later. (The animals were deprived of food and water during this period.)

DISCUSSION

Partial Blockade of Morphine Tolerance

Rats were assigned to one of three groups and received eight daily injections of either morphine (15 mg/kg), morphine plus naloxone, or naloxone alone. Naloxone (6 mg/kg) was administered both 10 minutes before and 110 minutes after morphine. On the ninth day, all rats received only morphine. All animals were tested for analgesia on days 1, 4 and 9 (see Table I). No analgesia was evident in the groups receiving morphine plus naloxone or naloxone alone on either day 1 or 4, and the areas obtained were no different than those customarily seen in our laboratory with rats treated with saline. On day 9, when the two naloxone-treated groups received only morphine, the response of the naloxone group was no different from the response of the morphine group on day 1. However, the rats that received morphine plus naloxone showed tolerance to morphine ($P < 0.05$ single-tail t-test). As an explanation for this tolerance, we believe that the naloxone blockade was not complete and that some morphine was reaching the receptor site.

To determine if tolerance to morphine could develop in the absence

Table II. Development of Morphine Tolerance in the Absence of Analgesia[1]

Treatment	Day 1	Day 5
Morphine (2 mg/kg)	125 ± 19 (10)	2373 ± 201 (10)*
Saline	142 ± 51 (10)	2956 ± 147 (8)

[1]See Table I
*Different from saline treated group on day 5 (P <0.05)

of detectable analgesia, an additional experiment was carried out. A group of rats received daily injections of 2 mg/kg of morphine for 4 days while a second group received saline. All animals were tested on the hot plate on day 1; there was no detectable analgesia in the group receiving morphine (see Table II). On day 5, both groups were again tested on the hot plate following 15 mg/kg of morphine. The low-dose morphine group exhibited a significant attenuation of morphine effect as compared to the saline group; there was tolerance development in the absence of detectable analgesia with our assay system.

Complete Blockade of Morphine Tolerance

Since it was evident that two injections of naloxone surrounding each daily morphine injection were insufficient to prevent the development of tolerance to morphine, we decided to give naloxone four times; 30 and 10 minutes before, 50, and 110 minutes after the morphine injection. Three groups of rats received the daily schedule of either morphine alone, morphine plus naloxone, or saline for eight days. Beginning on day 9, all rats received only morphine for nine additional days, for a total of seventeen days. Rats were tested on the hot plate on days 1, 4, 9, 12 and 17. No analgesia was evident on days 1 and 4 in the group receiving morphine plus naloxone, nor in the group receiving naloxone alone. The morphine-plus-naloxone group on day 9, the first day on which only morphine was given, was no different than the morphine group on day 1 (see Table III). It was evident, therefore, that the series of four naloxone injections had completely blocked the development of tolerance to morphine. Similarly, pretreatment with naloxone alone had no effect on subsequent morphine treatment; the two naloxone treated groups were equally as tolerant on day 17, their ninth day of morphine alone, as were the animals in the morphine group on day 9.

In another experiment, injections were given at weekly rather than daily intervals. Morphine, morphine plus naloxone, or naloxone

Table III. Complete Blockade of Morphine Tolerance by Naloxone: Daily Injections[1]

Treatment Group	Day 1	Day 4	Day 9	Day 12	Day 17
Morphine	1843 ± 238 (15)	307 ± 51 (15)	410 ± 82 (15)	140 ± 28 (15)	210 ± 65 (15)
Morphine plus Naloxone	91 ± 28 (16)	17 ± 24 (16)	1841 ± 186 (15)	675 ± 51 (15)	352 ± 48 (14)
Naloxone	84 ± 20 (16)	12 ± 26 (16)	2241 ± 97 (16)	807 ± 94 (16)	455 ± 52 (15)

[1]See Table I

alone were given the first two weeks and only morphine was administered to all groups the last three weeks. The results are comparable to those obtained with daily injections (see Table IV). The coadministration of naloxone blocked the morphine effect and the development of tolerance to morphine; treatment with naloxone alone had no effect on the subsequent development of tolerance to morphine. There was also no evidence of cross-tolerance to morphine induced by naloxone.

Concurrent Blockade of Morphine Tolerance and Dependence

The next question to be considered was whether the development of physical dependence to morphine would also be blocked by the same schedule of naloxone injections that completely blocked the development of tolerance. Four groups of rats were given a series of sixteen daily injections of either morphine, morphine plus naloxone (30 and 10 minutes before and 50 and 110 minutes after morphine), naloxone alone, or saline. Four hours after the last injection on day 16, all rats received an injection of either saline or 10 mg/kg of naloxone and were tested for precipitated abstinence by a modification of the method of Wei et al. (1973). Animals were observed for escape behavior, wet-dog shakes, diarrhea and ptosis for 15-minute periods immediately before and after the saline or naloxone injections. No abstinence signs were observed in any of the groups prior to the test injections, with the exception of one rat in the morphine group that demonstrated escape behavior (see Table V). Following the saline test injection, one rat in the morphine-naloxone group demonstrated wet-dog shakes; no other signs were seen. When the test injection of naloxone was given, wet-dog shakes were observed in one naloxone-pretreated rat, with no abstinence signs evident in either the saline or morphine-plus-naloxone pretreatment groups. Abstinence was precipitated, as would be expected, in the morphine group. During the 15-minute test period, 6 of the 17 rats attempted to escape and 15 showed evidence of diarrhea and ptosis. Additionally, 1 rat exhibited wet-dog shakes. All rats were weighed at the time of the test injection of saline or naloxone and again three hours later for the determination of acute weight loss. The percent of original weight was then calculated for each animal (see Figure 1). The only group exhibiting weight loss beyond control levels is the morphine group which received a naloxone injection; the naloxone-pretreated groups were no different than saline-pretreated controls.

Nine days after the animals were tested for evidence of precipitated abstinence, all rats received 15 mg/kg of morphine and were then tested on the hot plate for the presence of tolerance (see Table VI). Since no differences in morphine effect were evident due to the injections of

Table IV. Complete Blockade of Morphine Tolerance by Naloxone: Weekly Injections[1]

Treatment Group	Week 1	Week 2	Week 3	Week 4	Week 5
Morphine	2206 ± 196 (15)	1757 ± 162 (13)	736 ± 75 (13)	655 ± 122 (13)	418 ± 65 (13)
Morphine plus Naloxone	90 ± 20 (20)	70 ± 22 (20)	2162 ± 203 (16)	1323 ± 233 (14)	711 ± 175 (13)
Naloxone	71 ± 18 (20)	27 ± 19 (20)	2228 ± 224 (16)	1196 ± 157 (16)	726 ± 157 (15)

[1] See Table I

Table V. Abstinence Signs Observed in Chronically Pretreated Rats

16 Day Pretreatment (N)	Morphine (34)		Morphine & Naloxone (30)		Naloxone (30)		Saline (30)	
15 Minute Observation before test drug								
Escapes	1		0		0		0	
Shakes	0		0		0		0	
Diarrhea	0		0		0		0	
Ptosis	0		0		0		0	
Test Drug Treatment (N)	SAL* (17)	MOR$_i$** (17)	SAL (15)	NAX† (15)	SAL (15)	NAX (15)	SAL (15)	NAX (15)
15 Minute Observation after test drug								
Escapes	0	6	0	0	0	0	0	0
Shakes	0	1	1	0	0	1	0	0
Diarrhea	0	15	0	0	0	0	0	0
Ptosis	0	15	0	0	0	0	0	0

* Saline
** Morphine
†Naloxone, 10 mg/kg

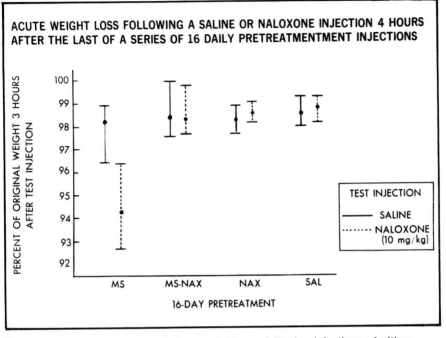

1 Acute 3-hour weight loss following injections of either saline (solid lines) or 10 mg/kg s.c. of naloxone (broken lines) in groups of rats pretreated for 16 days with either morphine (MS), morphine plus naloxone (MS-NAX), naloxone (NAX) or saline.

saline or naloxone nine days earlier, we have combined the saline and naloxone test group data in each case. As expected, the morphine-pretreated group shows a very high degree of tolerance as compared to the saline-pretreated group. The groups pretreated with naloxone or with morphine plus naloxone showed no evidence of tolerance; there were no differences from saline values. Thus, the coadministration of naloxone and morphine is capable of blocking both the development of physical dependence to morphine and the development of tolerance.

CONCLUSIONS

The experiments we have described in this paper indicate that access to the morphine receptor site and subsequent interaction with the receptor seem to be a prerequisite, a sine qua non, for the changes which result in tolerance and dependence. We believe that our results

Table VI. Results of Hot-Plate Assay Performed Nine Days after a Series of Sixteen Daily Pretreatment Injections[1]

Pretreatment	Response
Morphine	568 ± 129 (12)*
Morphine plus Naloxone	2273 ± 183 (22)
Naloxone	2146 ± 228 (17)
Saline	2488 ± 247 (17)

[1]See Table I
*Different from other three groups (P < 0.05)

indicate that the antagonists interact with or bind to the same receptor site as do the agonists. A number of investigators have postulated the existence of separate ligands for agonists and antagonists and have also postulated that chronic administration of antagonists results in an increase in receptor-site binding. We do not think that our work confirms the multiple receptor site hypothesis since our results would be extremely difficult to explain on this basis—one would expect some evidence of altered morphine effect after chronic administration of the pure antagonist. Nor do we see any pharmacological evidence of an increased number of binding sites; again on the basis of the lack of an alteration of morphine effect after the chronic administration of naloxone.

However, the absence of detectable pharmacological effect does not seem to preclude the development of tolerance or dependence. We have found that low doses of morphine that give no measurable evidence of analgesia are capable of producing tolerance. This simply means that our assay techniques are not sensitive enough to measure the minimal drug effect induced by low doses of agonist. There it no doubt in our minds, however, that complete blockade of agonist action by an appropriate schedule of antagonist administration, a schedule designed to take into account the diverse half-lives of agonist and antagonist, will prevent the subsequent development of tolerance and dependence. We also feel that our experiments lend further support to our belief that agonist interaction with the receptor site is necessary for tolerance and dependence, even though that interaction cannot be measured by present pharmacological assay techniques. Furthermore, we feel that there is a threshold dose below which no tolerance or physical dependence can be initiated. A minimum level of receptor-site binding seems to be essential. This is borne out by a large number of clinical studies with codeine where small doses of this drug given for relatively long periods of time appeared to induce neither tolerance nor dependence. Our own preliminary work with a 1 mg/kg dose of morphine, where no tolerance resulted, would seem to bear this out. It is obvious, of course, that much depends on the particular parameter of drug action being measured and the assay system that is being used.

ACKNOWLEDGMENTS

This work was supported in part by Research Grants # RO1-DA-00016 and PO1-DA-00257 from the National Institute on Drug Abuse.

We are grateful to Mrs. Rachelle Grell for her technical assistance.

REFERENCES

Cochin, J., and J. Axelrod. 1959. Biochemical and pharmacological changes in the rat following chronic administration of morphine, nalorphine and normorphine. *J. Pharmacol. Exp. Ther.* 125: 105–110.

Cochin, J., and C. Kornetsky. 1964. Development and loss of tolerance to morphine in the rat after single and multiple injections. *J. Pharmacol. Exp. Ther.* 145: 1–10.

Cochin, J., and B. E. Mushlin. 1972. The effect of Freund's adjuvant on morphine sensitivity and tolerance. *Fed. Proc.* 31: 528.

Deneau, G. A., and M. H. Seevers. 1960. Chronic administration of nalorphine, levallorphan and mixtures of levallorphan with morphine in the monkey. *Minutes 21st Meeting Committee on Drug Addiction and Narcotics, NRC-NAS,* App. 6. 2214–2220.

Eddy, N. B., M. Piller, L. A. Pirk, O. Schrappe, and S. Wende. 1960. The effect of the addition of a narcotic antagonist on the rate of development of tolerance and physical dependence to morphine. *Bull. Narc.* 12: 1–16.

Feinberg, M. P. and J. Cochin. 1972. Inhibition of development of tolerance to morphine by cycloheximide. *Biochem. Pharmacol.* 21: 3082–3085.

Mushlin, B., and J. Cochin. 1974. Effects of irradiation on the development of tolerance to morphine in the rat. *Fed. Proc.* 33: 502.

Mushlin, B. E., R. Grell, and J. Cochin. 1976. Studies on tolerance I. The role of the interval between doses on the development of tolerance to morphine. *J. Pharmacol. Exp. Ther.* 196: 280–287.

Orahovats, P. D., C. A. Winter, and E. G. Lehman. 1953. The effect of N-allylnormorphine upon the development of tolerance to morphine in the albino rat. *J. Pharmacol. Exp. Ther.* 109: 413–416.

Wei, E., H. H. Loh, and E. L. Way. 1973. Quantitative aspects of precipitated abstinence in morphine-dependent rats. *J. Pharmacol. Exp. Ther.* 184: 398–403.

Tissue Responses to Addictive Drugs
© 1976, Spectrum Publications, Inc.

Drug Induced Alterations on Alcohol Preference and Withdrawal

ANDREW K. S. HO
BENJAMIN KISSIN
Department of Basic Sciences

University of Illinois
Peoria School of Medicine
Peoria, Illinois

Division of Alcoholism and Drug Abuse
Department of Psychiatry
Downstate Medical Center
Brooklyn, New York

The mechanism involved in volitional consumption of ethyl alcohol in animals remains obscure in spite of numerous studies appearing in the literature. Recent studies in the neurochemical correlates of alcohol preference have been focused on various putative neurotransmitters in the brain. However, no single system appears to be responsible for alcohol preference although suggestions have been made on the possible roles of serotonergic, cholinergic and adrenergic systems. Myers and Veale (1968) suggested that serotonin (5-HT) may be involved in alcohol preference on the basis that when the synthesis of 5-HT in the brain of the rat was inhibited by p-chlorophenylalanine (pCPA), an inhibitor of tryptophan hydroxylase, volitional consumption of alcohol was found to be reduced. Frey et al. (1970) showed that p-chloro-amphetamine, an agent which depletes the brain content of 5-HT, also attenuated alcohol preference. However, other investigators

447

were unable to confirm the reduction of alcohol preference by *p*CPA. Nachman et al. (1970) contended that a conditioned aversion might be established through the pairing of ethanol or saccharin with the administration of *p*CPA; Geller (1973) showed that *p*CPA increased rather than decreased alcohol preference. Recently, we used 5,6-dihydroxytryptamine (5,6-DHT), an agent which depletes brain 5-HT, (Baumgarten et al., 1971) and observed that alcohol preference was significantly increased following an intracisternal injection of 5,6-DHT (75 μg/rat). The level of brain acetylcholine (ACh) was increased significantly at a time when alcohol preference also increased, i.e. approximately eight days after 5,6-DHT treatment. This 5,6-DHT-induced alcohol preference was antagonized by 4 (1-napthylvinyl)pyridine (NVP), an inhibitor of choline transferase (Ho et al., 1974). The 5,6-DHT-induced alcohol preference was also reported by Myers and Melchior (1975). The role of catecholamines in alcohol preference was not considered to be significant by Myers and Veale (1968) on the basis that α-methyl-*p*-tyrosine (αMpT), an inhibitor of tyrosine hydroxylase, produced no significant alteration in alcohol preference.

The possible involvement of the central cholinergic system in alcohol preference has been suggested (Ho and Kissin, 1975; Ho et al., 1974) on the basis that, in mice, a high alcohol-preferring strain, $C_{57}Bl/6J$, has a higher cholinergic activity than a poor alcohol-preferring strain, DBA/2J, as evidenced by the higher choline uptake and brain levels of ACh in $C_{57}Bl/6J$ mice. Many agents which interfere with the brain acetylcholine were also observed to alter alcohol preference.

In this chapter, we present some observations on the effects of NVP, 5,6-DHT, 6-hydroxydopamine (6–OHDA) and lithium on alcohol preference and withdrawal.

MATERIALS AND METHODS

Preference Studies

Adult male Sprague-Dawley rats weighing 200 to 250 g. were used. The animals were kept individually in standard wire-meshed cages in a constant temperature room (70°F), with a light-dark cycle of 12–12 hours. A period of four days was allowed for acclimatization of the rats before used for experiments. Two graduated glass drinking tubes (Kimax Instrument Co.) were fitted onto the outside of each cage: one filled with water and the other with varying concentrations of alcohol. The positions of the tubes were changed daily so as to prevent the development of a position habit, and also different tubes were used. The alcohol used was diluted from 95% ethanol with distilled water on a volume to volume basis to the required concentration. The preference-aversion cut-off concentration and the base-line consumption for each rat was determined as described previously (Ho et al., 1974). Food, water and alcohol were available ad libitum; the consumption and the body weight were recorded from 10 a.m. to 12 noon each day. Following treatment with drugs, the animals were given free choice between water and 5% (v/v) alcohol. In the case of 6-OHDA and 5,6-DHT, the animals were also given forced-drinking of alcohol in various concentrations. The rats with low alcohol preference were selected for both the 5,6-DHT and 6-OHDA experiments.

Chronic Alcohol Treatment and Withdrawal

Recently a procedure for the chronic ingestion of alcohol to produce physical dependence in rats was developed in our laboratory and was used in this study. A group of male Sprague-Dawley rats weighing between 120–150 g. at the start of the experiment was used. The rats were all individually housed as described. Alcohol solution was the sole fluid available. Initially, the concentration of alcohol available was 4% and the concentration was increased by 1% daily until it reached 20%; this was followed by an increment of 2% every two days until 40% was reached. The rats were maintained on 40% alcohol for four months. Physical dependence with characteristic withdrawal symptoms were observed. These included weight loss, tremor, hyperactivity, jumping, clonic-tonic convulsions, both provoked and spontaneous, coma and death. A modified arbitrary rating scale based on that described by Goldstein (1973) was used to assess the intensity of the withdrawal symptoms (see Table I). The effect of chronic alcohol exposure on volitional consumption of alcohol was tested at various periods up to 98 days. Each period of measurement of alcohol preference lasted for four days and the rats were given forced drinking afterwards.

Drug Treatment

5,6-DHT (75 μg/rat) or 6-OHDA (200 μg/rat) (supplied by Regis Chemical Co.) was administered i.c. under light ether anesthesia. In the withdrawal studies, the drug was given three days before withdrawal of alcohol. NVP was administered i.p. with doses of 5 or 10 mg/kg, twice daily. Similarly, lithium (as lithium carbonate) was given i.p. twice daily with doses varying from 0.3 mEq/kg to 2 mEq/kg.

Table I. An Arbitrary Rating Score on Ethanol Withdrawal Signs in Rats[1]

Signs	Score
a. Weight loss of 20% or more of the initial weight	1
b. Mild tremor, hyper-reflexia, compulsive drinking behavior	2
c. Continuous tremor, provoked or spontaneous jumping	3
d. Jumping, clonic-tonic convulsion, about 1 per hour	4
e. Severe clonic-tonic convulsions	5
f. Coma and death	6

[1] Ethanol dependent rats were withdrawn at 8 a.m. Withdrawal signs were observed 5 hours after withdrawal for up to 14 hours. Provoked jumping and convulsions were produced by ringing a bunch of keys around the rat for 60 seconds.

RESULTS

Alcohol Preference

NVP at a dose of 10 mg/kg i.p. twice daily in rats produced a significant decrease in the mean daily alcohol intake throughout the 7-day period of treatment, and the selection for alcohol recovered to the base-line level 5 days after the last treatment. Mean water intake was increased so that the total fluid intake appeared not to have been altered significantly. There was no significant change in food intake. Body weight loss was not significant until the sixth consecutive day after treatment (see Figures 1, 2). In rats pretreated with 5,6-DHT, alcohol preference was found to increase significantly and lasted about five-six days. The 5,6-DHT-induced alcohol preference was reduced significantly by NVP (5 mg/kg, twice daily) (see Figure 3). In rats treated with 6-OHDA, alcohol preference increased in a manner similar to 5,6-DHT treatment and this effect was antagonized by NVP.

Rats given lithium showed a marked reduction in the daily voluntary consumption of alcohol irrespective of their cut-off concentrations (see Figure 4). However, in animals with low alcohol preference, typical daily fluid consumptions for water and alcohol (5% v/v) were 103.0 ± 5.0 mg/kg and 6.0 ± 0.4 mg/kg (n= 20) respectively. In view of the small volume of alcohol intake in the rats showing poor alcohol preference, we selected rats which showed greater preference for 5% alcohol and tested the effect of lithium. In a group of eight rats which con-

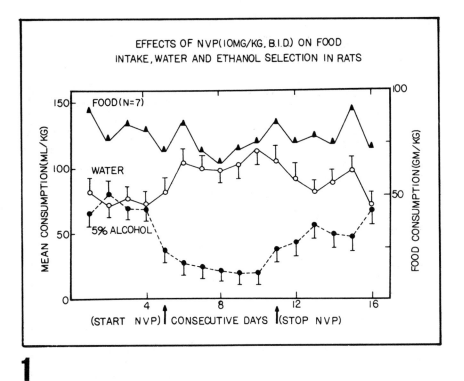

1

sumed a mean of 80 ml/kg/day of alcohol compared with an average consumption of 40 ml/kg/day approximately, lithium at 13 mg/kg i.p. given twice daily significantly ($p < 0.01$ to 0.001) reduced the voluntary consumption of alcohol throughout the course of treatment. The effect of lithium on alcohol preference was readily reversible when the treatment was terminated.

Chronic Alcohol Consumption and Withdrawal

In the chronic experiments, rats exposed to alcohol solution alone from two to four months, developed physical dependence to different degrees as characterized by their typical withdrawal symptoms. In the 15 rats exposed to alcohol alone, all the animals showed weight loss, hyperexcitability and tremor; about 60–70% of the rats showed withdrawal jumping, clonic and tonic convulsions and about 35–40% showed coma and a few rats died. These findings have been consistently observed in over 200 rats placed on a similar forced drinking schedule.

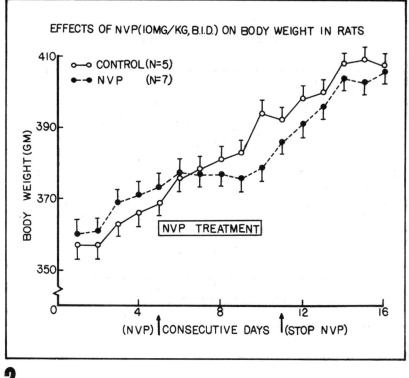

2

In rats pretreated with 6-OHDA and 5,6-DHT and exposed to a forced drinking schedule, total consumption of alcohol was increased markedly in rats treated with 5,6-DHT and to a lesser degree in rats treated with 6-OHDA, when compared with the saline control (see Figure 5). Consequently, over a period of 60 days on the forced-drinking schedule, the total consumption of alcohol was greater in the treated rats. Therefore, the degree of dependence as measured by their withdrawal symptoms appeared to be more severe. However, in rats previously made dependent on alcohol, and then given 5,6-DHT and 6-OHDA three days before withdrawal from alcohol, the severity of withdrawal was significantly decreased as measured by the arbitrary scores ($p < 0.01$, n = 8).

In the fourteen rats previously exposed to alcohol up to four months, daily consumption of 40% (v/v) alcohol was significantly reduced during the first and second days of treatment with 2 mEq/kg

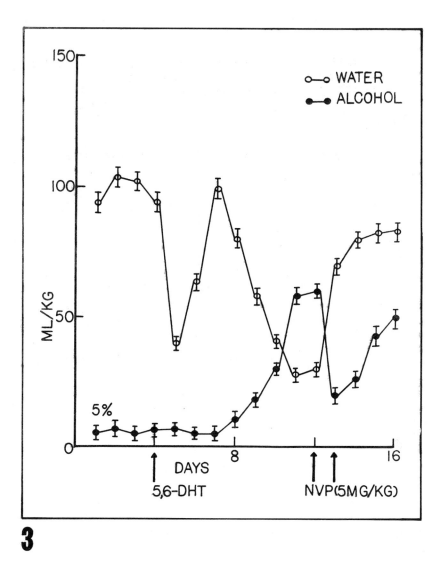

3

lithium twice a day (p< 0.001). Mean daily alcohol consumptions prior to lithium treatment were 62.4 ± 5.0 ml/kg and 37.9 ± 6.3 ml/kg during the first and second days after treatments respectively (see Figure 6). Because of the marked reduction in total fluid intake, the treatment was stopped after the second day so as to avoid further dehydration. In another experiment, we lowered the alcohol concentration to 30% (v/v) and examined the effect of oral lithium at 0.6 mEq/kg twice

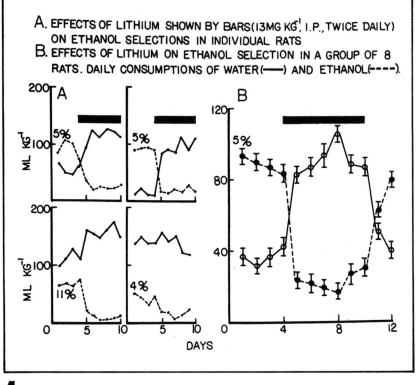

A. EFFECTS OF LITHIUM SHOWN BY BARS(13MG KG⁻¹, I.P., TWICE DAILY) ON ETHANOL SELECTIONS IN INDIVIDUAL RATS
B. EFFECTS OF LITHIUM ON ETHANOL SELECTION IN A GROUP OF 8 RATS. DAILY CONSUMPTIONS OF WATER(——) AND ETHANOL(----).

4

daily. There was no significant reduction in either alcohol or food consumption. However, when the oral dose of lithium was increased to 1.2 mEq/kg twice daily, both consumption of ethanol and food by the rats was reduced significantly. ($p < 0.02$, $n = 9$) on the first day, and returned to the base line level thereafter. There was no change in the mean body weight. Treatment with lithium at 1 mEq/kg dose produced no obvious change in withdrawal symptomatology. However, with a 4 mEq/kg dose for two days, the severity of withdrawal symptoms appeared to increase. Thus, in this group of seven treated rats, five out of seven rats went into coma compared to three in the controls, and all the lithium treated rats showed withdrawal jumping.

Volitional consumption of 5% alcohol during various periods of forced drinking were measured for up to 115 days. Results obtained showed that the volume of alcohol consumed increased progressively

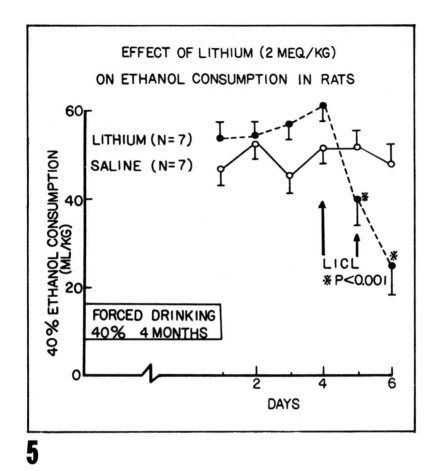

5

from 30 days onward and the corresponding consumption of water decreased resulting in no apparent change in total fluid intake (see Figure 7).

DISCUSSIONS

Alcohol Preference

There appears to be other mechanisms involved in the regulation of alcohol preference besides the central serotonergic activity originally suggested by Myers and Veale (1968). Our findings showed that both 5,6-DHT and 6-OHDA can induce alterations in alcohol preference

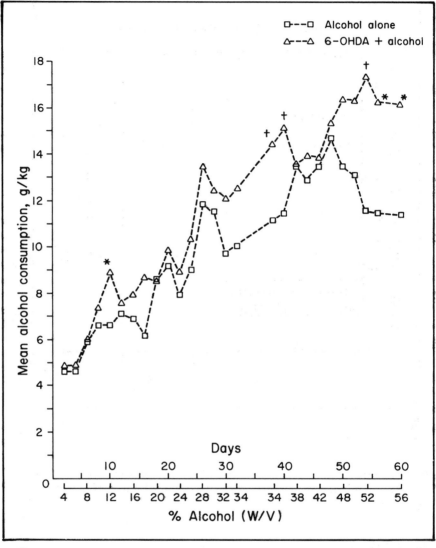

6

as well as other agents, such as pCPA, 5-HTP, paraldehyde, parachloro-amphetamine, etc. These findings suggest that several putative neuro-transmitter systems may be involved. The fact that the 5,6-DHT-induced increase in alcohol preference corresponded to an increase in brain ACh and that this increase could be antagonized by NVP suggests a possible

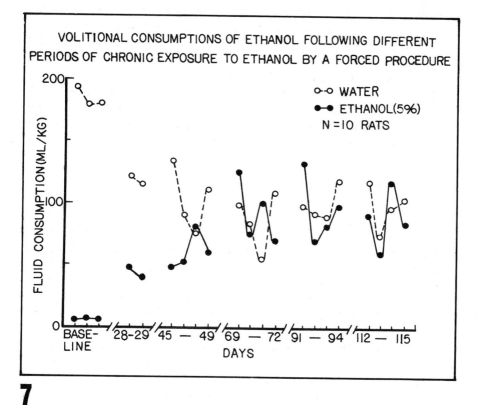

VOLITIONAL CONSUMPTIONS OF ETHANOL FOLLOWING DIFFERENT PERIODS OF CHRONIC EXPOSURE TO ETHANOL BY A FORCED PROCEDURE

7

cholinergic-serotonergic interaction in the regulation of alcohol preference (Ho et al., 1974). Recently, Myers and Melchoir (1975) reported
that intraventricular administration of 5,6-DHT resulted in an increase
in alcohol preference whereas 6-OHDA administration resulted in a
transient decrease, similar to the effect of αMpT. These investigators
suggested that an increase in the functional pool of 5-HT in the brain,
rather than a decrease, leads to a decline in alcohol preference. It would
appear that a delicate balance of one or more of the putative neurotransmitters may be responsible for alcohol preference. Thus, it may be
possible that alterations induced by 5,6-DHT on the serotonergic, or by
6-OHDA on the catecholaminergic systems may lead to a compensa-
tory change in the cholinergic systems resulting in a shift in the selection between alcohol and water. Results obtained on the reduction of
alcohol preference by lithium are interesting. Lithium has pharmacological properties in common with alcohol in that each compound

given alone produces diuresis and disturbance of electrolyte balance. In addition, lithium reduces the uptake of ^{14}C-choline and the brain level of ACh, as well as exerting its effects on the monoamines (Ho and Tsai, 1975; Schildkraut, 1973). Preliminary studies in our laboratory showed that other CNS stimulants, such as amphetamine, and depressants, such as morphine and other narcotic agents, interact with alcohol, leading to suppression or stimulation of alcohol preference (Ho et al., 1975). Common to all psychotropic drugs is their ability to exert influence on various putative neurotransmitter systems in the brain.

Alcohol Dependence

The results obtained in this study showed that drugs such as 6-OHDA and 5,6-DHT enhanced the consumption of alcohol under a forced drinking schedule. Using the ingestion method we have developed, the severity of physical dependence can be asssessed and its relationship to alcohol preference measured. Our data showed that chronic alcohol ingestion led to an increase in alcohol preference. The observation that 5,6-DHT or 6-OHDA administration three days before alcohol withdrawal suppressed some of the withdrawal symptomatology reinforces the suggestion that the central adrenergic mechanism may be involved in the expression of these various symptoms (Reis, 1973). On the basis of 5,6-DHT effects, it is possible that serotonergic mechanisms may also be involved. Preliminary neurochemical studies showed that 6-OHDA potentiated the alcohol-induced reduction in the uptake of ^3H-NE. In addition, ten hours after withdrawal from alcohol, the uptake of ^3H-NE rebounded above the control level. In the 6-OHDA pretreated alcohol-dependent rats, uptake of ^3H-NE remained suppressed. These findings correlate well with the behavioral observations that 6-OHDA suppressed the withdrawal symptomatology by reducing the adrenergic activity of the CNS.

ACKNOWLEDGMENTS

This work was supported in part by a grant-in-aid from the Distilled Spirits Council of America to A.K.S. Ho and MH-16477 to B. Kissin. The authors wish to thank Ms. Patricia Blair for typing the manuscript and Messrs. C. S. Tsai and R. C. A. Chen for technical assistance. Dr. Ho is a Career Teacher in Substance Abuse, NIDA TO1-DA00218-02.

REFERENCES

Baumgarten, H. G., A. Bjorklund, L. Lachenmayer, A. Nobin, and U. Stenevi. 1971. Long-lasting selective depletion of brain serotonin by 5,6-dihydroxytrpytamine. *Acta physiol scand.* Supp. 373.

Frey, H.-N., M. P. Magnussen, and C. Kaergaard Nielsen. 1970. The effect of p-chloramphetamine on the consumption of ethanol by rats. *Arch. Int. Pharm. Therap.* 183: 165.

Geller, I. 1973. Effects of para-chlorophenylalanine and 5-hydroxytryptophan on alcohol intake in the rat. *Pharmacol. Biochem. Behav.* 1: 361.

Goldstein, D. B., 1973. Relationship of alcohol dose to the intensity of withdrawal signs in mice. *J. Pharmacol. Exp. Therap.* 180: 203–210.

Ho, A. K. S., and B. Kissin. 1975. Evidence of a central cholinergic role in alcohol preference. In M. Gross, Ed. *Alcohol Intoxication and Withdrawal: Experimental Studies.* Vol. II. Plenum Publishers, New York, p. 303.

Ho, A. K. S., C. S. Tsai, R. C. A. Chen, and M. C. Braude. 1975. Drug interaction between alcohol and narcotic agents in rats and mice. In *Proc. Pharmacol. Exptl. Ther. Soc.* Fall Meeting, Davis, Calif.

Ho, A. K. S., C. S. Tsai, R. C. A. Chen, H. Begleiter, and B. Kissin. 1974. Experimental studies on alcoholism I.: Increase in alcohol preference by 5,6-dihydroxytryptamine and brain acetylcholine. *Psychopharmacologia* (Berlin) 40: 101.

Ho, A. K. S., and C. S. Tsai. 1975. Lithium and ethanol preference. *J. Pharm. Pharmac.* 27: 58.

Myers, R. D., and C. L. Melchior. 1975. Alcohol drinking in the rat after destruction of serotonergic and catecholaminergic neurons in the brain. *Res. Comm. Chem. Path. and Pharmacol.* 10: 363.

Myers, R. D., and W. L. Veale. 1968. Alcohol preference in the rat: Reduction following depletion of brain serotonin. *Science* 160: 1469.

Nachman, M., D. Lester, and J. LeMagnen. 1970. Alcohol aversion in the rat: Behavior assessment of noxious drug effects. *Science* 168: 1244.

Reis, D. J. 1973. A possible role of central noradrenergic neurons in withdrawal states from alcohol. *Annals N. Y. Acad. Sciences.* 215: 249.

Schildkraut, J. J. 1973. The effects of lithium on biogenic amines. In S. Gershon and B. Shopsin, Eds. *Lithium: Its Role in Psychiatric Research and Treatment.* Plenum Press, New York, pp. 51–74.

Tissue Responses to Addictive Drugs
© 1976, Spectrum Publications, Inc.

Brain Excitability Subsequent to Alcohol Withdrawal in Rats

B. PORJESZ
H. BEGLEITER
S. HUROWITZ

It has been postulated that a state of latent neural excitability develops during the alcoholization process, which is released upon termination of intake of the pharmacological agent (Seevers and Deneau, 1963; Kalent, et al., 1971; Mendelson, 1971). As a result of inherent methodological problems few studies have attempted to investigate withdrawal states in humans (Begleiter and Platz, 1972), making comprehensive animal research imperative.

Brain hyperexcitability in human alcoholics during alcoholization and withdrawal was examined using recovery functions of somatosensory evoked potentials by Begleiter et al. (1974). We found a progressive increase in brain excitability for each successive day of alcohol intake (during partial withdrawal), that reached a peak after one complete day of total abstinence. This finding was replicated in animals in a more recent study (Begleiter and Coltrera, 1975). Rats, implanted with recording electrodes at visual cortex and reticular formation received

461

intubated alcohol (or water) daily for 12 days. Visual evoked potentials obtained 24 hours after the last intubated dose indicated significant hyperexcitability in previously alcoholized rats. It was demonstrated that electrophysiological changes due to alcohol withdrawal far outlast overt behavioral aberrations.

It has been suggested by some investigators that central nervous system (CNS) disturbances persist far beyond the administration and removal of ethanol. In a study of human alcoholism, Mendelson, et al., (1966) found that when alcoholic and control subjects were subjected to an identical four-day period of alcoholization, only the alcoholics displayed withdrawal signs. In a similar study with animals, Branchey, et al., (1971) demonstrated that rats did not return to their pre-alcoholized state two-three weeks postwithdrawal; previously alcoholized animals exhibited severe withdrawal symptomatology when re-exposed to alcohol, unlike the naive matched-controls. Walker and Zornetzer (1974) studied both EEG and behavioral correlates of withdrawal from ethanol in mice. Withdrawal symptomatology was accompanied by abnormal EEG activity including spikes that often culminated in epileptic seizure discharges. Mice reintroduced and withdrawn from alcohol after an alcohol free interval, displayed more severe EEG disturbances than they had during their initial withdrawal episode. In another EEG experiment dealing with long-term CNS effects of alcohol, Gitlow et al. (1973) demonstrated that previously alcoholized animals displayed severe REM disturbances when re-exposed to alcohol after a six-month drug free period.

This chapter concerns itself with the attempt to investigate both short and long-term electrophysiological effects of chronic alcohol intake in rats.

MATERIALS AND METHODS

Twenty male hooded Long-Evans rats, with a mean weight of 358g were used in this experiment. They were housed individually in stainless steel cages, with ad lib access to food and water during the entire study.

Stereotaxic surgery was performed under Diabutal anesthesia (0.8cc/kg) for the purpose of recording visual evoked potentials (VEP's). Two monopolar teflon-coated stainless steel depth electrodes were implanted in the reticular formation and thalamus. Specific co-ordinates of the reticular formation placement were: 4.2 mm posterior to bregma, 2.2 mm lateral to the midline (left), and 7.0 mm from the surface of the brain; coordinates for the postventral nucleus of the thalamus were: 3.0 mm posterior to bregma, 2.2 mm lateral to the mid-line (right), and 6.5 mm deep, according to the stereotaxic atlas of Pellegrino and Cushman (1967). Stainless steel screw electrodes were placed in the skull overlying the visual cortex, 5.5 mm posterior to bregma and 4.0 mm lateral to the midline (left), and two similar screw electrodes placed bilaterally over the frontal cortex served as reference and ground. All leads were attached to a miniature connector and the assembly was fastened to the skull with acrylic cement. (Only data obtained from the visual cortex are presented in this chapter. Results from the other electrodes will be reported in a subsequent paper.)

The animals were allowed one to two weeks to recover from surgery, at which time they were placed in a sound-attenuated enclosure (IAC) and base line visual evoked potentials (VEP's) were recorded. During the recording sessions, the skull pedestal was attached to a cable con-nected to a mercury pool swivel, allowing the animals freedom of movement.

Photic stimulation was delivered with an Iconix stroboscopic light, set at a peak intensity of 1,000 lm and duration of 5 msec, at a rate of 1/2.5 sec for a total of 50 flashes. VEP's were amplified by a Grass Model 78 - B Polygraph and fed into a PDP 11/40 computer for on-line signal averaging of a 500 msec epoch. Amplitude measures were ob-tained between 100 - 180 msec at N_2-P_2 for the visual cortex recordings.

Base line evoked potentials were obtained for each animal individ-ually, following a habituation procedure. Throughout the experiment, each rat was tested on a carefully timed, staggered schedule such that only one rat was tested for base line, withdrawal, or challenge dose recordings per day.

Beginning on the morning following baseline determinations, 14 rats were intubated daily for 14 days, with an increasing progression of 20% (v/v) solution of 95% alcohol doses, (3 - 8g/kg) as follows: 3g/kg for the first two days; 4g/kg for the next two days; 5g/kg for two days, 6g/kg for two days, 7g/kg for the following four days, and 8g/kg for the remaining two days. Six control rats received an equivalent amount of water in the same fashion. VEP recordings were obtained beginning four hours after the last intubated dose, and were sampled every half hour, up to eight hours after the last intubation.

Following two weeks of abstinence, half of the experimental animals (N=7) and half of the controls (N=3) received an alcohol challenge-dose (2 ml/kg 20% (v/v) of 95% ethyl alcohol) i.p., while the remaining animals received the same challenge dose after five weeks. (In this chapter we are only reporting the results obtained from the two-week challenge-dose group.) VEP's were recorded immediately preceding the alcohol injection (base line) and were sampled every twenty minutes following the alcohol challenge for the first two hours. Thereafter, VEP's were recorded each hour for seven hours postinjection.

DISCUSSION

Rats in both the experimental and control groups gained an average of 22g during the two-week intubation period, and weighed 380.26 and 380.83g, respectively at that time.

There were no significant differences in base line VEP's recorded before intubation between the experimental and control groups (see Figure 1). Beginning 6.5 hours after the last intubated dose until the end of the testing period, significant differences between the two groups were obtained as follows: $p< .05$ at 6.5 hours ($U=16$), $p< .02$ at 7 hours ($U=9$), $p< .002$ at 7.5 hours ($U=4$) and $p< .02$ at 8 hours ($U=15$). The maximum withdrawal effect was found at 7.5 hours postwithdrawal and was manifested by a marked increase in VEP amplitude.

Following two weeks of abstinence, base line VEP's recorded from the experimental and control groups did not differ significantly from each other. However, significant differences were obtained 40 minutes after each group received a challenge dose of alcohol ($U=1$, $p< .01$). The naive animals displayed a marked decrease in VEP amplitude at this time, while the experimental animals began to show increases which rose progressively over the course of the experimental session (see Figure 2). Significant differences in VEP amplitude were obtained between the two groups for the seven hours they were sampled (see Table 1).

CONCLUSIONS

The results indicate an increase in central nervous system (CNS) hyperexcitability during withdrawal in rats previously exposed to chronic alcohol intake. This neural hyperactivity is manifested by a marked increase in visual evoked potential (VEP) amplitude in those animals with a two-week exposure to alcohol. These findings are consistent with our previous results in animals (Begleiter and Coltrera, 1975), and with humans (Begleiter, et al., 1974).

The time course of maximum CNS hyperexcitability obtained in the present study, namely 6.5 to 8 hours after the last alcohol intake, coincides with that reported by Hunter, et al. (1973) for rats, and Walker and Zornetzer (1974) for mice. In both studies, they monitored EEG in rodents that had received alcohol using a liquid diet technique,

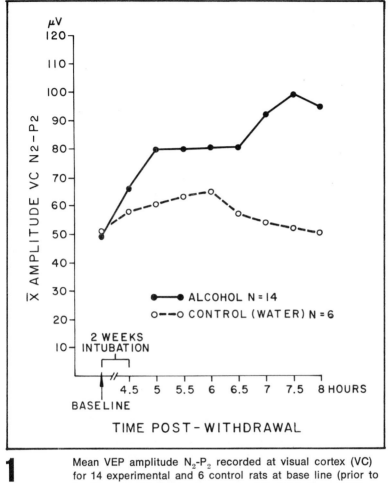

1 Mean VEP amplitude N_2-P_2 recorded at visual cortex (VC) for 14 experimental and 6 control rats at base line (prior to treatment) and following two weeks daily intubation of either alcohol or water, respectively. Base line recordings are identical for the two groups, while VEP's sampled at half hour intervals from 4.5 - 8 hours postwithdrawal, indicate increasing differences between the two groups that are maximal 6.5 - 8 hours postwithdrawal, due to the progressively increasing amplitude in the experimental group.

and found that EEG withdrawal signs were most severe from six to ten hours postwithdrawal. In addition, their electrophysiological correlates of withdrawal followed a similar time course of development as we obtained in the present experiment.

The present investigation is not only concerned with the immediate

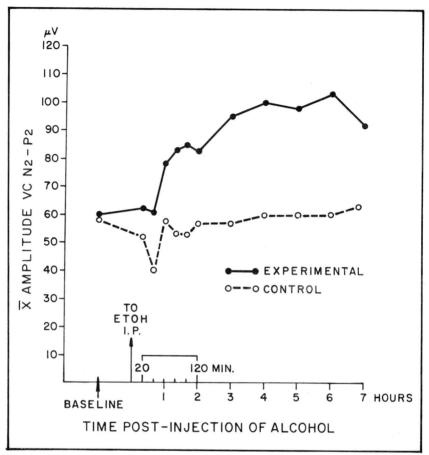

2 Mean VEP amplitude N_2-P_2 recorded at visual cortex in rats receiving a challenge dose of alcohol (2 g/kg i.p.) following two weeks of abstinence from either intubated alcohol (experimental) or water (control). Base line determinations obtained on the same day prior to the challenge injection indicate no difference between the two groups. Naive animals (controls) with no previous exposure to alcohol respond with a sharp decrease in VEP amplitude, reaching asymptote 40 minutes postinjection, while previously alcoholized animals (experimental) display marked increases in amplitude peaking three-seven hours postinjection.

effects of chronic alcohol intake, but is also interested in possible long-term CNS abnormalities. While VEP recordings obtained following two weeks of abstinence from alcohol do not indicate any apparent differences between previously alcoholized animals and control rats, more subtle differences were found to exist between the two groups.

Table I.

Time after injection	U-value	P	Significance
base line	18	—	NS
20 minutes	4	0.072	NS
40 minutes	1	0.012	*
60 minutes (1 hour)	3	0.042	*
80 minutes	4	0.072	NS
100 minutes	3	0.042	*
120 minutes (2 hours)	4	0.072	NS
3 hours	0	0.006	*
4 hours	1	0.012	*
5 hours	1	0.012	*
6 hours	2	0.024	*
7 hours	0	0.006	*

*Significant at less than 0.05

Mann-Whitney U-tests performed on amplitude N_2-P_2 recorded at visual cortex between previously alcoholized and alcohol-naive rats, following a challenge dose of alcohol injected two weeks after treatment. No significant difference exists between the two groups at this time, prior to the challenge injection (base line). Significant differences between the two groups immediately after the alcohol injection (time 40 minutes) are due to a decrease in VEP amplitude in the control group, while later significant differences between the two groups (three-seven hours post-injection) are attributed to the increase in VEP amplitude in the experimental group.

The neurophysiological responses of the postaddict rats to a challenge-dose of alcohol are readily distinguishable from those of naive animals. Naive rats responded to a challenge-dose of alcohol with a typical immediate depression in VEP amplitude, while postaddict rats not only did not manifest this VEP decrease, but displayed instead a progressive increase in VEP amplitude, reaching levels of neural hyperexcitability as high as they had during the initial withdrawal period. This finding suggests that a state of CNS latent hyperexcitability underlies the alcohol addiction syndrome, and becomes reactivated when the organism renews contact with the addictive pharmacological agent. A somewhat related finding has been reported by Walker and Zornetzer (1974), but with a very different approach, using two successive alcoholization and withdrawal periods, with one week of abstinence between them. They demonstrated that EEG aberrations accompanying withdrawal are more severe following a second, although shorter alcoholization period than they are following an initial, longer alcoholization period. In a previous experiment in our laboratory (Branchey, et al., 1971) we reported similar findings. The establishment of a state of physical dependence increased the incidence of withdrawal symptoms in a subsequent period of alcoholization. While no apparent withdrawal symptomatology was observed in naive animals, previously alcohol-dependent rats were prone to exhibit a severe withdrawal syndrome.

These findings, combined with those of the present investigation suggest the possibility that complex modifications in CNS responsivity occur in the addiction process. These changes can perhaps be considered as a form of long-term memory, an "addiction-memory," which lies dormant until it becomes reactivated by re-exposure to the addictive substance. In the present study, the mild dose of alcohol injected would normally not be sufficient to induce signs of hyperexcitability and, indeed, it did not in the naive animals. The full-blown excitability cycle that was elicited in the postaddict rats with this minimal dose of alcohol, suggests that a neurophysiological, adaptive change was already present in the postaddict rats, predisposing them to withdrawal symptoms. Evidence of a long-term biochemical change accompanying morphine addiction was reported by Sloan and Eisenman (1968). They demonstrated that postaddict rats secreted significantly less urinary norepinephrine than controls for a period of five months after morphine withdrawal, at which time adrenal norepinephrine levels were found to be elevated with considerable hypertrophy of the adrenal glands.

We are currently investigating the persistence of this neurophysiological dysfunction, its permanence, or possible irreversibility, by examining rats that are re-exposed to alcohol following various intervals of abstinence. In addition, the relationship between the length of exposure to alcohol, and the severity and persistence of neurophysiological aberrations are being presently examined by studying CNS hyperexcitability in rats subjected to chronic alcohol administration for different lengths of time. The mechanisms involved, and the manner in which this reactivation of CNS hyperexcitability is accomplished, remains to be investigated.

SUMMARY

In conclusion, our present data indicate that the effects of ethanol on an organism far outlast the administration and removal of the pharmacological agent; organisms appear to undergo adaptive modifications that directly affect CNS responsivity, and may be considered as a form of memory ("addiction-memory"). The nature, time course of development, and duration of this altered neurophysiological responsivity ("addiction-memory") remain to be examined during the induction, withdrawal, and postwithdrawal phases of alcohol addiction.

ACKNOWLEDGMENT

We would like to thank Mr. Adolfo Fecci for his helpful assistance throughout the experiment.

REFERENCES

Begleiter, H. and Coltrera, M. 1975. Evoked potential changes during ethanol withdrawal in rats. *The Amer. J. of Drug and Alcohol Abuse.* 1975.

Begleiter, H., and A. Platz. 1972. The effects of alcohol on the central nervous system in humans. In B. Kissin and H. Begleiter, Eds. *The Biology of Alcoholism.* Vol. 2, Plenum Press, New York, pp. 293–343.

Begleiter, H., B. Porjesz, and C. Yerre-Grubstein. 1974. Excitability cycle of somatosensory evoked potentials during experimental alcoholization and withdrawal. *Psychopharmacologia* (Berlin), 37: 15–21.

Branchey, M., G. Rauscher, and B. Kissin. 1971. Modifications in the response to alcohol following the establishment of physical dependence. *Psychopharmacologia* (Berlin) 22: 314–322.

Gitlow, S. E., S. H. Bentkover, S. W. Dziedzic, and N. Khazan. 1973. Persistence of abnormal REM sleep response to ethanol as a result of previous ethanol ingestion. *Psychopharmacologia* (Berlin) 33: 135–140.

Hunter, B. E., C. A. Boast, D. W. Walker, and S. F. Zornetzer. 1973. Alcohol withdrawal syndrome in rats: Neural and behavioral correlates. *Pharmacol. Biochem. and Behavior.* 1: 719–725.

Kalant, H., A. E. LeBlanc, and R. J. Gibbons. 1971. Tolerance to, and dependence on ethanol. In: Y. Israel and J. Mardones, Eds. *Biological Basis of Alcoholism.* John Wiley & Sons, New York, pp. 235–269.

Mendelson, J. H. 1971. Biochemical mechanisms of alcohol addiction. In B. Kissin and H. Begleiter, Eds. *The Biology of Alcoholism*, Vol. 1, Plenum Press, New York, pp. 513–544.

Mendelson, J. H., S. Stein, and M. T. McGuire. 1966. Comparative psychophysiological studies in alcoholic and non-alcoholic subjects undergoing experimentally induced ethanol intoxication. *Psychosom. Med.* 28: 1–12.

Pellegrino, L. J., and A. J. Cushman. 1967. *A Stereotaxic Atlas of the Rat Brain.* Appleton-Century Crofts, New York.

Seevers, M. H., and G. A. Deneau. 1963. Physiological aspects of tolerance and physical dependence. In W. S. Root and F. G. Hoffman, Eds. *Physiological Pharmacology.* Academic Press, New York.

Sloan, J. W., and A. J. Eisenman. 1968. Long persisting changes in catecholamine and metabolism following addiction and withdrawal from morphine. *The Addictive States, Ass. Res. Nerv. Dis. Proc.* 46: 96–105.

Walker, D. W., and S. F. Zornetzer. 1974. Alcohol withdrawal in mice: Electroencephalographic and behavioral correlates. *EEG. Clin. Neurophysiol.* 36: 233–243.

Tissue Responses to Addictive Drugs
© 1976, Spectrum Publications, Inc.

The Effect of Morphine on the Metabolic Transport of ^{3}H-lysine and Incorporation into Protein

M. A. LEVI
R. K. RHINES
D. H. FORD

*Downstate Medical Center
Brooklyn, New York*

Although public interest in the effects of opiates has only recently become significant with the increasing awareness of the social problems caused by the phenomena of tolerance and dependence, active scientific investigation in this field has been going on for nearly a century. Several hypotheses have been presented to explain the mechanism of cellular adaptation to morphine administration (Cochin, 1970; Cohen et al., 1965; Collier, 1968; Goldstein and Goldstein, 1961, 1968; Jaffe and Sharpless, 1968; Kerr and Pozuelo, 1971; Martin, 1968; Seevers and Deneau, 1968; Shuster, 1961). The interaction between morphine and protein synthesis in the CNS was the proposed site of action of four of these theories. Shuster (1961) and Goldstein and Goldstein (1961) have hypothesized similar mechanisms of morphine tolerance and physical dependence based on the phenomena of enzyme induction. Collier (1968)

471

has proposed that chronic morphine administration leads to an induction of protein drug receptors, while Cohen and et al. (1965) have proposed that morphine induces the production of a peptide which antagonizes morphine action. In support of these theories several investigators have shown that agents, which interfere with protein synthesis by inhibiting either transcription or translation, interfere with the development of tolerance to morphine (Cohen et al., 1965; Cox and Osman, 1970; Smith et al., 1967). However, the amount of these agents which must be given to block protein synthesis also causes unrelated side effects, which may actually be interfering with the development of tolerance.

Several investigators have examined the effect of morphine on the incorporation of labeled amino acids in protein with conflicting results. Using ^{14}C-leucine Clouet and Ratner (1968) observed that morphine had an effect on the accumulation of leucine in the free amino acid pool (FAA). Taking this effect into account, they found a significant decrease of incorporation of leucine into all brain fractions at three and four hours after morphine treatment. In addition, the specific activity of the microsomal protein was significantly decreased at 24 hours after morphine. However, when ^{14}C-lysine was used, 24 hours after morphine the incorporation of lysine into the brain proteins was increased over control levels (Clouet, 1970). In addition, both Hahn and Goldstein (1971) and Franklin and Cox (1972) have reported that morphine had no effect on the incorporation of labeled amino acids into electrophoretically separated brain proteins.

In the above and other studies, the effect of morphine has been related to protein synthesis of whole brain or various particulate cell fractions. Further, the labeled amino acids have been generally administered intraventricularly to bypass any effect of a blood-brain barrier. As suggested by several investigators (Clouet, 1972; Knapp and Mandell, 1973; Way, 1973), one possible explanation for the conflicting results in morphine related research has been the general lack of a regional approach to the study of morphine's biochemical effects. This study was undertaken in the expectation that a regional approach may demonstrate the as yet elusive theoretical increase in protein synthesis associated with the induction of morphine tolerance, and further pinpoint a specific region of the CNS for a concentrated search for the specific protein involved. Furthermore, studying the distribution of a labeled amino acid between the plasma FAA and the tissue FAA after intravenous administration of the label should produce information concerning the reported effect of morphine on amino acid transport into the CNS (Clouet and Neidle, 1970).

Table I. Duration of Analgesic Response after Acute Injection of Morphine Sulfate

Dose mg/kg	N*	% demonstrating analgesia at:			
		30 min.	60 min.	90 min.	120 min.
15	4	100	100	75	25
20	4	100	50	25	0
25	4	100	100	75	0
30	4	100	100	75	25
35	4	100	100	100[†]	67
40	5	100	100	100	100

[†]One animal died; values at 90 and 120 min. based on three animals.
*N = number of animals.

MATERIALS AND METHODS

Male Wistar rats (obtained from Carworth Farms) were kept in the departmental animal quarters until they had reached an appropriate weight. All animals weighed between 270 and 300 gms before intra-jugular cannulation. Rats were cannulated with a polyethylene cannula (PE 10), inserted into the left jugular vein under light ether anesthesia (Bleeker et al., 1969). After surgery the animals were placed in individual cages and given 24 hours to recover. They were supplied with food and water ad libidum.

The cannula was used for all injections. Morphine sulfate was dissolved in physiological saline and given at a dose of 40 mg/kg. Within seconds of administration of this dose the animals assumed a rigid posture in flexion of all limbs and showed the Straub tail response. In addition, (see Table I) using the hot plate procedure of Eddy and Leimbach (1953) this dose induced analgesia in 100% of the animals for 2 hours and induced a significant degree of tolerance 24 hours after a single injection (see Table II).

Tritiated l-lysine (4,5-^{3}H) monohydrochloride was obtained from Schwartz/Mann with a specific activity of 41.6 C/mm. The labeled lysine was injected without dilution using a dose of 0.1 mc/100 gms (2.92 μg of lysine/kg) and washed in with 0.1 ml of physiological saline.

All experimental animals received an i.v. injection of morphine either 2 or 24 hours before sacrifice, while control animals received a comparable volume of physiological saline. Animals were sacrificed

Table II. Duration of Analgesic Response to 40 mg/kg Morphine

Injection	N	Duration (mins)	S.E.	Sig.
Initial Injection	11	161	9.5	
				$p < 0.001$
2nd Injection 24 hours later	8	34	7.4	

15, 30, 45, and 60 minutes after an i.v. injection of labeled lysine. Just prior to death the animals were anesthetized with a 0.05 ml. injection of 50% phenobarbital. Their chests were then immediately opened, intracardiac blood samples were taken with heparinized syringes, and they were killed by exsanguination. The brain and a sample of pectoral muscle were quickly removed and placed in dry ice. The cerebral gray, hippocampus, and cerebellum were selected for study because they have been shown to have significantly different levels of narcotic receptors (Kuhar et al., 1973; Lowney et al., 1974). In addition, the hippocampus is one of the cortical structures of the limbic system which has been proposed as the level at which morphine induces both analgesia and tolerance (Erwin, 1968; Kukar et al., 1973; Levi, 1975; Mayer and Liebeskind, 1974).

The tissue samples were subjected to extraction procedures as previously described (Ford et al., 1974a; Henderson and Snell, 1948) (see Figure 1). The samples were analyzed so that at the end of the procedures the data concerning the metabolism of ^{3}H-lysine could be expressed as specific activity (S.A.) for the ^{3}H-lysine both accumulated in the FAA and incorporated into protein.

The results were tested for significance with a two-way analysis of variance. If a significant F ratio was found a Tukey Test was used to test for significance between paired means. Significance was taken at $p < 0.05$.

DISCUSSION

Total lysine content of precipitated proteins

Although it is possible to perceive different trends in the level of lysine in the proteins of the different tissues, an analysis of variance revealed no significant effect of morphine treatment (see Table III).

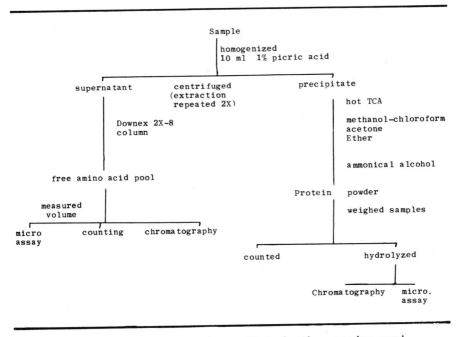

1 Flow sheet diagrm aillustrating the procedure used to obtain the free amino acid and protein fractions from the brain and muscle.

Specific Activity of ^{3}H-lysine in Precipitated Protein

Morphine had a similar pattern of effect in all four tissues studied (see Figures 2, 3, 4, 5). Two hours after morphine treatment the S.A. of ^{3}H-lysine tended to be significantly depressed and then 24 hours after morphine the S.A. returned to but did not exceed control values.

In the cerebral gray, when paired means were compared, the S.A. of ^{3}H-lysine in protein from animals killed 2 hours after morphine was significantly reduced at 15 ($p<0.05$) and 45 ($p<0.01$) minutes after the lysine injection. The S.A. of incorporated labeled lysine 24 hours after morphine was not signifcantly different than control values at any point, but was significantly higher ($p<0.05$) than 2 hours after morphine-treatment only in animals sacrificed 45 minutes after lysine injection.

In the cerebellum the SA of labeled lysine incorporated 2 hours after morphine treatment was significantly ($p< .01$) depressed 45 and 60 minutes after lysine. The S.A. then returned to control levels 24

Table III. The Total Amount of Lysine within the Protein Isolated from Areas of the CNS and Striated Muscle from Morphine-Treated and Control Rats

Treatment	Control	2 hours	24 hours
Tissue			
Cerebral Gray	0.67 ± .04	0.62 ± .05	0.64 ± .03
Cerebellum	0.81 ± .06	0.72 ± .04	0.73 ± .03
Hippocampus	0.68 ± .05	0.71 ± .05	0.65 ± .04
Muscle	0.85 ± .03	0.79 ± .05	0.90 ± .04

[1] Data is expressed as the mean ± the standard error in μmoles/mgm protein.

An analysis of variance revealed no significant differences due to morphine treatment, although there are significant regional differences.

hours after morphine and was significantly ($p < 0.01$) higher than the incorporation observed 2 hours after morphine at all time periods except the earliest.

In the hippocampus the S.A. of ^{3}H-lysine 24 hours after morphine was virtually identical to control values and they both were significantly higher ($p < 0.01$) than the corresponding values 2 hours after morphine except for 15 minutes after lysine.

In muscle tissue an analysis of variance revealed not only a significant effect of morphine on the absolute levels of ^{3}H-lysine incorporated ($p < 0.005$), but it also demonstrated a significant effect on the pattern of the level incorporated in relation to time ($p < 0.005$). The S.A. in the control animals demonstrated a biphasic increase into muscle protein over time, while both treatment groups demonstrated a relatively constant increase over time. The groups sacrificed 2 hours after morphine treatment tended to be below control levels ($p < 0.01$ at 30 and 45 minutes after lysine), while the S.A. in the 24-hour group returned to control levels except 45 minutes after lysine, when there was a significant increase ($p < 0.01$).

Lysine and the Free Amino Acid Pool

The actual S.A. of ^{3}H-lysine incorporated into protein is not only dependent on the level of protein synthesis, but is also dependent on the amount of amino acid which is available in the tissue FAA pool

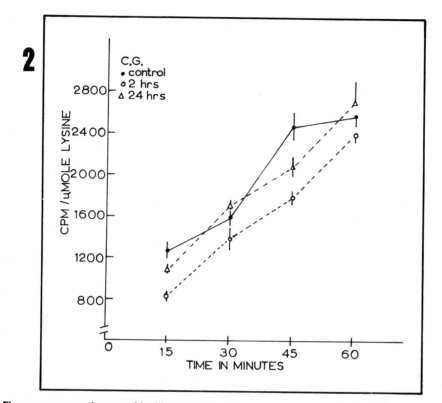

Figures representing graphic illustrations of the changes occurring in the specific activity of lysine (cpm/μmole) in the protein from the cerebral gray matter (C.G.), cerebellium (cereb.), hippocampus (hippo.) and muscle (mus.) at various time intervals after intravenous injection of ^{3}H-l-lysine into rats injected with saline (•) or morphine and killed 2 hours after drug administration (O) or 24 hours after drug administration (△).

for incorporation. Therefore, in order to accurately describe the effect of morphine on protein synthesis, it is necessary to measure the levels of lysine in the free pool (see Table IV). The values of the different treatment groups for any one tissue were fairly similar, and an analysis of variance revealed no significant differences.

Two hours after morphine injection, the S.A. of lysine in the three different neural FAA pools was significantly higher at all time periods studied than in comparable control pools (see Figures 6, 7, 8) and twenty-four hours after treatment the S.A. had generally returned to control levels. The only exceptions were in the cerebral gray of animals sacri-

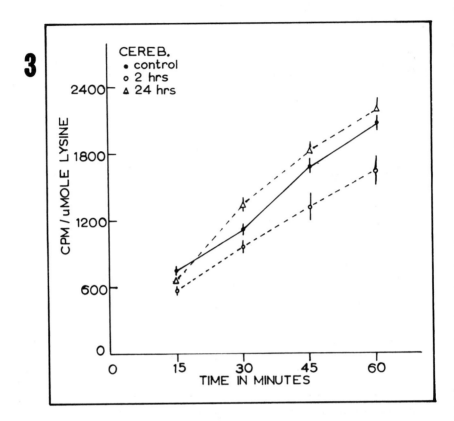

ficed 15 minutes after lysine injection, in which the S.A. was virtually equivalent to the 2-hour morphine group, and significantly higher than controls; and in the cerebellum of animals sacrificed 30 minutes after lysine injection, in which the S.A. was significantly lower than the 2-hour morphine group, but also significantly higher than in the controls. Changes in muscle, wherein the elevation in FAA was present 24 hours after morphine for the first half hour, and then returned to normal did not thus completely duplicate what was seen in the brain (see Figure 9).

The accumulation of amino acids into a tissue FAA pool is not solely dependent on the net rate of the transport processes, but is also dependent on the amount of amino acid present in the plasma for accumulation. Therefore, the increased levels of ^{3}H-lysine described above may not represent an effect of morphine on CNS amino acid transport, but rather an effect on the availability of amino acids in the plasma. Morphine did significantly increase the size of the plasma free lysine pool both 2 and 24 hours after treatment (see Table V). However, an equiva-

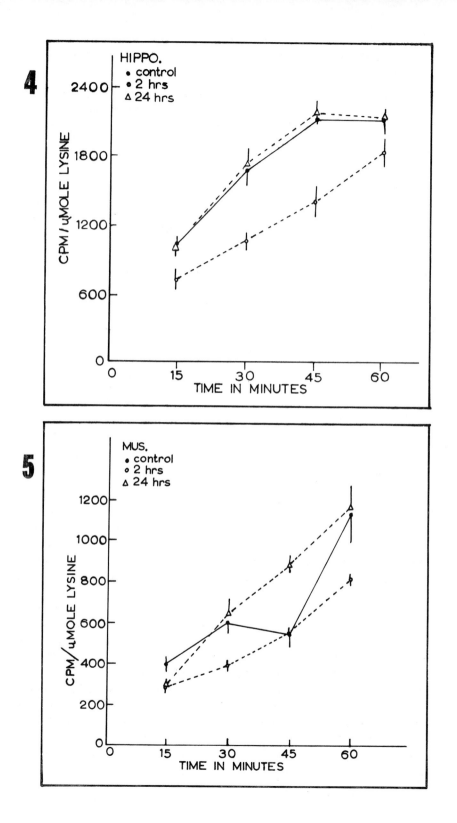

**Table IV. Total Amount of Lysine in the Free Amino Acid Pool
Extracted from Three Areas of the CNS and Striated Muscle from
Morphine-Treated and Control Rats**

Treatment	Control	2 hours	24 hours
Tissue			
Cerebral Gray	0.34 ± 0.03 (9)	0.34 ± 0.02 (9)	0.33 ± 0.04 (9)
Cerebellum	0.57 ± 0.03 (8)	0.60 ± 0.06 (8)	0.55 ± 0.06 (8)
Hippocampus	0.51 ± 0.04 (8)	0.51 ± 0.06 (9)	0.50 ± 0.06 (9)
Muscle	0.76 ± 0.06 (10)	0.80 ± 0.04 (10)	0.92 ± 0.08 (9)

[1]Data is expressed as the mean ± the standard error in μ mole of lysine/gm. of tissue.
(The number of animals is indicated in parenthesis.)

lent increase in the level of ^{3}H-lysine (cpm/ml) was also found (see Figure 10) so that when the data was expressed as S.A. (cpm/μmole), morphine was found to have no effect on the S.A. of tritiated lysine in the plasma FAA (see Figure 10), and therefore, no effect on the availability of lysine for transport into the CNS.

CONCLUSIONS

Morphine significantly inhibited the level of ^{3}H-lysine in the protein from the three brain regions and striated muscle, two hours after treatment. This depressive effect did not appear to be due to a decrease in the availability of labeled lysine for incorporation. The depressed uptake has also been shown to take place in the neuronal cell body as opposed to the surrounding neuropil (Ford et al., 1974b). This data expands the report by Clouet and Ratner (1967). The finding that the inhibitory effect appeared to be of approximately equal magnitude in the cerebellum and striated muscle, as well as in the cerebral gray and hippocampus is highly significant in view of the work on the regional distribution of morphine receptors (Kukar et al., 1973; Pert and Snyder, 1973). According to their data the cerebellum and striated muscle have virtually no receptors, yet both tissues demonstrated a similar response as did tissues where the effect may have been due to a drug:receptor interaction. Therefore, it appears that the inhibitory

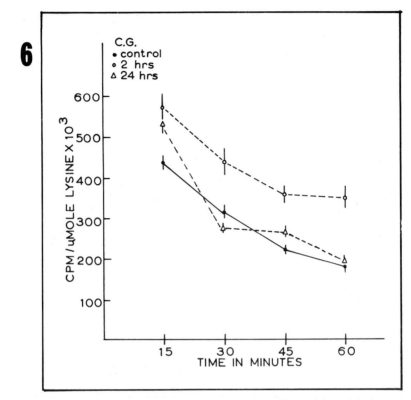

6

Figures representing graphic illustrations of the specific activity of lysine (cpm/μmole) in the free amino acid pool from the cerebral gray matter (CG.), cerebellum (cereb.), hippocampus (hippo.) and muscle (mus.) at varying time intervals after intravenous injection of ^{3}H-l-lysine into rats injected with saline (•), or morphine and killed 2 hours after drug administration (O) or 24 hours after drug administration ($\triangle$).

effect of morphine on the incorporation of ^{3}H-lysine into protein may be due to some type of nonspecific response, rather than to a specific drug:receptor effect.

Clouet and Ratner (1967) reported that this depressant effect of morphine was still present in the brains of rats made tolerant to the analgesic effect of morphine by five daily injections. The animals were sacrificed 1.5 hours after the last injection. However, in that type of study it is impossible to differentiate the acute effect of the last injection from the chronic effect of the total treatment schedule. This is a critical

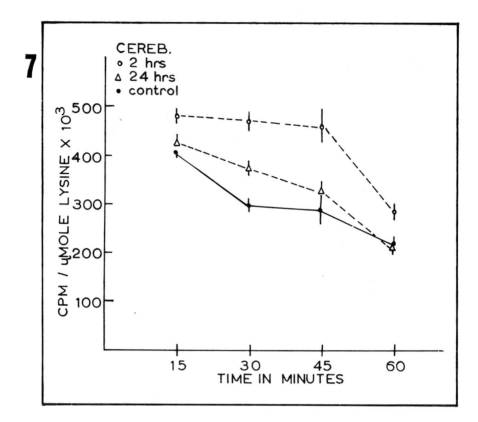

7

CEREB.
o 2 hrs
△ 24 hrs
• control

point when attempting to correlate the effect of morphine on protein synthesis with the development of tolerance, since tolerance is not being induced by the most recent injection, but rather by the entire previous treatment. In the present study an attempt was made to circumvent this problem by studying the animals 24 hours after a single injection at which time a second morphine injection (see Table II) in an additional group of rats, had demonstrated that a significant degree of tolerance had developed.

Morphine was found to significantly increase the size of the total pool of free lysine in plasma (see Table V), an effect which has not previously been described. Since lysine has been shown to be a potent competitive inhibitor of arginase in the Krebs' urea cycle (Hunter and Downs, 1945), this may have significance in terms of possible patho-

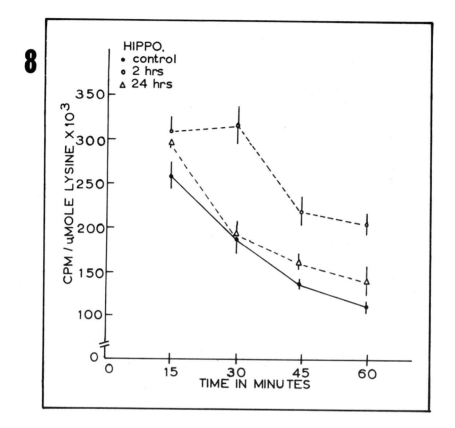

logical actions of morphine, if a similar effect is found in man.

In addition, morphine was found to significantly increase the level of free ^{3}H-lysine in all three brain regions (see Figures 6, 7, 8) investigated, after physiological transport of the labeled amino acid from blood into the brain. The increased levels were present 2 hours after morphine treatment, and tended to return to control levels 24 hours after treatment. This confirms the findings of Clouet and co-workers (Clouet and Ratner, 1967; Clouet and Neidle, 1970) who found increased levels of ^{14}C-leucine and lysine after intracisternal injection. In addition, our findings demonstrated that the increased tissue levels of labeled lysine were not due to an increase in availability of the molecule for transport, since morphine had no effect on the specific activity of ^{3}H-lysine in plasma. Therefore, since it has been previously shown that

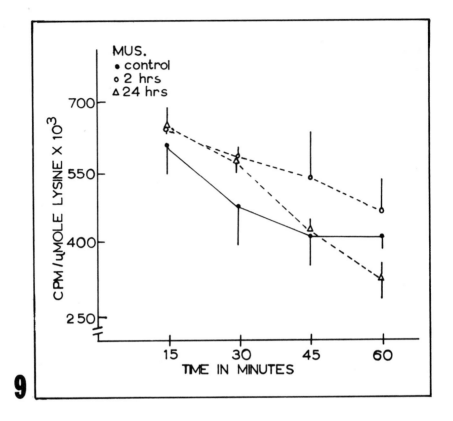

the amount of lysine transported into the brain is not affected by an increased plasma level of lysine, the increase in ^{3}H-lysine in the brain FAA after morphine probably represents decreased utilization.

SUMMARY

Two hours after morphine treatment the incorporation of ^{3}H-lysine into protein isolated from cerebral gray, hippocampus, cerebellum, and striated muscle was equally inhibited. In view of receptor isolation data, this paninhibitory effect was interpreted as representing a non-specific effect rather than a specific drug:receptor interaction effect.

Two hours after morphine treatment the amount of ^{3}H-lysine available for incorporation into protein was actually increased in the cerebral

Table V. The Effect of Morphine on the Level of Lysine in the Plasma Free Amino Acid Pool

Control	2 hours	24 hours
0.35 ± 0.03*	0.62 ± 0.03	0.57 ± 0.07

[1]Values represent the mean ± standard error in μ mole/ml derived from ten animals for each group.
*Significantly different from the other two groups at the 0.01 level.

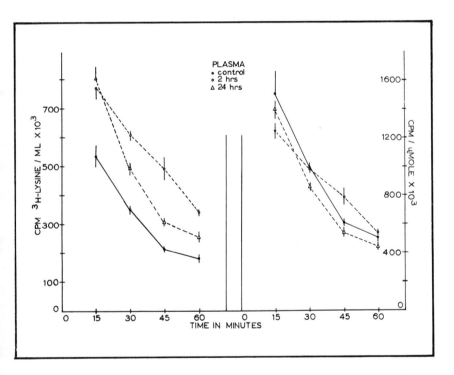

10   Graphic illustration of the levels of ^{3}H-lysine found in the plasma (cpm/ml) and the specific activity of plasma lysine (cpm/μmole) at various time intervals after intravenous injection of [3]H-*l*-lysine into control saline injected (•) rats and animals injected with morphine and killed 2 hours after drug administration (O) or 24 hours after drug administration (△).

gray, cerebellum, and hippocampus. Therefore, the morphine induced inhibition of lysine incorporation was due to an actual effect on protein synthesis, and not on the availability of the amino acid for incorporation.

Twenty-four hours after a single dose of 40 mg/kg of morphine, when the animals demonstrated a significant degree of tolerance to a second injection, the incorporation of lysine into protein had returned to, but not exceeded control levels in all three brain areas studied. This was interpreted as evidence against the hypothesis that a drug induced increase in protein synthesis was involved in the development of tolerance.

Morphine increased the level of free lysine in plasma, both 2 and 24 hours after treatment. This may have significant implications in view of the known pathological effects associated with congenital hyperlysinemia.

Morphine increased the accumulation of ^{3}H-lysine in the free amino acid pool of the cerebral gray, cerebellum, and hippocampus. Since morphine demonstrated no significant effect on the specific activity of ^{3}H-lysine in the plasma, this effect was not due to an increase in the availability but may reflect decreased utilization and (or) incorporation.

ACKNOWLEDGMENTS

This work was supported in part by a reseach grant from the NIDA, USPHS, DA 00114–04 and in part by a USPHS Training grant to the Department of Anatomy (SUNY), 5 TO1 GM 00379–15.

REFERENCES

Bleecker, M., D. H. Ford, and R. K. Rhines. 1969. A comparison of ^{131}I-triiodothyronine accumulation and degradation in ethanol--treated and control rat. *Life Sciences* (I) 8: 267–275.

Clouet, D. H. 1968. The effect of morphine administration on the incorporation of ^{14}C-leucine into protein in cell free systems from rat brain and liver. *J. Neurochem.* 15: 17–23.

Clouet, D. H. 1970. The effect of drugs on protein synthesis in the nervous system. In A. Lajtha, Ed. *Protein Metabolism of the Nervous System.* Plenum Press, New York, London, pp. 699–713.

Clouet, D. H. 1971. Protein and nuclei acid metabolism. In D. H. Clouet, Ed. *Narcotic Drugs, Biochemical Pharmacology.* Plenum Press, New York, London, pp. 216–228.

Clouet, D. H. 1973. Effects of narcotic analgesics on brain function. In G. E. Gaull, Ed. *Biology of Brain Disfunction.* Plenum Press, New York, pp. 115–149.

Clouet, D. H., and A. Neidle. 1970. The effect of morphine on the transport and metabolism of intracisternally injected leucine in the rat. *J. Neurochem.* 17: 1069–1074.

Clouet, D. H., and M. Ratner. 1967. The effect of the administration of morphine on the incorporation of ^{14}C-leucine into the proteins of rat brain in vivo. *Brain Res.* 4: 33–43.

Clouet, D. H., and N. Williams. 1974. The effect of narcotic analgesic drugs on the uptake and release of neurotransmitters in isolated synaptosomes. *J. Pharm. and Exp. Therap.* 188: 419–428.

Cochin, J. 1970. Possible mechanisms in the development of tolerance. *Fed. Proc.* 29: 19–27.

Cohen, M., A. S. Keats, W. Krivoy, and G. Ungar. 1963. Effect of actinomycin D on morphine tolerance. *Proc. Soc. Exp. Biol. Med.* 119: 381–384.

Collier, H. O. J. 1968. A general theory of the genesis of drug dependence by induction of receptors. *Nature* (London) 220: 228–231.

Eddy, N. B., and D. Leimbach. 1953. Synthetic analgesics II: Dithienybutenyl and dithienylbutylamines. *J. Phar. and Exp. Ther.* 107: 385–395.

Ervin, F. R. 1968. Effects of opioids on electrical activity of deep structures in the human brain. In A. Wikler, Ed. *The Addictive States.* Williams and Wilkins Company, Baltimore, pp. 150–156.

Ford, D. H., R. K. Rhines, and K. Voeller. 1974a. Morphine effects on neurons of the median eminence and on other neurons. In E. Zimmerman and R. George. *Narcotics and the Hypothalamus.* Raven Press, New York, pp. 51–66.

Ford, D. H., D. Weisfuse, M. Levi, and R. K. Rhines. 1974b. Accumulation of ^{3}H-lysine by brain and plasma in male and female rats treated acutely with morphine sulfate. *ACTA Neurol. Scandinav.* 50: 53–75.

Franklin, G. I., and B. M. Cox. 1972. Incorporation of amino acids into proteins of synaptosomal membranes during morphine treatment. *J. Neurochem.* 19: 1821–1823.

Goldstein, A., and D. B. Goldstein. 1968. Theory of drug tolerance and physical dependence. In A. Wikler, ed. *The Addictive States.* Williams and Wilkins Company, Baltimore, pp. 265–267.

Goldstein, A. 1961. Possible role of enzyme inhibition and repression in drug tolerance and addiction. *Biochem. Pharmac.* 8: 48.

Hahn, D. L., and A. Goldstein. 1971. Amounts and turnover of brain protein in morphine tolerant mice. *J. Neurochem.* 18: 1887–1893.

Henderson, L. M., and E. E. Snell. 1948. A uniform medium for the determination of amino acids with various microorganisms. *J. Biol. Chem.* 17: 15–29.

Hunter, A., and C. E. Downs. 1945. The inhibition of arginase by amino acids. *J. Biol. Chem.* 157: 427–446.

Jaffe, J. H., and K. S. Sharpless. 1968. Pharmacological denervation hypersensitivity in the nervous system: A theory of physical dependence. In A. Wikler, Ed. *The Addictive States.* Williams and Wilkins Company, Baltimore, pp. 226–246.

Kerr, F. L. W., and J. Pozuzlo. 1971. Suppression of physical dependence and induction of hypersensitivity to morphine by stereotaxic lesions in addicted rats. *Mayo Clinic Proc.* 46: 653–665.

Knapp, S., and A. J. Mandell. 1972. Narcotic drugs: Effects on the serotonin biosynthetic systems of the brain. *Science* 177: 1209–1211.

Kuhar, M. J., C. B. Pert, and S. M. Snyder. 1973. Regional distribution of opiate receptor binding in monkey and human brain. *Nature* (London) 245: 447–450.

Loh, H. H., and R. J. Mitzemann. 1974. Effect of morphine on the turnover and synthesis of ^{3}H-leu-protein and ^{14}C-phosphatidylcholine in discrete regions of the rat brain. *Biochem. Pharmac.* 23: 1753–1765.

Lowney, L. I., K. Schul, P. J. Lowery, and A. Goldstein. 1974. Partial purification of an opiate receptor from mouse brain. *Science* 183: 749–752.

Martin, R. W. 1968. A homeostatic theory of tolerance to and dependence on narcotic analgesics. In A. Wikler, Ed. *The Addictive States.* Williams and Wilkins, Baltimore, pp. 206–225.

Mayer, D. J., and J. C. Liebaskind. 1974. Pain reduction by focal electrical stimulation of the brain: An anatomical and behavioral analysis. *Brain Res.* 68: 73–93.

Pert, C. B., and S. M. Snyder. 1973. Properties of opiate receptor binding in rat brain. *Proc. Nat. Acad. Sci. USA.* 70: 2243–2247.

Seevers, M. M., and G. A. Denau. 1968. A critique of the dual action hypothesis of morphine physical dependence. In A. Wikler, Ed. *The Addictive States.* Williams and Wilkins Company, Baltimore, pp. 199–205.

Shuster, L. 1961. Repression and de-repression of enzyme synthesis as a possible explanation of some aspects of drug addiction. *Nature* (London 189: 315.

Smith, A., J. Gavitt, and M. Karmin. 1967. Blocking effect of puromycin, ethanol and chloroform on the development of tolerance to an opiate. *J. Pharmac. and Exp Therap.* 156: 85–91.

Takemori, A. E. 1971. Intermediary and energy metabolism. In D. H. Clouet, Ed. *Narcotic Drugs, Biochemical Pharmacology.* Plenum Press, New York, pp. 159–189.

Terenius, L., and A. Wahlstrom. 1974. Inhibition of narcotic receptor binding in brain extracts and cerebrospinal fluid. *Acta Pharm. et Toxicol.* 35: Suppl. 1, 55.

Way, E. L. 1973. Reassessment of brain 5-hydroxytryptamine in morphine tolerance and physical dependence. In W. W. Kosterlitz, M. O. J. Collier and J. E. Villarreal, Eds. *Agonist and Antagonist Actions of Narcotic Analgesic Drugs.* Macmillan Press Ltd., New York, pp. 153–163.

Tissue Responses to Addictive Drugs
© 1976, Spectrum Publications, Inc.

³H-lysine Accumulation into Brain and Plasma Proteins in Male Rats Treated with Morphine, Naloxone, or Naloxone Plus Morphine in Relation to Controls

D. H. FORD
R. K. RHINES
M. JOSHI
H. CHESLAK
H. SIMMONS
J. TOTH

*Downstate Medical Center
SUNY
Brooklyn, New York*

Numerous investigators have indicated that morphine inhibits protein synthesis in nontolerant animals wherein the effect of the opiate is determined within a few hours of its administration (Clouet, 1969, 1970, 1971; Clouet and Neidle, 1970; Ford et al., 1974; Clouet and Ratner, 1967, 1968). The interest of these investigators, as well as others, in protein synthesis is related to the possibility that tolerance to opiates is in some way associated with synthesis of protein (Cohen et al., 1965; Cox et al., 1968; Ho et al., 1972; Shen et al., 1970; Smith et al., 1967; and Way et al., 1968). Although this may be related to the formation of a new protein, the evidence for this has yet to be demonstrated. Attempts to identify the induction of a new protein in the brains of opiate-treated animals have been attempted by gel electrophoresis, but without success (Hahn and Goldstein, 1971). Perhaps, as suggested by Cox et al. (1968), the new species of protein represents such a small amount or is localized in so few neurons that it is easily overlooked when one examines masses of brain, even regionally.

Recently, Huidobro-Toro and Way (1975) have observed that there is an acetone extractable substance in the brains of morphine-tolerant mice that decreases the antinociceptive action of morphine. Since this active principle did not appear to be present in animals pretreated with cyclohexamide, the formation of this particular molecule may depend on a protein synthetic mechanism. Thus, while there are major interests in the roles of transmitters and receptors in relation to drug action, effects mediated via protein synthesis must still be considered.

In evaluating the effects of opiates, the responses of the animals to antagonists represent important models in attempting to discern the mode of action of a wide number of agents. Naloxone is a significant drug in this respect, since it is believed to block the effects of morphine and its congeners and has no agonistic or side effects of its own (Blumberg et al., 1961; Jasinski et al., 1967). This is apparently due to the capability of naloxone to block the specific receptors of morphine or displace morphine from the receptor if the opiate has been allowed to interact with such receptors prior to administering the naloxone. However, the observation by Catravas et al. (1975) wherein induction of epileptiform patterns in the amygdala with morphine was not reversed by naloxone suggest that this opiate antagonist may not block all of the responses caused by morphine. Further, naloxone, which blocks the analgesic effects of levallorphan, fails to block the disruption of operant conditioning caused by the drug (Wray and Cown, 1971). These findings, despite the more frequent reports on the efficacy of naloxone blockage of morphine, suggest that not all aspects of morphine action may be successfully or completely blocked. To what degree naloxone blocks the depression in protein synthesis induced by acute treatment with morphine is unknown, although it does block the effects of morphine in ^{14}C-dopamine and ^{14}C-norepinephrine synthesis (Smith et al., 1972). Thus, in view of the continued possibility that the development of tolerance and dependence on morphine and the production of the analgesic state may depend in some way on protein synthesis, it seemed useful to attempt to determine if naloxone would successfully block the morphine-depressed accumulation of a labeled amino acid into brain proteins and if it has any effect itself on protein synthesis.

MATERIALS AND METHODS

Sixty-eight male Sprague Dawley rats weighing approximately 300 gm were obtained from Spruce Tree Farms, Maryland for this study.

The left external jugular veins were cannulated with P.E. 10 polyethylene tubes as previously described (Bleecker et al., 1969) (see Figure 1). The animals were kept in individual cages after the surgical procdure and maintained on water and a standard laboratory chow (protein not less than 27%) ad libitum. There were 17 animals in each group. After the operative procedure, the animals were permitted 48 hours to recover before being injected with either saline, morphine, naloxone, or naloxone 5 minutes prior to morphine via the cannula. The two drugs and the ^{3}H-l-lysine were injected via the cannula while the animals were in an unanesthetized state. The injected material was flushed in with 0.2 ml of saline and the tubes heat-sealed to prevent backflow.

The labeled amino acid, ^{3}H-l-lysine monohydrochloride, was obtained from Schwarz/Mann, Orangeburg, New York. The specific activity was either 50 or 60 C/mM, depending on the batch used. The purity, as determined by ascending thin layer chromatography (Ford et al., 1974) was shown to be 92% lysine. The administered dose of ^{3}H-l-lysine was 1.0 MC/kg (2.92 ug/kg) in a volume of approximately 0.4 ml, depending on the body weight.

The animals were injected with 40 mg/kg of morphine sulfate (M) in saline, saline (S), or 10 mg/kg of naloxone (N) at time zero (see Figure 1). When N was given in conjunction with M, it was administered via the cannula 5 minutes prior to the opiate also at a dose level of 10 mg/kg. The dose of M selected was one which would produce analgesia as determined by the hot plate test (Eddy and Leimbach, 1953) in all of the animals for a period of two hours. The Straub tail response and catalyptic posturing also occurred in all animals treated only with M. What constitutes an effective dose of N appears quite varied, ranging from 1.0 mg/kg or less to 10.0 mg/kg. To ensure adequate blockage, we selected the higher dose of 10 mg/kg, as used by Holtzman (1974), since it invariably prevented the development of the usual responses to morphine. The relatively high dose of naloxone administered also would serve to ensure that an effective blood dose level would be maintained during the two-hour experimental period, despite its relatively short half life (see Figure 1). All morphine-treated naloxone and saline control animals were injected at time zero. The labeled lysine was injected 15, 30, 45, or 60 minutes before death by decapitation, and all rats were killed 2 hours after receiving the initial M injection at time zero. Five minutes prior to decapitation, all animals received an intraperitoneal injection of 0.5 ml of heparin to prevent clotting of the blood which was collected in centrifuge tubes from the cut vessels in the neck. While it is possible that the amino acid was injected after the time of maximal effect of naloxone (20 to 30 minutes

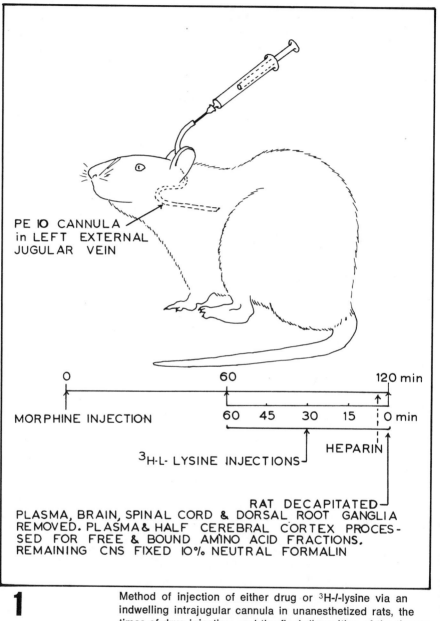

1 Method of injection of either drug or ^{3}H-*l*-lysine via an indwelling intrajugular cannula in unanesthetized rats, the times of drug injection, and the final disposition of the tissues after killing the animal by decapitation.

according to Smits and Takemori [1970]), it is not clear that the blocking capabilities of naloxone are restricted to this short a period Jasinski et al., 1967). Further, a recent observation by Mishlin et al. (1975) indicates that naloxone is still effective 110 minutes after administration of a dose of 6.0 mg/kg. Since our M + N treated animals showed no evidence of morphinization throughout the experimental period, we have concluded that there was sufficient blockage of morphine throughout the two-hour experimental period to interfere with morphine binding to receptors.

All extractions and tissue preparations to obtain free amino acid and protein fractions were performed as previously described (Ford et al., 1974). In addition, samples of brain were homogenized to obtain a protein extract which could be separated by gel electrophoresis.

The occipital lobe cortex of the brain (sample of approximately 50 mg) was dissected out and homogenized in 0.25 ml normal saline. 0.1 ml of the homogenate was mixed with 0.1 ml of sample buffer which contained 10% 2-mercaptoethanol, 4% sodium dodecyl sulfate (SDS), 0.08 M Tris-HCl buffer pH 6.8, 10% glycerol, and 0.001% bromophenol blue. This mixture was incubated in boiling water for 2 minutes. Of this mixture 5 μl (8–10 μg of protein) was layered on the polyacrylamide slab gel. The slab gels containing 5% (stacking) and 10% (separation) acrylamide were prepared from a stock solution of 30% acrylamide and 1% N-N'-bis-acrylamide. The final concentration of stacking gel was 0.13% N-N'-bis-acrylamide, 0.1% SDS, and 0.125M Tris-HCl buffer pH 6.8, and the final concentration of separation gel was 0.036M Tris-HCl buffer pH 8.7, 0.13% N-N'-bis-acrylamide, and 0.1% SDS. The gels were polymerized chemically by the addition of 0.03% tetramethylethylene diamine and ammonium persulfate. The running buffer (pH 8.3) contained 0.025M Tris, 0.192M glycine, and 0.1% SDS. The electrophoresis was carried out with a current of 50 mA constant current for about one and one-half hours. The gels were fixed for 15 minutes in 10% trichloracetic acid; stained for 3–4 hours with 0.25% Coomasie blue made in methanol acetic acid water (5:1:5) and destained with methanol acetic acid water (10:15:175).

Protein in the brain homogenate was determined by the method of Lowry et al. (1951), using bovine serum albumin as standard protein.

An amino acid analysis was also performed on the material in the free and bound acid containing fractions using a Technichon Analyzer to determine the total amount of lysine present in each fraction.

2

Changes in the specific activity (cpm/umole) of the lysine in the free amino acid fraction obtained from the plasma in saline-control (C), naloxine-treated (N), morphine-treated (M), and morphine+ naloxone-treated (M + N) rats at various time intervals after intravenous injection of ³H-*l*-lysine in unanesthetized animals. Vertical lines indicate the standard error of the mean in all figures. The comparisons listed under the figures indicate the points at which statistically significant differences occurred with P values < 0.01. The symbol = indicates there was no difference, while the arrows indicate the direction of change.

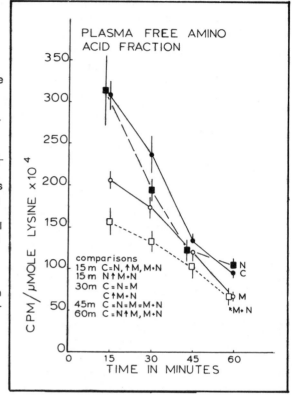

RESULTS

The data will be presented in terms of the specific activities, the specific accumulation of ³H-lysine (S. A. lysine in cerebral cortex/S. A. plasma lysine), and the specific incorporation (S. A. lysine in brain protein/S. A. brain lysine) in the free amino acid pool.

When the total sizes of the free lysine pools were determined by amino acid analysis, they were found to be in the brain: saline control 0.1139 μM/gm; naloxone-treated 0.1512 μM/gm; morphine-treated 0.1492 μM/gm; and in the morphine + naloxone-treated group 0.1300 μM/gm wet weight of cerebral cortex. In the plasma, the values were found to be: saline control 0.2118 μM/ml; Naloxone-treated 0.2291 μM/ml; morphine-treated 0.4291 μM/ml; and in the morphine + naloxone-treated group 0.3125 μM/ml. Using this data, the specific activity (S. A.) for lysine in the free pools was calculated and plotted (see Figure 2).

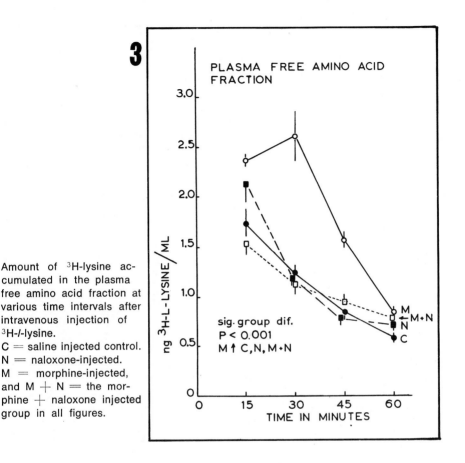

Amount of ^{3}H-lysine accumulated in the plasma free amino acid fraction at various time intervals after intravenous injection of ^{3}H-l-lysine.
C = saline injected control.
N = naloxone-injected.
M = morphine-injected, and M + N = the morphine + naloxone injected group in all figures.

It may be observed that the S. A. for lysine in the saline control and N-treated animals were essentially identical in the plasma at all time intervals (see Figure 2) and decreased with time. Moreover, there were several time intervals where the lysine S. A. was significantly higher than that observed in the M or M+N treated groups. Indeed, the pretreatment with N prior to administration of morphine seemed to cause an additional lowering of the lysine S. A. in plasma below that observed in animals receiving only M. The data presented in this figure depends not only on the size of the lysine pool but on the accumulation of labeled lysine in the pool (see Figure 3). Thus, the net lowering of the S. A. in the free pool in M-treated rats occurs because the very marked increase in pool size was of sufficient magnitude to overwhelm the net increases in labeled lysine in the pool. However, in the M + N group, there was no increase in labeled lysine in the pool as compared to

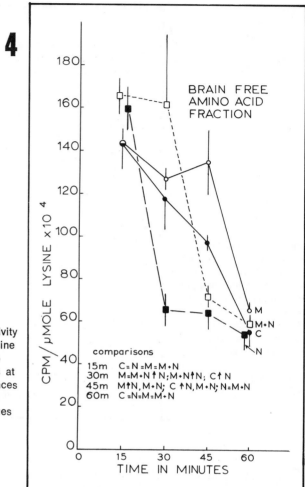

4

Changes in specific activity (cpm/umole) of the lysine in the brain free amino acid fraction. The times at which significant differences occurred are indicated below the graph. P values are all < 0.01.

controls. Therefore, since the pool size was also larger than in controls, the S.A. decreased even further than in the M-treated group. In the brain (see Figure 4) the relationship for the S. A. of lysine was somewhat different. As was expected, the S.A. for lysine in the M-treated group was higher than that observed for S-controls. Treatment with N, surprisingly, caused a marked drop in the lysine S. A. When N was combined with M, there was a shift to the right from the curve obtained by plotting the data obtained from animals receiving only N, and the effect was such that animals receiving N alone or in combination with M had a distribution of lysine which was significantly different from

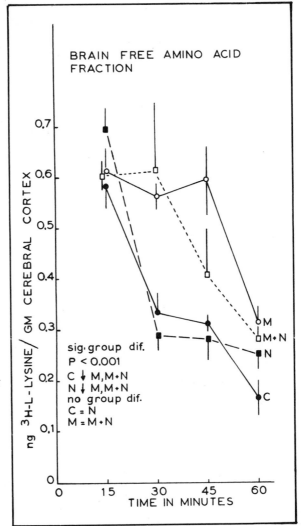

5

Amount of ³H-lysine accumulated in the brain free amino acid pool at various time intervals after intravenous injection of ³H/-lysine. Comparisons between groups are indicated below the graphs. C, N, M, and M + N are as previously indicated.

the combined effects of the changes in the size of the lysine pool and the degree to which the labeled lysine has entered it (see Figure 5). Thus, in the N-treated group, pool size has slightly enlarged over controls, but the accumulation of ³H-lysine remained similar to control values, leading to a decrease in S. A. In the M-treated group, pool size is slightly increased over controls, but the amount of labeled lysine in the pool is significantly higher than in controls. Therefore, the S. A. becomes greater. In the M + N treated group, the pool size was only

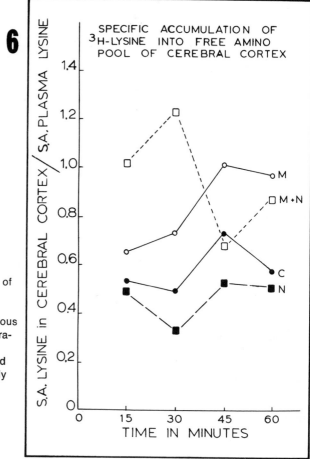

6

Specific accumulation of ³H-lysine into the free amino acid pool of the cerebral cortex at various time intervals after intravenous injection of ³H-*l*-lysine. C, N, M, and M + N are as previously indicated.

slightly greater than controls. However, again the accumulation of labeled lysine exceeds control values, leading again to a higher S. A.

An evaluation of the effect of the various treatments on the transport of ³H-lysine was determined by calculating the specific accumulation (see Figure 6). When the data is expressed in this manner, it appears that more ³H-lysine is accumulated in the free amino acid pool of the cerebral cortex from the M and M+N-treated groups.

Amino acid analysis of the lysine content in the protein obtained from the plasma and brain demonstrated that there was an average of 0.247 μmole of lysine/mg of plasma protein and 0.2528 μmole of lysine/mg of brain protein. By using thse figures, the S. A. of lysine in the plasma

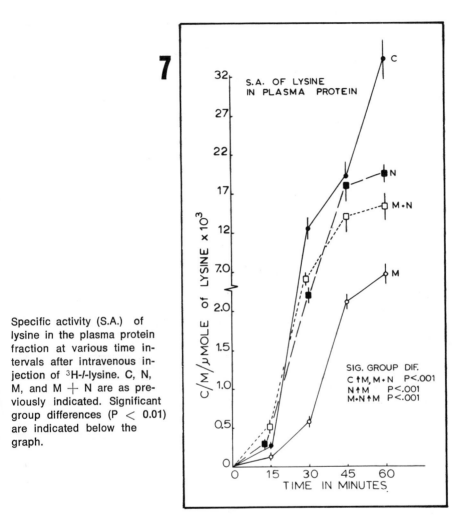

7

Specific activity (S.A.) of lysine in the plasma protein fraction at various time intervals after intravenous injection of ^{3}H-l-lysine. C, N, M, and M + N are as previously indicated. Significant group differences (P < 0.01) are indicated below the graph.

and brain protein fractions were calculated (see Figures 7 and 8). It is clear in the plasma protein that M-treatment causes a marked depression in the S. A. of the lysine fraction, indicating a decrease in incorporation of lysine as compared to the S-injected controls. The accumulation of ^{3}H-lysine into plasma proteins of N-treated animals was comparable to that observed in controls for the first 45 minutes after injecting the lysine. However, at 60 minutes, the level of accumulation was significantly lower than in controls (P<0.05). Despite this drop in uptake after 60 minutes, the levels of lysine accumulated into the

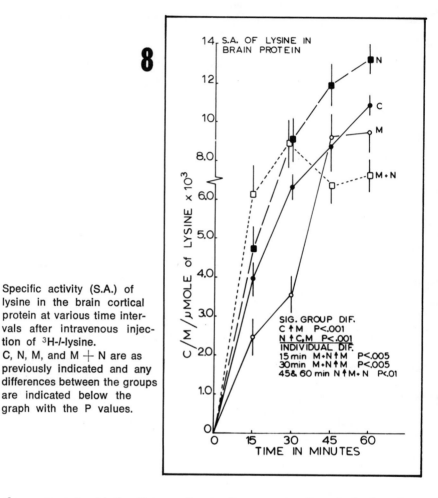

8

Specific activity (S.A.) of lysine in the brain cortical protein at various time intervals after intravenous injection of ^{3}H-*l*-lysine.
C, N, M, and M + N are as previously indicated and any differences between the groups are indicated below the graph with the P values.

plasma proteins in the N-treated animals were significantly higher than in the M-treated group and not significantly different from that observed in the M + N-treated group. Finally, the accumulation of ^{3}H-lysine into plasma protein was significantly higher in the M + N treated group than occurred in the morphinized animals. It may be noted in both the N and the M + N treated groups that there was a decreased rate of accumulation as compared to controls during the last 15 minutes of the study.

The data obtained by analysis of the S. A. of the lysine in the brain protein is less clear cut (see Figure 8). The marked inhibition in accumulation previously noted in morphine-treated Wistar animals

(Ford et al., 1974) was not as evident, although there was a highly significant depression in accumulation. (Note at 45 minutes the 2 groups are essentially identical in the levels of accumulation.) Further, the effect of naloxone on lysine accumulation into brain protein was stimulatory, causing a marked and highly significant increase in lysine accumulation as compared to the saline-injected controls. Obviously, the lysine accumulation in the N-treated animals has been influenced by the morphine antagonist. When combined with morphine, as in the M + N group, the antagonist appears to block the effect of morphine for the first 30 minutes and then fails during the last 30 minutes when the S. A. of lysine in the brain protein was significantly lower than in the N-treated group, approximating the levels of accumulation observed in the morphine and control groups. However, since the morphine and control groups were not dissimilar during the last 30 minute period, one cannot discuss the data in terms of a blockage of the morphine effect in inhibiting accumulation of lysine into brain protein.

When the specific incorporation of lysine into brain protein was calculated from the mean values of the S. A.'s (S. A. brain protein/S. A. of the brain free amino acid fraction), the effect of morphine given alone or in conjunction with naloxone on protein synthesis was more readily apparent (see Figure 9). The effect of M was to depress the incorporation of lysine into brain protein, while N had an enhancing effect which was marked at the 30 and 45 minute time intervals. When naloxone was given in conjunction with morphine, it blocked the depressive effect of morphine on protein synthesis during the first 45 minutes of the experiments, being comparable to the saline control group. However, at the 60 minute interval, the level of incorporation of lysine into brain protein was actually slightly lower than in the M-treated group.

Analysis of the electrophorograms (see Figures 10 and 11) of extractions of plasma and brain cerebral cortical proteins reveal no indication of any difference between any of the four groups studied. There was no indication of a change in the intensity of the staining reaction in any particular band which could suggest an increase or decrease in the amount of a particular protein present, nor was there a loss or addition of any bands.

CONCLUSIONS

In considering the effect of naloxone on the morphine depressive effect on brain protein synthesis, the final data (see Figure 9) on the

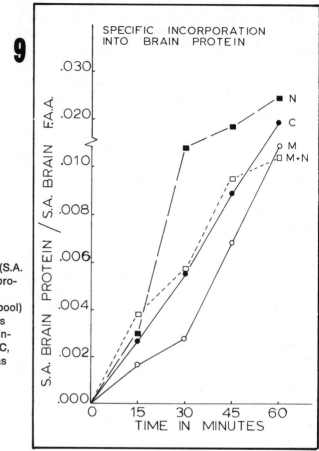

Specific incorporation (S.A. of lysine in the brain protein/S.A. lysine in the brain free amino acid pool) at various time intervals after the intravenous injection of ^{3}H-l-lysine. C, N, M, and M + N are as previously indicated.

specific incorporation of ^{3}H-lysine into brain protein demonstrates: (1) the expected depressed incorporation of the labeled amino acid into brain protein when animals are subjected to an acute treatment with morphine; (2) that naloxone itself appears to have an effect on the lysine incorporation, which is to increase it above control values when given at a dose level of 10 mg/kg i.v.; and (3) that naloxone successfully blocked the depression in lysine incorporation caused by morphine, but only for the first 45 minutes after injection of the amino acid. The slight drop in levels which are actually lower than for the M-treated group may be due to a decrease in the effectiveness of naloxone at this late interval, two hours after injection. However, this difference is probably not significant.

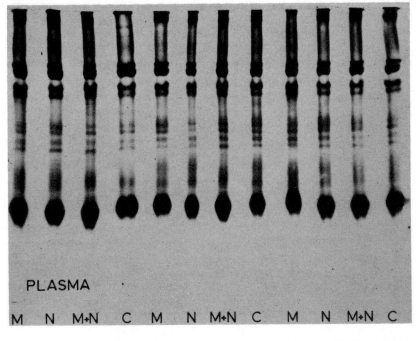

PLASMA

M N M+N C M N M+N C M N M+N C

10 Distribution of protein bands in a polyacrylimide gel slab obtained by separation of the proteins extracted from rat plasma. C, N, M, and M + N are as previously indicated.

The question as to whether or not naloxone would be effective in blocking the effect of morphine on lysine incorporation when given as early as 60 minutes before injecting the amino acid is to some degree answered by this figure in that N itself has caused an elevation of lysine incorporation for a long as 125 minutes after its injection (5 minutes before M). The more marked response observed at 95 and 110 minutes would appear to correspond to the observation of Mushlin et al. (1975) that naloxone is effective up to 110 minutes after its administration.

Thus, one may conclude that naloxone successfully blocks the morphine-induced depression of lysine incorporation into brain protein for the first 45 minutes after injection of labeled amino acid. If the amino acid had been injected earlier in relation to the naloxone injection there might very well have been complete blockade of the morphine-induced depression of incorporation throughout the experiment. What appears of particular interest is that a dose of 10 mg/kg of naloxone itself had an effect on ^{3}H-lysine incorporation into brain protein, which in consideration of the data (see Figure 6) is probably biochemically significant. To a degree, therefore, naloxone blockade of the morphine in-

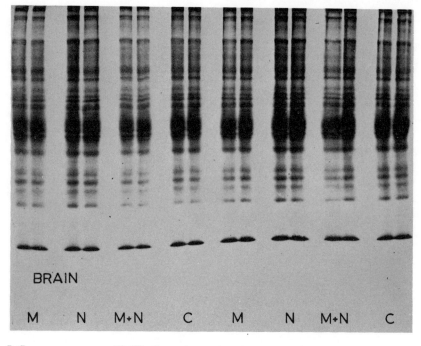

11 Distribution of protein bands in a polyacrylamide gel slab obtained by separation of the proteins extracted from rat cerebral cortex. C, N, M, and M + N are as previously indicated.

duced depression of protein synthesis may not be because it is an effective antagonist but because it has of itself a stimulatory effect on protein synthesis. Further, since the 10 mg/kg dose of naloxone is much higher than necessary to block the effect of morphine, it is possible that the increased incorporation of ^{3}H-lysine into brain protein is a pharmacologic effect which would not have occurred with a lower but effective blocking dose. Thus, as morphine depressed incorporation, naloxone augmented it. When combined together, the net effect of the agonist and the antagonist was to cause a degree of incorporation not greatly different from that observed in the saline-injected controls.

SUMMARY

Male Sprague-Dawley rats were injected with morphine, morphine + naloxone, naloxone, or saline via indwelling polyethylene cannulas and then with [3]H-*l*-lysine hydrochloride. The animals were killed at various intervals after receiving the labeled amino acid and the distribution of the ^{3}H-lysine determined in the free and bound lysine pools of the plasma and cerebral cortex.

Calculation of the specific accumulation and incorporation of lysine into the cerebral cortical free and bound pools indicated that morphine caused the expected inhibition of incorporation of the amino acid into the brain protein. Unexpectedly, the antagonist naloxone had a stimulatory effect on lysine incorporation when given alone which was of about equal magnitude to the depression in incorporation caused by morphine. When naloxone was given in conjunction with morphine, it blocked the depression in lysine incorporation normally caused by the opiate. However, this may not represent a true blockade of the morphine-effect, but a canceling out of the morphine depression of protein synthesis by its own stimulatory effect.

This demonstration of an effect on protein synthesis caused by naloxone indicates that further work must be performed to ascertain what are the full effects of naloxone before one can say that it not only blocks the physiological responses caused by opiates, but has no side effects of its own, at least at a moderately high dose.

ACKNOWLEDGMENTS

This work has been supported by a grant from the NIDA, USPHS DA 00114–04.

Naloxone was courteously supplied by the Endo Laboratories, Garden City, N. Y.

REFERENCES

Bleecker, M., D. H. Ford, and R. K. Rhines. 1969. A comparison of ^{131}I-l-triiodothyromine accumulation in ethanol-treated and control rats. *Life Sci.* 8: 267–275.

Blumberg, H., H. B. Dayton, M. George, and D. N. Rappaport. 1961. Counteraction of narcotic antagonist antagonist-analgesics by the narcotic antagonist, naloxone. *Proc. Soc. Exp. Biol. Med.* 123: 755–758.

Catravas, G. N., J. C. Blosser, J. R. Abbott, and H. Teitelbaum. 1975. Bilateral ESG response to unilateral administration of morphine: Development of unilatetral tolerance. *Fed. Proc.* 34: 758.

Clouet, D. H. 1969. Effect of morphine on protein and ribonucleic acid metabolism in brain. In J. O. Cole and K. Wittenborn, Eds. *Drug Abuse: Social and Psychopharmacological Aspects.* C. C. Thomas, Springfield, Ill. pp. 153–163.

Clouet, D. H. 1970. The effect of drugs on protein synthesis in the nervous system. In A. Lajtha, Ed. *Protein Metabolism of the Nervous System.* Plenum Press, New York, pp. 699–713.

Clouet, D. H. 1971. Protein and nucleic acid metabolism. In D. H. Clouet, Ed. *Narcotic Drugs, Biochemical Pharmacology.* Plenum Press, New York, pp. 216–228.

Clouet, D. H., and A. Neidle. 1970. The effect of morphine on the transport and metabolism of intracisternally injected leucine in the rat. *J. Neurochem.* 17: 1069–1074.

Clouet, D. H., and M. Ratner. 1967. The effect of the administration of morphine on the incorporation of (^{14}C) leucine into the proteins of rat brain *in vivo. Rrain Res.* 4: 33–43.

Clouet, D., and M. Ratner. 1968. The effect of morphine on the incorporation of ^{14}C-leucine into protein in cell free systems from rat brain and liver. *J. Neurochem.* 15: 17–23.

Cohen, M., A. S. Keats, W. Krivoy, and G. Ungar. 1965. Effect of actinomysin D on morphine tolerance. *Proc. Soc. Exp. Biol. Med.* 119: 381–384.

Cox, B. M., M. Ginsburg, and O. H. Osman. 1968. Acute tolerance to narcotic analgesic drugs in rats. *J. Pharm. Chemother.* 33: 157–170.

Eddy, N. B., and D. Leimbach. 1953. Synthetic analgesics. II: Dithienylbytenyl and dithienylbutylamines. *J. Pharm. and Exp. Ther.* 107: 385–393.

Ford, D. H., D. Weisfuse, M. Levi, and R. K. Rhines. 1974. Accumulation of ^{3}H-*l*-lysine by brain and plasma in male and female rats treated acutely with morphine sulfate. *Acta Neurol. Scandinav.* 50: 53–75.

Hahn, D. L., and A. Goldstein. 1971. Amounts and turnover of brain proteins in morphine tolerant mice. *J. Neurochem.* 18: 1887–1893.

Ho, I. K., S. E. Lu, S. Stulman, H. H. Loh, and E. L. Way. 1972. Influence of *p*-chlorophenylalanine in morphine tolerance and physical dependence and regional brain serotonin turnover studies in morphine tolerance-dependent mice. *J. Pharmacol. Exp. Ther.* 182: 155.

Holtzman, S. G. 1974. Interactions of pentazocine and naloxone on the monoamine content of discrete regions of the rat brain. *Biochem. Pharmacol.* 23: 3029–

Huidobro-Toro, and E. L. Way. 1975. Antagonism of morphine antinociception by brain extracts from tolerant mice. *Fed. Proc.* 34: 736.

Jasinski, D. R., W. R. Martin, and C. A. Haertzen. 1967. The human pharmacology and abuse potential of N-allyenorexy-morphinone (naloxone). *J. Pharmac. Exp. Ther.* 157: 420–426.

Lowry, O. H., W. J. Rosebrough, A. L. Farr, and R. J. Randall. 1951. Protein measurement with the folin phenol reagent. *J. Biol. Chem.* 193: 265–275.

Mushlin, B. E., P. Grittel, and J. Cochin. 1975. Blockade of the development of physical dependence to morphine by concurrent naloxone administration. *Fed. Proc.* 34: 735.

Ratner, M., and D. H. Clouet. 1964. The effect of morphine on ^{14}C-leucine incorporation by rat liver microsomes *in vitro. Biochem. Pharm.* 13: 1655.

Shen, F. H., H. H. Loh, and E. L. Way. 1970. Brain serotonin turnover in morphine tolerant and dependent mice. *J. Pharmacol. Exp. Ther.* 175: 427.

Smith, A., M. Karmin, and J. Gavitt. 1967. Tolerance in the lenticular effect of opiates. *J. Pharmacol. Exp. Ther.* 156: 85–91.

Smith, C. B., M. I. Sheldon, J. H. Bednarczyk, and J. E. Villarreal. 1972. Morphine-induced increases in the incorporation of ^{14}C-tyrosine into ^{14}C-dopamine and ^{14}C-norepinephrine in the mouse brain: Antagonism by naloxone and tolerance. *J. Pharmacol. Exp. Ther.* 180: 547–557.

Way, E. L., H. H. Loh, and F. Shen. 1968. Morphine tolerance, physical dependence and synthesis of brain 5-hydroxytryptamine. *Science* 162: 1290–1292.

Wray, S. R., and A. Cowan. 1971. The effects of naloxone, chlorpromazine and haloperidol pretreatment on levallorphan-induced disruption of rats' operant behavior. *Psychopharm.* (Brelin) 22: 261–270.

Tissue Responses to Addictive Drugs
© 1976, Spectrum Publications, Inc.

An Electrophoretic Study of Cerebrospinal Fluid Proteins in Humans Addicted to Heroin or Treated with Methadone

M. S. JOSHI
D. H. FORD

Department of Anatomy
Downstate Medical Center
Brooklyn, New York

Attempts have been made to correlate the biochemical events that take place following the interaction of the opiate and the opiate-receptor and the opiate specific pharmacologic effects. Many biochemical changes take place following opiate administration, but it is not yet clear whether any of these biochemical changes bring about the production of analgesia, or production of tolerance and physical dependence. Clouet (1971) has described an increase in protein synthesis that correlates with the addictive process. Ford et al. (1974) have demonstrated electron microscopic changes in the neuronal structures related to protein synthesis following morphine administration to rat. The presence of a unique acidic nonhistone protein which is synthesized in the brain of addicted mice has been recently demonstrated (Loh, 1975). Further, a role for a specific protein synthesis in the development of tolerance and physical dependence has been well emphasized.

Analysis of proteins in cerebrospinal fluid (CSF) by eletcrophoresis and by immunochemical techniques has been done in human subjects exhibiting many varieties of neurological disorders. Characteristic spinal fluid patterns are reported in inflammatory or degenerative disorders of the central nervous system (Kjellin and Stibler, 1974; Vandvik and Skrede, 1975; Clausen et al., 1964). The presence of CSF-specific proteins, not detected in blood serum, has been demonstrated by immunoelectrophoresis in rats (Macri et al., 1973) and humans (Clausen, 1961; Heitmann and Uhlenbruck, 1966; Macri et al., 1974). The presence or absence of the CSF-specific proteins did not correlate with the disease process (Heitmann and Uhlenbruck, 1966). The proteins in CSF were contributed by plasma proteins and also to some extent by brain tissue. The purpose of this chapter is to examine whether the altered protein metabolism following opiate addiction reflects on the protein composition of cerebrospinal fluid.

MATERIALS AND METHODS

The cerebrospinal fluid was obtained by spinal tap during routine diagnostic tests of patients who attended the neurology and neurosurgery clinics. Two of these samples were from patients who were heroin addicts, four samples were obtained from patients who were on methadone treatment and twenty samples were from "normal" patients who had not consumed opiate drugs.

Polyacrylamide slab gel electrophoresis (PAGE) was used to analyze proteins in serum, plasma, and CSF. PAGE without sodium dodecyl sulfate (SDS) was done on a 3% stacking gel in Tris-HCl buffer pH 6.8, and a 7.5% separation gel in Tris-HCl buffer pH 8.3. PAGE with SDS was done on a 5% stacking gel and a 10% separation gel containing 0.1% SDS. Tris-glycine buffer pH 8.3 containing 0.1% SDS was used as a running buffer. 8–20 μg protein was layered on the gel.

A 2- to 5-fold concentration of the macromolecules in the CSF was achieved by placing aquacide-II (Calbiochem) powder outside the dialysis bag containing CSF.

Protein estimations were done according to the method of Lowry et al. (1951), using bovine serum albumin as standard protein.

Stepwise precipitation of proteins from concentrated CSF by a saturated solution of ammonium sulfate was carried out at 0°C. The protein fractions thus obtained were extensively dialyzed against normal saline.

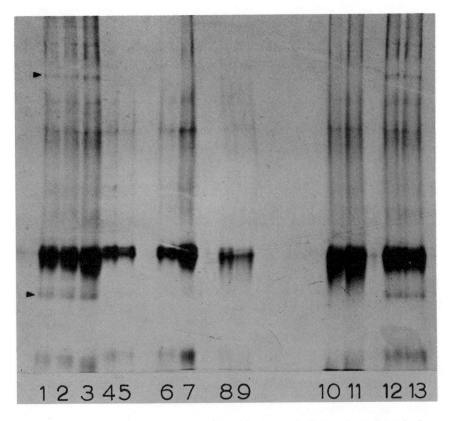

1   Polyacrylamide slab gel electrophoresis of cerebrospinal fluid. 1 and 2, unconcentrated CSF of heroin addicts; 3, 2-fold concentrated CSF of heroin addict (arrows indicate the slow- and fast-moving proteins); 4, 5, 6, 7, CSF of patients on methadone treatment; 8, 9, 10, 11, CSF of "normal" patients; 12 and 13, CSF of heroin addicts.

DISCUSSION

The protein concetnrations in CSF of two heroin addicts were 680 μg/ml and 445 μg/ml; the protein content of four methadone patients ranged between 350–385 μg/ml, while the protein content of "normal" CSF averaged 300 μg/ml.

PAGE of CSF of heroin addicts indicated the presence of two distinct additional protein bands (see Figure 1, arrows) as compared to methadone and "normal" CSF. One band, the slow-moving protein was closer to the cathode while the fast-moving protein was in the region of prealbumin.

511

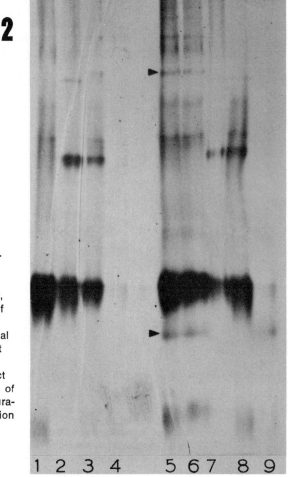

2

Polyacrylamide slab gel electrophoresis of cerebrospinal fluid and the ammonium sulfate saturation fractions. 1, normal CSF; 2, 0-40% saturation fraction of normal CSF; 3, 40-70% saturation fraction of normal CSF; 4, fraction soluble at 70% saturation of normal CSF; 5 and 6, heroin addict 7, 0-40% saturation fraction of heroin-CSF; 8, 40-70% saturation of heroin-CSF; 9, fraction soluble at 70% saturation of heroin-CSF.

Concentrated CSF obtained from a heroin addict and a normal patient was fractionated in three protein fractions by stepwise ammonium sulfate saturation. The first fraction was obtained at 0–40% saturation; the second fraction was obtained at 40–70% saturation and the third fraction was soluble in 70% saturated ammonium sulfate (see Figure 2). The slow-moving protein seen in CSF of heroin addicts seems to precipitate at 40–70% saturation while the fast-moving protein remains soluble at 70% saturation.

In order to determine the approximate molecular size of the two additional proteins in the CSF of heroin addicts, PAGE with SDS was done. CSF samples and standard proteins layered on the gel were previously incubated with 1% SDS and 5% 2-mercaptoethanol in boiling water for 2 minutes. The slow-moving specific protein in the CSF of heroin addicts was not detectable, while the fast-moving protein was detected in the prealbumin zone (see Figure 3). The approximate molecular weight of the fast-moving protein, calculated according to the method of Weber and Osborne (1969), was close to 45,000. Our inability to detect the slow-moving protein in SDS-gel may be due to the

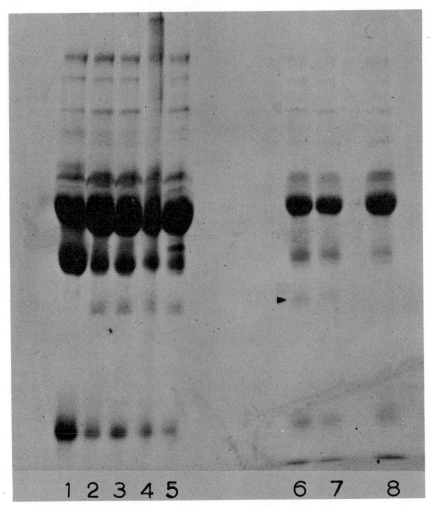

3

Polyacrylamide slab gel electrophoresis with SDS of 1, 2, 3, serum from patients on methadone; 4, normal serum; 5, normal plasma; 6 and 7, CSF of heroin addicts (the arrow indicates the fast-moving protein); 8, CSF of normal patient.

1 2 3 4 5   6 7   8

dissociation of this protein into subunits which merged with the other protein bands.

Comparison of the eletcrophoretic pattern of normal serum, normal plasma, serum obtained from methadone patients, CSF of heroin addicts, and "normal" patients was done by SDS-PAGE (see Figure 3). The fast-moving protein of CSF migrated differently than proteins in the prealbumin region of plasma or serum, suggesting that this protein may have been derived from sources other than blood. Further characterization of the protein detected in the CSF of heroin addicts by immunochemical methods is being pursued.

SUMMARY

Polyacrylamide slab gel electrophoresis of CSF of heroin addicts, CSF of patients treated with methadone, and the CSF of "normal" subjects was done. The CSF of heroin addicts showed the presence of two additional protein bands not detected in the CSF of methadone patients or "normal" subjects. The slow-moving protein was precipitable in 40–70% saturated ammonium sulfate solution, while the fast-moving protein which migrated in the prealbumin region remained soluble in a 70% saturated ammonium sulfate solution. The approximate molecular weight of the fast-moving protein, was determined by SDS-gel electrophoresis using standard proteins, was close to 45,000. The slow-moving protein was not detectable in SDS-gel. A comparison of the electrophoretic mobility of the fast-moving protein of CSF of heroin addicts with serum proteins in SDS-gel indicated that the CSF-protein may be derived from sources other than blood.

ACKNOWLEDGMENTS

We are thankful to Dr. J. Brown, Department of Neurosurgery and Dr. H. S. Schutta, Department of Neurology, Downstate Medical Center, Brooklyn, for their help in procuring the CSF samples.

REFERENCES

Clausen, J. 1961. Proteins in normal cerebrospinal fluid not found in serum. *Proc. Soc. Exp. Biol. Med.* 107: 170–172.
Clausen, J., J. Matzke, and W. Gerhardt. 1964. Agar-gel microelectrophoresis

of proteins in the cerebrospinal fluid: Normal and pathological findings. *Acta Neurol. Scand.* 40, Suppl. 10: 49–56.

Clouet, D. H. 1971. Protein and nucleic acid metabolism. In D. H. Clouet, Ed. *Narcotic Drugs: Biochemical Pharmacology.* Plenum Press, New York, pp. 216–228.

Ford, D. H., K. Voeller, B. Callegari, and E. Gresik. 1974. Changes in neurons of the median eminence-arcuate region of rats induced by morphine treatment: An electron microscopic study. *Neurobiology* 4: 1–11.

Heitmann, R., and G. Uhlenbruck. 1966. Uber den nachweis "spezifischer" proteine im liquor cerebrospinalis durch die immunoelektrophorese. *Deutsche Zeitschrift fur Nervenheilkunde* 188: 187–199.

Kjellin, K. G., and H. Stibler. 1974. CSF-protein patterns in extrapyramidal diseases. *Europ. Neurol.* 12: 186–194.

Loh. H. H. 1975. Biochemical process in addiction. In S. H. Snyder and S. Matthysse, Eds. *Opiate Receptor Mechanisms.* Neurosciences Research Program, Boston, pp. 102–103.

Lowry, O. H., N. J. Rosebrough, A. L. Farr, and R. J. Randall. 1951. Protein measurement with the folin phenol reagent. *J. Biol. Chem.* 193: 265–275.

Macri, J. N., M. S. Joshi, and M. I. Evans. 1973. An antenatal diagnosis of spina bifida in the Lewis rat. *Nature* (London) 246: 89–90.

Macri, J. N., R. R. Weiss, M. S. Joshi, and M. I. Evans. 1974. Antenatal diagnosis of neural-tube defects using cerebrospinal-fluid proteins. *The Lancet* 1: 14–15.

Vandvik, B., and S. Skrede. 1973. Electrophoretic examination of cerebrospinal fluid proteins in multiple sclerosis and other neurological diseases. *Europ. Neurol.* 9: 224–241.

Weber, K., and M. Osborn. 1969. The reliability of molecular weight determinations by dodecyl sulfate-polyacrylamide gel electrophoresis. *J. Biol. Chem.* 244: 4406–4412.

Tissue Responses to Addictive Drugs
© 1976, Spectrum Publications, Inc.

Acute Effects of Opiate Administration on Pituitary Gonadotropin and Prolactin Release

E. ZIMMERMANN
C. N. PANG

Department of Anatomy and
Brain Research Institute
UCLA School of Medicine
Los Angeles, California

In recent years it has become increasingly clear that opiate abuse is associated with profound changes in sexual and reproductive functioning. Menstural aberrations, altered sex drive, and diminished sex organ function are common clinical correlates of heroin addiction or methadone maintenance (Azizi et al., 1973; Bai et al., 1974; Cicero et al., 1975; Martin et al., 1973; Mendelson et al., 1975; Pelosi et al., 1974; and Santen, 1974). Despite growing awareness of these drug-related problems, effects of opiates on reproductive physiology have not been studied extensively in experimental animals. Twenty years ago Sawyer and his associates (Barraclough and Sawyer, 1955; Sawyer et al., 1955) demonstrated inhibition of ovulation in rats treated with morphine. They showed clearly that such treatment was effective only if administered prior to the "critical period" for the neurogenic stimulation of ovulation on the afternoon of the day of proestrus. Subsequent studies showed that morphine blockade of ovulation could be overcome by electrical stimulation of the hypothalamus (Everett, 1964). Although based upon indirect evidence, these early investigations clearly implicated a neural site of morphine inhibition of pituitary gonadotropin secretion. Our understanding of opiate effects on gonadotropin secretion has not advanced substantially beyond the conclusions drawn from these early studies although it is now possible to quantitate gonadotropin levels directly by radioimmunoassay.

Effects of opiate administration on pituitary secretion of prolactin are also not well understood. Years ago Meites et al. (1959) noted that morphine caused lactation in estrogen-primed rats. Galactorrhea has also been reported to occur in heroin addicts (Bai et al., 1974; Pelosi et al., 1974). Morphine-induced stimulation of prolactin release has recently been documented to occur in rats (Zimmermann et al., 1974) and man (Tolis et al., 1975) by direct radioimmunoassay of the hormone.

In view of the paucity of evidence regarding effects of opiate administration on pituitary secretion of gonadotropins and prolactin we undertook a series of experiments designed to determine, by radioimmunoassay, changes in circulating levels of luteinizing hormone (LH), follicle stimulating hormone (FSH), and prolactin in the rat following acute administration of morphine. This chapter is a brief review of these studies and of several reports which have appeared recently in the literature.

METHODS AND RESULTS

The first study was designed to determine the influence of various doses of morphine on the ovulatory surge of circulating levels of LH. Adult Sprague-Dawley female rats were maintained under conditions of cyclic illumination (lights-on from 5 a.m. to 7 p.m. alternated with darkness from 7 p.m. to 5 a.m.). Food and water were available at all times. Vaginal smears were obtained daily. Rats showing at least two normal 4-day cycles were given 0, 10, 20, 40, or 60 mg/kg morphine (free base) intraperitoneally, dissolved in isotonic saline, at 2 p.m. on the afternoon of proestrus. Four hours later blood was obtained by rapid jugular venipuncture under ether anesthesia and used for subsequent determination of plasma LH concentrations with the NIAMD rat LH radioimmunoassay kit. The time of blood collection coincides with the peak of the ovulatory surge of the LH concentrations in plasma under the lighting schedule used in our laboratory. To verify the occurance of ovulation all animals were sacrificed around noon the following day and uterine tubes were examined microscopically for the presence of ova.

Table I. Effects of Various Doses of Morphine on the Proestrous Surge of Plasma LH in Female Rats

Treatment	Dose (mg/kg)	No. of Rats	Plasma LH (ng/ml)
Saline	—	13	1157 ± 133*
Morphine	10	6	1842 ± 234†
Morphine	20	6	908 ± 405
Morphine	40	15	854 ± 197
Morphine	60	9	99 ± 22†

* Mean ± S.E.
† p $<$ 0.01 compared to saline-treated controls.

Compared with saline-treated controls, animals receiving 10 mg/kg morphine showed apparently enhanced levels of LH and all rats in this group ovulated. In contrast, rats given 60 mg/kg morphine showed marked suppression of LH levels and failure to ovulate. Groups receiving either 20 or 40 mg/kg morphine showed intermediate levels of LH which did not differ from that of saline-treated controls but were less ($p < 0.05$) than that of rats given 10 mg/kg and greater ($p < 0.05$) than that of rats given 60 mg/kg morphine (see Table I). Inspection of the data from individual animals in the 20 and 40 mg/kg groups revealed a strong correlation between the level of LH and the presence of tubal ova suggesting that these intermediate doses may block, in an all-or-none fashion, neural mechanisms responsible for triggering the proestrous surge of LH in the rat.

A similar pattern of changes in plasma levels of FSH was observed in proestrous rats 4 hours after intraperitoneal administration of various doses of morphine at 2 p.m., just prior to onset of the critical period. The results, obtained using the NIAMD rat FSH radioimmunoassay kit, are presented in Table II. As expected on the evening of proestrus, control levels of circulating FSH were quite high. Whereas administration of 10 mg/kg morphine had no apparent effect on these high levels, 20 mg/kg appeared to cause a striking elevation of FSH levels. This observation is based upon responses of only 3 animals and is therefore regarded as merely tentative evidence of morphine-induced stimulation of FSH release. In contrast, administration of 40 or 60 mg/kg morphine resulted in significant suppression of FSH levels.

These studies indicate that morphine exerts dose-dependent effects on the proestrous surge of LH and FSH in the rat. Lower doses appear to facilitate the ovulatory discharge of gonadotropins from the pituitary but in our experience such effects are variable and await verification.

Table II. Effects of Various Doses of Morphine on the Proestrous Surge of Plasma FSH in Female Rats

Treatment	Dose (mg/kg)	No. of Rats	Plasma FSH (ng/ml)
Saline	—	13	686 ± 56*
Morphine	10	6	637 ± 130
Morphine	20	3	1483 ± 453†
Morphine	40	10	400 ± 38†
Morphine	60	6	327 ± 55†

* Mean ± S.E.
† p < 0.01 compared to saline-treated controls.

Higher doses of morphine inhibit the cyclic discharge of gonadotropins which in the rat occurs in response to a spontaneous periodic neural triggering mechanism. The specificity of the inhibitory action of morphine on the proestrous surge of LH and FSH is not known but administration of 10 mg/kg of naloxone just prior to 60 mg/kg morphine in a protocol similiar to that described above completely antagonized the action of the opiate. Although the exact site of the inhibitory action of morphine is not known it is presumed to be at the level of the hypothalamus. This presumption is based in part upon the fact that rats treated with 60 mg/kg morphine showed an intact plasma LH response to administration of LH releasing hormone (LHRH) on the evening of proestrus (Pang et al., in preparation).

It is well established that gonadectomy leads to sustained enhancement of gonadotropin secretion. To further explore effects of opiates on mechanisms regulating gonadotropin release the influence of morphine on elevated levels of LH and FSH following ovariectomy was studied. Rats ovariectomized 7 weeks previously received intraperitoneal injections of 60 mg/kg morphine or saline. One hour later the animals were rapidly decapitated, trunk blood was collected and the plasma separated for subsequent radioimmunoassay of LH and FSH concentrations. In addition it was of interest to study effects of morphine on prolactin release in ovariectomized rats, thus prolactin levels in plasma samples obtained in this study were also determined by radioimmunoassay (see Table III).

Saline-injected control animals showed relatively high circulating levels of LH and FSH which are characteristic of those found in rats several weeks after ovariectomy. Animals treated with 60 mg/kg morphine one hour earlier showed suppression of LH and FSH levels to

Table III. Effects of Morphine on Plasma Levels of
LH, FSH and Prolactin on Ovariectomized Rats

Treatment	No. of Rats	LH (ng/ml)	FSH (ng/ml)	Prolactin (ng/ml)
Saline	5	595 ± 79*	1935 ± 197	341 ± 107
Morphine (60 mg/kg)	5	385 ± 32†	1492 ± 42†	3442 ± 874**

* Mean ± S.E.
† p < 0.05
** p < 0.01

approximately 65% and 75%, respectively, of control levels. In contrast to the suppression of gonadotropin levels, plasma levels of prolactin were highly elevated one hour after injection of morphine. These findings suggest that morphine inhibits the tonic hypersecretion of LH and FSH and stimulates release of prolactin in ovariectomized rats. These contrasting actions of morphine may involve suppression of hypothalamic release of LHRH and of prolactin inhibiting factor.

To clarify the temporal characteristics of the stimulatory effect of morphine on prolactin release a final study was performed. Adult male Sprague-Dawley rats were injected intraperitoneally with 30 mg/kg morphine and decapitated 0, 30, 60, or 120 min later. Plasma was collected and subsequently used for radioimmunoassay of prolactin concentrations. Plasma levels of prolactin were markedly elevated (p < 0.01) above initial levels at 30 and at 60 min following morphine injection. By 120 min following drug injection prolactin concentrations had returned to initial levels (see Table IV).

CONCLUSIONS

The results of these studies confirm the findings of Barraclough and Sawyer (1955) and demonstrate that large doses of morphine block spontaneous ovulation in the rat by suppressing the ovulatory surge of LH and FSH. In addition these studies indicate that morphine inhibits mechanisms underlying tonic elevation of gonadotropin secretion following ovariectomy in the rat. These observations may help explain the diminished seminal vesicle and prostate gland weights observed in morphine-treated rats (Cicero et al., 1974) and the reduced levels of circulating testosterone (Azizi et al., 1973; Cicero et al., 1975; Mendelson and Mello, 1975; Mendelson et al., 1975), reduced secondary sex

Table IV. Plasma Levels of Prolactin at
Various Intervals Following
Morphine Administration in Male Rats

Min. After Injection of Morphine (30 mg/kg, ip)	No. of Rats	Prolactin (ng/ml)
0	5	167 ± 14*
30	6	350 ± 71†
60	6	248 ± 23†
120	5	155 ± 11

* Mean ± S.E.
† $p < 0.01$ compared to initial levels (0 min).

organ secretions (Cicero et al., 1975), and diminished libido (Cushman, 1973; Martin et al., 1973) in male heroin and methadone addicts. Opiate-induced suppression of cyclic release of gonadotropins might also help explain the high incidence of infertility, amenorrhea, oligomenorrhea, and other menstrual aberrations among women addicted to narcotics (Bai et al., 1974; Pelosi et al., 1974; Santen, 1974).

The prolactin results obtained in these studies are consistent with our earlier findings that morphine stimulates prolactin release (Zimmermann et al., 1974) and could explain the observation of Meites et al. (1959) that morphine administration causes milk secretion in rats. Likewise the galactorrhea observed in female heroin addicts (Pelosi et al., 1974; Santen, 1974) might also be accounted for on the basis of morphine-induced release of prolactin. A preliminary report by Tolis et al. (1975) indicates that therapeutic doses of morphine stimulate prolactin release in women. A single report indicates that large doses of morphine may also inhibit secretion of prolactin in male rats (Shin et al., 1975). Since the interval between morphine administration and blood sampling was not given in their report it is not certain whether the findings of Shin et al. (1975) conflict with those noted above. Morphine may cause initial stimulation followed by suppression of circulating levels of prolactin.

Morphine may act at a variety of sites to influence neuroendocrine functions (George, 1971). However, based upon a review of the available evidence it seems reasonable to conclude that the narcotic acts primarily at a hypothalamic level to inhibit gonadotropin release and to stimulate release of prolactin. Evidence supporting this conclusion includes the findings that: (1) electrical stimulation of the hypothalamus causes ovulation in the morphine-blocked rat (Everett, 1964); (2) morphine acts directly on hypothalamic neurons to alter their rate of spontaneous discharge and these effects are antagonized by naloxone (Eidelberg and Bond, 1972); (3) direct implantation of morphine into the hypothalamus elicits other neuroendocrine responses (George, 1971); and (4) small amounts of morphine administered intraventricularly cause marked stimulation of prolactin release in rats (Ojeda et al., 1974) whereas it lacks this effect when applied to pituitary tissue *in vitro* (Shin et al., 1975). The most probable explanation consistent with these diverse findings is that acute administration of morphine results in diminished release of hypothalamic gonadotropin releasing hormone(s) and prolactin inhibiting factor.

The precise neurochemical mechanism(s) by which morphine acts acutely to alter hypothalamic control of gonadotropin and prolactin secretion is not known. Nevertheless considerable evidence suggests that some alteration of hypothalamic neurotransmitter metabolism and/or release may be involved. This evidence has recently been reviewed and summarized by De Wied et al. (1974) who suggest that more than one transmitter participates in the neural regulation of cyclic and tonic secretion of LH, FSH, and prolactin. Convincing evidence indicates that the dopaminergic tuberoinfundibular system plays an important role in the tonic inhibition of prolactin secretion and stimulation of gonadotropin secretion (Collu et al., 1973; Kamberi, 1973; Schneider and McCann, 1969; and De Wied and De Jong, 1974). A single large dose of morphine decreased norepinephrine (Johnson and Clouet, 1973) and increased dopamine content (De Wied et al., 1974) in the hypothalamus of the rat. The present studies indicate that such treatment is associated with reduced release of LH and FSH and increased release of prolactin. These findings cannot easily be reconciled without additional information regarding effects of morphine on rates of turnover and release of hypothalamic norepinephrine and dopamine. Morphine administration reportedly increases the turnover of serotonin in the rat brain (Haubrich and Blake, 1973; Yarbrough et al., 1971). Since this transmitter has been shown to inhibit release of LH and FSH while stimulating release of prolactin (Kamberi, 1973), the results of the present studies might be attributed to an increase in the activity of serotonergic mechanisms in the hypothalamus. Atropine has long been known to block ovulation in the rat (Sawyer et al., 1955) and more recent studies have shown it to suppress the proestrous surge of LH and FSH levels when administered to rats intraventricularly (Kamberi and Bacleon, 1973). Several cholinergic drugs have been shown to inhibit prolactin release in the rat (Grandison et al., 1975). In view of the well-known inhibitory effect of morphine on acetylcholine release

and antagonists on rat brain acetylcholine. *J. Pharm. Exp. Therap.* 184: 18–32.

Eidelberg, E., and M. L. Bond. 1972. Effects of morphine and antagonists on hypothalamic cell activity. *Arch. Int. Pharmacodyn.* 196: 16–24.

Everett, J. W. 1964. Central neural control of reproductive functions of the adenophypophysis. *Rev. Physiol.* 44: 373–431.

George, R. 1971. Hypothalamus: Anterior pituitary gland. In D. H. Clouet, Ed. *Narcotic Drugs Biochemical Pharmacology.* Plenum Press, New York, pp. 283–299.

Grandison, L., M. Gelato, and J. Meites. 1974. Inhibition of prolactin secretion by cholinergic drugs (37988). *Proc. Soc. Exp. Biol. Med.* 145: 1236–1239.

Haubrich, D. R., and D. E. Blake. 1973. Modification of serotonin metabolism in rat brain after acute or chronic administration of morphine. *Biochem. Pharmacol.* 22: 2753–2759.

Johnson, J. C., and D. H. Clouet. 1973. Studies on the effect of acute and chronic morphine treatment on catecholamine levels and turnover in discrete brain areas of rats. *Fed. Proc.* 32: 757.

Kamberi, I. A. 1973. The role of brain monoamines and pineal indoles in the secretion of gonadrotrophins and gonadotrophin-releasing factors. *Prog. Brain Res.* 39: 261–278.

Kamberi, I. A., and E. S. Bacleon. 1973. Cholinergic pathways and gonadotropin releasing factors. (Abstract) *Fed. Proc.* 32: 240.

Martin, W. R., D. R. Jasinski, C. A. Haertzen, D. C. Kay, B. E. Jones, P. A. Mansky, and R. W. Carpenter. 1973. Methadone—A reevalution. *Arch. Gen. Psychiat.* 28: 286–295.

Meites, J., C. S. Nicoll, and P. K. Talwalker. 1959. Induction and maintenance of lactation in rats by eletcrical stimulation of uterine cervix. *Proc. Soc. Exp. Biol. Med.* 102: 127–131.

Mendelson, J. H., and N. K. Mello. 1975. Plasma testosterone levels during chronic heroin use and protracted abstinence. *Clin. Pharm. Ther.* 17: 529–533.

Mendelson, J. H., J. E. Mendelson, and V. D. Patch. 1975. Plasma testosterone levels in heroin addiction and during methadone maintenance. *J. Pharmacol. Exp. Ther.* 192: 211–217.

Ojeda, S. R., P. G. Harms, and S. M. McCann. 1974. Possible role of cyclic AMP and prostaglandin E_1 in dopaminergic control of prolactin release. *Endocrinology* 95: 1694–1703.

Pang, C. N., and E. Zimmermann. 1975. Effects of morphine on plasma levels of luteinizing hormone (LH), thyroid stimulating hormone (TSH) and prolactin in ovariectomized rats. *Anat. Rec.* 181: 444.

Pang, C. N., E. Zimmermann, and C. H. Sawyer. 1974. Effects of morphine on the proesterous surge of luteinizing hormone in the rat. *Anat. Rec.* 178: 434.

Pelosi, M. A., J. C. Sama, H. Caterini, and H. A. Kaminetzky. 1974. Galactorrhea-amenorrhea syndrome associated with heroin addiction. *Am. J. Obstet. Gynec.* 118: 966–970.

Santen, R. J. 1974. How narcotics addiction affects reproductive function in women. *Contemp. Ob. Gyn.* 3: 93–96.

Sawyer, C. H., B. V. Critchlow, and C. A. Barraclough. 1955. Mechanism of blockade of pituitary activation in the rat by morphine, atropine and barbiturates. *Endocrinology* 57: 345–354.

Schneider, H. P. G., and S. M. McCann. 1969. Possible role of dopamine as transmitter to promote discharge of LH-releasing factor. *Endocrinology* 85: 121–132.

Shin, S. H., W. J. Hay, M. O'Connor, and K. Jhamandas. 1975. Morphine effect on prolactin secretion in male rats. *Fed. Proc.* 34: 251.

Tolis, G., J. Hickey, and H. Guyda. 1975. Effects of morphine on serum growth hormone (GH), prolactin (PRL), cortisol and thyroid stimulating hormone (TSH) in man. *Abs. 57th Ann. Meeting, The Endocrine Soc.* No. 55.

Yarbrough, G. G., D. M. Buxbaum, and E. Sanders-Rush. 1971. Increased serotonin turnover in the acutely morphine treated rat. *Life Sci.* 10: 977–983.

Zimmerman, E., C. N. Pang, and C. H. Sawyer. 1974. Morhpine-induced prolactin release and its suppression by dexamethasone in male rats. *Abs. 56th Ann. Meeting, The Endocrine Soc.* No. 526.

Tissue Responses to Addictive Drugs
© 1976, Spectrum Publications, Inc.

The Effects of Narcotics on Growth Hormone, ACTH and TSH Secretion

ROBERT GEORGE

*Department of Pharmacology
and Brain Research Institute
University of California
Los Angeles, California*

NORIO KOKKA

*Department of Pharmacology
and Therapeutics
California College of Medicine
University of California
Irvine, California*

It is well documented that narcotic analgesics may alter pituitary activity. Although the mechanisms by which narcotics influence pituitary function are not clear, there is much evidence that indicates these effects are mediated via the central nervous system (CNS) and, more specifically, the hypothalamus. The hormones of the anterior pituitary have been shown to be under the control of releasing factors (RF) that are synthesized in the hypothalamus and then are transported to the pituitary by the hypophyseal portal blood supply (Blackwell and Guillemin, 1973).

However, the mechanisms underlying the control of these hypothalamic neurons have not been clearly elucidated. It has been suggested that 'transmitter' substances (dopamine, norepinephrine, serotonin and acetylcholine) found in the hypothalamus play an essential role in the regulation of the secretions of the neurosecretory neurons (Fuxe

527

and Hökfelt, 1969; Wurtman, 1970; de Wied and de Jong, 1974). In addition, the hypothalamus, because of its many afferent connections and its anatomical relationship with the pituitary, acts as a 'final common path' or 'nodal point' through which impulses that arise from the periphery or from other brain regions can depress or activate anterior pituitary function.

The brain regions most commonly associated with modulation of hypothalamic activity are the structures of the limbic system (hippocampus, amygdala, septal area, olfactory tubercle, anterior thalamic nuclei, mammillary bodies of the hypothalamus, cingulate gyrus, hippocampal gyrus, entorhinal cortex and pyriform lobe) and the midbrain. These limbic system structures have rich interconnections with the hypothalamus and midbrain reticular formation. The hypothalamic relationships suggest a role for these structures in the control of motivation and emotion. The midbrain relationships suggest a role in the regulation of arousal and attention.

Thus it would not be surprising to see that drugs which affect emotion, motivation and arousal can also alter pituitary activity via their effects on the limbic-midbrain system.

This chapter will deal only with the effects of narcotics on pituitary secretion of adrenocorticotropin (ACTH), growth hormone (GH), and thyrotropin (TSH).

ADRENOCORTICOTROPIN (ACTH)

In most of the studies cited below adrenal corticosteroids (CS) were used as index for ACTH secretion since no reliable radioimmunoassay is presently available. Acute administration of morphine has been reported to significantly elevate plasma CS levels in the rat, mouse, and dog but not in man or guinea pig (George, 1971; Sloan, 1971). Recent reports indicate that the cat also responds to morphine with elevated plasma CS levels (Borrell, et al., 1974; French, et al., 1974).

In the rat, low doses of morphine (5 or 10 mg/kg) do not elevate CS levels whereas doses of 20 mg/kg or higher significantly elevate CS levels and the response is dose related. Preadministration of naloxone (antagonist:agonist ratios of 1:2 or 1:4) completely block this effect of morphine and methadone but not apomorphine (Kokka, et al., 1973; Kokka and George, 1974). These data clearly indicate that morphine and apomorphine increase plasma CS by different mechanisms.

The ACTH releasing effect of morphine is chiefly mediated via the hypothalamus. George and Way (1959) showed that lesions which destroyed at least one half of the anterior median eminence abolished the adrenal cortical response to morphine. In a later study it was shown that lesions in the basomedial hypothalamus, without damage to the median eminence, partially blocked adrenal cortical stimulation by morphine (Kokka and George, 1974). However, since morphine exerts many of its pharmacologic actions by acting on structures in the central nervous system and, since the hypothalamus contains numerous connections from many rostral and caudal regions of the CNS, it is conceivable that morphine stimulates corticotropin secretion by acting on some extrahypothalamic area. Thus studies were initiated by Lotti, et al. (1969) to determine what effects morphine would have on CS secretion following intrahypothalamic administration. They localized an area in the middle region of the hypothalamus where focal injection of morphine (5-50 μg) produced both a marked reduction of adrenal ascorbic acid and an elevation of plasma corticosterone.

Chronic administration of morphine reduces adrenal cortical steroid secretion in man (Eisenman, et al., 1961), rats (Paroli and Melchiorri, 1961), and guinea pigs (Sobel, et al., 1958). Tolerance to the CS releasing effect of morphine and methadone has been noted within 24 to 48 hours in the rat (Kokka and George, 1974). Methadone maintained patients have been reported to have normal resting plasma cortisol and most of them respond normally to insulin hypoglycemia (Cushman, 1974).

Either abrupt withdrawal in rats and man (Sloan, 1971) or naloxone precipitated withdrawal in rats (Kokka and George, 1974) results in marked elevation of plasma CS levels.

GROWTH HORMONE (GH)

The factors controlling immunoassayable growth hormone secretion vary considerably from man to other species. In man many stimuli that cause an increase in GH secretion also stimulate ACTH secretion. However, in most subprimate species the stimuli that elevate CS secretion simultaneously inhibit GH secretion. In the rat this inverse relationship has been clearly demonstrated when comparing stressed to nonstressed rats (Takahashi, et al., 1971; Kokka, et al., 1972) and when comparing diurnal rhythms of these hormones (Simon and George, 1975).

Thus far the only stimulus that has been reported to elevate both hormones simultaneously is morphine. Administration of small doses of morphine, 5 or 10 mg/kg, significantly elevates plasma GH levels. Larger doses, 20 or 40 mg/kg, elevate both GH and CS. Pretreatment with dexamethasone or naloxone blocks the CS rise but not that of GH produced by morphine (Kokka and George, 1974; Kokka, et al., 1973).

Martin et al. (1975) have shown the GH response to morphine to be dose dependent and exquisitely sensitive. There is a log dose response over a range of 10 to 10,000 μg/kg when morphine is injected intravenously. They also reported that preinjection of somatostatin, somatotropin-release inhibiting factor (SRIF), completely blocked the GH releasing effect, while large hypothalamic lesions involving the entire ventromedial nucleus (VMN) and part of the arcuate nucleus produced a partial blockade. However, in an earlier study Kokka and George (1974) reported that similar large lesions involving the VMN did not alter the normal GH response to morphine.

In methadone and heroin addicts the GH response to insulin hypoglycemia and arginine administration has been found to be impaired (Cushman, 1972).

THYROTROPIN

The primary action of the opiates on thyrotropin secretion is an inhibitory one. The acute administration, one hour following morphine injection, produces a prompt reduction in plasma levels of immunoassayable TSH. This effect can be seen with low doses, 5 or 10 mg/kg, of morphine. The administration of a larger dose, 20 mg/kg, produces a greater fall in TSH (Simon, et al., unpublished data). The latter effect may be due to the release of CS or stress of the larger dose of morphine since CS administration or a variety of stresses are known to inhibit thyroid activity (Brown-Grant, et al., 1954a,b) (see Table I).

Interestingly, TSH has a diurnal rhythm that closely parallels GH and like GH this rhythm is inversely related to CS (Simon, et al., unpublished data). Other similarities in the secretory patterns of TSH and GH are that their secretions may be inhibited by stresses and that their secretory rates are altered by low doses of morphine.

Chronic studies in rats with morphine and codeine also indicate that they have an inhibitory effect on TSH secretion. Histological studies have shown that chronic morphine administration (30 and 60 mg/kg twice daily) for 3 weeks decreased thyroid weights and pituitary TSH content, and prevented the appearance of thyroidectomy cells in the pituitaries (Hohlweg, et al., 1961). Administration of morphine for 12 days (10 and 20 mg/kg twice daily) reduces thyroid and pituitary weights and pituitary TSH content as measured by bioassay (Bakke, et al., 1974). Chronic administration of codeine or morphine, 14 and 12 days respectively, lowers basal thyroid function, but does not influence

Table I. Effects of Morphine on Plasma Corticosterone,
GH and TSH at 4 pm, 60 min Post Injection

	Dose mg/kg	Corticosterone μg/100 ml	GH ng/ml	TSH μU/ml
Saline	—	(30) 24.3 ± 1.59*	(30) 8.9	(20) 109.0 ± 9.0
Morphine	5	(30) 20.9 ± 1.89	(30) 74.5^A	(30) 62.98 ± 8.99**
	10	(30) 21.0 ± 1.50	(30) 83.7^A	(20) 63.01 ± 10.2**
	20	(30) 34.3 ± 2.56†	(30) 62.0^A	(15) 36.6 ± 6.01**

* Mean ± S.E.M.
(—) Number of rats
Student's t test used for comparison of CS and TSH drug groups with saline
† p 0.01
** p 0.001
^{A} = 0.001
Rank — Sum vs saline. Since GH data deviate from a normal distribution within groups, nonparametric statistics were used to compare medians of GH values (Simon & George, 1975).

TSH hypersecretion due to methyl- or propylthiouracil administrations.

The first studies in which ^{131}I was used for assessing pituitary-thyroid activity during morphine administration were reported by Sámel (1958). He found that injecting rats with morphine (10 mg/kg) daily subcutaneously inhibited ^{131}I uptake and release of ^{131}I-labeled hormone by the thyroid. George and Lomax (1965), also using ^{131}I-labeled hormone to assay TSH secretion, noted that repeated administration of small doses of morphine (5-10 mg/kg) inhibited thyroid hormone release within 24 hours following the initial injection. ·This inhibition persisted throughout the injection period of 66 hours and for 24-30 hours following the last injection.

In an effort to localize this inhibitory site of morphine action, Lomax and George (1966) investigated the effects of systemic morphine administration in rats with hypothalamic lesions. Bilateral electrolytic lesions were made in two groups of rats: in one the region of the anterior hypothalamic/ventromedial nuclei and the other in the medial mammillary nuclei. Repeated injections of morphine (5-10 mg/kg) produced a marked inhibition in thyroid activity in rats with anterior lesions. The inhibition was comparable to that found in intact animals. On the other hand, lesions in the mammillary nuclei completely blocked the thyroid inhibitory effect of morphine and the release curves were virtually identical with those of untreated controls (see Table II). The lesion sites, on histological examination were found to involve, rostrally, the paraventricular and anterior hypothalamic nuclei and, caudally, all or part of the medial mammillary nuclei. Most importantly, the median

Table II. Summary Table of the Effects of Systemic Administration of
Morphine on Thyroid [131] I Release Rates
in Intact and Hypothalamic Lesioned Rats

	Number of Animals	Mean Initial Release Rate ± S.E.M. (% per 24 hr)	Mean Release Rate after Morphine (%)	P
Intact	10	16.9 ± 0.7	3.0 ± 0.8	<0.01
Rostral hypothalamic lesions	9	14.8 ± 0.6	3.0 ± 1.1	<0.01
Caudal hypothalamic lesions	9	13.4 ± 0.8	13.0 ± 1.0	<0.5

eminence and the infundibular tract were left intact. From these data it would appear that the thyroid inhibitory effect of morphine is mediated via the caudal hypothalamus in the region of the medial mammillary nuclei (see Table II).

It is well established that the anterior region of the median eminence of the hypothalamus is concerned with the regulation of pituitary TSH secretion. Electrolytic lesions in this area reduce the basal level of thyroid secretion and prevent propylthiouracil-induced goiter formation while electrical stimulation of this region increases plasma TSH levels as measured by radioimmunoassay in rats (Martin and Reichlin, 1970). And finally, the presence of thyrotrophin-releasing factor (TRF) in this region has been clearly documented.

Morphine is a compound which has a dual action on the CNS, i.e. it may act as a stimulant or a depressant. The dose of morphine used in these studies (5 mg/kg) was found to cause an elevation in body temperature in the rat in contrast to higher doses which produced a marked hypothermia. These temperature changes are due to a direct action of morphine on the thermoregulatory centers in the anterior hypothalamus (Lotti et al., 1965a). Also, injection of morphine into rats pretreated with nalorphine, or into rats made tolerant to morphine, frequently produced a rise in their body temperature (Lotti et al., 1965b; 1966).

If one assumes that tolerance develops to the depressant and not the stimulant effects of morphine (Seevers and Deneau, 1963), and that nalorphine antagonizes, primarily, the depressant effects of morphine (Woods, 1956), then the increase in core temperature in the rats studied by Lotti et al. (1965a,b) must be due to a stimulant effect of morphine on the thermoregulatory centers in the hypothalamus. Thus, if we can extrapolate from these studies to the effect of morphine on thyroid activity, it would seem possible that the dose of morphine used (5 mg/kg) could have had an excitatory effect on the hypothalamic neurons resulting in a reduction in thyroid activity by activation of inhibitory areas in the posterior hypothalamus.

To test this hypothesis, studies were undertaken to determine the effects of microinjection of morphine into various regions of the hypothalamus on thyroid function in the rat (Lomax et al., 1970). Doses of 5 or 10 μg of morphine were injected and a total of 36 rats received bilateral injections of morphine sulfate into various regions of the hypothalamus. They were injected with 5 μg in each site at 48 and 56 hr, then 10 μg at 72 and 80 hr after the onset of thyroid counting. Of the animals so treated, 14 exhibited marked inhibition of thyroid ^{131}I release during the period of injections. The injection sites in these 14 rats were found to lie in two principal areas: between the preoptic nuclei and the chiasma, or in the region of the posterior and the supramammillary nuclei. In the 6 rats with rostral injection sites, morphine completely arrested the release of ^{131}I, but the release returned to normal after the 72nd hr, before the final injection of morphine. In contrast to these animals, the release of ^{131}I was abolished throughout the period of morphine administration in the 8 animals injected into the caudal hypothalamic regions. Injection of morphine into other hypothalamic sites failed to alter normal thyroid activity.

The inhibition of thyroid secretion following morphine injection into the rostral hypothalamus was a rather unexpected finding and indicates that the drug does not have a single site of action. These data pointed out that morphine has a more complex action on pituitary-thyroid function than we had visualized from our earlier experiments.

As mentioned previously, morphine has a dual action on the CNS. Both stimulation and depression of neurons can occur. Tolerance develops to the depressant but not to the stimulant action of morphine. Therefore, it is interesting to note that in the case of injections into the rostral hypothalamic sites, there was a reversion to the normal thyroid release rate even during the period of morphine administration. This suggests the development of tolerance to morphine. A similar type of tolerance was seen to the hypothermic effect of morphine by Lotti et al. (1966). In contrast to this, tolerance was not detected when morphine was injected into the caudal hypothalamus. It would seem that there are two target sites for morphine in the hypothalamus: both activation of a caudal site and depression of a rostral site leading to decreased pituitary-thyroid activity. This possibility is further supported by the studies of Lotti et al. (1965a) who found that injection of microquantities of morphine into the rostral hypothalamus produced hypothermia, catatonia, respiratory depression, and an increase in pain threshold, effects which are commonly noted after a large systemic dose of morphine. Conversely, injection of morphine into the caudal hypothalamus produced hyperthermia and marked excitation, associated with increased motor activity and aggressive behavior.

Recent experiments in our laboratory, using immunoassay, show that tolerance to the TSH-inhibiting effect of morphine does not occur. Rats injected for 2 weeks with a 40 mg/kg dose twice daily showed a 60% reduction in plasma TSH levels 1 hour after their last injection when compared with saline injected controls. Also, these TSH levels were found to be significantly lower than levels found in rats with 17 hour withdrawal. These data indicate that the greater inhibitory effect on TSH secretion by chronic morphine administration is more specific than the stress of withdrawal (Simon et al., unpublished observations).

In 6 methadone maintained addicts normal TSH responses to a large dose of TRH (400 μg i.v.) have been reported although the authors state "that more subtle alterations in either pituitary or thyroidal response might be demonstrated with the administration of smaller amounts of TRH." Also basal levels of T_4, T_3 and TSH were found to be in the normal range (Shenkman et al., 1972).

MORPHINE AND BRAIN AMINES

There are many conflicting reports in the literature regarding the effects of morphine and brain biogenic amines. In a review by Way (1972), he cites evidence that clearly links serotonin to many morphine effects, i.e., analgesia, tolerance and physical dependence. However, he carefully points out that "it should be recognized that morphine affects other neurohormones and the functions of these brain substances very likely are enmeshed." This view is supported by Collier et al. (1972), who found that atropine, para-chlorophenylalanine and indomethacin, a prostaglandin inhibitor, modify some effects of morphine withdrawal in the rat.

Morphine also has been shown to deplete brain catecholamines, an effect probably reflected by increased turnover, since the drug increases the incorporation of ^{14}C-tyrosine into ^{14}C-dopamine and ^{14}C-norepinephrine (Smith, 1972).

Data on morphine's effect on brain acetylcholine levels are in discord too. However, Cheney, et al., (1975) studying the rate of acetylcholine (ACh) turnover, reported that the single injection of morphine (140 μ moles/kg i.p.) reduced synthesis of ACh in occipital cortex but not in striatum. Chronic morphine administration, with implanted pellets, decreased ACh turnover in striatum without affecting occipital cortex ACh. Naloxone reversed both turnover changes. These interrelationships have been reviewed recently by de Wied, et al. (1974).

Effects of morphine on anterior pituitary and brain amines

In view of morphine's effects on brain biogenic amines, anterior pituitary hormone activity and the modulating effect brain amines have on the pituitary, studies were undertaken to determine whether correlations could be found between the amines (5-HT, NE, DA) in different brain regions and hormones in male rats as a result of acute and chronic morphine treatment.

Acute morphine effects

In this study, late afternoon was chosen for amine and hormone measurements because striking diurnal shifts occur at this time period (Simon and George, 1975). GH levels at 4:00 p.m. are in the declining phase while CS levels were rising. In addition, regional brain amine levels undergo diurnal shifts in late afternoon. The brain regions were striatum, septum, cortex, amygdala pons, midbrain and hypothalamus. Also, we felt that the amines and hormones might be most vulnerable to disruption by morphine if injected at a time when levels were changing.

Morphine was injected in doses of 5, 10, and 20 mg/kg. All injections were given at 3:00 p.m. and the rats were sacrificed an hour later. The low doses, 5 and 10 mg/kg, elevated GH levels only. Administration of 20 mg/kg increased both CS and GH plasma levels. The only significant change in brain amine level was an increase in striatal dopamine (Simon, George and Garcia, 1975a).

Chronic morphine effects

This study was designed to examine the relationship between regional levels of brain amines (norepinephrine, NE; dopamine, DA; and serotonin, 5-HT) and plasma hormone levels (corticosterone, CS; and growth hormone, GH) in rats following chronic morphine administration (40 mg/kg twice daily). Rats were sacrificed at 4:00 p.m. (and the final injection was made at 9:00 a.m.). Amine and hormone levels were determined after 1, 2, and 6 weeks of daily injections of morphine. Increased plasma CS was found after 1 and 2 weeks of injections and decreased GH levels were present after 2 and 6 weeks. In another 2 week study when morphine was administered 1 hour before sacrifice, plasma levels of CS were decreased and GH increased. Serotonin levels were decreased in all brain regions after 2 and 6 weeks of morphine administration and DA was decreased in the amygdala after 6 weeks. In 2 weeks treated rats injected 1 hour before sacrifice 5-HT levels had returned to control levels and DA was decreased. Inverse correlations were found to relate with 5-HT and CS levels, CS with GH levels and GH with brain DA. A direct correlation was present in GH and 5-HT levels (Simon, George and Garcia, 1975b).

SUMMARY

It is apparent from the evidence cited above that morphine and methadone alter hypothalamic-pituitary function.

The secretions of the anterior pituitary gland have been found to be under the control of polypeptide releasing factors (RF) which are released into a capillary system in the median eminence at the base of the hypothalamus. The releasing factors are carried down the pituitary stalk by the hypophyseal portal vessels which form sinusoids in the anterior pituitary and allow the releasing factors to act on the hormone synthesizing cells. Evidence suggests that RF release is regulated, at least in part, by the action of several neurotransmitter pathways known to be present in the hypothalamus. In addition, the influence of several other brain areas on hormone secretion has been studied by electrical stimulation and lesioning techniques. The influence of areas such as the midbrain and limbic system is believed to be exerted through excitatory and inhibitory inputs to the hypothalamus, which may be mediated by one or more of the transmitters found there in high concentration. Among those transmitters that have been proposed to have influence over the hormone secretions are acetylcholine, serotonin (5-HT), norepinephrine (NE), and dopamine (DA).

The effects of morphine and methadone on pituitary function are probably mediated via their actions on the limbic-midbrain circuit, (this circuit has been reported to contain the highest concentration of opiate receptors, Kuhar et al., (1973); Hiller et al., (1973) which in turn alters the levels of transmitter substances in the hypothalamus.

Morphine, acutely administered, produces a distinct pattern of effects on anterior lobe function that is dose related. Low doses increase GH and inhibit TSH secretion. High doses increase both GH and CS plasma levels while inhibiting TSH release. Preadministration with naloxone completely blocks the rise in plasma CS while enhancing the GH releasing effect.

Chronic administration of morphine produces adrenal cortical hypertrophy, although CS levels return to normal. TSH secretion remains below normal control levels while the GH releasing effect persists.

In contrast to the effects of chronic morphine administration, abstinence or naloxone precipitated withdrawal markedly elevated plasma CS levels while lowering GH and TSH levels.

Although the behavioral effects of morphine may vary in different species (cat shows excitement, rat shows depression) the hormonal changes are alike. During withdrawal the cat becomes catatonic while the rat is hyperactive, however the hormonal pattern again remains the same in both species. Thus by measuring hormonal changes as well as behavioral effects during an addiction cycle it is possible to quantify more precisely the transmitters and identify those circuits that are involved in the phenomena of tolerance, physical dependence and abstinence.

In conclusion, it would seem from these studies that there are at least two distinct types of neurons that are affected by morphine. One type is activated by small doses of morphine and this effect is not antagonized by naloxone nor does tolerance occur to this effect. The second type is depressed by high doses of morphine. This depressant effect is blocked by naloxone preadministration or by chronic morphine administration.

ACKNOWLEDGMENT

The preparation and part of the work reported in this manuscript were supported by a research grant from USPHS, DA01006.

REFERENCES

Bakke, J. L., N. L. Lawrence, and S. Robinson. 1974. The effect of morphine on pituitary-thyroid function in the rat. *Eur. J. Pharmacol.* 25: 402–406.

Blackwell, R. E., and R. Guillemin. 1973. Hypothalamic control of adenohypophysial secretions. *Ann. Rev. Physiol.* 35: 357–390.

Borrell, J., I. Llorens, and S. Borrell. 1974. Study of the effects of morphine on adrenal corticosteroids, ascorbic acid and catecholamines in unanesthetized and anesthetized cats. *Hormone Res.* 5: 351–358.

Brown-Grant, K., G. W. Harris and S. Reichlin. 1954a. The effect of emotional and physical stress on thyroid activity in the rabbit. *J. Physiol.* (London) 126: 29–40.

Brown-Grant, K., G. W. Harris, and S. Reichlin. 1954b. The influence of the adrenal cortex on thyroid activity in the rabbit. *J. Physiol.* (London) 126: 41–51.

Cheney, D. L., M. Trabucchi, C. Racagni, C. Wang, and E. Costa. 1975. Effects of acute and chronic morphine on regional rat brain acetylcholine turnover rate. *Life Sciences* 15: 1977–1990.

Collier, H. O. J., D. L. Francis, and C. Schneider. 1972. Modification of morphine withdrawal by drugs interacting with humoral mechanisms: Some contradictions and their interpretation. *Nature* (London) 237: 220–223.

Cushman, P. Jr. 1972. Growth hormone in narcotic addiction. *J. Clin. Endocrinol. Metab.* 35: 352–358.

Cushman, P. Jr., and M. J. Kreek. 1974. Some endocrinologic observations in narcotic addicts. In E. Zimmerman and R. George, Eds. *Narcotics and the Hypothalamus.* Raven Press, New York, pp. 161–173.

de Wied, D., and W. de Jong. 1974. Drug effects and hypothalamic-anterior pituitary function. *Ann Rev. Pharmacol.* 14: 389–412.

de Wied, D., J. M. van Ree, and W. de Jong. 1974. Narcotic analgesics and the neuroendocrine control of anterior pituitary function. In E. Zimmerman and R. George, Eds. *Narcotics and the Hypothalamus.* Raven Press, New York, pp. 251–264.

Eisenman, A. J., H. F. Fraser, and J. W. Brooks. 1961. Urinary excretion and plasma levels of 17-hydroxycorticosteroids during a cycle of addiction to morphine. *J. Pharmacol. Exp. Ther.* 132: 226-231.

French, E. D., J. F. Garcia, and R. George. 1974. Intracerebral morphine and naloxone effects on growth hormone and cortisol in naive and morphine dependent cats. *Proc. West. Pharmacol. Soc.* 17: 159–163.

Fuxe, K., and T. Hökfelt. 1969. Catecholamines in the hypothalamus and the pituitary gland. In W. F. Ganong and L. Martini, Eds. *Frontiers in Neuroendocrinology.* 1969. Oxford University Press, New York, pp. 47–96.

George, R. 1971. Hypothalamus: Anterior pituitary gland. In D. H. Clouet, Ed. *Narcotic Drugs, Biochemical Pharmacology.* Plenum Press, New York, pp. 283–299.

George, R., and P. Lomax. 1965. The effects of morphine, chlorpromazine and reserpine on pituitary-thyroid activity in rats. *J. Pharmacol. Exp. Ther.* 150: 129–134.

George, R., and E. L. Way. 1959. The role of the hypothalamus in pituitary-adrenal activation and antidiuresis by morphine. *J. Pharmacol. Exp. Ther.* 125: 111–115.

Hiller, J. M., J. Pearson, and E. J. Simon. 1973. Distribution of stereospecific binding of the potent narcotic analgesic etorphine in the human brain: Predominance in the limbic system. *Res. Commun. Chem. Pathol. Pharmacol.* 6: 1052–1063.

Hohlweg, V. W., G. Knappe, and G. Dörmer. 1961. Tierexperimentelle

Untersuchunger über den Einfluss von Morphin auf die Gonadotrope und Thyrotrope Hypophsenfunktion. *Eudokr. Bd.* 40: 152–159.

Kokka, N., J. F. Garcia, and H. W. Elliott. 1973. Effects of acute and chronic administration of narcotic analgesics on growth hormone and cortico-' trophin (ACTH) secretion in rats. *Prog. Brain. Res.* 39: 347–358.

Kokka, N., J. F. Garcia, R. George, and H. W. Elliott. 1972. Growth hormone and ACTH secretion: Evidence for an inverse relationship in rats. *Endocrinology* 90: 735–743.

Kokka, N., and R. George. 1974. Effects of narcotic analgesics, anesthetics, and hypothalamic lesions on growth hormone and adrenocorticotrophic secretion in rats. In E. Zimmerman and R. George, Eds. *Narcotics and the Hypothalamus.* Raven Press, New York, pp. 137–157.

Kuhar, M. J., C. B. Pert, and S. H. Snyder. 1973. Regional distribution of opiate receptor binding in monkey and human brain. *Nature* (London) 245: 447–450.

Lomax, P., and R. George. 1966. Thyroid activity following administration of morphine in rats with hypothalamic lesions. *Brain Res.* 2: 361–367.

Lomax, P., N. Kokka, and R. George. 1970. Thyroid activity following intracerebral injection of morphine in the rat. *Neuroendocrinology* 6: 146–152.

Lotti, V. J., Kokka, N., and R. George. 1969. Pituitary-adrenal activation following intrahypothalamic microinjection of morphine. *Neuroendocrinology* 4: 326–332.

Lotti, V. J., P. Lomax, and R. George. 1965a. Temperature responses in the rat following intracerebral microinjection of morphine. *J. Pharmacol. Exp. Ther.* 156: 135–139.

Lotti, V. J., P. Lomax, and R. George. 1965b. N-allylnormorphine antagonism of the hypothermic effect of morphine in the rat following intracerebral and systemic administration. *J. Pharmacol. Exp. Ther.* 156: 420–425.

Lotti, V. J., P. Lomax, and R. George. 1966. Acute tolerance to morphine following systemic and intracerebral injection in the rat. *Int. J. Neuropharmacol.* 5: 35–42.

Martin, J. B., A. Audet, and A. Saunders. 1975. Effects of somatostatin and hypothalamic ventromedial lesions on GH release induced by morphine. *Endocrinology* 96: 839–847.

Martin, J. B., and S. Reichlin. 1970. Thyrotropin secretion in rats after hypothalamic electrical stimulation or injection of synthetic TSH-releasing factor. *Science* 168: 1366–1368.

Paroli, E., and P. Melchiorri. 1961. Urinary excretion of hydroxy-steroids, 17-ketosteroids and aldosterone in rats during a cycle of treatment with morphine. *Biochem. Pharmacol.* 6: 1–17.

Sámel, M. 1958. Blocking of the thyrotropic hormone secretion by morphine and chlorpromazine in rats. *Arch. Int. Pharmacodyn.* 117: 151–157.

Schreiber, V., V. Zbusek, and V. Zbuzkova-Kmentova. 1968. Effect of codeine on thyroid function in the rat. *Physiol. Bohemoslov.* 17: 253–258.

Seevers, M. H., and G. A. Deneau. 1963. Physiological aspects of tolerance and physical dependence. In W. S. Root and F. G. Hofman, Eds. *Physio-logical Pharmacology*, Vol. 1. Academic Press, New York, pp. 565–640.

Shenkman, L., B. Massie, T. Mitsuma, and C. S. Hollander. 1972. Effects of chronic methadone administration on the hypothalamic-pituitary-thyroid axis. *J. Clin. Endocrinol. Metab.* 35: 169–170.

Simon, M. L., and R. George. 1975. Diurnal variations in plasma cortico-sterone and growth hormone as correlated with regional variations in norepinephrine, dopamine and serotonin content of rat brain. *Neuro-endocrinology* 17: 125–138.

Simon, M. L., R. George, and J. F. Garcia. 1975a. Acute morphine effects on regional brain amines, growth hormone and corticosterone. *Europ. J. Pharmacol.* 34: 21–26.

Simon, M. L., R. George, and J. F. Garcia. 1975b. Chronic morphine effects on regional brain amines, growth hormone and corticosterone. *Europ. J. Pharmacol.* 34: 27–38.

Sloan, J. W., 1971. Corticosteroid hormones. In D. H. Clouet, Ed. *Narcotic Drugs, Biochemical Pharmacology*. Plenum Press, New York, pp. 262–282.

Smith, C. B. 1972. Neurotransmitters, and the narcotic analgesics. In S. J. Mulé and H. Brill, Eds. *Chemical and Biological Aspects of Drug Depen-dence*. CRC Press, Cleveland, pp. 495–504.

Sobel, H., S. Schapiro, and J. Marmorston. 1958. Influence of morphine on urinary corticoid excretion by guinea pigs following exposure to cold and administration of Pitressin. *Amer. J. Physiol.* 195: 147–149.

Takahashi, K., W. H. Daughaday, and D. M. Kipnis. 1971. Regulation of immunoreactive growth hormone secretion in male rats. *Endocrinology* 88: 909–917.

Way, E. L. 1972. Role of serotonin in morphine effects. *Fed. Proc.* 31: 113–120.

Woods, L. A. 1956. The pharmacology of nalorphine. *Pharmacol. Rev.* 8: 175–198.

Wurtman, R. J. 1971. Brain monoamines and endocrine function. *Neurosci. Res. Progr. Bull.* 9(2): 172–297.

Tissue Responses to Addictive Drugs
© 1976, Spectrum Publications, Inc.

Effect of Morphine on the Ulstrastructure of the Pituitary Gland in Normal and Ovariectomized Rats

EVA B. CRAMER
DONALD H. FORD

Department of Anatomy
State University of New York
Downstate Medical Center
Brooklyn, New York

Considerable physiological evidence has accumulated which indicates that morphine affects hormonal secretion from the anterior pituitary gland of many species (George, 1971).

In humans acute morphine administration (as in morphine anesthesia) inhibits cortisol and growth hormone (GH) response to surgical stress (George et al., 1974). Similarly, in chronic morphine administration, as in heroin or methadone addicts, adrenal corticosteroid (CS) secretion is reduced (Eisenman et al., 1961) and the GH response to insulin hypoglycemia is impaired (Cushman, 1972). Heroin addiction also causes amenorrhea and menstrual dysfunction in women (Stoffer, 1963; Gaulden et al., 1964; Bai et al., 1974) and impotence or decreased libido (Cushman, 1973) and a lowered plasma testosterone level in men (Mendelson et al., 1974; Mendelson and Mello, 1975). However, serum thyroxine and triiodothyronine concentrations have been reported to be normal in heroin (Cushman, 1972) and methadone addicts (Shenkman et al., 1972).

In an attempt to understand morphine induced hormonal abnormalities seen in humans, investigators have been studying the effects of opiates on laboratory animals. Acute administration of morphine to rats significantly elevates plasma CS (Hirai et al., 1970; Kokka et al., 1973; Yamamoto, 1973; Sable-Amplis, 1974), GH (Kokka et al., 1973; Martin et al., 1975) and prolactin (LTH) levels (Zimmerman et al., 1974; Zimmermann and Pang, 1976), while plasma levels of thyrotrophin (TSH) (George and Kokka, 1976), lutenizing hormone (LH) and f°llicle-stimulating hormone (FSH) (Zimmerman and Pang, 1976) are lowered.

On the other hand, chronic administration of morphine to rats results in a decrease in CS secretion (Munson and Briggs, 1955; Paroli and Melchiorri, 1961), an increase in plasma levels of GH (Kokka et al., 1973), a decrease in pituitary TSH content (Bakke e tal., 1974), and a threefold increase in pituitary FSH, while pituitary content of LH is not altered (Rennels, 1960).

Despite the growing physiological evidence of altered pituitary function cited above, there have been few histological studies of the anterior pituitary glands of morphine-treated animals. Fourteen years ago Holweg et al. (1961) reported chronic morphine administration prevented the appearance of thyroidectomy cells, and Rennels (1961), also using chronic morphine treatment, indicated an increase in what he believed were FSH cells in male rats. Recently, Yano et al. (1973) reported a dilation of the endoplasmic reticulum in ACTH producing cells after acute morphine administration.

To determine if ultrastructural changes occur in other pituitary cells, the anterior pituitary glands of normal rats chronically treated with morphine were examined with the electron microscope. In an attempt to more dramatically demonstrate the morphological effect of chronic morphine treatment on hormone secretion, the anterior pituitary glands of animals producing and secreting increased quantities of gonadotrophic hormone (ovariectomized rats) were also studied with the electron microscope.

MATERIALS AND METHODS

Six normal adult female rats and eight, four-week ovariectomized rats of the Sprague Dawley strain from Charles River, weighing approximately 300 grams were used in this study. Half the animals were injected via chronic indwelling venous catheters with increasing doses of morphine (30, 45-50, 60-70, 90 mg/kg) twice daily for four days and 120 mg/kg once in the morning of the fifth day. Equal volumes of saline were injected into pair-fed control rats maintained under similar conditions (14 hours light, 10 hours dark). Approximately 2-2½ hours after the last injection the animals were killed by guillotine and the anterior pituitary gland quickly removed and fixed in 2% glutaraldehyde in 0.1 M phosphate buffer pH 7.3. Two and one-half to four hours later the tissues were then rinsed in 0.1 M phosphate buffer, postfixed in 1% osmium tetroxide in 0.1 M phosphate buffer, dehydrated and embedded in Epon 812. Thin sections were stained with uranyl acetate and lead citrate and examined with the Phillips 300 electron microscope. Vagina smears were taken from the non-castrate animals and the weights of the thyroids, adrenals and ovaries of all animals determined.

DISCUSSION

In general the animals in both the intact and ovariectomized groups had a similar reaction to the intravenous injections of morphine. A short time after the initial 30 mg/kg dose the rats manifested muscular rigidity, catalepsy, exophthalmia and the Straub tail effect. After the afternoon injection the animals were no longer rigid or cataleptic, although they still exhibited exophthalmia and the Straub tail effect. The 45-50 and 60 mg/kg doses caused exophthalmia and the Straub tail effect after both the morning and afternoon injections. The 70 and 90 mg/kg dose caused the same type of reaction as the 30 mg/kg dose and the one dose of 120 mg/kg on the morning of the last day also resulted in marked muscular rigidity, catalepsy, exophthalmia and Straub tail effect.

Endocrine weights

There was no significant difference in the absolute or relative weight of the adrenals or thyroids in either the intact or ovariectomized experimental and control animals. Likewise, there was no significant difference in ovarian weight of intact, morphine-, or saline-injected rats.

Vaginal Smears

While the saline pair-fed intact controls were in various stages (proestrus, estrus, metestrus) of the estrous cycle at the time of death, the intact animals in the morphine-injected group were all in diestrus.

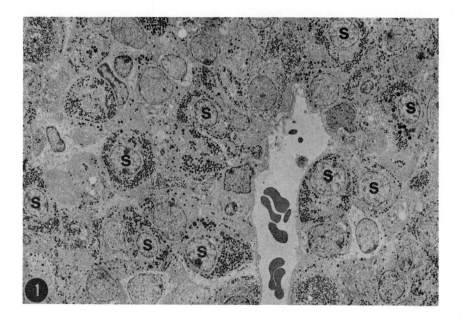

Low magnification of the anterior pituitary gland of a saline-injected intact control rat. Note the relative number of secretory granules in the somatotrophs (s). (×1,800.)

Anterior Pituitary Gland

Intact

Examination of the anterior pituitary of intact control and morphine-injected animals revealed some differences. Scanning of pituitary cells at low magnification revealed that the morphine injected rats had anterior pituitary glands which appeared to have fewer secretory granules (see Figures 1 and 2). This difference seemed to be due to a decrease in the number of secretory granules in somatotrophs. Closer examination of somatotrophs revealed normal appearing endoplasmic reticulum and a Golgi complex with newly forming secretory granules. There was no obvious increase in lysosomes or change in the mitochondria or nuclei. However, round or oval areas resembling areas of extracted lipid were seen with increased frequency in the cytoplasm of morphine-treated animals (see Figure 3). Similar structures were seen with equal frequency in nongranular pituitary cells (chromophobes) of both saline- and morphine-injected animals. Examination of cells producing prolactin, gonadotrophin, and thyroid-stimulating hormone revealed cells in different stages of secretion but without significant

544

differences from controls. Golgi complexes with newly forming secretory granules were apparent. There was no obvious change in the number of secretory granules, dilation of the endoplasmic reticulum, change or increase in lysosomes, or variations in the mitochondria or nucleus.

Ovariectomized

Scanning of the anterior pituitary gland of control and morphine-treated ovariectomized animals revealed similar numbers of gonadectomy cells in both groups. There was no obvious ultrastructural effect on secretion. The gonadectomy cells were in various stages of transition into signet ring cells. Consequently, there was no apparent inhibition of the dilation of ER or its ability to coalesce. The Golgi complexes were large and contained newly forming secretory granules. Since release of secretory granules is difficult to observe in gonadectomy cells (Mendoza et al., 1973; unpublished observations), no attempt was made to quantitate this phenomenon. The nucleus and mitochondria of these cells appeared normal. Initially it seemed that there was an increased number of lysosomes in the experimental gonadectomy cells but further inspection revealed no significant differences from controls.

Low magnification of the anterior pituitary gland of a morphine-treated intact rat. Note that the somatotrophs (s) have fewer secretary granules than controls. (g) gonadotroph. ($\times$2,200).

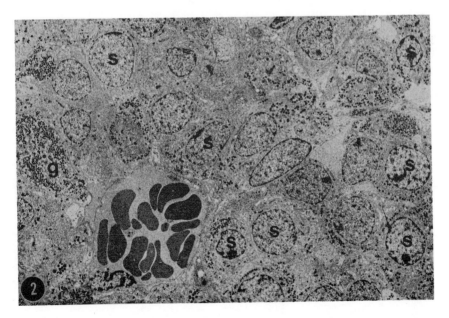

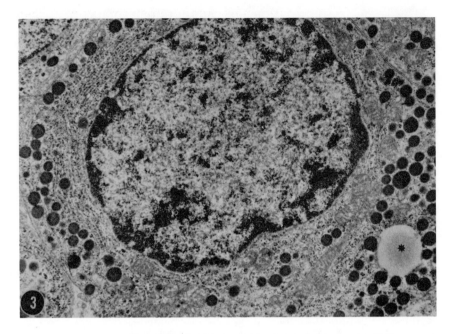

Somatotroph of a morphine-treated intact rat which contains a lipid droplet (star) among its secretory granules. (×11,900.)

As in the intact animals chronically treated with morphine, there appeared to be an increase in lipid in the pituitary cells of morphine-treated ovariectomized animals. However, the presence of lipid seemed more common in the morphine-treated ovariectomized rats (see Figure 4). Lipid was found with increased frequency in somatotrophs (see Figures 5 and 6) and luteotrophs (see Figure 7). It was usually found in close association with secretory granules or near the Golgi apparatus. Again, as in the normal rats, lipid was seen in similar amounts in non-granular cells (chromophobes) of control and experimental ovariectomized animals (see Figure 8). However, in the ovariectomized group of animals the lipid droplets in each cell type frequently appeared more electron opaque than those seen in the intact group of experimental and control animals. This difference may be due to the longer time (hour to one and a half hour) the pituitary glands of the ovariectomized rats were in the glutaraldehyde fixative.

CONCLUSIONS

The results of these studies reveal that chronic morphine treatment causes an increased accumulation of lipid in the somatotrophs of intact female rats. The cause of the increased accumulation of lipid in these cells is uncertain, however it is further accentuated in the ovariectomized rat. In these castrate animals lipid is now also found in prolactin-producing cells. From these observations it would appear that the female sex steroids may have a modifying effect on the action of morphine.

Low magnification of the anterior pituitary gland of a morphine-treated ovariectomized rat. Castration increases the number of lipid droplets (arrows) in pituitary cells. (×3,200.)

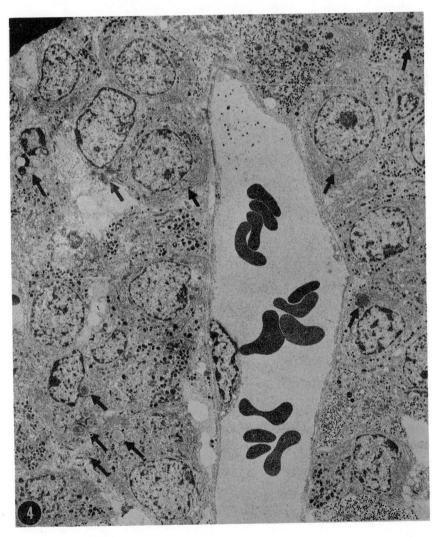

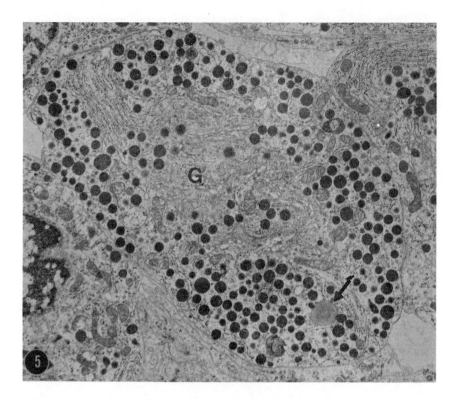

Somatotroph of a morphine-treated ovariectomized rat which contains a lipid droplet (arrow) among its secretory granules. Note the large Golgi complex (G). (×7,800.)

Morphine treatment has been reported to cause structural changes in cell organelles of two other areas of the endocrine system. The first reported change was a transformation of the shape of the mitochondrial cristae of the cells of the zona fasiculata of the adrenal cortex six hours after a single dose of morphine (Yano et al., 1973). The second reported change was an increase in the incidence of whorled bodies of endoplasmic reticulum (rough endoplasmic reticulum changing to smooth endoplasmic reticulum) in neurons of the hypothalamus of male rats. This was observed after both acute and chronic morphine administration (Ford et al., 1974). Hence morphine has been shown to alter the appearance of endoplasmic reticulum and mitochondria and in this study to cause lipid accumulation in cells of the endocrine system. Perhaps these ultrastructural findings will provide some clue to its metabolic site of action.

Examining pituitary cells with the electron microscope is a way to observe extreme changes in pituitary secretion, whereas subtle changes would be much more difficult to detect. The reasons for these limitations are: observations of a limited area of pituitary tissue; normal variation in the relative number of secretory granules in pituitary cells which produce the same hormone; and the inability to kill control and experimental animals at the exact time of a pulsatile burst of hormone release of each cell type. From this study the only apparent effect on secretion was a relative degranulation of somatotrophs. Whether this reflects a decrease in synthesis, an increase in release, or some other alteration in cellular metabolism is unclear. However, Kokka et al. (1973) have reported an increase in plasma GH after chronic morphine treatment which may indicate that the fewer numbers of secretory granules seen in these cells is due to an increase in hormone release. Although the estrous cycle in intact morphine-treated animals appeared to be interrupted, no obvious changes in gonadotrophs occurred. And again, after ovariectomy, no changes in gonadectomy cells were observed. The possible reasons why more morphological changes in secretion were not detected may be that: the animals had become tolerant to morphine; morphine does not have a sustained effect on secretion and its influence is gone by 2-2½ hours after administration; and/or the

Somatotroph of a morphine-treated ovariectomized rat which contains three large lipid droplets (stars). Newly forming secretory granules can be seen in the Golgi complex (G). (×11,900.)

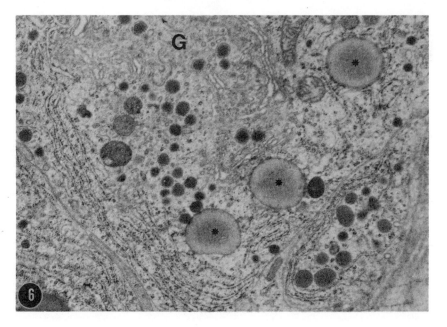

alterations in secretion are too subtle to be detected by this technique alone. To eliminate these problems the best way to continue this investigation would be to first monitor changes in the pituitary and plasma levels of pituitary hormones by radioimmunossay and then to study the process of secretion with electron microscopic autoradiography.

SUMMARY

Intact and ovariectomized adult female Sprague Dawley rats were chronically injected two times daily with increasing doses of morphine (30, 45-50, 60-70, 90, and 120 mg/kg). After 5 days the anterior pituitary glands of morphine and saline injected rats were removed and embedded for electron miscroscopy. Ultrastructural inspection of the anterior pituitary gland of morphine-treated intact animals appeared to reveal

Luteotrophs of morphine-treated ovariectomized rats. A lipid droplet (star) can be seen in the cytoplasm of a degranulated luteotroph. Newly forming secretory granules (arrows) can be seen in the Golgi region. (×10,200.) Inset. An example of lipid accumulation (star) in a granulated luteotroph. (×8,500.)

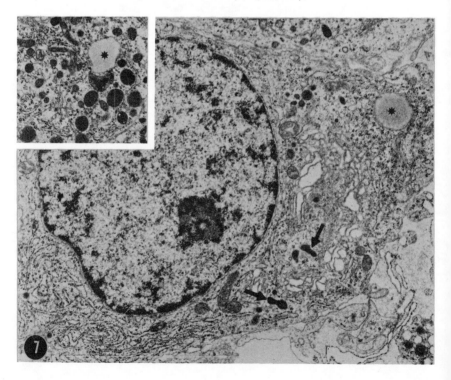

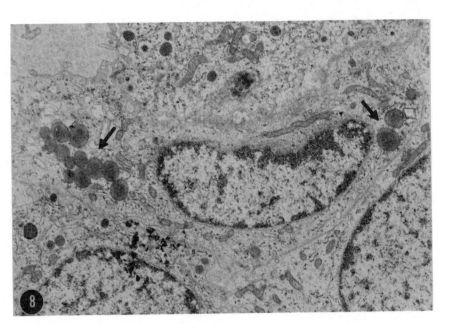

Lipid droplets (arrows) in a chromophobe of a morphine-treated ovariectomized rat. (×9,200.)

a decrease in the number of secretory granules in somatotrophs and an increase in the number of lipid droplets in the cytoplasm of these cells. Following ovariectomy there was a further increase in the amount of lipid in the anterior pituitary gland of morphine-treated animals. More lipid droplets were seen in somatotrophs and lipid accumulation in luteotrophs was now apparent. No definitive change in the ultrastructure of gonadectomy cells was noted.

ACKNOWLEDGMENT

The preparation and work reported in this manuscript was supported by a grant number DA 00114–04 from the USPHS National Institute of Drug Abuse.

REFERENCES

Bai, J., E. Greenwald, H. Catering, and H. A. Kaminetzky. 1974. Drug related menstrual aberrations. *Obstetr. Gynecol.* 44: 713–719.
Bakke, J. L., N. L. Lawrence, and S. Robinson. 1974. The effect of morphine on pituitary-thyroid function in the rat. *Eur. J. Pharmacol.* 25: 402–406.

Cushman, P., Jr. 1972. Growth hormone in narcotic addiction. *J. Clin. Endocrinol. Metab.* 35: 352–358.

Cushman, P. Jr. 1973. Plasma testosterone in narcotic addiction. *Amer. J. Med.* 55: 452–458.

Eisenman, A. J., H. F. Fraser, and J. W. Brooks. 1961. Urinary excretion and plasma levels of 17-hydroxycorticosteroids during a cycle of addiction to morphine. *J. Pharmacol. Exp. Ther.* 132: 226–231.

Ford, D. H., K. Voeller, B. Callegari, and E. Gresik. 1974. Changes in neurons of the median eminence-arcuate region of rats induced by morphine treatment: An electronmicroscopic study. *Neurobiology* 4: 1–11.

Gaulden, E. C., D. C. Littlefield, O. E. Putoff. 1964. Menstrual abnormalities associated with heroin addiction. *Amer. J. Obstet. Gynecol.* 90: 155–160.

George, J. K., C. E. Reier, R. R. Lanese, and J. M. Rower. 1974. Morphine anesthesia blocks cortisol and growth hormone response to surgical stress in humans. *J. Clin. Endocrinol. Metab.* 38: 736–741.

George, R. 1971. Hypothalamus: Anterior pituitary gland. In D. H. Clouet, Ed. *Narcotic Drugs, Biochemical Pharmacology.* Plenum Press, New York, pp. 283–299.

George, R., and N. Kokka. The effects of narcotics on growth hormone, ACTH and TSH secretion. (This text)

Heyden, S. 1969. Epidemiology. In F. G. Schettler, and G. S. Boyd, Eds. *Atherosclerosis.* Elsevier Publishing Company, Amsterdam, pp. 289–301.

Hirai, M., L. K. Nan, and T. Nakao. 1970. Acute effect of morphine administration on secretion of adrenal corticosterone in rats. *Endocrinol. Japon.* 17: 65–81.

Holweg, W., G. Knappe, and G. Dörner. 1961. Investigation of experimental animals on influence of morphine on gonadotrophin and thyrotrophin hypophyseal function. *Endokrinologie* 40: 152–159.

Kokka, N., J. F. Garcia, and H. W. Elliott. 1973. Effects of acute and chronic administration of narcotic analgesics on growth hormone and corticotrophin (ACTH) secretion in rats. *Prog. Brain Res.* 39: 347–360.

Martin, J. B., J. Audet, and A. Saunders. 1975. Effects of somatostatin and hypothalamic ventromedial lesions on GH release induced by morphine. *Endocrinology* 96: 839–847.

Mendelson, J. H., and N. K. Mello. 1975. Plasma testosterone levels during chronic heroin use and protracted abstinence. *Clin. Pharm. Ther.* 17: 529–533.

Mendelson, J. H., J. E. Mendelson, and V. D. Patch. 1974. Effect of heroin and methadone on plasma testosterone in narcotic addicts. *Fed. Proc.* 33: 232 (Abstract)

Mendoza, D., A. Arimura, and A. V. Schally. 1973. Ultrastructure and light microscopic observations of rat pituitary LH-containing gonadotrophs following injection of synthetic LH-RH. *Endocrinology* 92: 1153–1160.

Munson, P. L., and F. N. Briggs. 1955. The mechanism of stimulation of ACTH secretion. *Rec. Prog. Horm. Res.* 11: 83–117.

Paroli, E., and P. Melchiorri. 1961. Urinary excretion of hydroxysteroids, 17-ketosteroids and aldosterone in rats during a cycle of treatment with morphine. *Biochem. Pharmacol.* 6: 1–17.

Rennels, E. G. 1960. The effect of morphine on the pituitary content of FSH and LH in the rat. *Anat. Rec.* 136: 264 (Abstract)

Rennels, E. G. 1961. Effect of morphine on pituitary cytology and gonadotrophic levels in the rat. *Texas Rep. Biol. & Med.* 19: 646–657.

Sable-Amples, R., R. Agid, and D. Abadie. 1974. Reversal of the action of morphine on the secretory activity of the adrenal cortex. *Biochem. Pharm.* 23: 2111–2118.

Shenkman, L., B. Massie, and T. Mitsuma. 1972. Effects of chronic methadone administration on the hypothalamic-pituitary-thyroid axis. *J. Clin. Endocrinol. Metab.* 35: 352–358.

Stoffer, S. S. 1963. A gynecologic study of drug addicts. *Amer. J. Obstet. Gynecol.* 101: 779–783.

Yamamoto, H., S. Mikita, I. Yano, Y. Masuda, and T. Murano. 1973. Studies on the physical dependence liability of analgesics. 2. Relationship between transformation of intramitochondrial structures in adrenocortical cells and corticosterone biosynthesis in morphine addicted rats. *Jap. J. Pharmacol.* 23: 217–225.

Yano, I., H. Nishino, H. Yamamoto, and T. Murano. 1973. Studies on the physical dependence liability of analgesics. 1. Electron microscopic studies on the ultrastructural transformation of mitochondria in the cells of zona fasciculata of the adrenal cortex in morphine addicted rats. *Jap. J. Pharmacol.* 23: 201–215.

Zimmerman, E., and C. N. Pang. Acute effects of opiate administration on pituitary gonadotrophin and prolactin release. (This text)

Zimmermann, E., C. N. Pang, and C. H. Sawyer. 1974. Morphine-induced prolactin release and its suppression by dexamethadone in male rats. *56th Ann. Meeting, The Endocrine Soc.* No. 526. (Abstract)

Tissue Responses to Addictive Drugs
© 1976, Spectrum Publications, Inc.

Psychotropic Drug-stress Interaction Effects on the Hypothalamic-pituitary-adrenal Axis in Man and a Nonhuman Primate

J. MARK ORDY
K. R. BRIZZEE
M. B. KAACK

Data Regional Primate Research Center
Tulane University
Covington, Louisiana

J. L. CLAGHORN

Texas Research Institute of Mental Sciences
Houston, Texas

DRUG EFFECTS ON NEUROENDOCRINE REGULATION

Adaptation to aversive and noxious stimuli in a changing environment is one of the basic homeostatic requirements for the survival of animals and man. Although the nervous and endocrine systems may have fundamentally different modes of operation, both are involved in the defense of the organism against noxious stimuli and stress. Homeostatic adjustment and equilibrium are maintained by the integrated activity of the hypothalamus and neuroendocrine system. New concepts and interdisciplinary research approaches, starting from different points of view, have now converged to examine the effects of various psychotropic drugs on the brain with particular emphasis on the hypothalamus and on neuroendocrine regulation of adaptation to deviations

555

from steady state environmental conditions, stress and other environmental challenges.

During the past ten years some very remarkable and rapid progress has been made in clarification of basic mechanisms and of drug effects on neuroendocrine regulation. This rapid progress can be attributed in part to concurrent advances in the following areas: 1) neuropsychology; recent developments include relating behavioral adaptations to stress to physiological, neurochemical, and morphological changes in the limbic system, neuroendocrines, the hypothalamic-pituitary-adrenal axis, and the autonomic system; 2) neuroendocrinology; increasing evidence has been presented for a role of neurotransmitters and releasing/inhibitory substances of neuroendocrine transducer cells in the hypothalamus as regulators of endocrine function; 3) neuropharmacology; there has been continuing clarification of drug effects on neurotransmitters and neuroendocrine regulation; and 4) psychopharmacology; increasing evidence has been reported for inhibition by psychotropic drugs of stress-induced release of hypothalamic monoamines, CRF, pituitary ACTH, adrenal corticosteroids, and catecholamines. The aims of this chapter are to provide a brief synopsis of current concepts and research findings on the structural and functional organization of: the limbic, neuroendocrine, and autonomic systems, with particular emphasis on the hypothalamic-pituitary-adrenal axis; on hypothalamic control through monoamines and releasing or inhibiting factors of pituitary-adrenal secretions; and on stress-induced release of hypothalamic monoamines, corticotrophic releasing factors (CRF), pituitary ACTH, adrenal cortisol, and catecholamines, and their inhibition by psychotropic drugs. After a brief review of current work on limbic and neuroendocrine regulation of pituitary and adrenal hormones, experimental evidence will be presented from some acute and chronic experiments with normal and psychiatric subjects, and nonhuman primates on stress-induced release of hypothalamic norepinephrine, serotonin, pituitary ACTH, adrenal cortisol, and catecholamines, and their inhibition by two major tranquilizers, chlorpromazine (CPZ) and haloperidol (HPD).

ROLE OF THE BRAIN AND ENDOCRINES IN LEARNING AND HOMEOSTASIS

The brain plays a unique role in adaptation to the physical and social environments through reflexes, conditioning and learning. Learning and homeostasis are attained and maintained by the coordinated activities of the brain and endocrines. There has been increasing evidence that the hypothalamus, neuroendocrine and limbic components of the CNS, integrate by intricate homeostatic feedback mechanisms the responses to deviations from steady state conditions, stress and various environmental challenges (Michael, 1968; Ganong, 1970; Smelik, 1970). The "language" of neurons consists of electrochemical codes. Neuroendocrine homeostatic feedback regulation appears to be maintained by both hypothalamic neurotransmitters and hormones. The integration between the brain and endocrines is most apparent in the hypothalamus. In response to converging neural stimuli, hypothalamic neuroendocrine "transducer" cells secrete factors or hormones that stimulate or inhibit the release of pituitary hormones (Wurtman, 1971). Pituitary-adrenal hormones in turn have a profound influence on the brain through the median eminence (Ganong, 1970; de Wied, 1970).

Whereas psychopharmacological studies of learning have focused on the neocortex and drugs that influence learning through cholinergic mechanisms (Carlton, 1969), the limbic system, the hypothalamic-pituitary-adrenal axis and drugs that affect biogenic amines have received increasing attention in relation to emotions or affective states, drives, arousal and reactivity to stress. As part of the adaptation to acute and chronic aversive or noxious stimuli, "fear motivated" learning and levels of arousal or affective states have now been "linked" through the limbic system and the hypothalamic-pituitary-adrenal axis (Kety, 1967, 1972; de Wied, 1970). The potential role of catecholamines which mediate the actions of hallucinogenic, narcotic drugs, antidepressants and anti-psychotic drugs has also been examined (Friedhoff, 1975).

LIMBIC SYSTEM, NEUROENDOCRINES, HYPOTHALAMIC-PITUITARY-ADRENAL AXIS, AUTONOMIC RELATIONS

The limbic system includes structures of the forebrain that are anatomically interconnected with one another and with the hypothalamus. The neuroendocrine system is broadly defined as those structures in the CNS that are concerned with the regulation of endocrine function. With the known exceptions of the direct innervations of the adrenal medulla and pineal gland, CNS influences on endocrine functions appear to be mediated by the hypothalamo-hypophysial neurovascular connections. A widely used classification of limbic structures subdivides the limbic regions into three systems: the rhinal system with direct connections from the olfactory bulb; the Paleo system which includes a portion of the old cortex and the amygdala; and the hippocampal-cingulate system, with the hippocampus and related regions of the old cortex (Papez, 1937; MacLean, 1949; Hockman, 1972). The limbic influences on the hypothalamic-pituitary-adrenal axis occur through a corticotrophic releasing factor (CRF), presumably localized in a "pool" of neuroendocrine transducer neurons of the hypothalamus. It has been proposed that the limbic-hypothalamic and, subsequently, the pituitary-adrenal regulation of homeostatic adaptation is based on excitatory and inhibitory pathways. The hippocampus and amygdala of the limbic system have been implicated in short term memory and expression of emotions, respectively. The amygdaloid complex and the hippocampus seem to be major limbic structures that regulate the CRF-neuron pool in the hypothalamus (Schadé, 1970). Firing patterns of neurons in the CRF-pool are low under basal conditions. Disturbances of the internal or external environments significantly enhance their tonic activity and result in CRF release (Cross and Silver, 1966). It has been proposed that afferent impulses from the limbic system mediate the significant increases in pituitary ACTH secretion in response to emotional stimuli and stress (Ganong, 1970). Recent research developments include clarification of higher cortical control of limbic and autonomic functions (Hockman, 1972), the possible identification of hypothalamic monoamines and releasing factors and their responsiveness to a wide range of stimuli and to drugs (Martini and Meites, 1970; de Wied and de Jong, 1974), neurochemical aspects in neuroendocrine regulation of adaptation to environmental challenges (Siegel and Eisenman, 1972), and the mode of excitatory-inhibitory influences of hypothalamic monoamines in regulation of neuroendocrine transducer cells and endocrine function (Ganong, 1970; Wurtman, 1971; Frohman and Stachura, 1975).

Negative or inhibitory feedback loops are general endocrine characteristics for maintaining the particular level of hormone output in response to acute and chronic disturbances. A change in the endocrine gland secretory activity is detected by control mechanisms. This information is used to adjust the control mechanism. The control of neuroendocrine secretory activity also involves "feedback loops." For many of the neuroendocrine secretions, receptor cells sensitive to the levels of various hormones in the general circulation have been proposed in the pituitary, hypothalamus and limbic systems (Ganong, 1970, 1974). "Short and long" negative closed, as well as positive "open" feedback loops for emergency "overrides" have been proposed for the control of neuroendocrine functions (Ganong, 1970). ACTH-cortisol interactions represent a closed-loop feedback for the rate of basal ACTH secretion. However, converging neural inputs in the hypothalamus represent open-loop feedback for overriding basal secretions and providing increased ACTH output in response to stress (Ganong, 1970) (see Figure 1).

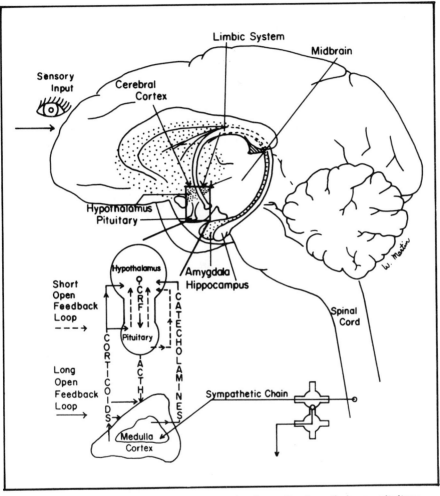

1 Limbic system, neuroendocrines, the hypothalamus-pituitary-adrenal axis and autonomic system relations.

Several key concepts are essential for the interpretation of any integrated activity produced by acute and chronic drug-stress interaction effects in the limbic system, neuroendocrines, the hypothalamic-pituitary-adrenal axis and the autonomic nervous system. With acute or chronic stress, it may be essential to "override" the negative and closed feedback control loop level and "set" the hormone concentrations to different levels. A "set-point" theory of neuroendocrine control has been proposed for pituitary ACTH released under acute or chronic as opposed to basal conditions (Ganong, 1970; Siegel and Eisenman, 1972). The law of initial value (LIV) has also been proposed for assessment of autonomic lability or refractoriness in response to arousal and stress. According to this so-called law, for autonomic lability, it is necessary to equate treatment or stress effects for pretreatment or basal differences within and among subjects in the assessment of homeostasis (Wilder, 1950; Lacey, 1956). More recent trends include behavioral biofeedback conditioning of autonomic responses in normal subjects and in some psychosomatic disorders (Lacey, 1972; Birk, 1973).

STRESS ACTIVATION OF THE LIMBIC SYSTEM, NEUROENDOCRINES, HYPOTHALAMIC-PITUITARY-ADRENAL AXIS

It is now widely accepted that stress induced activation of the limbic system and the hypothalamic-pituitary-adrenal axis in mammals involves changes in neuronal excitability in the limbic system, hypothalamic monoamines, releasing or inhibiting factors, pituitary ACTH, adrenal corticosteroids, and catecholamines (Harris and George, 1969; Ganong, 1970; Smelik, 1970; Siegel and Eisenman, 1972). Stimulus variables used for the activation of the neuroendocrine system have ranged from subtle psychological factors to more direct effects produced by electric shock, temperature, surgical trauma, and various chemical agents. Response variables have included such diverse categories as behavioral disorganization and autonomic arousal, alterations in biogenic amines and corticotrophic releasing factors (CRF) in the hypothalamus, changes in the pituitary secretions of ACTH, and the adrenal output of corticosteroids and medullary catecholamines (Ganong, 1966, 1970, 1972; Siegel and Eisenman, 1972). Some remarkable progress has been made in recent years in relating behavioral adaptation to stress to physiological, biochemical, and morphological changes in the limbic system (Rick and Thompson, 1965; Nauta, 1972) and the hypothalamic-pituitary-adrenal axis (de Wied et al., 1968; Fuxe et al., 1970; Mirsky, 1970; Wurtman, 1971; Mason, 1972). Pituitary ACTH and related peptides have been reported to facilitate learning, whereas corticosteroids appear to facilitate extinction of fear-motivated behavior (de Wied et al., 1970; McEwen and Weiss, 1970). Aversive stimuli, changes in psychosocial relations, and drugs have been reported to change hypothalamic monoamines (Ordy et al., 1966; Welch and Welch, 1969; Wurtman, 1971), monoamine oxidase (MAO) activity (Eleftheriou and Boehlke, 1967), releasing factors (Meites, 1970), and also lead to increased secretions of adrenal corticosteroids (Mason, 1972) and catecholamines (Henry et al., 1971; Goldberg and Welch, 1972). Single unit electrical and microchemical studies have identified hormone-sensitive neurons in the limbic system and hypothalamus as part of the "short and long, closed negative and open positive feedback loops" that are involved in neuronal and hormonal interactions during behavioral adaptation to stress (Ganong, 1970; de Wied, 1970). Ablations and stimulations of, or steroid implants in the limbic system and reticular formation have also been reported to alter adrenal secretions (Siegel and Eisenmen, 1972). Stress-induced increases in circulating corticosteroid levels have been related to emotional states and to Na-K activated ATPase in the brain (Maas, 1972); to single unit neuronal excitability in the limbic system (Steiner, 1970; to increased nuclear size of neurons in hypothalamic regions (Palkovits and Mitro, 1968) and also to increased nuclear size of cells in adrenals (Kotby et al., 1971; Palkovits and Stark, 1972). In some neurochemical interpretations of the etiology of affective disorders including schizophrenia, it has been proposed that biogenic amine "reward" mechanism may be damaged in the limbic system and the diencephalon (Wise and Stein, 1973). It has also been proposed that biogenic amines may play not only an important role in mood, motivation, and memory but that they may be significantly altered in some affective disorders (Kety, 1972; Friedhoff, 1975). However, some investigators have questioned the exclusive reliance on the "catecholamine hypothesis" of affective disorders (Grote et al., 1974).

MAJOR HYPOTHESES CONCERNING CONTROL OF PITUITARY-ADRENAL HORMONES

Due to the rapid effects elicited by sensory stimuli and emotional arousal, it has been widely accepted that the CNS must play a major role in regulating the synthesis and release of pituitary ACTH. It is now generally accepted that the hypothalamus is the focal point at which neural stimuli converge to regulate pituitary secretions. However, at various times, the following three major hypotheses have been proposed for control of pituitary ACTH secretion: Pituitary ACTH secretion is regulated by blood levels of epinephrine; ACTH secretion depends upon the level of circulating adrenocortical hormones; and ACTH secretion is regulated by neurotransmitters acting on excitatory or inhibitory factors of neuroendocrine transducer cells in the hypothalamus (Harris and George, 1969; Ganong, 1970, 1974).

According to the hypothesis of epinephrine release of pituitary

ACTH, stress results in hypothalamic stimulation, transmission of neural impulses through the brainstem to the adrenal medulla, release of epinephrine, and the triggering of pituitary ACTH by increased circulating epinephrine (Harris and George, 1969). Increases in blood ACTH concentrations after an epinephrine infusion have been observed in the rat (Farrell and McCann, 1952) and in man (Vernikos-Danellis and Marks, 1962). However, in other studies, increases in blood ACTH were not observed in the dog or in man (Nelson et al., 1952; Arner et al., 1963; Vance and Shioda, 1964). These conflicting findings have suggested that the role of epinephrine in the release of ACTH in man remains questionable. The extensive use of tranquilizers in neuropsychiatric disorders has also prompted considerable interest in their role as blocking agents for inhibiting the pituitary output of ACTH in response to stress (Harwood and Mason, 1957; Munson, 1963; de Wied and de Jong, 1974; Frohman and Stachura, 1975). However, while some animal studies have indicated inhibition of stress-induced release of pituitary ACTH (Mahfouz and Ezz, 1958), other studies have shown hypersecretion of ACTH into circulation and a significant reduction of pituitary ACTH by phenothiazines independent of stress (Smith et al., 1963). Significant increases in catecholamines in the blood of normal subjects have been reported after stress (von Euler, 1964) and in neuropsychiatric patients (Pscheidt et al., 1964). Other studies have reported significant differences in cardiovascular responses to epinephrine infusion between normal subjects and psychiatric patients (Cardon et al., 1961; Jus, 1964; Cardon and Mueller, 1964; Albin et al., 1965). The reported differences in circulating catecholamines between normal subjects and neuropsychiatric patients have suggested that there should also be significant differences in blood ACTH concentrations if epinephrine plays a role in the release of ACTH. However, basal blood ACTH concentrations of psychiatric patients or after an epinephrine infusion and tranquilizers have not been examined previously.

In order to test the hypothesis of stress-induced epinephrine release of pituitary ACTH, a study was undertaken to compare ACTH concentrations in samples of blood obtained from normal and psychiatric subjects before and after an epinephrine infusion. Specific aims of the study were as follows: to compare blood ACTH concentrations before and after a one-minute epinephrine infusion between normal female subjects and acute schizophrenic female patients; to examine the effects of a one-minute saline infusion and of the blood withdrawal on blood ACTH concentrations of normal female subjects; and to examine blood ACTH levels and the effect of chlorpromazine on blood ACTH concentrations in acute schizophrenic female patients before and after three weeks of CPZ treatment.

Twenty-four normal and 24 acute schizophrenic females ranging in age from 21 to 40 years were assigned to 4 groups. Group 1 with 12 normal subjects received a one-minute epinephrine infusion (0.25 μg/kg) and the second group of 12 Ss served as control for a one-minute saline infusion and blood withdrawal. Group 3, with 12 schizophrenic patients, was infused for one minute with epinephrine, and Group 4, with 12 Ss, received 3 weeks of chlorpromazine treatment (100/400 mg per day oral CPZ). Estimates of ACTH concentrations in the pre- and post-infusion and the pre- and post drug groups were made by the adrenal ascorbic acid depletions (AAAD) produced by the 25 ml human blood samples in hydrocortisone-blocked assay rats. The 2 blood samples were separated by a 2.5-minute interval. Blood was collected into heparinized syringes. The AAAD values were converted to ACTH concentrations by a log-dose relationship obtained by 3 blood volumes and three ACTH reference standards and expressed as mU ACTH/100 ml (Vernikos-Danellis and Marks, 1962).

The one-minute epinephrine infusion did not result in a significant increase in blood ACTH of the 12 normal (pre-epi 7.94; postepi 4.57) or 12 psychiatric (pre-epi 11.58; postepi 9.55) subjects. Blood ACTH concentrations were, in fact, significantly lower in the second blood sample of the 12 normal females after the one-minute epinephrine infusion and in the second blood sample of 12 normal saline-infused and blood withdrawal female controls (preSal 9.12; postSal 6.32) ($p < .01$). The first blood samples of the 12 psychiatric females in the epinephrine-infusion group and the 12 patients in the CPZ treatment group contained significantly higher concentrations of ACTH than those of the 24 normal subjects. Compared to blood ACTH levels at the time of admission, blood ACTH levels in the 12 psychiatric patients after three weeks of CPZ decreased significantly (preCPZ 10.96; postCPZ 6.03) ($p < .01$) (see Figure 2).

Assay of blood ACTH was made on male albino Wistar rats weighing 90–120 g. The adrenal ascorbic acid depletion (AAAD) of each 25 ml blood sample was established by the i.v. injection of the whole human blood at 3 ml/100 g rat body weight into six hydrocortisone-blocked rather than hypophysectomized assay rats (Vernikos-Danellis and Marks, 1962). The AAAD values were converted into ACTH estimates by a log-dose relationship determined by three blood samples (1.5, 3.0, 6.0 ml/100 g rat) and three ACTH reference standards (.05, .20, .80 mU ACTH/ml Armour, 25 units/mg, lyophilized) (see Figure 3).

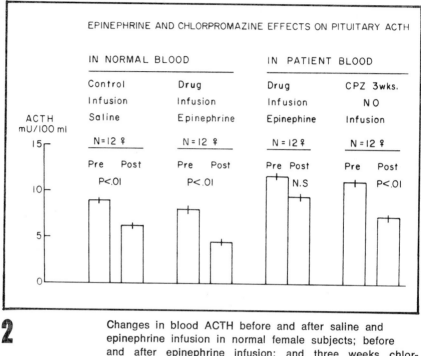

EPINEPHRINE AND CHLORPROMAZINE EFFECTS ON PITUITARY ACTH

2 Changes in blood ACTH before and after saline and epinephrine infusion in normal female subjects; before and after epinephrine infusion; and three weeks chlorpromazine in female psychiatric patients.

HYPOTHALAMIC NEUROTRANSMITTERS AS REGULATORS OF NEUROENDOCRINE TRANSDUCER CELL FACTORS AND PITUITARY ACTH

It is now widely accepted that terminals of hypothalamic neuroendocrine transducer cells lie in close approximation to the primary capillary plexus, and secrete specific factors or hormones into it that travel through the portal system to stimulate or inhibit the release of anterior pituitary hormones. There are an increasing number of studies on neurotransmitter control by dopamine, norepinephrine and serotonin over these neuroendocrine transducer cell releasing or inhibiting factors that are involved in regulation of pituitary ACTH secretion (Ganong, 1974; Frohman, 1975; Frohman and Stachura, 1975). The convergence of various cholinergic and monoaminergic neural stimuli upon CRF-secreting neurons involves some complex patterns of CRF output based on ongoing basal levels, new set-points, circadian rhythms, circulating steroids, metabolic constituents, and acute and chronic stress. The three

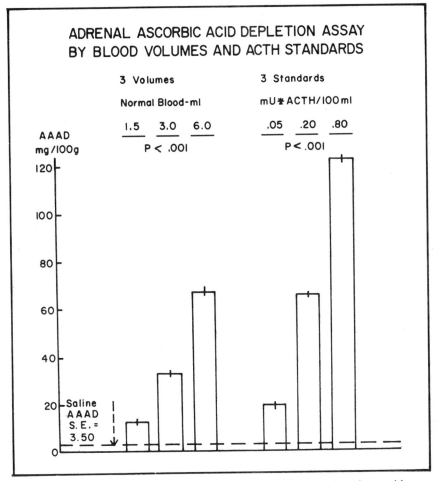

**ADRENAL ASCORBIC ACID DEPLETION ASSAY
BY BLOOD VOLUMES AND ACTH STANDARDS**

3 Assay of blood and pituitary ACTH by adrenal ascorbic acid depletion (AAAD) by i.v. injection of whole human blood at 3 ml/100 g rat body weight in six hydrocortisone-blocked assay rats. AAAD values were converted into ACTH estimates by a log-dose relationship based on three blood samples and three ACTH reference standards.

monoamines, dopamine, noreprinephrine and serotonin, have received increasing attention in regulation of CRF and other neuroendocrine secretions (Ganong, 1974). Some experimental evidence obtained in rats and dogs has suggested that the release of pituitary ACTH as regulated by CRF may be under inhibitory control of hypothalamic nor-

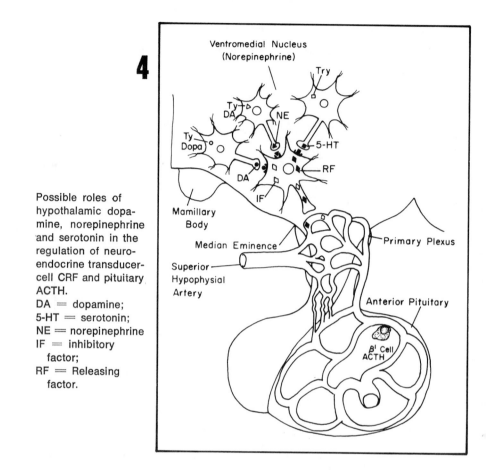

Possible roles of hypothalamic dopamine, norepinephrine and serotonin in the regulation of neuroendocrine transducer-cell CRF and pituitary ACTH.
DA = dopamine;
5-HT = serotonin;
NE = norepinephrine
IF = inhibitory factor;
RF = Releasing factor.

epinephrine (Ganong, 1970, 1971, 1972, 1974; de Wied and de Jong, 1974). Dopamine (DA), norepinephrine (NE) and Serotonin (5-HT) have been proposed for the regulation of CRF and other releasing (RF) or inhibitory (IF) factors of neuroendocrine transducer cells involved in the regulation of pituitary ACTH and other hormones (see Figure 4).

ACUTE AND CHRONIC DRUG-STRESS INTERACTION EFFECTS ON HYPOTHALAMIC MONOAMINES, PITUITARY ACTH, ADRENAL CORTISOL AND CATECHOLAMINES IN THE SQUIRREL MONKEY

A variety of drugs including chlorpromazine, haloperidol, nembutal, etc., as well as ether anesthesia have been reported to be potent inhibitors of stress-induced pituitary ACTH release through their possible effects on hypothalamic monamines (Guillemin, 1957, 1974; Maynert and Levi, 1963; de Wied and de Jong, 1974; Frohman and Stachura, 1975). Studies with human subjects are scarce and provide only indirect, fragmentary, and inconclusive evidence concerning drug inhibition of neurotransmitter control over stress-induced increases of pituitary ACTH secretions. Some conflicting findings have also been reported concerning the role of norepinephrine in the output of CRF since some studies have reported it to be inhibitory in the rat and dog but stimulatory in the baboon (Ganong, 1974; Frohman and Stachura, 1975).

Acute experiments on drug-stress interaction effects on the hypothalamic-pituitary-adrenal axis in the squirrel monkey

Studies with higher diurnal primates are also extremely scarce. A number of acute experiments were undertaken to examine the effects of brief social isolation, electric shock, chlorpromazine (CPZ), haloperidol (HPD) and reserpine on hypothalamic norepinephrine as well as the inhibition of electric shock-induced decreases in NE concentration by pretreatment with a single dose of chlorpromazine and haloperidol in the squirrel monkey (Ordy et al., 1966). In these acute experiments, 12 hours of social isolation resulted in significant hypothalamic norepinephrine depletion to .60 μg/g compared to basal levels of 1.60 μg/g in non-handled controls. A single injection of CPZ (15 mg/kg i.p.) had no effect 2 hours after injection on hypothalamic norepinephrine levels. A single injection of reserpine (10 mg/kg i.p.) reduced NE levels significantly to .20 μg/g after 12 hours. Pretreatment with a single dose of CPZ (15 μg/kg i.p.) and HPD (2.5 mg/kg, i.p) one hour before a 1-hour electric shock exposure effectively inhibited the electric shock depletions of hypothalamic norepinephrine (see Figure 5).

The concentrations of ACTH in pituitary tissue of nonhandled control, saline injected stress, chlorpromazine- and haloperidol-treated monkeys were also obtained by the adrenal ascorbic acid depletion in (AAAD) assay rats with i.v. injection of pituitary tissue extracts at 0.02 μg/ml. In 6 nonhandled controls, basal pituitary ACTH levels were 17.3 mU ACTH/mg of pituitary tissue. In a study with only 3 monkeys, 12 hours after capture, handling stress and a single injection of saline, ACTH tissue levels increased but not quite significantly to 25.0 mU ACTH/mg. Consequently, the critical acute experiments on stress, CPZ and HPD drug effects alone, and whether pretreatment with CPZ or HPD would inhibit stress-induced changes in pituitary tissue ACTH remain to be carried out. These acute drug-stress interaction effects on hypothalamic CRF and monoamine levels and pituitary tissue ACTH need

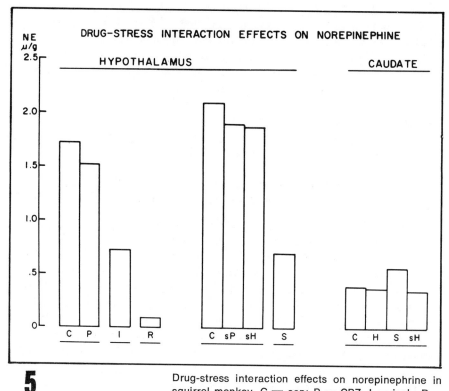

5 Drug-stress interaction effects on norepinephrine in squirrel monkey. C = con; P = CPZ, I = isol.; R = reserpine; H = HPD; S = shock; sP = shock and chlorpromazine sH = interaction.

to be carried out concurrently in the same subjects under carefully controlled temporal conditions to establish the direct role of hypothalamic monoamines on CRF and ACTH. Turnover studies of monoamines are also essential since tissue concentrations may not provide accurate assessment of the dynamic changes in synthesis and release in acute or chronic experiments. In this context, it should be noted that some studies have reported stress-induced increases in rate of synthesis of brain monoamines without affecting their levels (Smookler and Buckley, 1968).

In these acute experiments, the objectives were not only to examine drug-stress interaction effects on hypothalamic norepinephrine and pituitary ACTH but also to evaluate the output of adrenal cortisol and catecholamines in the squirrel monkey under basal conditions, saline injection, reserpine, and following isolation, handling and capture. The same biochemical procedures used for evaluation of hypothalamic catecholamines were also used to determine the norepinephrine and

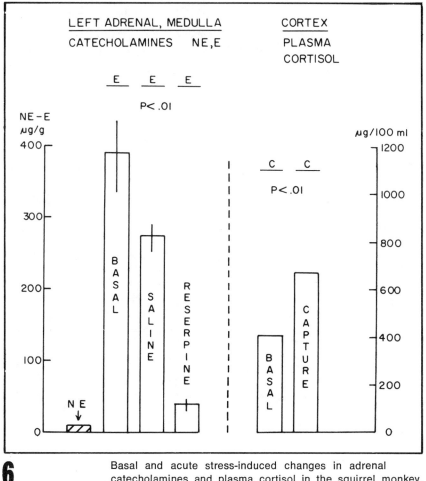

6 Basal and acute stress-induced changes in adrenal catecholamines and plasma cortisol in the squirrel monkey. Cortisol data from Brown, 1970.

epinephrine content in the adrenals of the squirrel monkey. Surprisingly, only epinephrine (E) was localized in the adrenals, indicating that the adrenal medulla of the squirrel monkey contained no measurable quantities of norepinephrine. It has been reported that cortisol (C) is the major steroid in squirrel monkey plasma. Extremely high resting or basal values of 405 μg/g/100 ml have been reported. One hour following capture and handling stress, cortisol values increased significantly to 672 and following chair restraint, to 1024 μg/g/100 ml (Brown et al., 1970, 1971) (see Figure 6).

7

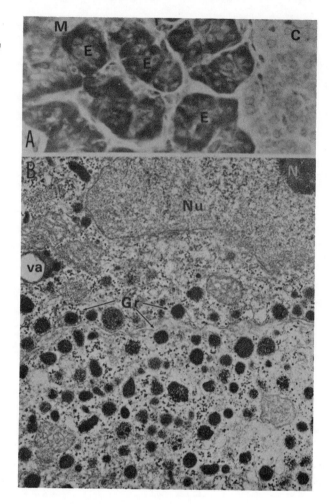

A. Histochemical localization of epinephrine-containing cells (E) in the adrenal medulla of the squirrel monkey.
M = medulla;
C = cortex.
×600.
B. Electron micrograph of epinephrine-containing cells with dense core granules (Gr) in the adrenal medulla of the squirrel monkey.
Nu = nucleus;
N = nucleolus;
Va = vacuole.
×14,000.

To verify the biochemical findings, histochemical and ultrastructural evaluations were also made to determine the cellular distribution of epinephrine and norepinephrine within chromaffin cells in the adrenal medulla of the squirrel monkey (Wood, 1963; Coupland and Hopwood, 1966) (see Figure 7). No norepinephrine-containing cells were demonstrable with these differential staining and electron microscopic procedures for the two catecholamines in the adrenal medulla of the squirrel monkey.

Light and electron microscopic evaluations were also made of the topography, morphological organization and the ultrastructure of the hypothalamus and neurovascular link between the hypothalamus and anterior pituitary in the median eminence of the squirrel monkey (Rinne and Arstila, 1965). Hypothalamic control of anterior pituitary lobe activity is mediated entirely through the factors carried by the hypophyseal portal circulation to the pituitary gland from the hypothalamic neuro-endocrine transducer cells which lie in close approximation to the primary capillary plexus. Granules and vesicles can be observed in nerve ter-minals adjacent to the capillary endothelium of the median eminence (see Figure 8).

Chronic drug-stress interaction effects on hypothalamic monoamines, pituitary ACTH and adrenal ascorbic acid in the squirrel monkey

Although many acute studies have been reported, few studies in-volving prolonged or chronic stress have been reported in the literature.

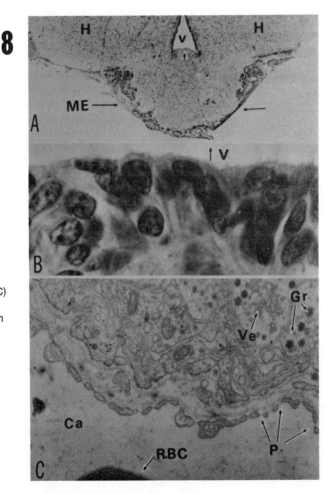

Morphology of hypothalamus in squirrel monkey: (A) topography, × 100; (B) cellular structure, × 600; (C) ultrastructure of neurovascular link in median eminence (ME), ×14,000. Ca = capillary; Gr = dense core vesicles; P = pores, Ve = vesicles; V = ventricle.

Table I. Chronic 30-day Drug-Stress Interaction Effects on
Norepinephrine (NE) in Ventromedial and Serotonin (5-HT)
in Dorsal Hypothalamus of the Squirrel Monkey

Monoamines	Non-handled	Saline	HPD .10 μg/kg	1 Hr. Elec. Shock	HPD .10 μg/kg Elec. Shock
Ss, n	n = 6	n = 6	n = 6	n = 6	n = 6
NE, M ± S.E.	1.60 − .17	.58 − .08*	.39 − .08*	.73 − .10*	.40 − .06†
5-HT, M ± S.E.	2.47 − .06	2.25 − .08	1.43 − .12*	1.74 − .15*	1.27 − .03†

* Group means significantly different from means of non-handled controls.
† One hr previous pretreatment with HPD and 1 hr electric shock interaction means are significantly lower than electric shock alone.

In one chronic 30-day study of drug-stress interaction effects on hypothalamic norepinephrine (NE) in the ventromedial region and serotonin (5-HT) in the dorsomedial region, 30 adult female squirrel monkeys were assigned to 1 nonhandled control group, 1 saline-injected stress group, 1 HPD (haloperidol) (.10 μg/kg) group, 1 electric shock group, and 1 electric shock-pretreated 1 hour with .10 μg/kg HPD group. Six Ss were in each group. The stress and drug treatment were carried out for 30 days. Thirty days of saline injection stress decreased NE significantly from 1.70 to 0.58 μg/g compared to nonhandled controls. HPD decreased NE to 0.39, electric shock to 0.73, and electric shock with pretreatment of HPD to 0.40 μg/g. This low dose level of HPD (.10 μg/kg), compared to the significant inhibition of stress effects by a higher dose of 2.5 μg/kg in the acute experiment, did not inhibit chronic stress effects on NE levels.

In contrast to decreased NE, 30 days of saline injection-stress did not decrease serotonin significantly (2.05 μg/g) compared to nonhandled 5-HT levels (2.47 μg/g). The 5-HT levels in the .10 μg/kg HPD, electric shock, and pretreatment with HPD (.10 μg/kg) followed by shock were 1.43, 1.74, and 1.27 μg/g, respectively (see Table I).

In another 30-day chronic study, drug-stress interaction effects were examined on escape-avoidance behavior, pituitary tissue ACTH, and adrenal ascorbic acid levels. Thirty-six adult female squirrel monkeys were assigned to 2 control and 4 drug groups and subjected to 30 days of handling and saline injection stress, behavioral testing, and drug treatment. One of the 2 control groups served as nonhandled controls and the second group received daily saline injections for 30 days. Group 3 received 5 mg/kg and group 4, 15 mg/kg CPZ. Group 5 received 0.1 and Group 6, 1.0 mg/kg HPD. Six Ss were assigned to each of the 6 groups. All Ss were tested 1 hour after i.m. saline or drug injection for

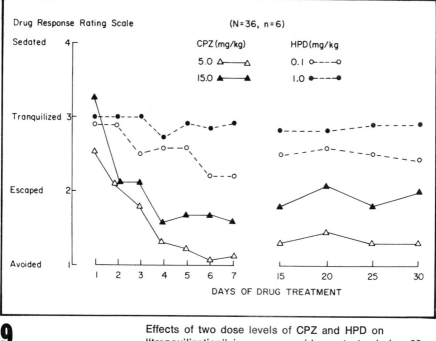

Drug Response Rating Scale   (N=36, n=6)

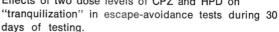

9

Effects of two dose levels of CPZ and HPD on "tranquilization" in escape-avoidance tests during 30 days of testing.

30 days on a four-point behavioral escape-avoidance test. The 2 dose levels of HPD resulted in a continuous average rating of "tranquilization" during 30 days of testing. The 2 dose levels of CPZ resulted in a comparable drug response primarily on day one with a rapid development of behavioral tolerance from day two onward at the lower CPZ dose level (see Figure 9).

All 36 monkeys were sacrificed by decapitation and the pituitary and adrenals were dissected in less than 2 minutes. Estimates of pituitary tissue ACTH in the 2 control, 2 CPZ and 2 HPD groups were obtained by the AAAD assay in rats by i.v. injection of 0.02 mg/ml pituitary extract (see Figure 10). The mean of the nonhandled control group (0) for pituitary ACTH was 17.3 mU ACTH/mg. Thirty days of saline injection and handling stress (PL) increased pituitary ACTH significantly to 93.0 mU ACTH/mg. Pituitary ACTH in the 30-day 5 mg/kg CPZ group was 37.1 and in the 15 mg/kg CPZ group, 16.2 mU ACTH/mg. Pituitary ACTH of both CPZ groups was significantly lower than the saline-injected stress group but the 15 mg/kg CPZ value of 16.2 did

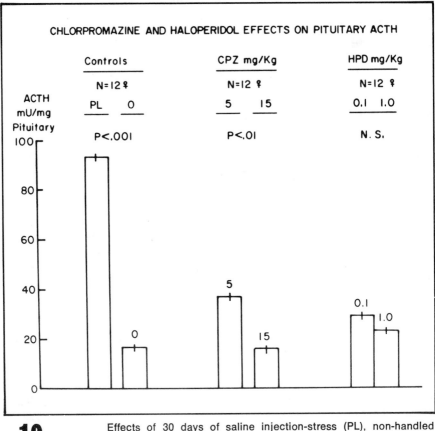

CHLORPROMAZINE AND HALOPERIDOL EFFECTS ON PITUITARY ACTH

Effects of 30 days of saline injection-stress (PL), non-handled control conditions (O), and two dose levels of CPZ and HPD on pituitary tissue ACTH in the squirrel monkey.

not differ significantly from the 17.3 value of the nonhandled control. Both CPZ groups differed significantly from each other. Pituitary ACTH of the 0.1 mg/kg HPD was 28.8 and of the 1.0 mg/kg HPD was 22.9 mU ACTH/mg. Pituitary ACTH in both HPD drug groups was significantly lower than in the saline-injected stress group but the 2 dose levels did not differ from each other nor from the nonhandled controls (see Figure 10).

The adrenals from the 36 monkeys were also evaluated for changes in adrenal ascorbic acid (AAA) concentration. Of the 2 control groups, the AAA mean of the nonhandled control group was 172 and of the saline-injected stress group, the mean was 209 mg/100 g adrenal tissue. The group mean of the 0.1 mg/kg HPD group was 216 and of the 1.0

mg/kg HPD group it was 200 mg/100 g. The group mean of the 5.0 mg/kg group was 174 and of the 15.0 mg/kg CPZ group it was 158 mg/100 g. As combined treatment groups, the two dose levels of HPD increased significantly, whereas the two dose levels of CPZ decreased significantly AAA compared to controls ($p < .05$).

USE OF THE SQUIRREL MONKEY AS A PRIMATE MODEL IN PSYCHOPHARMACOLOGY

For a variety of comparative and logistical reasons, the squirrel monkey has rapidly become one of the most widely used nonhuman primates in basic and biomedical research (Rosenblum and Cooper, 1968). The most frequently cited advantages for the use of the squirrel monkey in neurobiological research are the extensive sensory, learning and motor capacities in phylogenetic perspective and the very large size and weight of the brain relative to low body weight. Increasing use of the squirrel monkey has been reported in pharmacology (Hansen, 1968). Several neuroendocrinological studies have examined the effects of lesions, drugs, and stress on the hypothalamic-pituitary-adrenal axis in the squirrel monkey (Ordy et al., 1966; Brown et al., 1970, 1971). Since the squirrel monkey is highly responsive to its physical and social environments, considerable care has to be exercised in the housing, maintenance and handling of animals included in neuroendocrinological research. As in the case of man, particular attention is required to the selection and treatment of saline-injected and nonhandled control groups since it is apparent that the past history, conditioning, learning and conditioned expectancies interact with drug effects, particularly at lower dose levels, in the squirrel monkey, as they do in man. In order to identify sources of variance and draw conclusions at statistically acceptable levels of confidence in neuroendocrinological research with the squirrel monkey, at least two control groups and two drug levels appear essential in any experimental design in which attempts are made to examine drug-stress interaction effects on behavior in relation to electrical, chemical, and morphological variables in the brain and endocrines (see Figure 11).

GENERAL SUMMARY AND CONCLUSIONS

The limbic system and the hypothalamic-pituitary-adrenal axis are critically involved in the integration of responses to environmental stress and other challenges. An increasing number of studies have indicated

DRUG-STRESS INTERACTION PSYCHOPHARMACOLOGY DESIGN

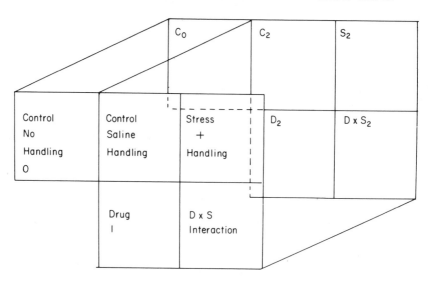

11

Schematic illustration of the minimum requirements of six subjects (squirrel monkeys) per group, at least two types of control groups, and two drug levels in a psychopharmacology experimental design for identifying sources of variance in drug-stress interaction effects, at statistically acceptable levels of confidence.

hypothalamic neurotransmitter control of neuroendocrine transducer cell CRF and pituitary ACTH secretions in response to stress (Wurtman, 1971; Ganong, 1974; Frohman and Stachura, 1975). Intricate interrelationships have been established among neurotransmitter-mediated impulses of limbic origin in the hypothalamus, their regulation of CRF and pituitary secretions, and various feedback influences from adrenal hormones on the neuroendocrine system. Three major hypotheses have been proposed for control of pituitary ACTH secretions: according to the "epinephrine hypothesis," stress increases systemic epinephrine which triggers release of pituitary ACTH; stress induced increases in circulating adrenocortical hormones influence ACTH secretions; neural impulses from limbic pathways convergence through hypothalamic monoamines to regulate CRF and pituitary ACTH secretion. Drug-stress interaction studies have indicated psychotropic drug inhibition of stress-induced release of hypothalamic monoamines, pituitary ACTH and adrenal hormones (Krieger, 1973; de Wied and de Jong, 1974). Pertinent studies were reviewed in this chapter briefly and some experimental evidence was also presented on acute and chronic drug-stress interaction effects on the hypothalamic-pituitary-adrenal axis in man and the squirrel monkey. Whereas some remarkable and rapid progress has been made on psychotropic drug effects on neuroendocrine functions, a number of gaps or points of conflict require clarification.

Pituitary ACTH secretion under basal and stress conditions

Studies with human subjects are scarce and provide only limited, fragmentary and indirect evidence of neuroendocrine control of ACTH secretion. In man, it has not been established whether pituitary ACTH secretions into circulation are continuous under basal conditions or occur only intermittently with arousal and stress (Ganong, 1963; Ney et al., 1963). Estimates of basal levels have ranged from 0.1 to 2.0 mU ACTH/100 ml in normal human blood (Vernikos-Danellis et al., 1966). Using a radioimmunoassay for ACTH, concentrations of 0.5 mU/100 ml, with a range of 0.3 to 0.7 mU/100 ml have also been reported (Demura, 1966). However, so-called basal blood ACTH can increase very significantly in normal and clinical conditions. In 8 patients with partial adrenalectomy for Cushing's syndrome, significant increases, ranging from 1.2 to 90.0 mU/100 ml have been reported (Nelson, 1966). In psychiatric patients, 1.5 mU ACTH/100 ml was estimated in 2 of 11 patients. No detectable corticotrophic activity was found in the 9 other patients, or in 15 normal controls tested under the same conditions (Persky, 1962).

Effects of epinephrine, saline infusion, blood withdrawal and tranquilizers on blood ACTH in human subjects.

The lability of neuroendocrine responses to diverse stimuli and methodological problems of reliability and sensitivity have precluded assessment of whether basal ACTH concentrations are continuous or intermittent in human blood. A variety of pharmacological agents have been proposed for the rapid release of ACTH from the pituitary to establish an "activation range" or secretory capacity for normal subjects and some clinical categories (Vernikos-Danellis, 1965). Significant transient increases of 40 to 45 mU ACTH/100 ml have been reported in the blood of normal females and 10 to 15 mU ACTH/100 ml in normal males, 2.5 minutes after the onset of a 1-minute epinephrine (0.5 μg/kg) infusion (Vernikos-Danellis and Marks, 1962). However, in another study, no significant increases were observed with the same dose in 6 normal males after a comparable 1-minute epinephrine infusion (Vance and Shioda, 1964).

In the study reported in this chapter, the 1-minute lower dose epinephrine (.25 µg/kg) infusion did not result in a significant increase in blood ACTH in 12 normal or 12 acute schizophrenic females. A significantly lower postepinephrine ACTH in the second blood sample was observed. This may be attributed to the anticipated blood withdrawal, saline and epinephrine infusions. Maximum physiological responses have been reported to occur in naive subjects on first exposure to the laboratory test condition while the subject is awaiting the onset of the test procedure (Sabshin et al., 1957). Significant differences have been reported in psychological and physiological responses to an epinephrine injection depending upon the subject's differential expectation of a drug or a placebo (Penick and Fisher, 1965). In view of the significant interaction of blood withdrawal and different test expectancies with saline and drugs, it seems apparent that the magnitude of the increases in blood ACTH should be interpreted in relation to each subject's initial basal blood ACTH in accordance with the law of initial value (LIV).

Physiologically, ACTH concentrations represent a balance between pituitary secretion and removal from the blood stream. The significantly lower blood ACTH in the second blood sample of the epinephrine and control groups may also be related in part to the extremely rapid inactivation of endogenous circulating ACTH after acute stress. Studies with timed hypophysectomy in adrenalectomized rats have shown that 75% of the circulating ACTH may disappear within 3 minutes (Syndor and Sayers, 1953).

The pre- and postepinephrine infusion blood ACTH of psychiatric patients was higher than of normal females. The higher blood ACTH and lack of a prompt reduction of ACTH in the second blood sample following epinephrine infusion represent a significant neuroendocrine difference between the normal and psychiatric subjects. There was a wide range of individual differences among normal and psychiatric subjects. Basal ACTH concentrations in normal subjects were also higher than have been reported previously in some studies. However, similar wide individual differences have been reported in circulating catecholamines in response to different test conditions and various forms of stress in normal human subjects (von Euler, 1964; O'Hanlon, 1965) and nonhuman primates (Mason et al., 1961).

Animal experiments have suggested inhibition of ACTH secretion to stress by tranquilizers. Experiments with human subjects have provided conflicting findings (Munson, 1963; de Wied, 1967). In this study, the second blood sample from the 12 acute schizophrenic females after 3 weeks of phenothiazines resulted in significantly lower blood ACTH than the first blood samples obtained before drug treatment. However, the reduction of blood ACTH after drug treatment may have been confounded with hospitalization.

According to the "epinephrine hypothesis," stress-induced systemic epinephrine triggers the release of pituitary ACTH. Obviously, conflicting findings have been reported with human subjects. Animal studies have also failed to confirm the hypothesis. Adrenal denervated, medullectomized, sympathectomized, and completely adrenalectomized animals still respond with pituitary ACTH secretions to a variety of stresses (Harris and George, 1969). Increased circulating epinephrine also does not appear to stimulate pituitary ACTH secretion in the dog.

In summary, the clinical and experimental findings indicate that stress-induced release of circulating epinephrine alone may not play a critical role in triggering pituitary ACTH secretions in response to stress.

Acute drug-stress interaction effects on hypothalamic norepinephrine, pituitary ACTH, adrenal cortisol and catecholamines in the squirrel monkey.

In acute studies, psychotropic drugs have been reported to be inhibitors of stress-induced pituitary ACTH release through their possible effects on hypothalamic monoamines and neuroendocrine transducer cell releasing or inhibitory factors. Studies with rats and dogs have suggested that pituitary ACTH may be under inhibitory control of hypothalamic norepinephrine. However, some studies have reported hypothalamic norepinephrine to be inhibitory in the rat and dog but stimulatory in the baboon. Acute experiments were undertaken to examine drug-stress interaction effects on hypothalamic norepinephrine, pituitary ACTH, adrenal cortisol and catecholamines in the squirrel monkey. Compared to nonhandled controls, 12 hours of social isolation, 1 hour of electric shock and a single dose of reserpine produced significant depletion in hypothalamic norepinephrine. Pre-treatment with chlorpromazine (15 μg/kg, i.p.) and haloperidol (2.5 μg/kg, i.p.) 1 hour before stress, effectively inhibited electric shock depletion of norepinephrine. Basal pituitary tissue ACTH levels were established in nonhandled controls. Handling and saline injection stress raised ACTH in pituitary tissue. However, acute experiments on stress, CPZ and HPD drug effects alone and whether pretreatment with these psychotropic drugs would inhibit concurrent stress induced increases in pituitary ACTH and decreases in hypothalamic CRF, norepinephrine, dopamine and serotonin remain to be carried out.

Plasma cortisol increased significantly from basal levels one hour after capture, handling, and chair restraint. Biochemical and morphological evaluations indicated that epinephrine was the predominant catecholamine within chromaffin cells of the adrenal medulla. Light and electron microscopic evaluations were also made of the topography, morphological organization and ultrastructure of the hypothalamus and the neurovascular link in the median eminence of the squirrel monkey. Presumed neurosecretory granules and vesicles were observed in nerve terminals adjacent to the capillary endothelium of the median eminence.

Chronic drug-stress interaction effects on hypothalamic norepinephrine, serotonin, pituitary ACTH and adrenal ascorbic acid

Two studies were undertaken on chronic 30-day drug-stress interaction effects on behavior, hypothalamic norepinephrine, serotonin, pituitary ACTH, and adrenal ascorbic acid in the squirrel monkey. In 1 chronic study, 2 dose levels of HPD resulted in a continuous tranquilization whereas 2 dose levels of CPZ produced comparable effects only on day 1, with a rapid development of behavioral tolerance at the lower CPZ dose level. Compared to nonhandled controls, 30 days of saline injection stress increased pituitary ACTH significantly. Pituitary ACTH in both CPZ and HPD drug groups were significantly lower than in the saline-injected stress group but they did not differ from nonhandled controls. These results suggested that pretreatment with both doses of CPZ and HPD 1 hour each day before 1 hour of electric shock effectively inhibited the saline stress induced increases in pituitary tissue ACTH concentrations. Another study was undertaken to determine whether saline-stress induced increases in pituitary ACTH were correlated with concomitant decreases in hypothalamic norepinephrine and serotonin. Thirty days of saline injection decreased hypothalamic norepinephrine significantly whereas serotonin levels were not decreased significantly, although a considerable but not significant decline was also apparent. A low dose level of HPD (.10 μg/kg) did not produce significant inhibition of saline-injected stress decreases in hypothalamic norepinephrine.

The acute and chronic experiments with the squirrel monkey have provided some provocative but also incomplete findings on psychotropic drug inhibition of stress induced increases in pituitary ACTH and concomitant decreases in hypothalamic CRF, norepinephrine, dopamine and serotonin. According to some earlier studies, hypothalamic serotonin does not seem to be the mediator for pituitary ACTH release in response to stress (Guillemin, 1967). It has been reported that morphine decreases norepinephrine in the hypothalamus, brainstem and adrenals (Holzbauer and Vogt, 1954; Maynert and Levi, 1964). Whereas chlorpromazine and phenobarbital inhibited the stress induced decreases in norepinephrine, morphine did not have this action. Stress induced decreases in brain NE were prevented with MAO but not with COMT inhibitors. Cholinergic mechanisms were also excluded since atropine, phenoxybenzamine, mecamylamine, and pyrobutamine did not inhibit stress induced decreases in brain NE (Maynert and Levi, 1964).

Some major unresolved problems in psychotropic drug effects on neuroendocrine functions

Remarkable progress has been made in clarification of neuroendocrinological control of pituitary-adrenal secretions in response to stress. Considerable progress has also been made on psychotropic drug effects on hypothalamic-pituitary-adrenal functions. However, several unresolved major problems remain for experimental clarification. These include: 1) the identity and mode of hypothalamic monoamine neurotransmitter regulation of CRF; 2) the isolation and chemical analysis of CRF; 3) the site and mechanisms of CRF release; 4) the site at which cortisol and ACTH feedback interactions inhibit ACTH; 5) the effects of psychotropic drugs on rate of impulse frequency in monoaminergic neurons and the synthesis of neurotransmitters; 6) the relationship of psychotropic drug receptor binding to their pharmacological activity; 7) multiphasic differences between acute and chronic drug-stress interaction effects on hypothalamic CRF, monoamines, pituitary ACTH and adrenal hormones and 8) establish the role of catecholamines and hormones in learning, motivation and emotions.

The squirrel monkey as a primate model in psychopharmacology

Increasing use of the squirrel monkey has been reported in neuroendocrinological research. Particular attention is required to the selection and treatment of saline-injected and nonhandled control groups; since it is apparent that the past history, conditioning, learning and expectancies interact with drug effects, particularly at lower dose levels, in the squirrel monkey as they do in man. In order to identify sources of variance and draw conclusions concerning drug effects at statistically acceptable levels of confidence, at least six subjects per group, and at least two control groups and two drug levels are essential in any experimental design in which attempts are made to examine drug-stress interaction effects on behavior in relation to electrical, chemical and morphological variables in the brain and endocrines.

ACKNOWLEDGMENTS

The studies with the normal and psychiatric subjects were conducted at the Cleveland Psychiatric Institute, 1708 Aiken Avenue, Cleveland, Ohio. Sincere thanks are due to T. Samorajski, J. Claghorn, H. Kretchmer, D. Schroeder, C. Meliska, and the West "B Group" for their participation in this research program with the human subjects and nonhuman primates. Supported by NIH grants RR00164-14, MH-07591 and NB-3853.

REFERENCES

Albin, M. S., J. M. Ordy, R. L. Collins, and H. E. Kretchmer. 1965. A comparison of chlorpromazine effects on cardiovascular response to epinephrine in surgical and psychiatric patients. Anesth. and Analg. 44: 392.

Arner, B., P. Hedner, T. Karlefors, and H. Wrestling. 1963. Hemodynamic changes and adrenal function in man during hyperglycemia. Acta Endocrinol. 44: 430.

Birk, L. Ed. 1973. Biofeedback: Behavioral Medicine. Grune and Stratton, New York.

Brown, G. M., L. J. Grota, D. P. Penney, and S. Reichlin. 1971. Pituitary-adrenal function in the squirrel monkey. Endocrinology 86: 519–529.

Brown, G. M., D. S. Schalch, and S. Reichlin. 1971. Hypothalamic mediation of growth hormone and adrenal stress response in the squirrel monkey. Endocrinology 89: 694–703.

Cardon, P. V., L. Sokoloff, T. S. Vates, and S. S. Kety, 1961. The physiological and psychological effects of intravenously administered epinephrine and its metabolism in normal and schizophrenic men. J. Psychiat. Res. 1: 37.

Cardon, P. V., and P. S. Mueller. 1964. Effects of norepinephrine on the blood pressure, glucose and free fatty acids of normal and schizophrenic men, with reference to heart rate and to indices of physical fitness and of thyroid and adrenal cortical function. J. Psychiat. Res. 2: 11.

Carlton, P. L. 1969. Brain-acetylcholine and inhibition. In J. T. Tapp, Ed. Reinforcement and Behavior. Academic Press, New York.

Coupland, R. E., and D. Hopwood. 1966. Mechanism of a histochemical reaction differentiality between adrenaline- and noradrenaline-storing cells in the electron microscope. Nature (London) 209: 590–591.

Cross, B. A., and I. A. Silver. 1966. Electrophysiological studies on the hypothalamus. Brit. Med. Bull. 22: 254–260.

Demura, H. 1966. A sensitive radioimmunoassay for plasma ACTH levels. *J. Clin. Endo. Med.* 26: 1297.

de Wied, D. 1967. Chlorpromazine and endocrine function. *Pharmacol. Rev.* 19: 251.

de Wied, D. 1970. Pituitary control of avoidance behavior. In L. Martini, M. Motta, and F. Fraschini, Eds. *The Hypothalamus.* Academic Press, New York.

de Wied, D., B. Bohus, and H. M. Greven. 1968. Influence of pituitary and adrenocortical hormones on conditioned avoidance behavior in rats. In R. P. Michael, Ed. *Endocrinology and Human Behavior.* Oxford University Press, New York.

de Wied, D., and W. DeJong. 1974. Drug effects and hypothalamic-anterior pituitary function. *Ann. Rev. Pharmacol.* 14: 389–412.

de Wied, D., A. Witter, and S. Lande. 1970. Anterior pituitary peptides and avoidance acquisition of hypophysectomized rats. In D. de Wied and J. A. Weijnen, Eds. *Progress in Brain Research* Vol 32: *Pituitary, Adrenal and the Brain.* Elsevier, Amsterdam.

Eleftheriou, B. E., and K. W. Boehlke. 1967. Brain monoamine oxidase in mice after exposure to aggression and defeat. *Science* 155: 1693–1694.

Farrell, G., and S. M. McCann. 1952. Detectable amounts of adrenocorticotropic hormone in blood following epinephrine. *Endocrinology* 50: 274.

Friedhoff, A. J., Ed. 1975. *Catecholamines and Behavior* Vols. I and II. Plenum Press, New York.

Frohman, L. A. 1975. Neurotransmitters as regulators of endocrine function. *Hospital Practice* April: 54–67.

Frohman, L. A., and M. E. Stachura. 1975. Neuropharmacologic control of neuroendocrine function in man. *Metabolism* 25: 211–234.

Fuxe, K., H. Carrodi, T. Hokfelt, and G. Jonsson. 1970. Central monoamine neurons and pituitary-adrenal activity. In D. de Wied and J. A. Weijnen, Eds. *Progress in Brain Research* Vol. 32: *Pituitary, Adrenal and the Brain.* Elsevier, Amsterdam.

Ganong, W. F. 1963. The central nervous system and the synthesis and release of adrenocorticotrophic hormone. In A. V. Nalbondov, Ed. Advances in Neuroendocrinology. University of Illinois Press, Urbana.

Ganong, W. F. 1966. Neuroendocrine integrating mechanisms. In L. Martini and W. F. Ganong, Eds. *Neuroendocrinology* Vol. 1. Academic Press, New York.

Ganong, W. F. 1970. Control of adrenocorticotropin and melanocyte-stimulating hormone secretion. In L. Martini, M. Motta, and F. Fraschini, Eds. *The Hypothalamus.* Academic Press, New York.

Ganong, W. F. 1972. Evidence for a central noradrenergic system that inhibits ACTH secretion. In K. M. Knigge, D. E. Scott, and A. Weindl, Eds. *Brain-Endocrine Interaction.* Karger, Basel.

Ganong, W. F. 1974. Brain mechanisms regulating the secretion of the pituitary gland. In F. O. Schmitt and F. G. Worden, Eds. *The Neurosciences: Thirdy Study Program.* MIT Press, Cambridge.

Goldberg, A. M., and B. L. Welch. 1972. Adaptation of the adrenal medulla: Sustained increase in choline acetyltransferase by psychosocial stimulation. *Science* 178: 319–320.

Grote, S. S., S. G. Moses, E. Robins, R. W. Hudgens, and A. B. Croninger. 1974. A study of selected catecholamine metabolizing enzymes: A comparison of depressive suicides and alcoholic suicides with controls. *J. Neurochem.* 23: 791–802.

Guillemin, AR. 1957. Centrally acting drugs and pituitary-adrenal responses to stress. In W. S. Fields, Ed. *Brain Mechanisms and Drug Action.* Charles C. Thomas, Springfield.

Guillemin, R. 1974. In D. F. Swaab and J. P. Schadé, Eds. *Progress in Brain Research* Vol. 41: *Integrative Hypothalamic Activity.* Elsevier, Amsterdam.

Hansen, H. M. 1968. Use of the squirrel monkey in pharmacology. In L. A. Rosenblum and R. W. Cooper, Eds. *The Squirrel Monkey.* Academic Press, New York.

Harris, G. W. and R. George. 1969. Neurohumoral control of the adenohypophysis and the regulation of the secretion of TSH, ACTH and growth hormone. In W. Haymaker, E. Anderson, and W. J. H. Nauta, Eds. *The Hypothalamus.* Charles C. Thomas, Springfield.

Harwood, C. T., and J. W. Mason. 1957. Acute effects of tranquilizing drugs on the anterior pituitary-ACTH mechanism. *Endocrinology* 60: 239.

Henry, J. P., P. M. Stephens, J. Axelrod, and R. A. Mueller. 1971. Effect of psychosocial stimulation on the enzymes involved in the biosynthesis and metabolism of noradrenaline and adrenaline. *Psychom. Med.* 33: 227–236.

Hockman, C. H., Ed. 1972. *Limbic System Mechanisms and Autonomic Function.* Charles C. Thomas, Springfield.

Holzbauer, M., and M. Vogt. 1954. The action of chlorpromazine on diencephalic sympathetic activity and on the release of adrenocorticotrophic hormone. *Brit. J. Pharmacol.* 9: 402.

Jus, A., K. Jus, and J. Kakalewski. 1964. The action of intravenously administered noradrenaline on the polygraphic reactions of schizophrenic patients. In D. Bente and P. B. Bradley, Eds. *Neuro-Psychopharmacology.* Elsevier, Amsterdam.

Kety, S. S. 1967. The central physiological and pharmacological effects of the biogenic amines and their correlations with behavior. In G. C. Quarton, T. Melnechuk, and F. O. Schmitt, Eds. *The Neurosciences: A Study Program.* Rockefeller University Press, New York.

Kety, S. S. 1970. The biogenic amines in the central nervous system: Their possible roles in arousal, emotion and learning. In F. O. Schmitt, Ed. *The Neurosciences: Second Study Program.* Rockefeller University Press, New York.

Kety, S. S. 1972. Catecholamines and affective behavior. In J. L. McGaugh, Ed. *Advances in Behavioral Biology:* Vol. IV. *The Chemistry of Mood, Motivation and Memory.* Plenum Press, New York.

Kotby, S., H. D. Johnson, H. D. Dellman, and N. H. McArthur. 1971. Adreno-cortical nuclear size and function in response to high environmental temperature. *Life Sci.* 10: 387–396.

Krieger, D. T. 1973. Neurotransmitter regulation of ACTH release. *Mt. Sinai J. Med.* 40: 302–314.

Lacey, J. I. 1956. The evaluation of an autonomic response: Toward a general solution. *Ann. N. Y. Acad. Sci.* 67: 123–164.

Lacey, J. I. 1972. Some cardiovascular correlates of sensorimotor behavior: Examples of visceral afferent feedback. In C. H. Hockman, Ed. *Limbic System Mechanisms and Autonomic Function.* Charles C. Thomas, Springfield.

Maas, J. W. 1972. Adrenocortical steroid hormones, electrolytes and the dis-position of the catecholamines with particular reference to depressive states. *J. Psychiat. Res.* 9: 227–241.

MacLean, P. D. 1949. Psychosomatic disease and the "visceral brain": Recent developments bearing on the Papez theory of emotion. *Psychosom. Med.* 11: 338–353.

Mahfouz, M., and E. A. Ezz. 1958. The effect of reserpine and chlorproma-zine on the response of the rat to acute stress. *J. Pharmacol. Exp. Ther.* 123: 39.

Martini, L., and J. Meites, Eds. 1970. *Neurochemical Aspects of Hypothal-amic Function.* Academic Press, New York.

Mason, J. W. 1972. Organization of psychoendocrine mechanisms: A review and reconsideration of research. In N. S. Greenfield and R. A. Sternbach, Eds. *Handbook of Psychophysiology.* Holt, Rinehart and Winston, New York.

Mason, J. W., G. Mangan, J. V. Brady, D. Conrad, and D. McK. Roich. 1961. Concurrent plasma epinephrine, norepinephrine and 17-hydroxycorti-costeroid levels during conditioned emotional disturbances in monkeys. *Psychosomat. Med.* 23: 344.

Maynert, E. W., and R. Levi. 1964. Stress-induced release of brain nor-epinephrine and its inhibition by drugs. *J. Pharmac. Exp. Ther.* 143: 90–95.

McEwen, B. S., and J. M. Weiss. 1970. The uptake and action of corticoster-one: Regional and subcellular studies on rat brain. In D. de Wied and J. A. Weijnen, Eds. *Progress in Brain Research.* Vol. 32. *Pituitary, Adrenal and the Brain.* Elsevier, Amsterdam.

Meites, J. 1970. Modification of synthesis and release of hypothalamic releas-ing factors induced by exogenous stimuli. In L. Martini and J. Meites, Eds. *Neurochemical Aspects of Hypothalamic Function.* Academic Press, New York.

Michael, R. P., Ed. 1968. *Endocrinology and Human Behaviour.* Oxford Uni-versity Press, New York.

Mirsky, I. A. 1970. Effects of ACTH and corticosteroids on animal behavior. In D. de Wied and J. A. Weijnen, Eds. *Progress in Brain Research.*

Vol. 32: *Pituitary, Adrenal and the Brain.* Elsevier, Amsterdam.

Munson, P. L. 1963. Pharmacology of neuroendocrine blocking agents. In A. V. Nalbandov, Ed. *Advances in Neuroendocrinology.* University of Illinois Press, Urbana.

Nauta, W. J. H. 1972. The central visceromotor system: A general survey. In C. H. Hockman, Ed. *Limbic System Mechanisms and Autonomic Function.* Charles C. Thomas, Springfield.

Nelson, D. H. 1966. Plasma ACTH determinations in fifty-eight patients before or after adrenalectomy for Cushing's syndrome. *J. Clin. Endocrinol. Med.* 26: 722.

Nelson, D. H., A. A. Sandberg, J. G. Palmer, and E. M. Glenn. 1952. Levels of 17-hydroxycorticoids following intravenous infusion of epinephrine in normal men. *J. Clin. Endocrinol. Med.* 12: 936.

Ney, R. L., N. Shimizu, W. E. Nicholson, D. P. Island, and G. W. Liddle. 1963. Correlation of plasma ACTH concentration with adrenocortical response in normal human subjects, surgical patients and patients with Cushing's disease. *J. Clin. Invest.* 42: 1669.

O'Hanlon, J. F. 1965. Adrenaline and noradrenaline: Relation to performance in a visual vigilance task. *Science* 150: 507.

Ordy, J. M., T. Samorajski, and D. Schroeder. 1966. Concurrent changes in hypothalamic and cardiac catecholamine levels after anesthetics, tranquilizers and stress in a subhuman primate. *J. Pharmac. Exp. Ther.* 152: 445.

Palkovits, M., and A. Mitro. 1968. Morphological changes in the rat hypothalamus and adrenal cortex in the early postnatal period after ACTH and hydrocortisone administration, stress and adrenalectomy. *Neuroendocrin.* 3: 200–210.

Palkovits, M., and E. Stark. 1972. Qualitative histological changes in the rat hypothalamus following bilateral adrenalectomy. *Neuroendocrin.* 10: 23–30.

Papez, J. W. A. 1937. A proposed mechanism of emotion. *Arch. Neurol. Psychiat.* 38: 725–743.

Penick, S. B., and S. Fisher. 1965. Drug-set interaction: Psychological and physiological effects of epinephrine under differential expectations. *Psychosom. Med.* 27: 177.

Persky, H. 1962. Adrenocortical function during anxiety. In R. Roessler and N. S. Greenfield, Eds. *Physiological Correlates of Psychological Disorder.* University of Wisconsin Press, Madison.

Pscheidt, G. R., H. H. Berlet, C. Bull, J. Spaide, and H. E. Himwich. 1964. Excretion of catecholamines and exacerbation of symptoms in schizophrenic patients. *J. Psychiat. Res.* 2: 163.

Rick, I., and R. Thompson. 1965. Role of the hippocampo-septal system, thalamus and hypothalamus in avoidance conditioning. *J. C. C. P.* 59: 66–72.

Rinne, U. K., and A. V. Arstila. 1965. Ultrastructure of the neurovascular link between the hypothalamus and anterior pituitary gland in the median eminence of the rat. *Neuroendocrinology* 1: 214–227.

Rosenblum, L. A., and R. W. Cooper, Eds. 1968. *The Squirrel Monkey*. Academic Press. New York.

Sabshin, M., D. A. Hamberg, R. R. Grinker, H. Persky, H. Basowitz, S. J. Korchin and J. A. Chevalier. 1957. Significance of pre-experimental studies in the psychosomatic laboratory. *AMA Arch. Neurol. Psychiat.* 78: 207.

Schadé, J. P. 1970. The limbic system and the pituitary-adrenal axis. In D. de Wied and J. A. Weijnen, Eds. *Progress in Brain Research*. Vol. 32. *Pituitary, Adrenal, and the Brain*. Elsevier, Amsterdam, pp. 2–11.

Siegel, G. J., and J. S. Eisenman. 1972. Hypothalamic-pituitary regulation. In R. W. Albers, G. J. Siegel, R. Katzman, and B. W. Agranoff, Eds. *Basic Neurochemistry*. Little, Brown and Co., Boston.

Smelik, P. G. 1970. Integrated hypothalamic responses to stress. In L. Martini, M. Motta and F. Fraschini, Eds. *The Hypothalamus*. Academic Press, New York.

Smith, R. L., R. P. Maickel, and B. B. Brodie. 1963. ACTH-hypersecretion induced by phenothiazine tranquilizers. *J. Pharmac. Exp. Ther.* 139: 185.

Smookler, H. H., and J. P. Buckley. 1969. Relationships between brain catecholamine synthesis, pituitary adrenal function and the production of hypertension during prolonged exposure to environmental stress. *Int. J. Neuropharmacol.* 8: 33.

Steiner, F. A. 1970. Effects of ACTH and corticosteroids on single neurons in the hypothalamus. In D. de Wied and J. A. Weijnen, Eds. *Progress in Brain Research* Vol 32. *Pituitary, Adrenal and the Brain*. Elsevier, Amsterdam.

Sydnor, K. L., and G. Sayers. 1953. Biological half-life of endogenous ACTH. *Proc. Soc. Exptl. Biol. Med.* 83: 729.

Vance, V. K., and Y. Shioda. 1964. Effect of intravenous epinephrine on blood ACTH concentration as measured by steroidogenesis in the hypophysectomized rat. *Endocrinology* 74: 807.

Vernikos-Danellis, J. 1965. The regulation of the synthesis and release of ACTH. *Vitamins and Hormones*. Academic Press, New York.

Vernikos-Danellis, J., E. Anderson, and L. Trigg. 1966. Changes in adrenal corticosterone concentration in rats: Method of bio-assay for ACTH. *Endocrinology* 79: 624.

Vernikos-Danellis, J., and B. H. Marks. 1962. Epinephrine-induced release of ACTH in normal human subjects. *Endocrinology* 70: 525.

von Euler, U. S. 1964. Quantitation of stress by catecholamine analysis. *Clin. Pharmacol. Ther.* 5: 398.

Welch, B. L., and A. S. Welch. 1969. Sustained effects of brief daily stress (fighting) upon brain and adrenal catecholamines and adrenal, spleen and heart weight of mice. *Proc. Nat. Acad. Sci.* 64: 100–107.

Wilder, J. 1950. The law of initial values. *Psychosomat. Med.* 12: 392.

Wise, C. D., and L. Stein. 1973. Dopamine-β-hydroxylase deficits in the brains of schizophrenic patients. *Science* 181: 344–347.

Wood, J. G. 1963. Identification of and observations on epinephrine and norepinephrine containing cells in the adrenal medulla. *Am. J. Anat.* 112: 283–303.

Wurtman, R. J. 1971. Brain monoamines and endocrine function. *Neurosci. Res. Bull.* 9: 177–297.

Tissue Responses to Addictive Drugs
© 1976, Spectrum Publications, Inc.

Persistent Effects of Neonatal Narcotic Addiction in the Rat

THEO SONDEREGGER

Department of Psychology
University of Nebraska
Lincoln, Nebraska

EMERY ZIMMERMANN

Department of Anatomy and
Brain Research Institute
UCLA School of Medicine
Los Angeles, California

The problem of neonatal narcotic addiction is now widely recognized as a tragic correlate of opiate abuse among women of childbearing age. Early diagnosis and management have greatly improved the survival rate of addicted infants (Naeye and Blanc, 1973; Naeye et al., 1973; Wilson et al., 1973; and Krause et al., 1958), but any long-term effects of narcotic addiction and withdrawal early in life remain to be identified and analyzed. In this connection an experimental animal model is needed and is being developed in this and in other laboratories (Friedler and Cochin, 1972; Friedler, 1972; Bakke, Lawrence, and Bennett, 1973; Banerjee, 1975; and Steele and Johannesson, 1975a, 1975b) for the systematic study of short-term and long-term effects of exposure to narcotics during development and early life.

The rat is a popular subject for such studies for several reasons, including its convenient life span, the existing fund of information regarding various aspects of its development and because it is relatively immature at birth and is therefore ideally suited for the study of late and early neonatal administration of opiates without simultaneously dosing the mother. Taking advantage of this fact, we conducted a series of studies in which newborn rats were injected with morphine during the first week of life, which is developmentally equivalent to the third trimester in human development. Animals treated during the second and third postnatal weeks were also studied since various physical and chemical treatments during that period are known to affect adult behavior in the rat (Denenberg and Zarrow, 1971) and are therefore relevant to understanding long-lasting effects of early opiate addiction.

The results of our initial study are presented in detail elsewhere (Zimmermann et al., 1974). In that study rats received twice daily injections of morphine throughout the first 3 weeks of life. The prolonged growth deficit, tolerance to morphine, and sensitivity to naloxone obtained in that study suggested that exposure of the immature female rat to morphine resulted in a protracted, morphine-specific alteration of neuroendocrine and nociceptive brain mechanisms. We reasoned that such long-term effects might be correlated with developmental periods of differing sensitivity to morphine. This report describes our findings in two subsequent studies in which newborn rats received morphine injections for restricted periods. In the first study pups were treated during either the first, second, or third weeks of life. In the second study animals received morphine either on days 3-12 or 12-21 following birth.

METHODS AND RESULTS

In the first study pregnant Sprague-Dawley rats (Simonsen) were maintained under constant temperature ($24° \pm 1°C$) and standardized conditions of illumination (light 4 a.m. to 6 p.m., alternating with dark) with food and tap water available at all times. The day after birth (day 1) male pups were discarded and females were randomly assigned within litters of 8 to 1, of six treatment groups. During week 1, two pups from each litter (M_1 group) were subcutaneously injected twice daily with morphine (increased to reach a dose of 4 mg/kg on day 6, tapered to 1 mg/kg on day 7, and stopped on day 8). One control pup from each litter (S_1) received comparable injections of 0.9% saline. Groups M_2, M_3, S_2 and S_3 animals, 1 pup in each litter per group, received a similar series of morphine or saline injections during weeks 2 or 3. Maximum concentrations reached on the sixth injection day were 8 or 16 mg/kg for groups M_2 and M_3, respectively. The pups

Table I. Mortality of Female Rats Treated Neonatally with Morphine or Saline

Treatment Group	Time of Neonatal Treatment (Week)	Initial Number of Pups	Number of Deaths			Total	% of Group
			Treatment Week				
			1	2	3		
Morphine	1	18	2	6	0	8	44
Saline	1	9	0	2	0	2	22
Morphine	2	9	0	2	0	2	22
Saline	2	9	0	0	0	0	0
Morphine	3	11	0	0	0	0	0
Saline	3	10	0	0	0	0	0

were weaned at 22 days of age and housed by random selection in pairs under the conditions described above.

Marked differences were found in the mortality rates. The groups differed greatly during the treatment periods and shortly thereafter (see Table I). Forty-four % (8/18) of the M_1 animals died, but 6 of the 8 deaths occurred in the week immediately following cessation of treatment in this group. Two deaths also occurred in the S_1 and 2 in the M_2 groups, but the latter deaths occurred during the treatment period.

On day 15, 53% of morphine-treated animals had eyes open whereas 89% of other animals had undergone eyes opening. The difference was significant ($\chi^2=14.48$, df=1, $p<0.001$), suggesting some developmental retardation in the morphine-treated animals.

Animals were weighed weekly throughout the experiment. Body weights of the morphine-treated groups were lower than those of their saline-treated controls at the end of their respective treatment periods and remained lower ($p<0.05$) until the rats were 28 days-of-age. Thereafter, body weights of M_1 and M_2 animals were not significantly different than their controls although the M_3 weights were depressed through day 49 ($p<0.05$). In all groups the body weights of morphine-treated animals were generally lower than those of their controls throughout the remainder of the experiment (day 103). In our previous study (Zimmermann et al., 1974), morphine-treated animals evidenced depressed body weights for 105 days.

When body weights were translated into growth rates, i.e. weight increase each week as percentage of the starting weight for the week, all groups showed a rebound growth effect ($p<0.05$) for a week or two after cessation of treatment even though the body weights were

Table II. Onset of Vaginal Opening in Rats
Addicted to Morphine Early in Life

Neonatal Treatment	(Week)	No. of Rats	Onset of Vaginal Opening (Days)		
Morphine	1	10	37.00	±	1.02*
Saline	1	7	39.00	±	0.95
Morphine	2	7	37.28	±	0.97
Saline	2	9	38.22	±	0.85
Morphine	3	10	39.09	±	0.85
Saline	3	10	39.60	±	0.70
Morphine Treated by Week 2		17	37.14	±	1.00 †
Saline or No. Treatment by Week 2		36	38.98	±	0.77

* Mean ± S.E.
† $p < 0.07$

still lower than those of the controls. For the M_3 animals this effect persisted through day 49.

Although the onset of eye-opening was delayed in the M_1 and M_2 groups, both of these groups appeared to be precocious with respect to the time of vaginal opening (see Table II). Average times for the M_1 and M_2 groups were 37.00 and 37.28 days respectively, whereas those for all other groups ranged from 38.22 to 39.60 days. These data suggest that morphine may advance the onset of vaginal opening by 1 to 2 days and are consistent with the 2.8 day advancement reported by Weiner and Scapagnini (1974) in female Sprague-Dawley rats treated with morphine (2 mg/kg/day) during the late prepuberal period. They observed no difference in the estrous cycles between control and treated animals following the onset of vaginal opening. Examination of the vaginal smears in the present study from days 49-58 similarly indicated that all animals were cycling. The failure of M_3 animals in this study to exhibit advancement in the time of vaginal opening does not agree with the findings of Weiner and Scapagnini (1974) and the difference remains to be explained.

Traditionally, the open field test has been used to differentiate among behavioral effects of early treatment in both young and adult rats. On day 26, the rats were tested in the open field for 2 min on 3 consecutive days using a procedure and an apparatus similar to that of Quadagno et al. (1972). The order of testing was randomized each day. At the beginning of a trial, a rat was placed in a closed container, transported to the darkened room containing the apparatus, and placed in the center square. Animals were not identified until after testing.

Statistical comparisons between the means of the various measures in morphine and saline groups were not significant except that the M_3 group was less active, i.e. crossed fewer lines ($p < 0.05$) than the S_3 group (see Table III). Activity changes over trials showed no consistent direction. Other workers (Davis and Lin, 1973) have reported that pups of rat mothers injected with morphine during gestation days 5-18 were significantly more active and exhibited more rearing than their saline controls in the open field test. Since there were some trends, i.e. the M_2 and M_3 groups were less active, it is not clear whether the lack of behavioral effects were due to treatment procedures or to the greater variability in the responses of some of the morphine-treated animals.

Several parameters of pituitary-adrenal function in rats treated with morphine early in life were compared to their appropriate controls. On day 30, resting levels of plasma corticosterone were ascertained, using standardized procedures developed previously (Zimmermann and Critchlow, 1967). Due to the small numbers of animals in each group, only afternoon levels were measured. The rats were subjected to ether anesthesia and rapid jugular venipuncture (3 min) beginning at 4 p.m., a time which corresponds to the diurnal peak in circulating corticosterone levels in rats maintained under the lighting conditions used in our laboratory. Plasma was frozen for subsequent fluorometric determination of corticosterone (Glick et al., 1964). Resting levels of corticosterone in animals treated with morphine or saline during each neonatal treatment period did not differ significantly (see Table IV). These findings are consistent with those obtained previously in rats exposed to morphine during the entire 3 weeks of postnatal life (Zimmermann et al., 1974).

On day 44, the neonatal treatment groups were compared with respect to their corticosterone responses to a challenge dose of the morphine antagonist, naloxone. Although at the dose used this agent does not stimulate the pituitary-adrenal axis in the naive rat, it causes a striking increase in circulating levels of corticosterone in rats made dependent on morphine by subcutaneous implantation of a morphine pellet (Zimmermann et al., 1975). Beginning at 4 p.m., animals were injected intraperitoneally with naloxone (5 mg/kg). Thirty min later, each animal was quickly anesthetized with ether, and a sample of jugular venous blood collected and analyzed as described above. Corticosterone levels in neonatal morphine- and saline-treated animals were comparable suggesting an absence of protracted dependence as a result of neonatal exposure to morphine for a limited period (see Table IV).

On day 62, the rats were challenged with morphine to determine

Table III. Means of Open Field Measures Obtained on Days 26, 27, and 28 in Female Rats Addicted to Morphine Early in Life

Neonatal Treatment	(Weeks)	No. of Rats	Lines Crossed	Center Squares Entered	Latency (sec)	Grooming Episodes	Rearing (sec)	Defecation (%)
Morphine	1	10	45.2 ± 9.2*	3.9 ± 0.9	3.4 ± 0.6	2.6 ± 0.4	13.0 ± 3.1	60
Saline	1	7	43.1 ± 3.4	3.4 ± 0.7	3.8 ± 0.3	2.0 ± 0.3	12.1 ± 1.2	43
Morphine	2	7	28.5 ± 8.1	3.3 ± 0.7	3.1 ± 0.5	1.6 ± 0.4	10.0 ± 2.3	42
Saline	2	9	30.3 ± 3.4	3.3 ± 0.5	3.6 ± 0.3	1.7 ± 0.4	10.3 ± 1.4	67
Morphine	3	11	30.1 ± 5.3†	3.6 ± 1.6	5.4 ± 1.1	2.5 ± 0.3	9.0 ± 1.2	55
Saline	3	10	45.7 ± 6.4†	4.1 ± 0.7	4.0 ± 0.3	2.1 ± 0.2	14.5 ± 2.1	40

* Mean ± S. E.
† p < 0.05

Table IV. Plasma Corticosterone Levels under Resting Conditions and in Response to Naloxone Challenge in Adult Female Rats Addicted to Morphine Early in Life

Neonatal Treatment	(Week)	Resting Level Corticosterone (μg %) (Day 30)	Response to Naloxone (5 mg/kg) Corticosterone (μg %) (Day 44)	Response to Naloxone (5 mg/kg) 36 hr after Morphine Pellet Implant Corticosterone (μg %) (Day 120)
Morphine	1	16.67 ± 2.10†	20.19 ± 1.76	45.42 ± 2.60
Saline	1	18.85 ± 2.59	19.36 ± 3.60	46.95 ± 7.03
Morphine	2	15.26 ± 1.44	18.51 ± 2.58	47.00 ± 2.18
Saline	2	19.15 ± 3.25	23.35 ± 3.41	49.71 ± 2.80
Morphine	3	23.58 ± 4.01	24.81 ± 1.72	50.83 ± 3.54
Saline	3	17.56 ± 2.08	21.29 ± 2.74	46.25 ± 3.38

† Mean ± S. E., each group represents 7-11 rats.

Table V. Plasma Corticosterone Levels after Morphine Challenge (30 mg/kg) in 62-Day-Old Female Rats Addicted to Morphine Early in Life

Neonatal Treatment	(Week)	No. of Rats	Corticosterone Levels (μg %)		
Morphine	1	8	75.21	±	6.14*
Saline	1	7	60.71	±	7.95
Morphine	2	7	56.19	±	7.95
Saline	2	9	71.30	±	6.32
Morphine	3	11	52.39	±	7.81†
Saline	3	10	81.67	±	4.95†

* Mean ± S.E.

† $P < 0.005$ one-tailed "t" comparison

whether tolerance to morphine persisted as a consequence of limited early morphine treatment. Beginning at 4 p.m., animals were injected intraperitoneally with morphine (30 mg/kg) and 30 min later blood was obtained and prepared for corticosterone analysis, as described above (see Table V). Although the steroid levels of both the M_2 and M_3 groups were lower than those of their respective controls, only the M_3 vs S_3 difference was significant ($p < 0.005$). This finding confirms our earlier results showing protracted tolerance to the ACTH releasing action of morphine in rats addicted to morphine early in life (Zimmermann et al., 1974).

As a final pituitary-adrenal test, on day 120, animals were challenged with naloxone (5 mg/kg) 36 hrs after they had been implanted with 2 morphine pellets. Since morphine pellet implantation is sufficient to produce measurable dependence on morphine (Way et al., 1969) it was of interest to determine whether previous neonatal morphine dependence would modify the degree of dependence achieved by a standardized exposure to morphine in adulthood. All neonatal treatment groups showed a similar rise in steroids (see Table IV), thus early exposure to morphine could not be differentiated from saline on the basis of this dependence test.

In summary, this study replicated some but not all of the findings made in our previous study (Zimmermann et al., 1974). The differences in results may be attributable to differences in the neonatal treatment conditions. During the 21-day period of morphine injections in our earlier study each rat pup received a total dose of morphine equal to twice that given to the animals in the present study. Other workers (Bakke et al., 1973) reported that a depressed weight was not observed in female rats injected with morphine (4 mg/kg) on days 1-5 but was found with 7.7 mg/kg injected during the same period. Their lower morphine dosage is analagous to our M_1 dose. The high mortality rate among the M_1 group was probably due to effects of withdrawal rather than concentration of morphine since most deaths occurred during the week following cessation of treatment. The effect of this considerable loss of morphine-sensitive subjects on the results of subsequent tests is only speculative. We conclude that the limited neonatal treatment periods and/or dosage levels in the present study were inadequate to reproduce all of the effects observed in our earlier study except possibly a prolonged tolerance to morphine, as indicated by the corticosterone responses of the M_3 group to the morphine challenge (Table V).

Based upon these earlier studies a third study was undertaken. We elected to increase the morphine dosage and to lengthen the period of treatment so that the earlier period occurred prior to eye-opening (days 3-12) and the latter one after that time (days 12-21). Again the focus of the experiment was to identify certain long-lasting neuroendocrine and pharmacological effects of neonatal narcotic addiction in female rats and to correlate these effects with developmental periods of differential sensitivity to narcotic treatment. In addition, 2 behavioral tests were performed and an additional control group was included to evaluate injection effects per se.

Sprague-Dawley female rat pups (Simonsen) were obtained when 2 days old. Animals were randomly divided into 5 treatment groups, each represented within each litter of 8 pups. The following treatment ages and morphine dosages were used: M_1 group (days 3-12), morphine increased to 8 mg/kg on days 5-10 and tapered on days 11 and 12; M_2 group (days 12-21), morphine increased to 16 mg/kg on days 14-19, and tapered on days 20-21. All animals thus received 10 days of injections. S_1 and S_2 controls received comparable schedules of 0.9% saline; a no treatment (NT) group was handled but not injected. All pups were weighed daily and injections adjusted accordingly. On day 22 the subjects were weaned, housed in pairs and weights obtained weekly thereafter.

On day 14, 88% of the M_1 group and 85% of the other animals had their eyes open. These findings are not consistent with those of our previous study where eye opening was delayed in the groups treated with morphine before day 14. One possible explanation is the difference of onset of treatment time in the two studies.

The mortality rate of the M_1 group was only 8%, in contrast with the 44% observed in the preceding study. The most likely explanation for this discrepancy is that 13-day-old animals are better able to tolerate withdrawal than 8-day-old animals; sensitivity to morphine per se does not appear to change markedly prior to 16 days of age (Kupferberg, 1963).

In both morphine treatment groups, body weights were depressed soon after treatment began and they remained comparable to those of the saline and no treatment control groups throughout the experiment (see Table VI). M_1 body weights were significantly lower than those of the S_1 group only through day 20 ($p<0.05$); M_2 weights were depressed below those of the S_2 group through day 63 ($p<0.05$).

Examination of growth rates, computed as described, presents additional information. For both morphine-treated groups, growth rates dropped significantly below those of the control groups ($p<0.025$) at the beginning of their treatment period but rapidly accelerated even while the morphine treatment was continuing and surpassed those of the control groups when the dose of the narcotic was reduced. These growth rates, particularly for the M_2 group, look remarkably similar to those shown by rats underfed for 1 week by placement in an oversized litter (Kennedy, 1968).

On days 29-31 all animals were tested in the open field apparatus as described above. Two observers were used and response measures extended to include the time spent in locomotor (forward motion) activity as well as the time spent grooming (see Table VII). Data were examined in a one-way analysis of variance with repeated measures. No significant main effects were found. However, over the course of the trials, animals became more active, spent more time in locomotion, defecated less, and surprisingly, groomed more ($p<0.05$). These findings are different from those in the second study where no consistent changes over trials were observed.

The open field behavioral test, as used in these studies, did not seem to be sensitive to early morphine treatment effects or alternatively, the twice daily handling of the animals possibly completely obscured any treatment effects. Consequently, we introduced another behavioral test which has detected differences in effects of drug treatment in rats, a conditioned suppression test. In this test, the animals must acquire an instrumental response for a positive reward, and experience a noxious stimulus, e.g., electric shock, which is not contingent upon behavior. The resultant conditioned emotional response (fear), if learned, suppresses the acquired instrumental response. The specific task used was a modification of Berger and Stein's procedure (1969).

For this test, animals were placed on a 23-hr food deprivation schedule and concomitantly learned to drink a sweetened milk solution (1 part Borden's Eagle Brand sweetened condensed milk: 2 parts tap water) in daily 5-min home cage trials prior to feeding. Animals were

Table VI. Mean Weekly Weight (grams) for Female Rats Addicted Early in Life to Morphine

Group		1	2	3	4	5	6	7	8	9	10	11
							Weeks					
NT	M	16.0	28.5	47.9	87.0	127.0	—	177.3	199.5	214.3	231.6	240.3
	SE	±0.7	±1.7	±2.3	±3.3	± 3.5	—	± 4.1	± 4.3	± 4.7	± 4.5	± 5.0
(N = 20)												
M$_1$	M	16.5	26.8*	46.7	85.1	125.0	—	183.8	205.7	222.2	238.1	246.9
	SE	±0.5	±0.9	±1.3	±1.9	± 2.3	—	± 2.7	± 3.0	± 3.3	± 3.7	± 4.0
(N = 36)												
S$_1$	M	17.4	30.0	49.7	89.2	128.4	—	183.6	204.7	219.9	234.3	244.3
	SE	±0.4	±1.2	±1.7	±2.2	± 2.9	—	± 3.5	± 3.9	± 4.3	± 4.7	± 4.6
(N = 24)												
M$_2$	M	15.6	27.1	39.4*	77.4†	117.3	—	172.1*	194.5*	207.6†	223.0	233.5
	SE	±0.8	±1.3	±2.3	±2.8	± 3.0	—	± 3.1	± 3.9	± 4.0	± 6.1	± 5.7
(N = 11)												
S$_2$	M	15.2	27.1	46.8	85.0	123.4	—	182.6	204.8	217.1	232.2	242.9
	SE	±0.6	±1.9	±2.2	±3.1	± 3.0	—	± 2.9	± 3.1	± 3.2	± 5.1	± 4.5
(N = 11)												

* p $<$ .025 "t" comparison, one-tailed
† p $<$ .05 "t" comparison, one-tailed

NT = No Treatment
M$_1$ Morphine (days 3-12)
S$_1$ Saline (days 3-12)
M$_2$ Morphine (days 12-21)
S$_2$ Saline (days 12-21)
SE = Standard error

Table VII. Means of Open Field Measures Obtained on Days 29, 30, and 31 in Female Rats Addicted to Morphine Early in Life

Neonatal Treatment	(days)	No. of Rats	Lines Crossed	Center Squares Entered	Latency (sec)	Locomotion (sec)	Rearing (sec)	Grooming (sec)	Defecation
Morphine	3-12	36	37.8 ± 5.7*	0.3 ± 0.2	18.4 ± 6.0	18.8 ± 2.6	15.5 ± 1.9	1.6 ± 0.3	0.6 ± 0.2
Saline	3-12	24	41.4 ± 5.5	0.4 ± 0.2	19.1 ± 7.3	22.1 ± 2.8	18.1 ± 2.8	1.6 ± 0.4	0.7 ± 0.3
Morphine	12-21	11	39.1 ± 8.3	0.7 ± 0.9	18.1 ± 11.8	15.5 ± 4.3	13.7 ± 2.2	1.7 ± 0.4	0.7 ± 0.4
Saline	12-21	11	34.2 ± 9.3	0.3 ± 0.3	17.8 ± 8.0	18.5 ± 4.3	12.5 ± 2.2	2.1 ± 0.8	0.6 ± 0.5
Not Treated		20	44.6 ± 6.2	0.4 ± 0.4	6.7 ± 2.5	23.6 ± 2.9	14.7 ± 1.8	1.6 ± 0.3	0.7 ± 0.5

* Means and S. E.'s

Table VIII. Conditioned Suppression Test Criterion Times of
Female Rats Addicted to Morphine Early in Life

Group	No. of Rats	Logarithm of Training Trial		Logarithm of Test Trial		"t" comparisons of training and test trials	
		M	SE	M	SE		
M_1 NS	11	1.7821	0.2021	1.6765	0.1744	1.41	NS
M_1 S	11	1.7856	0.2773	2.0091	0.3731	1.910	NS
S_1 NS	12	1.6781	0.1892	1.4828	0.3785	1.89	NS
S_1 S	10	1.6758	0.2318	2.2170	0.2829	−4.72	p < .01
NTNS	10	1.8475	0.2656	1.5755	0.4847	1.75	NS
NT S	9	1.7644	0.2583	2.2831	0.2425	−4.37	p < .01
M_2 NS	5	1.7754	0.2450	1.6782	0.3207	2.21	NS
M_2 S	6	1.9009	0.2014	2.3236	0.2887	−2.70	p < .05
S_2 NS	5	1.7656	0.2084	1.5953	0.1356	−2.30	NS
S_2 S	6	1.7840	0.3965	2.5327	0.2883	−5.75	p < .01

[1] Time to make 100 licks
M_1 = Morphine (days 3-12)
M_2 = Morphine (days 12-21)
NT = No Treatment

S_1 = Saline (days 3-12)
S_2 = Saline (days 12-21)
S = Shock
NS= No Shock

given daily trials beginning on day 90, in a standard, Lafayette operant box equipped with a drinkometer and a bottle containing the sweetened milk solution. When an animal was placed in the box, clocks were activated to measure the latency of drinking, as well as the time to reach criterion, 100 licks of solution. Animals not reaching criterion were removed after 20 min.

Rats were given 4 days of training. On training day 4, they were given a training trial as described, returned to the operant box, from which the drinking spout had been removed, and allowed to remain for 15 sec. At the beginning of the 15th second, half of the animals in each neonatal treatment group received 1 sec of 0.6 mA current delivered through the floor by means of a scrambler and constant current device. All animals squealed while receiving shock. The other rats were in the nonshock groups and simply remained in the box an extra second. Rats were immediately returned to their home cages. For the day 5 test trial, animals were treated as in the training procedures. Training and testing orders were determined by a randomized block design.

These data were transformed into logarithms to reduce variability, which was large in the shocked groups (see Table VIII). Means between the last training trial and the test trial for each group were compared,

Table IX. Plasma Corticosterone Responses to Naloxone (5 mg/kg) Administered on Day 40 or Day 145 in Female Rats Addicted to Morphine Early in Life

Treatment	Corticosterone Levels (μg %) Day 40	30 min After Naloxone Day 145
Morphine (days 3-12)	14.25 ± 3.87 (11)*	17.47 ± 1.50 (25)
Saline (days 3-12)	11.10 ± 1.20 (11)	18.35 ± 2.95 (10)
Untreated	11.97 ± 1.26 (13)	18.19 ± 2.84 (7)
Morphine (days 12-21)	11.15 ± 1.09 (10)	—
Saline (days 12-21)	9.70 ± 0.76 (11)	—

* Mean ± S. E., numbers in parentheses denote number of rats

using a one tailed "t" test for dependent measures. In all groups, except the M_1 group, animals receiving shock took longer on the test trial ($p < 0.01$) and showed longer latencies than their control groups receiving no shock. The latter animals, i.e. those who received no shock were faster on the test trial. The no shock M_1 animals speeded up on the test trial, indicating that they had learned the drinking response. Although the M_1 group receiving shock were on the average slightly slower on the test trials, differences between training and test scores were not significant as had been the case with the other neonatal treatment groups. Thus, the shocked M_1 animals failed to show the conditioned suppression exhibited by all other shocked groups; they failed to show the same fear of shock. Latency changes were also significant ($p < 0.01$) and were consistent with the trials to criterion data.

Failure to suppress the response in the M_1 animals was probably not due to a decreased sensitivity to pain since these animals showed no deficit in pain threshold when tested for control responses in a hotplate test to be discussed below. Thus, the data from the conditioned suppression test suggest that treatment with morphine from days 3-12 may cause lasting impairment of the animal's ability to acquire fear.

Protocols similar to those used in the preceding study were used to compare corticosterone responses of the animals to naloxone and to morphine. Half of the neonatally treated animals and their controls were injected with naloxone at 8:30 a.m. on day 40 and the remaining animals at that time on day 145 (see Table IX). The M_1 group, which received morphine days 3-12, showed the highest steroid levels compared to the controls and the untreated groups on day 40, but the differences were not significant. Likewise, corticosterone levels were comparable in all groups on day 145. These findings are consistent with those of the preceding studies and indicate that early addiction to morphine is compatible with normal resting pituitary-adrenal function in adulthood.

At 156 days of age, the influence of early morphine treatment on the analgesic response to morphine was tested with the hotplate technique (Eddy and Leimbach, 1953). Compared with S_1, S_2, or NT animals receiving saline, other S_1, S_2, or NT animals showed a typical marked increase in response latency ($p < 0.01$) 30 and 60 min after injection of the test dose of morphine (10 mg/kg). By 90 min after injection the effect had disappeared. Rats treated prepuberally with morphine, M_1 and M_2 groups, showed a smaller ($p < 0.01$) increase in response latency at 30 and 60 min which disappeared after 60 min. Injection of the M_1 and M_2 groups with saline instead of the test morphine produced no change in response latency. Both the M_1 and M_2 groups, thus, evidenced protracted tolerance to the analgesic effect of morphine as a consequence of neonatal addiction to morphine (see Table X). This observation is consistent with our earlier findings using this test (Zimmermann et al., 1974).

DISCUSSION AND CONCLUSIONS

The results of these three studies demonstrate that certain long-lasting changes in behavioral and neuroendocrine functioning in the rat occur consequent to morphine treatment early in life. These effects appear, in some instances, to depend upon the time of treatment, as well as upon the amount of morphine administered. Obviously, the study of critical developmental or organizational periods is complex and likely involves interactions between interdependent processes, e.g., in the present study, an age-dependent change of susceptibility to morphine toxicity (Kupferberg, 1963), as well as maturation events, are operational stimuli.

Our findings included depressed body weights in morphine-treated animals. These phenomena were of variable duration, and there was a rebound growth effect during, as well as right after, treatment. Depressions of body weights have been observed previously in studies dealing with early morphine injections (Bakke et al., 1973; Banerjee, 1974; Friedler and Cochin, 1968; Friedler, 1972; Johannesson et al., 1972; and Weiner and Scapagnini, 1974). Malnutrition during early growth periods can also produce long-term body weight depression (Kennedy, 1968), as well as other effects (Sobotka, 1974). Unfortunately, our work cannot separate the effects of malnutrition from the effects of morphine. Bakke, et al. (1973), however, have raised calorie-restricted

Table X. Effect of Neonatal Administration of Morphine on the Analgesic Action of Morphine (10 mg/kg, i.p.) in Adult Female Rats

Treatment	No. of Rats	Change in Response Latency (sec) at Various Intervals after Morphine Injection			
		30 min	60 min	90 min	120 min
Days 3-12 / Day 156					
Morphine / Saline	17	−0.47 ± 0.34*	−0.37 ± 0.23	−0.23 ± 0.53	0.61 ± 0.51
Morphine / Morphine	17	3.53 ± 1.05†	1.19 ± 1.11†	−2.25 ± 0.84	−3.35 ± 0.91
Saline / Morphine	13	9.55 ± 2.25†	7.42 ± 2.58†	−0.09 ± 0.85	−2.26 ± 0.62
Saline / Saline	10	−0.56 ± 0.49	−2.10 ± 0.85	−1.26 ± 0.78	−2.94 ± 1.17
Untreated / Saline	10	−1.57 ± 0.44†	−0.91 ± 0.40†	−0.41 ± 0.55	−1.19 ± 0.47
Untreated / Morphine	10	7.35 ± 3.03†	8.53 ± 3.50†	0.61 ± 1.06	−2.77 ± 0.44
Days 12-21 / Day 156					
Morphine / Saline	5	−2.66 ± 1.06	−1.36 ± 0.53	0.76 ± 2.31	−1.68 ± 1.05
Morphine / Morphine	5	4.98 ± 2.35†	1.10 ± 1.39†	−0.02 ± 0.91	−0.74 ± 1.40
Saline / Morphine	5	15.68 ± 2.94†	14.24 ± 4.48†	3.32 ± 2.59	−1.88 ± 0.40
Saline / Saline	6	0.22 ± 1.66	−0.45 ± 5.06	−3.82 ± 3.01	−4.08 ± 3.05

* Mean ± S. E.
† p < 0.01

rats as controls for their young morphine-treated rats and found that both groups had depressed body weights which did not differ significantly from one another.

Relatively few studies of long-term behavioral consequences of early morphine treatment have been conducted, but the implications from such studies are extremely important, particularly if deficits are identified which may be modified. Fishbein and Ford (1973) demonstrated that morphine treatment of rat mothers influenced the protein and RNA content of the brains of their offspring, and Steele and Johannesson (1975b) also showed that infusion of maternal rats at near term effects protein synthesis, possibly by interfering with the availability of mRNA. As alterations in proteins have long been thought to be associated with changes in long-term memory, it seems feasible that learning could be affected by early morphine treatment.

Banerjee (1975) showed that rats exposed to morphine prenatally and neonatally exhibited faster acquisition of a conditioned avoidance response if given a low concentration of morphine (.01%) and an impaired acquisition with higher concentrations (0.02%). He concluded that "prenatal and neonatal exposure to potentially addictive drugs" effected rates of learning to a lesser degree than if the drugs were first administered during the training period. In our work, animals in treatment groups exhibited no differences in rates of acquisition of the appetitive response, but the animals treated during days 3-12 with morphine failed to acquire an emotional response. The relation of neonatal morphine injection to avoidance learning certainly merits more attention.

In some instances, early morphine treatment has produced changes in later open field behavior in rats; Davis and Lin (1972) reported higher activity scores on days 30 and 70 in the pups of mothers treated with morphine during pregnancy. Animals in our last study showed increased activity over trials, indicating that asymptotic activity levels had not been reached on the initial trial. However, since open field activity has been shown to be affected monotonically by the amount of handling or stimulation rather than by the age of handling in the immature rat, and since all animals in all of our studies were handled daily during the preweaning period, it is likely that treatment effects may be masked by the stimulation of handling. Also, the mothers rather than the pups were treated in the Davis and Lin study. Observations of the animals' behavior in the open field did suggest differences of a qualitative nature among the treatment groups, and perhaps a cataloging of stereotyped behaviors (Charness et al., 1975) would be appropriate.

Protracted tolerance appears to be a prominent effect of early addiction to morphine. This phenomenon has now been demonstrated with respect to both the analgesic and the pituitary-adrenal stimulating actions of morphine. Cochin and Kornetsky (1964) produced evidence that morphine tolerance may last for more than one year in the rat. Several investigators have demonstrated persistent tolerance to morphine analgesia as a result of prenatal or early postnatal administration in rats (Huidobro and Huidobro, 1973; Nicak and Masnyk, 1966; Nicak, 1971; Kokka et al., 1973; and Johannesson et al., 1972). Our previous study has been confirmed and extended by .the present findings and it appears that the duration of the protracted tolerance to morphine may be more than 156 days. The implications of persistent tolerance in the clinical management of pain in individuals addicted to narcotics in childhood are considerable and should be explored systematically.

SUMMARY

Developmental, neuroendocrine, and behavioral effects of early morphine addiction in female rat pups were investigated in a series of studies in which treatment ages were varied to include: days 1-7, 8-14, 15-21, 3-12, 12-21, and 1-21. Compared with controls, body weights of morphine-injected animals, regardless of treatment age, were depressed during treatment and remained depressed for periods up to 105 days. Delayed eye-opening and early vaginal openings occurred in some of the animals administered morphine before day 14. Behaviorally, animals treated with the narcotic from days 3-12 showed impaired ability to learn a conditioned suppression response; all animals, in any early morphine treatment group, showed a reduced analgesic response to morphine, some even when 156 days old. Neonatally narcotic-treated rats also showed a decreased steroid rise in response to morphine challenges in adulthood. The persistence of these effects suggests that exposure of the immature female rat to morphine results in prolonged, possibly permanent morphine-specific alteration of brain mechanisms concerned with behavioral and neuroendocrine phenomena and supports the feasibility of using a rat model to study long-term effects of neonatal narcotic addiction.

ACKNOWLEDGMENTS

This work was supported by USPHS grant DA 826, and by University of Nebraska Research Council funds.
We also wish to thank Dr. Anna Taylor, Dr. C. N. Pang, Dr. Bruce

NEONATAL NARCOTIC ADDICTION 607

Bromley, John Young, and Dave Barrows for their suggestions and aid in some phases of data collection and analyses; Berilyn Branch and Valerie New for their excellent technical assistance; and Lynda Gelaude and Fedora Liner for their secretarial help.

REFERENCES

Bakke, J. L., N. Lawrence, and J. Bennett. 1973. Late effects of perinatal morphine on pituitary-thyroidal and gonadal function. *Biol. Neonate.* 23: 59–77.

Banerjee, U. 1974. Programmed self-administration of potentially addictive drugs in young rats and its effects on learning. *Psychopharmacologia* (Berlin) 38: 111–124.

Banerjee, U. 1975. Conditioned learning in young rats born of drug-addicted parents and raised on addictive drugs. *Psychopharmacologia* (Berlin) 41: 113–116.

Berger, B. D., and L. Stein. 1969. An analysis of the learning deficits produced by Scopolamine. *Psychopharmacologia* (Berlin) 14: 271–283.

Charness, M., Z. Amit, and M. Taylor. 1975. Morphine induced stereotypic behavior in rats. *Behav. Biol.* 13: 71–80.

Cochin, J., and C. Kornetsky. 1964. Development and loss of tolerance to morphine in rat after single and multiple injections. *J. Pharmacol. Exp. Ther.* 145: 1–10.

Davis, W. M., and C. H. Lin. 1972. Prenatal morphine effects on survival and behavior of rat offspring. *Res. Com. In Chem. and Pharmacol.* 3: 205–214.

Denenberg, V. H., and M. X. Zarrow. 1971. Effects of handling in infancy upon adult behavior and adrenocortical activity: Suggestions for a neuroendocrine mechanism. In D. N. Walcher and D. N. Peters, Eds. *Early Childhood.* Academic Press, New York, pp. 39–71.

Eddy, N. E., and D. Leimbach. 1953. Synthetic analgesics. II Diethienylbutenyl and dithienylbutylamines. *J. Pharmacol. Exp. Ther.* 107: 385–393.

Fishbein, J. O., and D. H. Ford. 1973. The effect of maternal morphine administration on the offspring. *ISPNE Abstracts.*

Friedler, G. 1972. Growth retardation in offspring of female rats treated with morphine prior to conception. *Sci.* 175: 654–655.

Friedler, G., and J. Cochin. 1968. The effect of cross-fostering on growth patterns in offspring of morphinized and withdrawn female rats. *Fed. Prod.* 27: 754.

Glick, D. D. von Redlish, and S. Levine. 1964. Fluorometric determination of corticosterone and cortisol in 0.02–0.05 milliliters of plasma or submilligram samples of adrenal tissue. *Endocrinology* 74: 652–655.

Huidobro, J. P., and F. Huidobro. 1973. Acute morphine tolerance in newborn and young rats. *Psychopharmacologia* (Berlin) 28: 27–34.

Johannesson, T., W. J. Steele, and B. A. Becker. 1972. Infusion of morphine in maternal rats at near-term: Maternal and foetal distribution and effects on analgesia, brain DNA, RNA and protein. *Acta Pharmacol. et Toxicol.* 31: 353–368.

Kennedy, C. C. 1968. Interactions between feeding behavior and hormones during growth. *Annals N. Y. Acad. Sci.* 68: 1049–1060.

Kokka, N., J. F. Garcia, and H. W. Elliott. 1973. Effects of acute and chronic administration of narcotic analgesics on growth hormone and corticotrophin (ACTH) secretion in rats. *Prog. Brain Res.* 39: 347–360.

Krause, S. O., P. M. Murray, J. B. Holmes, and R. E. Burch. 1958. Heroin addiction among pregnant women and their newborn babies. *Am. J. Obst. & Gynec.* 75: 754–758.

Kupferberg, J. H. 1963. Pharmacologic basis for the increased sensitivity of the newborn rat to morphine. *J. Pharmacol.* 141: 105–112.

Naeye, R. L., W. Blanc, W. Leblanc, and M. A. Khatamee. 1973. Fetal complications of maternal heroin addiction: Abnormal growth, infections and episodes of stress. *J. Pediatrics* 6: 1055–1061.

Naeye, R. L., and W. Blanc. 1973. Fetal growth in offspring of heroin addicts: A quantitative study. *Amer. J. Path.* 70: 85a.

Nicak, A., and S. Masnyk. 1966. Modification of the analgetic effect in relation to the developmental stage in rats. *Med. Pharmacol. Exp.* 14: 273–275.

Nicak, A. 1971. Pethidine-induced inhibition of nociceptive stimuli in young and aged rats. *Agents and Actions* 2: 18–20.

Quadagno, D. M., J. Shryne, C. Andersen, and R. A. Gorski. 1972. Influence of gonadal hormones on social, sexual, emergence and open field behavior in the rat: Rattus norvegicus. *An. Behav.* 20: 732–740.

Sobotka, T. S., M. Cook, and R. Brodie. 1974. Neonatal malnutrition: Neurochemical, hormonal and behavioral manifestations. *Brain Res.* 65: 443–457.

Steele, W. J., and T. Johannesson. 1975a. Effects of morphine infusion in maternal rats at near-term on ribosome size distribution in foetal and maternal rat brain. *Acta Pharmacol. et Toxicol.* 36: 243–256.

Steele, W. J., and T. Johannesson. 1975b. Effects of prenatally-administered morphine on brain development and resultant tolerance to the analgesic effect of morphine in offspring of morphine treated rats. *Acta Pharmacol. et Toxicol.* 36: 243–256.

Way, E. L., H. Loh, and F. H. Shen. 1969. Simultaneous quantitative assessment of morphine tolerance and physical dependence. *J. Pharmacol.* 167: 1–8.

Weiner, R., and Scapagnini. 1974. Effect of central acting drugs on the onset of puberty. In E. Zimmermann and R. George, Eds. *Narcotics and the Hypothalamus.* Raven Press, New York, pp. 175–183.

Wilson, G. S., M. M. Desmond, and W. M. Verniaud. 1973. Early development of infants of heroin-addicted mothers. *Amer. J. Dis. Child.* 123: 457–462.

Zimmermann, E., and V. Critchlow. 1967. Effects of diurnal variation in plasma corticosterone levels on adrenocortical response to stress. *Proc. Soc. Exp. Biol. Med.* 125: 658–663.

Zimmermann, E., B. Branch, A. N. Taylor, J. Young, and C. N. Pang. 1974. Long-lasting effects of prepuberal administration of morphine in adult rats. In E. Zimmermann and R. George, Eds. *Narcotics and the Hypothalamus.* Raven Press, New York, pp. 183–194.

Zimmermann, E., C. N. Pang, B. Branch, and A. Newman Taylor. 1975. ACTH secretion in rats bearing subcutaneous morphine pellets. *Fed. Proc.* 34: 301.

Tissue Responses to Addictive Drugs
© 1976, Spectrum Publications, Inc.

The Effects of Maternal Morphine or Methadone Intake on the Growth, Reflex Development and Maze Behavior of Rat Offspring

JACQUELINE F. McGINTY
DONALD H. FORD

Department of Anatomy
State University of New York
Downstate Medical Center
Brooklyn, New York

Urban obstetricians commonly treat pregnant women who are addicted to narcotics or being maintained on methadone. In 1971, 1 out of every 60 infants born at the State University or Kings County Hospital was born to a heroin-addicted mother (Harper, et al., 1973). The addictive effects of opiates taken by a woman during pregnancy often manifest themselves in the newborn within 72 hours of birth. The neonatal withdrawal syndrome is well documented (Blatman, 1971, 1973; Cobrinik, et al., 1959; Goodfriend, et al., 1956; Hill and Desmond, 1963; Lewis, et al., 1973; Perlmutter, 1967; Reddy, et al., 1971; Zelson, et al., 1971). However, there are less data on the association between narcotic intake and infant viability, birth weight, or complications. What is reported is often contradictory. For example, Blatman (1973) reported birth weights of babies born to heroin addicts to be lower than those born to methadone-treated women although both groups had a mean birth weight which was less than that of the rest of the clinic population evaluated. Contrarily, Newman (1973) reported no correlation between methadone dosage or duration of intake and neonatal birth weights, complications, or malformations.

Even less is known about the effects of narcotics on the long-term growth and development of the child. Postnatal follow-up studies on such children are often nonexistent, very short, or unsatisfactory due to lack of parental cooperation (Lewis, 1973). Observations which have been made on children from the age of eight months until four years have shown normal mental and physical development (Blatman and Lipsitz, 1970) or, on the contrary, a slow growth rate in the first year followed by a slight but measurable lag in the expression of physical and psychological development up to three years of age (Hill and Desmond, 1963). Since environmental factors as well as prenatal exposure to opiates may influence growth and development, it is impossible to attribute a lag in either to any one factor in the clinical situation.

In order to determine the effects of maternal opiate intake on the growth and development of offspring, we are endeavoring to design an experimental model for study using laboratory animals. Previous attempts in this laboratory using intravenous morphine injections during the third trimester have resulted in either resorption of the fetuses or a 20-30 gram weight loss of the gravid rat during the last days of gestation. Consequently, another route of administration was tried on a pair of female Wistar rats who were given 0.5 mg/ml morphine sulfate in their drinking water. Both animals resorbed their fetuses. Another pregnant Wistar rat was given 0.3 mg/ml morphine in her water. She delivered but did not lactate. Although morphine is not supposed to be as effective orally as when it is injected, these detrimental results suggest that the morphine was having an effect on reproduction. Based on the experience with these trials, the following model was established with the hope of obtaining surviving litters to study throughout development.

MATERIALS AND METHODS

We divided 8 Sprague-Dawley rats into 4 groups of 2 animals each on the fifteenth day of their 21 day gestation. Group 1 received 0.3 mg/ml morphine sulfate in the drinking water. Group 2 received 0.5 mg/ml (d)*l*-methadone in the drinking water. However, this latter dosage proved to be sufficiently distasteful to these rats that they reduced their water intake markedly with a similar drop in food intake also. Therefore, on the third day of treatment, the methadone dosage was dropped to 0.35 mg/ml and was maintained at this level. Group 3 was pair fed to the morphine-treated animals; that is, they were fed the same amount of food on day two of treatment as the Group 1 animals had eaten on day one and so forth throughout pregnancy and lactation. Group 4 constituted a normal or ad lib control with free access to food and water. The rats were housed individually in a temperature controlled room with a 12 hour light:12 hour dark cycle. Each rat was weighed at the start of treatment and three times per week thereafter.

At delivery, all pups were weighed and the litters were reduced to eight infants apiece. The extra pups were sacrificed on day one of life for histological analysis of brain tissue. These pups were decapitated, the brains were dissected out, fixed in formalin, embedded in paraffin, and sectioned for staining with hematoxylin and eosin. Cortical thicknesses were measured with a micrometer. Cell and nuclear volumes of the hypoglossal nucleus were calculated by the formula of Schadé and Harreveld (1961) for the volume of ventral horn cells. The nuclear volumes of the cells of the inferior olivary nucleus were also calculated, using the formula for the volume of a sphere.

The remaining pups in each litter started behavioral testing on the second day of life. They were weighed on testing days which continued three times per week for 35 days. Seven categories of development were followed as described below.

1. *Spontaneous behavior*. The pup was placed individually in an open field marked off in 3 in x 3 in squares where any behavior exhibited during 1 min was recorded.

2. *Light touch response*. A Von Frey hair was used to touch the animal lightly on its muzzle, shoulder, hind leg, and forepaw and the response to each touch was recorded.

3. *Righting reflex*. The animal was placed on its back and the time and ease of turning onto the ventral surface were recorded.

4. *Contact placing*. The dorsum of the animal's paw was brushed lightly against a stable surface and the development of a reflex withdrawal of the limb and placement on the surface for support was noted.

5. *Vestibular drop reaction*. The rat was held high off a table and was brought down swiftly. Development of a pronounced extension of all four limbs in a protective posture was noted.

6. *Climbing*. The rat was placed between the experimenter's thumb and index finger, hanging by its forelimbs. Strength of grip and subsequent hoisting of the body up onto the dorsum of the hand was recorded.

7. *Pain response*. The animal's response to compression of the tail was recorded.

Any relevant comments and additional observations were recorded with the above information on an infant rat evaluation form.

Upon weaning, offspring were separated by sex and housed by litter. They were weaned at age 26 days except for those of the Pair Fed 2 group whose mother died of unknown causes on the twentieth day postpartum. These animals quickly foraged for themselves without any observably ill effects. At weaning, the Morphine 1 group was placed on 0.3 mg/ml morphine sulfate in the drinking water. The Morphine 2 group did not receive any further drug treatment. The Methadone group received 0.35 mg/ml in its drinking water after weaning. All animals were fed ad libitum.

At age 54 days, after all animals exhibited the tested patterns of adult behaviors, 6 of each group were killed by an ether overdose. The cerebral hemispheres, cerebellum, diencephalon-brain stem, pituitary and endocrine organs were removed, fixed in formalin, and weighed. The remaining 2 animals of each litter were spared to begin a problem solving task which was undertaken to attempt to determine if the morphine or methadone treatment had affected the learning ability of the rat offspring. Only females were used because the only 2 males in the Methadone group died within 24 hours of each other at 21 days of age.

The test apparatus for the learning task and the training procedure used were described by Rabinovitch and Rosvold (1951). It consisted of a simple maze-learning design taught to the animals with a suitable adaptation period, preliminary runs, and numerous test trials. On completion of the learning task, time records and the number of mistakes made in the maze were subjected to an analysis of variance. The rats were killed on day 66 by an ether overdose. The same tissues as described above were removed, fixed, and weighed. Analyses of variance were performed on all tissues removed from both age groups to determine any significant differences in weights among treatment groups.

RESULTS

Figure 1 illustrates the changes in maternal body weight from the initiation of treatment on day 15 of gestation until parturition on day twenty-one. The Ad Lib Control mother gained 100 grams during this time. The Pair Fed 1 animal gained only 45 grams and the Pair Fed 2 animal gained only 35 grams with an initial weight loss of 5 grams. The Morphine 1 rat gained 65 grams and the Morphine 2 rat gained 78 grams. The only other weight loss was evident in the Methadone groups.

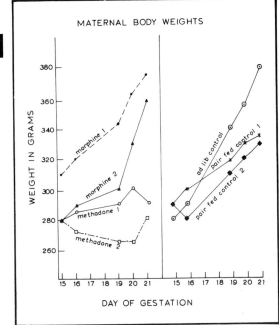

The effect of morphine or methadone on the weights of gravid rats from the initiation of treatment on day 15 of gestation until parturition on day 21. Each curve represents the weight change of one animal.

The Methadone 1 animal showed slow gains up to 20 grams with a final 5 gram weight loss which may have been indicative of the subsequent loss of her entire litter. The Methadone 2 animal lost 15 grams initially and just regained that amount by delivery.

The Methadone-treated mothers ate an average of 12 grams of food per day and drank a mean 18 ml of water as compared to the Morphine-treated mothers' mean intake of 20 grams of food and 40 ml of water per day—approximately double the intake of the Methadone animals. Decreasing the dosage of methadone on the third day of treatment did not appreciably improve food and water intake during the last days of gestation.

All the Morphine, Methadone, and Pair Fed rats, and one of the Ad Lib Control rats delivered litters. The other Normal Control rat did not show any signs of pregnancy and was excluded from the study when she did not deliver. The Methadone 2 animal delivered 10 pups. Five died immediately and 5 died within 24 hours of birth. This mother slowly and incompletely cleaned up the afterbirth. She showed no signs of lactation and her breast tissue was undeveloped. The other mother rats all showed normal maternal and nesting behaviors (see Table I).

Table I.   The effect of prenatal exposure to morphine or methadone on litter size, sex of offspring, and incidence of mortality among offspring.

LITTER	SIZE	♂	♀	DEATHS
MORPHINE 1	13	7	6	0
MORPHINE 2	8	5	3	0
METHADONE 1	10	not sexed		10-at birth
METHADONE 2	10	2	8	3-day 20, 21
PAIR FED 1	11	4	6	1-at birth
PAIR FED 2	12	5	7	0
AD LIB 1	8	5	3	0
AD LIB 2	0	-	-	-

There were no significant size differences between the litters of different treatment groups. The largest litter size difference occurred between the two Morphine groups. However, this difference did not correlate with a significant difference in birth weights between the 2 Morphine litters. The sex distribution among litters was unremarkable except for that of the viable Methadone litter which had 2 males and 8 females. Both of the males died within 3 weeks along with 1 female. The mortality rate was extremely high only in the Methadone litters.

Tables II and III show the results of histological analysis on the brains of one day old rats taken from each treatment group. Table II shows the cytoplasmic and nuclear volumes of cells of the hypoglossal nuclei and nuclear volumes of inferior olivary nuclei. Each value represents the mean of ten cells from one animal. In the hypoglossal nucleus, the cytoplasmic volume is greater among the control groups than in that of the experimentals generally, while the nuclear volume of cells remains relatively constant across all groups. Thus, the increased cytoplasmic to nuclear volume ratio (CV/NV) among both control groups means that there is a greater amount of cytoplasm in relation to the

Table II. Cytoplasmic and nuclear volumes of cells from the hypoglossal nuclei and nuclear volumes of cells from the inferior olivary nuclei of one day old rats exposed to morphine or methadone in utero. CV/NV = the cell to nuclear volume ratio. Each value represents the mean for ten cells from one animal. Cell volumes were calculated from the formula of Schade and Harreveld for ventral horn cells (1961).

TREATMENT GROUP	HYPOGLOSSAL NUCLEUS			INFERIOR OLIVE
	CELL VOL. (μ^3cv)	NUCLEAR VOL. (μ^3nv)	CV/NV	NUCLEAR VOL. (μ^3nv)
MORPHINE	879±113	353±34	2.24±.36	114±114
METHADONE	672±68	253±26	2.81±.77	140±23.8
PAIR FED	866±84	294±25	3.12±.45	105±6.0
	1015±73	260±27	4.38±.60	122±9.2
	1210±69	313±35	4.40±.64	172±26.5
	1062±85	325±11	3.29±.26	128±10.1
AD LIB	1238±171	312±24	4.08±.32	68±11.2

volume of the cell's nucleus. Not enough cytoplasm was available to measure in the inferior olive. Table III depicts the thickness of the cerebral cortices from the one day old rats. The cortices of controls are thicker than those of the experimental animals. The data also suggest a more orderly columnar organization among control cortices. Disruption of the cell columns in the cortices of the Methadone animals was similar to that seen in irradiated fetuses.

Table IV shows the mean birth weight of each litter and the results of an analysis of variance performed on these data. At birth, the Ad Lib Control group weighed significantly more, and the Methadone offspring weighed significantly less, than all other groups. The Morphine litter weights were equivalent but the Pair Fed 1 weights were significantly heavier than the Pair Fed 2 weights. Recall that the Pair Fed 2 mother lost 5 grams at the initiation of treatment which may account for a setback in the growth of her litter in utero. The Morphine offspring

Table III.   Thickness of the cerebral cortices from one day old rats exposed to morphine or methadone in utero. Each number represents the value for one animal.

LITTER	CORTICAL THICKNESS	OBSERVATIONS
MORPHINE	417μ	CELLS LESS
	417μ	DENSELY PACKED
	417μ	THAN CONTROLS
METHADONE	334μ	CELL COLUMNS
	417μ	DISRUPTED AND
		LESS DENSE
		THAN CONTROLS
PAIR FED	540μ	
	500μ	
AD LIB	500μ	
	500μ	
	542μ	

were significantly smaller than the Ad Lib and Pair Fed 1 groups but larger than the Pair Fed 2 and Methadone litters. There were no significant differences between weights of males and females at birth.

Throughout development, the Methadone rats remained smaller and developed more slowly than all other offspring. Analyses of variance were performed for days 19, 30, 43, and 54. The weights of the Ad Lib Control group remained significantly heavier than the Methadone and Morphine animals' weights on the days analyzed. The Pair Fed animals' weights did not differ from the Ad Lib Controls'; nor did the Pair Fed litters' weights differ from the Morphine groups' weights. The Methadone animals weighed significantly less than the Pair Fed and Morphine groups on days 43 and 54 (see Figures 2 and 3). Analyses were performed on the same days as described for the female data. The Pair Fed and Ad Lib Control weights were equivalent. The Morphine litters weighed significantly less than the Pair Fed litters on days 43 and 54 and less than the Ad Lib Control animals at all periods measured.

Table IV.   The mean birth weights of control rats and rats exposed to morphine or methadone in utero and the results of an analysis of variance performed. Each number represents the mean weight of eight pups in each litter.

LITTER	MORPHINE 1	MORPHINE 2	METHADONE
X̄ WGT. & S.E.	6.40±.119	6.26±.112	5.16±.102
	=MORPHINE 2 >METHADONE p<.001 >PAIR FED 2 p<.05 <PAIR FED 1 p<.025 <AD LIB p<.001	=MORPHINE 1 >METHADONE p<.001 >PAIR FED 2 p<.005 <PAIR FED 1 <AD LIB p<.05	<MORPHINE 1 <MORPHINE 2 <PAIR FED 1 <AD LIB p<.001 <PAIR FED 2 p<.05

LITTER	PAIR FED 1	PAIR FED 2	AD LIB
X WGT. & S.E.	7.00±.032	6.08±.104	7.40±.087
	>MORPHINE 1 p<.025 >MORPHINE 2 >PAIR FED 2 >METHADONE p<.001 <AD LIB p<.05	<MORPHINE 1 p<.05 <MORPHINE 2 <PAIR FED 1 p<.001 <AD LIB p<.001 METHADONE p<.05	>MORPHINE 1 >METHADONE >PAIR FED 2 p<.001 >MORPHINE 2 >PAIR FED 1 p<.05

With regard to other parameters of development, the Methadone animals again lagged the most. Their fur appeared two days later than that of Normal animals and remained sparse and uneven throughout life. Their eyes and ears opened one day later than the Ad Lib Controls'. Neither the vaginas of the Morphine or Methadone animals opened until 100% of the vaginas of the Pair Fed and Ad Lib Control animals had opened (see Figures 4 and 5).

Of the developmental reflexes and motor skills which were followed, no significant differences emerged between groups. However, there were trends which were apparent and can be summarized as follows. The neonatal rat's only purposive behavior consists of approaching the mother to suckle followed by sleeping. Because its eyes and ears are not open at birth, the neonate must be able to locomote toward its mother by sensing her warmth and her smell. It is able to creep a short distance

---

2

The growth from day 1 to day 54 of female rats from control litters or from litters exposed to morphine or methadone. Analyses of variance were performed on data for days 19, 30, 43, and 54. Significant differences were found between the Ad Lib Control group and the Morphine group at the .01 level. Differences between the Ad Lib group and the Methadone group were significant at the .001 level and between the Methadone and Pair Fed and Morphine groups at the .01 level, the latter on days 43 and 54. Numbers in parentheses refer to the number of rats in each group.

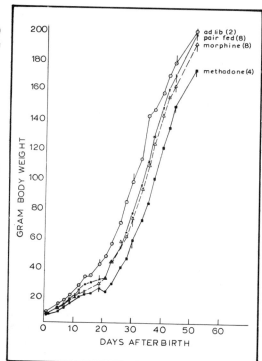

with the help of reciprocally flexing forelimbs and it drags its hindlimbs. At all other times it lies on its belly with its legs sprawled out to the side. The neonate responds to regional tactile and painful stimuli with a whole body startle response and prolonged convulsions. When placed on its back, the rat cannot right itself initially, then gradually shows a struggling, segmental effort with much rocking back and forth which may or may not be successful in turning the infant over. Few other overt signs of behavior are present in the neonate.

The eleventh day of the rat pups' life was selected to illustrate one point of reflex and motor skill development at a time when differences between treatment groups were maximal. At this age, the normal rat began to show vigorous behavior beyond the approach–suckle–sleep cycle. The three other groups showed different stages of retardation. In an open field marked off in three inch squares, the Ad Lib Control rats traversed an average of 15 squares per minute, the Pair Fed rats traversed a mean of 9 squares, the Morphine rats a mean of 4 squares, and the Methadone animals tended to stay within the square where

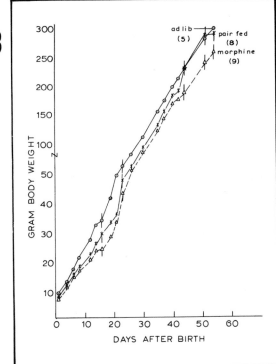

3

The growth from day 1 to day 54 of male rats from control litters or from litters exposed to morphine. The Morphine animals weighed signifiicantly less than the Pair Fed animals on days 43 and 54 at the .01 level and less than the Ad Lib animals at the .01 level on days 19, 30, 43, and 54. Numbers in parentheses refer to the number of rats in each group.

they were initially placed (see Table V). All animals showed exploratory sniffing and head turning. The Ad Lib animal was able to support the weight of its body on its forelimbs at this age as well as to walk in a coordinated, quadrupedal fashion. The animals of both the Pair Fed and Morphine groups could only partially support their bodies on their limbs and walked with some reciprocal limb movement and some hind-limb dragging. At 11 days of age the Methadone rats could not support their bodies on their limbs and they did not show reciprocal limb movements. In the Ad Lib Control animals, a definite increase in loco-motor speed and agility accompanied active exploration whereas the other animals were more limited by their less developed locomotor abil-ities at this age (see Table VI). When the Ad Lib Control rats were placed upon their backs, they immediately righted themselves and started to move away. The Pair Fed and Morphine animals showed less seg-mentation and struggling than the neonate. The Methadone rats showed the most difficulty and segmentation. When touched lightly with a

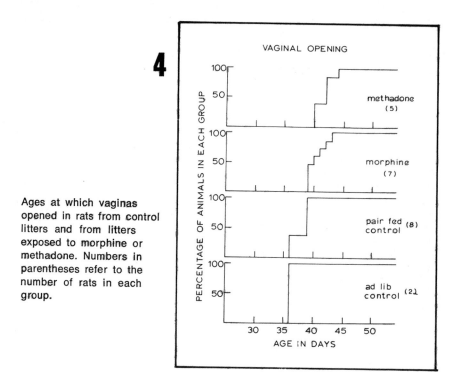

4

VAGINAL OPENING

Ages at which vaginas opened in rats from control litters and from litters exposed to morphine or methadone. Numbers in parentheses refer to the number of rats in each group.

brush, the Ad Lib Controls and the Pair Fed rats scratched or withdrew the area stimulated. The Morphine and Methadone rats still showed a whole body startle response to touch. The Ad Lib, Pair Fed, and Morphine animals all showed the same response to compression of the tail; they squeaked, wagged their tails and made attempts to escape. The Methadone rats still showed a whole body startle with twisting of the pelvis, prolonged tail wagging, and a squeal. At 11 days, only the normal controls were successful climbers. Contact placing by all groups was evident at this age and the vestibular drop reaction was not. This hierarchy of maturation persisted throughout the developmental period. The experimental animals showed the same pattern of adult behaviors as the controls but the appearance of these behaviors was delayed. This delay was most apparent in the Methadone rats and less so in the Morphine and Pair Fed animals.

The results of the maze-learning task showed no significant differences between groups but certain trends were noted. The Ad Lib Control animals made the fewest mistakes and ran the maze in the shortest amount of time. The Methadone animals performed almost as well according to both criteria. Subjectively, these animals did not seem

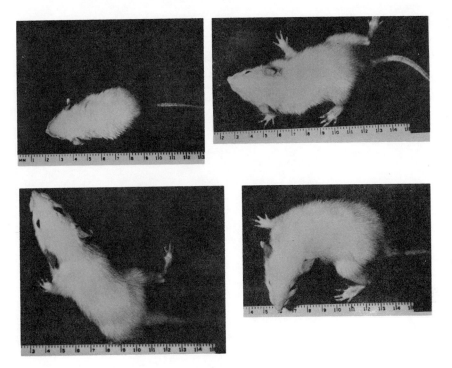

5 Photographs of a representative rat from each treatment group at age 28 days. Upper left: Methadone-exposed. Upper right: Morphine-exposed. Lower left: Ad Lib control. Lower right: Pair Fed control.

to be as distracted and did not spend as much time exploring the test apparatus during trials as did the Morphine or Pair Fed rats.

In general, the Morphine animals' absolute brain weights (at 54 days) were less than those of either control (see Table VII). Conversely, the brain tissue from the Morphine rats comprised a greater percentage of body weight than did that of the Pair Fed or Ad Lib animals. The brain tissue from the female rats who were killed on day 66 after running the maze showed less consistent results in the smaller sample available (see Table VIII). However, the general hierarchical trend of heavier brain weight, lower percentage of body weight for the control compared to the experimental animals tended to be evident. The endocrine organs showed little variation in size.

CONCLUSIONS

This work represents the preliminary results of an experimental model in the process of being revised. Revisions are necessary primarily

Table V.   The pattern of spontaneous behaviors exhibited by 11-day-old rats from control litters or from litters exposed to maternal intake of morphine or methadone.

	Ad Lib	Pair Fed
Spontaneous Behavior	Traversed fifteen squares per minute	Traversed nine squares per per minute
	Sniffing, head turning	Sniffing, head turning
	Body supported on limbs	Body partially supported on limbs
	Coordinated quadrupedal walk	Some reciprocal limb movement; some dragging
	Active exploration	Moderate exploration
	Morphine	**Methadone**
Spontaneous Behavior	Traversed four squares per minute	Stayed in 3″ square
	Sniffing, head turning	Sniffing, head turning
	Body partially supported on limbs	Body not supported on limbs
	Some reciprocal limb movement; some dragging	Non-reciprocal limb use; hindlimb dragging

to unravel drug effects from the effects of fetal undernourishment in a larger sample of animals. Any significant differences which have been reported at this time must be attributed to a compound interaction between fetal undernourishment and drug effects. Information derived from this pilot study indicates that there are real differences between the experimental treatment groups and the normal control group with respect to birth, growth, and brain weights, histological analysis of brain tissue, and reflex development. If a nutritional deficiency alone were responsible for the deficits in the drug-treated animals, one would expect to find no differences between the morphine-treated litters and the litters pair fed against the Morphine litters. However, differences between these two groups are suggested particularly in body weights and in cerebral cortical thicknesses at birth.

The data on the methadone-treated animals are more difficult to interpret in the absence of an adequate pair fed control. However, there is a clue that an independent effect of methadone may be operating if one considers the histological analysis of cerebral cortex. While differences in cortical thickness may be nutritionally derived, the disruption of the columnar organization of the cells in the cortices of the methadone-

Table VI. Various developmental patterns of behavior exhibited by 11-day-old rats from control litters or from litters exposed to maternal intake of morphine or methadone.

	Ad Lib	Pair Fed
Righting	Immediate; moves away.	Less segmental.
Light	Local response.	Local response.
Touch	Scratch or withdrawal	Scratch or withdrawal
Pain	Squeak Tail wag Escape	Squeak Tail wag Escape
Climbing	Spontaneous Successful	Not spontaneous Unsuccessful

	Morphine	Methadone
Righting	Less segmental	Segmental; struggling
Light	Whole body startle	Whole body startle
Touch		
Pain	Squeak Tail wag Escape	Squeal Prolonged pelvic twisting Whole body startle
Climbing	Unsuccessful	Unsuccessful

treated animals alone does not appear to be a nutritionally related phenomenon. Further investigation of these variables in a larger sample of rats may be worthwhile.

Recently, we have injected both morphine and methadone subcutaneously into a group of Sprague-Dawley rats in graduated dosages for one month. The animals appeared to be well nourished and they gained weight during this treatment period. We are planning to try this route of administration on pregnant rats with the hope of separating the effects of fetal undernourishment from the possible teratological effects of these narcotics.

SUMMARY

A pilot study was undertaken on the effects on offspring of chronic morphine or methadone in the drinking water of pregnant, and subsequently, nursing rats. Experimental animals, beginning drug treatment on day 15 of gestation, were compared to rats pair fed with the Morphine mothers and to Normal Controls who had free access to food and water.

Table VII.   The wet weights of brain tissue expressed as the mean absolute value and as the percentage of body weight from male rats 54 days old from control litters or from litters exposed to morphine. Numbers in parentheses refer to the number of rats in each group. Analyses of variance were performed on the weights and p values are given where significant differences were found.

LITTER	WHOLE BRAIN		HEMISPHERES		CEREBELLUM		BRAIN STEM	
	ABSOL. WGT.	% BODY WGT.	ABSOL. WGT.	% BODY WGT.	ABSOL. WGT.	% BODY WGT.	ABSOL. WGT.	% BODY WGT.
MORPHINE 1 (4)	2584±20	1.017±.032	1606±21 >MOR2 p<.01	.632±.017	336±4	.132±.001	642±9	.253±.013
MORPHINE 2 (5)	2475±14	1.022±.04	1494±14	.617±.025	358±6	.148±.006	623±6	.257±.009
PAIR FED (8)	2626±26 >MOR1 p<.01 >MOR2 p<.005	.914±.072	1604±18 >MOR2 p<.001	.558±.01 <MOR1 <MOR2 p<.005	357±5 >MOR1 p<.05	.124±.002 <MOR1 <MOR2 p<.05	665±12	.227±.01
AD LIB (5)	2616±34 >MOR1 >MOR2 p<.01	.940±.05	1583±39	.568±.03	363±8 >MOR1 p<.05	.130±.008 <MOR2 p<.005	671±7	.238±.011

One methadone-treated litter of 10 pups died within 24 hours of birth. The second methadone-treated litter lost its 2 male pups and 1 female within 3 weeks of birth.

The Methadone offspring weighed significantly less than all other offspring at birth and throughout life. Their overall development occurred more slowly than that of the other groups. Their fur appeared later, and, with few exceptions, their eyes, ears, and vaginas opened at a later date. Their reflexes and motor skills developed later than those of any other group, but eventually the Methadone rats exhibited all the tested patterns of normal adult behavior.

The Morphine litters were significantly smaller than the Normal and one Pair Fed Control group at birth. They weighed less than the Normal Controls and their reflex development lagged behind normal throughout development, but not as much as the Methadone animals'.

The Normal Control rats were the most robust, most heavily and evenly furred, the largest, and the first to open their eyes, ears, and

Table VIII. The wet weights of brain tissue expressed as the mean absolute value and as the percentage of body weight from female rats 66-days-old from control litters or from litters exposed to morphine or methadone. Numbers in parentheses refer to the number of rats in each group. P values are given where significant differences were found.

LITTER	WHOLE BRAIN		HEMISPHERES		CEREBELLUM		BRAIN STEM	
	ABSOL. WGT.	% BODY WGT.	ABSOL. WGT.	% BODY WGT.	ABSOL. WGT.	% BODY WGT.	ABSOL. WGT.	% BODY WGT.
MORPHINE 1 (2)	2413±49 <MOR 2 PAIR AD LIB p<.05	1.48±.03	1446±7 <PAIR p<.005 <AD LIB p<.05	.886±.01 >AD LIB p<.01	316±10 <AD LIB p<.05	.194±.007	651±21	.398±.014 <MOR 2 p<.05
MORPHINE 2 (2)	2569±31	1.67±.02	1529±18	.994±.01	328±3 <AD LIB p<.025	.231±0	712±11	.462±0 >PAIR p<.05
METHADONE (2)	2431±70	1.46±0	1429±11	.859±.04	295±15 <AD LIB p<.05	.177±0	707±57	.427±.05
PAIR FED (2)	2598±12	1.38±.01	1548±5	.819±.01	340±22	.180±.01	710±39	.375±.03
AD LIB (2)	2593±13	1.36±.07	1487±3	.784±0	366±4	.193±0	740±0	.390±0

vaginas, as well as to develop all the tested reflexes and motor skills.

The Pair Fed animals' growth and development fell between that of the Normal Controls and the Morphine animals in all respects.

In a series of mazes run by a small sample of females taken 'from each group at 60 days of age, the Normal Controls traversed the field fastest and with the fewest mistakes. The Methadone animals performed almost as well according to both criteria.

Of the tissues removed and weighed at death, the endocrine organs varied little in size whereas whole brain wet weights from normal animals were significantly heavier than those from methadone or morphine-treated groups. Significant differences in whole brain wet weight as a percentage of body weight tended to vary inversely with the absolute body weights in each group.

The above findings are considered in relation to fetal undernourishment and the possible teratological effects of morphine and methadone which warrant further study.

ACKNOWLEDGMENTS

We would like to thank Dr. Caroline Ware for her assistance in evaluating the behavior of the infant rats and Dr. Jacqueline Jakway for her helpful suggestions and critical appraisal of the manuscript.

This work was supported by a U. S. Public Health Service Grant (DA 00114–04).

REFERENCES

Blatman, S. 1971. Commentaries. *Pediatrics* 48 (2): 173–175.

Blatman, S. 1973. Methadone effects on pregnancy and the newborn. In *National Conference on Methadone Treatment*, No. 5, vol. 2. National Association for the Prevention of Addiction to Narcotics, New York, pp. 842–845.

Blatman, S., and P. Lipsitz. 1970. Infants born to heroin addicts maintained on methadone: Neonatal observations and followup. In *National Conference on Methadone Treatment*, No. 3, National Association for the Prevention of Addiction to Narcotics, New York, pp. 175–176.

Cobrinik, R. W., T. R. Hood, and E. Chusik. 1959. Effects of maternal narcotic addiction on the newborn. *Pediatrics* 24: 288.

Goodfriend, M. J., I. A. Shey, and M. D. Klein. 1956. Effects of maternal narcotic addiction on the newborn. *Am. J. Obstet. Gynec.* 71: 29–36.

Harper, R. G., G. I. Solish, E. Sang, H. Purow, and W. Panepinto. 1973. The effect of a methadone treatment program upon pregnant addicts and their infants. In *National Conference on Methadone Treatment*, No. 5, vol. 2. National Association for the Prevention of Addiction to Narcotics, New York, pp. 1133–1137.

Hill, R. M., and M. M. Desmond. 1963. Management of the narcotic withdrawal syndrome in the neonate. *Pediatric Clinics of North America* 10 (1): 67.

Lewis, B. W., and J. K. Stothers. 1973. Congenital narcotic addiction. *Postgrad. Med. J.* 49: 83–85.

Newman, R. G. 1973. Results of 120 deliveries of patients in the New York City Methadone Maintenance Treatment Program. In *National Conference on Methadone Treatment*, No. 5, vol. 2. National Association for the Prevention of Addiction to Narcotics, New York, pp. 1114–1121.

Perlmutter, J. F. 1967. Drug addiction in pregnant women. *Am. J. Obstet. Gynec.* 99: 569.

Rabinovitch, M. S., and H. E. Rosvold. 1951. A closed field intelligence test for rats. *Canadian J. Psychol.* 5: 122.

Reddy, A. M., R. G. Harper, and G. Stern. 1971. Observations on heroin and methadone withdrawal in the newborn. *Pediatrics* 48: 353–358.

Schadé, J. P., and A. Van Harreveld. 1961. Volume distribution of moto- and interneurons in the peroneus-tibialis neuron pool of the cat. *J. Comp. Neurol.* 117: 387–398.
Zelson, C., E. Rubio, and E. Wasserman. 1971. Neonatal narcotic addiction: A ten year observation. *Pediatrics* 48: 178–189.

Tissue Responses to Addictive Drugs
© 1976, Spectrum Publications, Inc.

The Sea Urchin Egg as a Model System to Study Effects of Narcotics on Secretion

CONSTANCE CARDASIS
HERBERT SCHUEL

Departments of Anatomy and Biochemistry
State University of New York
Downstate Medical Center
Brooklyn, New York

The sea urchin egg affords a model system for studying the effects of narcotics. There is evidence that many of the actions of narcotics may not be limited to neurons but can be considered as cellular phenomena. For example, single cell systems such as cultured fibroblasts, protozoa, and even bacteria have been studied (Simon, 1971).

The fertilized sea urchin egg can be used to study narcotic affects on many cellular processes including the initiation of protein and nucleic acid synthesis, chromosome replication, differentiation, the assembly and function of microtubules, cell division, etc. This chapter deals with the effects of narcotics on the process of secretion, in particular the actual release of secretory granules. Narcotics may affect discharge of secretory granules in mammalian cells, particularly at synapses (Cox and Weinstock, 1966; Ford et al., 1974; Sharkawi and Schulman, 1969) and possibly at endocrine glands. The fertilized sea urchin egg offers numerous advantages for the study of the mechanism of narcotic effect on release.

631

The mature unfertilized sea urchin egg is surrounded by a plasma membrane and a vitelline layer. The latter is similar to the glycocalyx surrounding many other types of cells. Under the surface of the egg is a single layer of cortical (secretory) granules, separated from the plasma membrane by 200 Å. These granules are similar to secretory granules in other kinds of cells. They are surrounded by a membrane and contain substances such as calcium (Cardasis et al., 1974), sulfated acid mucopolysaccharides (Schuel et al., 1974) and proteases (Schuel et al., 1973), which are common to secretory granules of many cell types. Development of the cortical granules occurs during oogenesis when they are pinched off from the Golgi apparatus and migrate to the surface (Anderson, 1968). The cortical granules in the mature egg are all fully formed and ready to be released when stimulated.

Discharge of the cortical granules and detachment of the vitelline layer to form the fertilization membrane begin immediately after insemination. The release begins at the site of sperm penetration and spreads around the entire surface of the egg, all the cortical granules being released within a period of 60 seconds. The mechanism of release is by exocytosis. There appears to be a series of membrane fusions between the cortical granule membranes and plasma membrane. The granule contents are expelled into the perivitelline space (Anderson, 1968).

Calcium has been implicated in this process (Epel, 1975) as it has been in release of secretory granules of many other types of cells (Poste and Allison, 1973; Rubin, 1970). Pyroantimonate has been used as an electron dense stain to determine the ultrastructural location of calcium in mammalian cells (Herman, et al., 1973). We have applied this technique to sea urchin eggs. Calcium can be seen complexed to antimonate before (see Figure 1) and 30 seconds following fertilization (Figure 2). The use of EGTA and X-ray microprobe analysis has verified the presence of calcium in these deposits (Cardasis et al., 1974; Schuel et al., 1975). Calcium-antimonate complex deposits can be seen on the plasma and vitelline membranes, the cortical granule membrane and within the egg cytoplasm prior to fertilization (see Figure 1). There are large deposits in the lumen of the discharging cortical granules and in the perivitelline space at 30 seconds following fertilization (see Figure 2).

The release of secretory products from the cortical granules (see Figure 2) is essential for the full elevation of the fertilization membrane and for changes in its structure (Anderson, 1968; Epel, 1975; Longo and Schuel, 1973; Longo et al., 1974). The fertilization membrane is essential for establishing a permanent and complete block to the entry of extra sperm. Should the release of the cortical granules be slowed down or inhibited, the full elevation of the fertilization membrane and

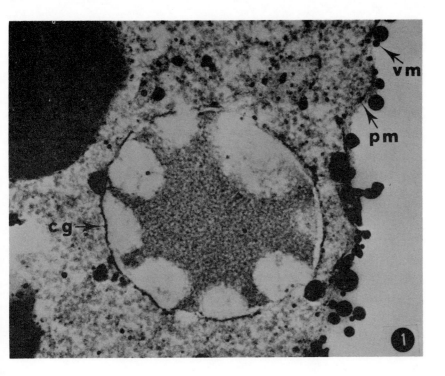

The cortex of an unfertilized sea urchin, *Arbacia punctulata,* egg fixed in glutaraldehyde and postfixed in osmium-pyroantimonate. Antimonate deposit is seen on the cortical granule membrane (cg), plasma membrane (pm), vitelline membrane (vm) and within the egg cytoplasm. X-ray microprobe analysis and the use of EGTA has determined that the antimonate deposit contains calcium. ×73,000.

changes in its structure will not occur, thereby resulting in polyspermy.

The number of polyspermic eggs can be used as a simple, rapid way to indicate that the normal secretory release process has been altered. Fixation of the eggs at one hour following fertilization, a time when most eggs have undergone their first cleavage, allows the determination of the number of polyspermic eggs with the light microscope. The polyspermic eggs will have cleaved into more than two cells or, if they have not cleaved, multiple sperm asters or multiple spindles may be seen as clear space within the egg. Thus, if release is impaired or delayed (i.e., by drug treatment), polyspermy occurs and can be used as an index of altered secretion. The ease with which this may be observed by light microscopy makes this a model system with numerous advantages in the study of the effects of narcotics on the process of secretion.

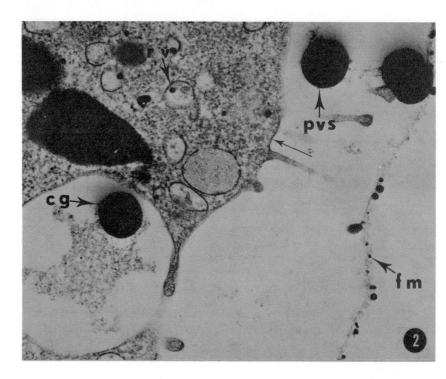

The cortex of a sea urchin, *Arbacia punctulata*, egg, 30 seconds postfertilization, fixed in glutaraldehyde and postfixed in osmium-pyroantimonate. Antimonate deposit is seen in the perivitelline space (pvs), lumen of discharging cortical granule (cg), fertilization membrane (fm), and lumen of rod-containing vesicles (rv). X-ray microprobe analysis and the use of EGTA has determined the deposit contains calcium. Note the absence of deposit on the plasma membrane (small arrow). ×33,800.

It is a simple and convenient culture system. The effects of narcotics on a living cell may be observed without elaborate tissue culture techniques. The medium is sea water, which is the normal site of fertilization for these eggs. Furthermore, many of the affects of narcotics such as polyspermy and interference with cleavage can be seen quickly and easily with the light microscope, without histological preparation. Drug action on a single cell population can be studied. The complex interactions existing between different cell types and organs which occur in adult multicellular organisms cannot occur.

The process of release of secretory granules is highly synchronized. Interference with release can be easily determined as all granules would normally be released within 60 sec after insemination. Secretion granules are all fully formed in the mature egg thereby isolating the process of release from other stages of secretion. Not only is release

634

Table I. Effects on Sea Urchin Eggs of Various Narcotics and Other Drugs That Act on the Human Nervous System

Drug	Polyspermy	Cleavage Inhibition or Delay	Reference
Morphine	Yes	—	Hertwig and Hertwig (1887)
	Yes	Yes	Clark (1936)
	—	No	Krahl (1950)
Cocaine	Yes	No	Clark (1936)
	Yes	No	Schuel, et al., (personal communication)
Barbiturates	—	Yes	Krahl (1950)
Fat Solvent Anesthetics (Alcohol, chloral hydrate, ether, urethan, etc.)	Yes	Yes	Hertwig and Hertwig (1887) Lillie (1914); Harvey (1932); Clark (1936); Heilbrunn (1956); Lonning (1967); Mateyko (1967); Longo and Anderson (1970)

not complicated by other cells acting as intermediaries, but it is not complicated by other phases of secretion within a particular cell being affected by narcotics, i.e. rates of protein synthesis, packaging of granules, etc.

The use of the sea urchin egg in the study of narcotic effects is actually a very old model. Investigators began looking at whether narcotics caused polyspermy in sea urchin eggs as early as 1887 (Hertwig & Hertwig), before the relationship between polyspermy and the cortical reaction was clear. Morphine, cocaine, and certain fat solvent anesthetics all cause polyspermy in the fertilized sea urchin egg (see Table I). Some of these investigators also demonstrated an inhibition or delay in cleavage of the eggs. Some of the more recent investigations demonstrated with the electron microscope that the actual release process was affected by certain of the fat solvent anesthetics (Longo and Anderson, 1970; Lonning, 1967).

METHODS AND DISCUSSION

Induction of polyspermic fertilization by morphine and methadone

Five ml of various dosages of either morphine sulfate (10^{-3}, 10^{-5} and 10^{-7}M or methadone HCl (10^{-3}, 10^{-5} and 10^{-7}M) dissolved in sea

Table II. Induction of Polyspermy by Morphine and Methadone in Sea Urchin Eggs

Drug	Percent of Fertilized Eggs Showing Polyspermy
None (Sea water control)	5
Morphine Sulphate	
10^{-3} M	46
10^{-5} M	33
10^{-7} M	26
Methadone HCl	
10^{-3} M	Toxic
10^{-5} M*	71
10^{-7} M	25

* 52% of eggs at this dose were unfertilized.

water were added to 2 ml of unfertilized sea urchin, *Arbacia punculata,* eggs in petri dishes. Ten minutes later the eggs were fertilized with 1 drop of sea water containing about 4% sperm (v/v) and allowed to develop for one hour in the presence of the drug. Control eggs were processed in the same manner but in sea water which did not contain either drug. All fertilized eggs were fixed with formalin and the number of polyspermic eggs counted with the light microscope. One hundred eggs were counted per dish and 2 dishes were set up for each dosage, resulting in a total of 200 eggs counted per dose (see Table II).

The percentage of polyspermic eggs decreased with decreasing concentrations of morphine. Methadone, unlike morphine, was toxic to the eggs at the higher concentrations. At 10^{-3} M methadone the eggs died immediately. At 10^{-5} M, while there was a high amount of polyspermy, the drug was still fairly toxic as 52% of the eggs were not fertilized. There was polyspermy without toxicity at 10^{-7} M methadone.

Effects of naloxone on morphine and methadone induced polyspermy

Naloxone is used clinically to antagonize the effects of narcotics (Mora et al., 1969). Pilot experiments have been conducted to determine the naloxone effect on morphine and methadone induced polyspermy in sea urchin eggs.

One group of eggs was treated with various concentrations of naloxone (6 x 10^{-4}, 3 x 10^{-5}, 6 x 10^{-7} M) for 15 minutes, fertilized, and

Table III. Effects of Naloxone on Morphine and Methadone Induced Polyspermy in Sea Urchin Eggs

	% Fertilized Eggs Showing Polyspermy		
Drug	Naloxone Alone	Narcotic Alone	Naloxone + Narcotic
6×10^{-4} M Naloxone	75	—	—
3×10^{-5} M Naloxone	22	—	—
6×10^{-7} M Naloxone	20	—	—
10^{-3} M Morphine	—	14	—
10^{-6} M Methadone	—	26	—
10^{-3} M Morphine + 6×10^{-4} M Naloxone	—	—	75
10^{-3} M Morphine + 3×10^{-5} M Naloxone	—	—	26
10^{-6} M Methadone + 6×10^{-4} M Naloxone	—	—	71
10^{-6} M Methadone + 6×10^{-7} M Naloxone	—	—	11
Sea water control egg	2%	—	—

handled in the same manner as the eggs in the previous experiment. Control eggs were fertilized in sea water.

Another group was treated with either 10^{-3} M morphine or 10^{-6} M methadone in the same manner as the naloxone group.

A third group of eggs was treated with the above concentrations of naloxone for 5 minutes. This was followed by the addition of either 10^{-3} M morphine or 10^{-6} M methadone to the naloxone. Following 15 minutes of exposure to the narcotic the eggs were fertilized and treated in the same manner as the preceding 2 groups (see Table III).

The naloxone alone has an effect on polyspermy which decreases with decreasing concentration. The effects of naloxone plus narcotic are never an addition of the individual drug effects. There is an indication of a blockage of the effect of methadone when in combination with the lower dose of naloxone.

CONCLUSIONS

Both methadone and morphine cause polyspermy in sea urchin eggs. The percentage of polyspermic eggs decreases with decreasing drug concentration, indicating that release of secretory granules may be affected by both these drugs. Methadone is far more toxic to the eggs than equal doses of morphine and can only be used at low doses (10^{-6}, 10^{-7} M) to study the effect on secretory granule release.

Naloxone also has a concentration dependent effect on the percentage of polyspermic eggs. This is not necessarily at variance with *in vivo* mammalian work, as high doses of naloxone are now being shown to affect certain processes (Ford et al., this text). Since the effect on polyspermy of the agonist and antagonist drugs are never additive, some type of complex interaction between the drugs may be occurring. There is an indication of a blockade of the methadone effect on polyspermy by the lowest concentration of naloxone employed. Further variations in the drug concentrations and duration of exposure, or the use of the stereoisomeric forms of the narcotics may elucidate these relationships.

The sea urchin egg is a simple model which enables one to study the direct effects of narcotics on the process of secretion. Using this model it may be possible to determine the mechanism of the narcotic effect on secretory granule discharge. For example, whether narcotic inhibits secretory granule discharge by interference with calcium levels or binding within the cell.

SUMMARY

The sea urchin egg offers numerous advantages in the study of the effects of narcotics on the process of release of secretory granules. It is a simple and convenient culture system in which drug action on a single cell population can be studied. The process of release of secretory granules is highly synchronized. Secretion granules are all fully formed in the mature egg, thereby isolating the process of release from other stages of secretion.

Determination of the percentage of polyspermic eggs following fertilization is a simple and rapid method of indicating interference with the release process. If the release of cortical granules is inhibited or retarded, the fertilization membrane will not form a complete block against the entry of extra sperm. Both morphine and methadone resulted in an increase in polyspermic eggs, which was concentration dependent, suggesting that release of secretory granules is affected by these drugs. Methadone was far more toxic than morphine at the higher concentrations (10^{-3} M, 10^{-5} M).

A pilot experiment demonstrates that naloxone used in high concentrations also increases polyspermy. This effect is less noticeable at lower concentrations of naloxone. The combination of naloxone plus either morphine or methadone suggests that some type of complex interaction occurs between the drugs as their effects are never simply additive. There is an indication of a blockage of the methadone increase in polyspermy by the lowest concentration of naloxone employed.

ACKNOWLEDGMENTS

Supported in part by grants from SUNY Research Foundation, grants 012 7122 A and 12–7125–A, NIDA-USPHS Grant DA 00114–04, the Population Council Grant M75.034, American Cancer Society Grant P-616, and the National Science Foundation Grant BMS 75–16126.

REFERENCES

Anderson, E. 1968. Oocyte differentiation in the sea urchin, *Arbacia punctulata*, with particular reference to the origin of cortical granules and their participation in the cortical reaction. *J. Cell Biol.* 37: 514–539.

Cardasis, C., H. Schuel, and L. Herman. 1974. Ultrastructural localization of calcium in unfertilized sea urchin eggs. *J. Cell Biol.* 63: 49a.

Clark, J. M. 1936. An experimental study of polyspermy. *Biol. Bull.* 70: 361–384.

Cox, B. M., and W. Weinstock. 1966. The effect of analgesic drugs on the release of acetylcholine from electrically stimulated guinea-pig ileum. *J. Pharmac. Chemother.* 27: 81–92.

Epel, D. 1975. The program and mechanisms of fertilization in the echinoderm egg. *Amer. Zool.* 15: 507–522.

Ford, D. H., R. K. Rhines, M. Joshi, and H. Cheslak. ^{3}H-*l-l*ysine accumulation into brain and plasma proteins in male rats treated with naloxone or naloxone-morphine. This text.

Ford, D. H., K. Voeller, C. Callegari, and E. Gresik. 1974. Changes in neurons of median eminence-arcuate regions of rats induced by morphine treatment. An electron microscope study. *J. Neurobiol.* 4: 1–11.

Harvey, E. N. 1932. Physical and chemical constants of the egg of the sea urchin *Arbacia punctulata*. *Biol. Bull.* 62: 141–154.

Heilbrunn, L. V. 1956. *The Dynamics of Living Protoplasm*. Academic Press, New York.

Herman, L., T. Sato, and C. N. Hales. 1973. The electron microscopic localization of cations to panceatic islets of Langerhans and their possible role in insulin secretion. *J. Ultrastruct. Res.* 42: 298–311.

Hertwig, O., and R. Hertwig. 1887. Über den Befruchtungs-und Teilungsvorgang des tierischen Eies unter dem Einfluss äusserer Agentieng. *Jena Zietsch, N. F.* 13 (20): 120–241 and 477–510.

Krahl, M. E. 1950. Metabolic activities and cleavage of eggs of the sea urchin *Arbacia punctulata*. A review, 1932–1949. *Biol. Bull.* 89: 175–217.

Lillie, R. S. 1914. The action of various anesthetics in suppressing cell division in sea urchin eggs. *J. Chem. Biol.* 17: 121–140.

Longo, F., and E. Anderson. 1970. A cytological study of the relation of the cortical reaction to subsequent events of fertilization in urethane treated eggs of the sea urchin, *Arbacia punctulata*. *J. Cell Biol.* 47: 646–665.

Longo, F. J., and H. Schuel. 1973. An ultrastructural examination of polyspermy induced by soybean trypsin inhibitor in the sea urchin *Arbacia punctulata*. *Dev. Biol.* 34: 187–199.

Longo, F. J., H. Schuel, and W. L. Wilson. 1974. Mechanism of soybean trypsin inhibitor induced polyspermy as determined by an analysis of refertilized sea urchin (*Arbacia punctulata*) eggs. *Dev. Biol.* 41: 193–201.

Lonning, S. 1967. Electron microscopic studies on the block to polyspermy. *Sarsia* 30: 107–116.

Mateko, G. M. 1967. Developmental modifications of *Arbacia punctulata* by various metabolic substances. *Biol. Bull.* 133: 184–228.

Mora, A., A. Bruner, S. Levit, and A. Freedman. 1969. Naloxone in heroin dependence. *Clin. Pharm. & Ther.* 9: 568–577.

Poste, G., and A. C. Allison. 1973. Membrane fusion. *Biochem. Biophys. Acta* 300: 421–465.

Rubin, R. P. 1970. The role of energy metabolism in calcium-evoked secretion from the adrenal medulla. *J. Physiol.* 206: 181–192.

Schuel, H., C. Cardasis, L. Herman, and W. Wilson. 1975. Ultrastructural localization of calcium in early stages of fertilization in Arbacia eggs. *Biol. Bull.* 149: 446.

Schuel, H., W. L. Wilson, K. Chen, and L. Lorand. 1973. A trypsin-like proteinase localized in cortical granules isolated from unfertilized sea urchin eggs by zonal centrifugation. Role of the enzyme in fertilization. *Devel. Biol.* 34: 175–186.

Schuel, H., J. W. Kelly, E. R. Berger, and W. L. Wilson. 1974. Sulfated acid mucopolysaccharides in the cortical granules of eggs. Effects of quarternary ammonium salts on fertilization. *Exp. Cell Res.* 88: 24–30.

Sharkawi, M., and M. P. Schulman. 1969. Inhibition by morphine of the release of (^{14}C) acetylcholine from rat brain cortex slices. *J. Pharm. Pharmac.* 21: 546–547.

Simon, E. J. 1971. Single cells. In D. H. Clouet, Ed. *Narcotic Drugs Biochemical Pharmacology.* Plenum Press, New York, pp. 310–341.

Tissue Responses to Addictive Drugs
© 1976, Spectrum Publications, Inc.

Ultrasonic Evaluation of the Lateral Ventricles in Addicts, Their Children, and Neonates: Preliminary Findings

M. TENNER
G. WODRASKA
C. MONTESINOS

Department of Radiology
Downstate Medical Center
State University Hospital
Brooklyn, New York

We have been unable to find literature devoted to echoencephalographic studies of the lateral ventricles in drug addicts. D. Von Zerssen et al. (1970) hypothesized that addiction to drugs can lead to irreversible brain damage. He measured, by ultrasound, the lateral diameter of the third ventricle in 34 drug addicts and found enlargement of the third ventricle in these patients in comparison with a control group. Cerebral atrophy demonstrated by air encephalography in young cannibis smokers has been communicated by A. M. G. Campbell et al. (1971) in 10 patients in which amphetamines and LSD had also been taken. Further, there are several communications relating to cerebral angiographic changes in drug abuse patients (C. L. Rumbaugh et al., 1971).

The purpose of this chapter is to evaluate by echoencephalography the lateral ventricles in addicts, their children, and neonates. The patients are on the Methadone Maintenance Program in Kings County Hospital

641

and Downstate Medical Center. The project is still in preparation and we are now communicating our preliminary findings.

METHODS

Ultrasound evaluation of the lateral ventricles requires the stepwise anatomic delineation of anatomic structures guided by external reference landmarks. Three portions of each lateral ventricle are evaluated as is the third ventricle. A 2.25 MHz transducer is used in infants and young children and a 1.0–1.5 MHz transducer is used in older children and adults. The ventricular measurement is made from the acoustic midline to the ultrasonic reflection of the superolateral corner of the lateral ventricle. This measurement does not exceed 20 mm with a ± 10% range. In the infant with a transverse biparietal diameter of less than 12 cm, the lateral ventricle measurement can be expected to be less than 20 mm and no greater than one-sixth of the biparietal diameter. A full description of the technique has been previously given (Tenner, M. S. et al., 1974 and Tenner, M. S. and Wodraska, G., 1975).

DISCUSSION

The first group of patients (see Table I) is primarily an adult female addict population on the methadone maintenance program. Their ages and drug histories are listed. If they gave birth during the study period, the child's date of birth is listed and these infants are also evaluated and included in this group. A small group of children born prior to the study but accompanying the parent were also available for evaluation and their findings are also listed. A summary of the evaluation of ventricular size in adult addicts and their children is as follows:

		Ventricular Evaluation In Adult Addicts	*Ventricular Evaluation of Children of Adult Addicts*
NORMAL	20 mm	1	11
BORDERLINE	20–22 mm	4	3
ENLARGEMENT			
1+	20–24 mm	6	4
2+	24–28 mm	6	0

The second group of 29 patients are neonates who had withdrawal symptoms (see Table II). The ages at which they were studied, the position, and size of the ventricular system and the maternal drugs are also listed. Several of these neonates were available for serial follow-up

Table I. Adult Addicts (Children Evaluated When Possible)

Name	Age (Years)	No. Years on Drugs	Heroine	Cocaine	Bar- biturate	Multiple Drugs	Amount of Drugs Daily	Meth- adone Main- tenance	III V.	Ultrasound Lat Vent. RT	LT	Clinical Findings
H V	25	4½	x	x	x	x	6½ bags (b)	x	M	24 22 20	24 22 20	
M F	42	20	x				20-25 (b)	x	M	26 24 24	26 24 24	
A T	23	2	x				4 (b)	x	3 mm L-R	26 26 22	24 22 22	
A A	7/12/73 (2 yrs.)								M	norm.	norm.	
M V	25	5	x					x	3-4 mm R-L	22 22 22	22 22 22	
S Z	24	4	x	x		x	8 (b)	x	M	26 26 24	26 26 24	
B B	24	3	x				up to 10 (b)	x	2 mm L-R	22 22 24	norm.	
W A	28	2	x				1 (b)	x	2 mm R-L	20 20 20	22 20 22	
W K	12/12/72 (2.5 yrs.)							x	M	norm.	norm.	

Table I. *Continued*

Name	Age (Years)	No. Years on Drugs	Heroine	Cocaine	Barbiturate	Multiple Drugs	Amount of Drugs Daily	Methadone Maintenance	Ultrasound III V.	Lat Vent. RT	Lat Vent. LT	Clinical Findings
M M	23	5	x				50 mg	x	2 mm L-R	22 22 22	norm.	
M J	7/27/73 (2 yrs.)								M	norm.	norm.	
V Y	21	2	x				5 (b)	x	3 mm L-R	22 22 20	20 18 18	
W T	19	2	x				40 mg	x	M	24 24 24	24 24 24	
T M	19	3	x		x	x	5 (b)	x	M	24 26 24	24 26 24	
S S	27	2	x	x	x	x	4-5 (b)	x	M	24 26 24	24 26 24	
S T	1/5/73 (2.5 yrs.)								M	20 20 18	22 20 20	
L R	21	2½	x	x	x	x		x	2-3 mm R-L	26 24 24	26 24 24	

Pt	Date / Age	History								(b)		Shift		
L D	10/25/72 (2.7 yrs.)	born with heroin "withdrawal"					×	×			×	M	20 20 18	20 20 18 norm.
C J	26	1 yr 2 mo	×	×	×		×	×	×	30 (b)	×	1-2 mm L-R	20 22 24	26 26
M V	19	5	×	×	×				×		×	2 mm R-L	22 22	22 20
M T	1.5 yrs.											M	22 20	22 20
H L	24	2½	×					×				M	26 26 26	26 26 26
H C	8/17/73 (2 yrs.)				×							M	18 20 18	18 20 18
S E	22		×					×			×	M	20 20 20	20 20 20
S G	8/16/73 (2 yrs.)											2 mm L-R	18 18 18	16 16 16
S G	"											1-2 mm L-R	16 16 16	14 14 14
B S		2 yrs. × 4 yrs.								4 (b) 5-6 day	×	no shift	24 24 22	24 24 22

645

Table I. *Continued*

Name	Age (Years)	No. Years on Drugs	Heroine	Cocaine	Bar-biturate	Multiple Drugs	Amount of Drugs Daily	Meth-adone Main-tenance	Ultrasound III V.	Lat Vent. RT	Lat Vent. LT	Clinical Findings
						CHILDREN						
D T	0.6 yrs.								no shift	22 / 24 / 22	22 / 24 / 22	
V D	0.85 yrs.									norm.	norm.	
A P	0.6 yrs.									norm.	norm.	
C H	0.62 yrs.								1-2 mm L-R asym	norm.	norm.	
S R	1.6 yrs.								no shift	24 / 24 / 24	22 / 22 / 22	
A M									10 mm 1-2 L-R	20 / 20 / 20	18 / 20 / 18	
T B	1.2 yrs.								2 mm L-R	20 / 20 / 20	20 / 20 / 20	
D S										18 / 18 / 18	18 / 18 / 18	*
M K	1.9 yrs.								1-2 mm L-R	20 / 20 / 20	22 / 22 / 22	**

* Microcephalic. Ventricles are enlarged for head diameter.   ** Microcephalic & retarded. Ventricles are enlarged for head diameter.

Table II. Withdrawal Neonates

Patient #	Age Studied	III V.	RLV	LLV	Maternal Drug
4653	6 days	1-2 mm L-R	16 mm	14 mm	Methadone
			16 mm	14 mm	
			14 mm	12 mm	
"	2 weeks	no shift	16 mm	16 mm	
			16 mm	16 mm	
			16 mm	16 mm	
4384	22 days	2 mm L-R	18 mm	16 mm	Methadone
			18 mm	16 mm	
			18 mm	16 mm	
"	33 days	1-2 mm L-R	16 mm	14 mm	
			16 mm	14 mm	
			16 mm	14 mm	
4370	3 weeks	2 mm L-R	18 mm	16 mm	Methadone
			18 mm	16 mm	
			16 mm	14 mm	
"	11 mos.	2-3 mm L-R assym.	20 mm	20 mm	
			20 mm	20 mm	
			20 mm	20 mm	
4369	3 weeks	no shift	16 mm	16 mm	Methadone
			16 mm	16 mm	
			16 mm	16 mm	
"	11 mos.	no shift	20 mm	20 mm	
			20 mm	20 mm	
			20 mm	20 mm	
4534	24 days	no shift	16 mm	16 mm	Heroin
			16 mm	16 mm	
			16 mm	16 mm	
4867	4 days	2 mm L-R	16 mm	14 mm	Heroin
			16 mm	14 mm	
			16 mm	14 mm	
4729	14 days	no shift	16 mm	16 mm	Methadone
			16 mm	16 mm	
			16 mm	16 mm	
5427	11 days	2 mm L-R	16 mm	14 mm	
			18 mm	16 mm	
			16 mm	14 mm	
4314	19 days	2 mm L-R	18 mm	16 mm	Methadone
			18 mm	16 mm	
			18 mm	16 mm	
5626	2 days	2 mm L-R	16 mm	14 mm	Heroin
			16 mm	14 mm	
			14 mm	12 mm	

Table II. *Continued*

Patient #	Age Studied	III V.	RLV	LLV	Maternal Drug
5547	0 days	2 mm L-R	18 mm	16 mm	Methadone
			18 mm	16 mm	
			18 mm	16 mm	
5629	1 day	2 mm L-R	18 mm	14 mm	Heroin
			18 mm	14 mm	
			16 mm	12 mm	
6154	8 days	no shift	10 mm	10 mm	Methadone
			12 mm	12 mm	
			12 mm	12 mm	
"	7 weeks	2-3 mm L-R	14 mm	14 mm	
			14 mm	14 mm	
			12 mm	12 mm	
"	3½ mos.	1-2 mm L-R	18 mm	14 mm	
			18 mm	14 mm	
			18 mm	14 mm	
"	7 mos.	1-2 mm L-R	18 mm	18 mm	
			18 mm	18 mm	
			18 mm	18 mm	
G G		no shift	14 mm	14 mm	Heroin
			14 mm	14 mm	
			14 mm	14 mm	
6753	10 days	no shift	18 mm	18 mm	Methadone
			18 mm	18 mm	
			18 mm	18 mm	
6664	17 days	2 mm L-R	16 mm	12 mm	Heroin
			16 mm	14 mm	
			16 mm	12 mm	
G M	4 days	1-2 mm L-R	18 mm	14 mm	Methadone
			18 mm	14 mm	
			18 mm	14 mm	
G S	5 days	2 mm L-R	16 mm	14 mm	Methadone
			16 mm	14 mm	
			16 mm	14 mm	
7848	22 days	2 mm L-R	16 mm	14 mm	Heroin
			16 mm	14 mm	
			16 mm	14 mm	
7861	18 days	1-2 mm L-R	16 mm	14 mm	Drug Free
			16 mm	14 mm	
			16 mm	12 mm	
8000	9 days	no shift	16 mm	16 mm	Methadone
			16 mm	16 mm	
			16 mm	16 mm	

Table II. *Continued*

Patient #	Age Studied	III V.	RLV	LLV	Maternal Drug
8073	6 days	no shift	16 mm 16 mm 14 mm	16 mm 16 mm 14 mm	Methadone
017	7 days	L-R asym	16 mm 18 mm 16 mm	14 mm 16 mm 14 mm	
B B	12 days	1-2 mm L-R	normal normal normal	normal normal normal	
0708	9 days	no shift	16 mm 16 mm 16 mm	14 mm 14 mm 14 mm	
0496	15 days	1-2 mm L-R	14 mm 14 mm 14 mm	12 mm 12 mm 12 mm	
0644	12 days	2 mm L-R	16 mm 16 mm 16 mm	14 mm 14 mm 12 mm	
B H	2 days	no shift	14 mm 12 mm 14 mm	14 mm 12 mm 16 mm	
B J		1-2 mm L-R	16 mm 16 mm 16 mm	14 mm 14 mm 14 mm	
0547	3 days	1-2 mm L-R	14 mm 14 mm 14 mm	12 mm 12 mm 12 mm	
0757	7 days	2-3 mm L-R	16 mm 16 mm 16 mm	12 mm 12 mm 12 mm	
9954	1 mo. 3 wk.	2 mm L-R	16 mm 16 mm 14 mm	12 mm 12 mm 10 mm	
G S	1½ mos.	no shift	16 mm 16 mm 14 mm	16 mm 16 mm 14 mm	
0301	5 weeks	no shift	16 mm 16 mm 16 mm	14 mm 14 mm 14 mm	Methadone

examination. A summary of the withdrawal neonates and the follow-up studies when available is as follows:

WITHDRAWAL NEONATES
NORMAL = 7
ABNORMAL = 27
LEFT VENTRICULAR COMPRESSION = 21
BILATERAL VENTRICULAR COMPRESSION = 6
FOLLOW-UP = 5
    RETURN TO NORMAL –
        1 = two weeks
        1 = 11 weeks
        1 = remained compressed bilateral at 7 weeks
            left compression at 14 weeks
            normal at 7 months
    BORDERLINE –
1 = left compression gone but third ventricular asymmetrical
    REMAINED ABNORMAL –
1 = 33 days

CONCLUSIONS

Ventricular size in adult methadone maintained addicts showed a much greater degree of enlargement than the normal population with 70% showing definite enlargement. The children of the addicts showed a lesser percentage of enlarged ventricles in relation to their addicted mothers, but still significantly beyond the normal population. It cannot be stated with certainty what the etiology is of the enlargement of the lateral ventricles. These findings would seem to indicate a mild degree of brain atrophy. Although a recent postmortem study shows that the brains are pathologically not grossly atrophied (Sher, J.), it is possible that a mild degree of atrophy was masked by post mortem swelling. An alternate explanation is that the enlargement may be the result of increased cerebrospinal fluid pressure. However, no corroborating evidence for this could be found in the literature. In the children, at least two of the four definitely enlarged lateral ventricles were associated with microcephaly and so are felt to be part of a definite structural brain deficiency.

The withdrawal neonates showed a surprising finding with evidence of lateral ventricular compression, mostly left sided. This was manifested by finding lateral ventricle measurements smaller than anticipated associated with a third ventricle shifted away from the compressed ventricle. In the follow-up study, most of these patients' ventricular system returned to normal. The significance of the left sided preponderance is not known but is probably related to the slightly greater volume of cerebral tissue normally found in the left hemisphere. The etiology of the compressed ventricles is not known. It may be the result of cerebral edema on an ischemic basis from a combination of both birth trauma and physiologic depression from the addictive drug. This is obviously not the complete explanation as the compression was found well beyond the immediate period of delivery. A study to evaluate normal newborns, using our methods, to see if a similar finding of compressed ventricles is present is currently being undertaken. Ventricular measurements of newborns done by T. Valkeakari (1973) showed no evidence of compression.

REFERENCES

Campbell, A. M. G., M. Evans, J. L. G. Thompson, and J. M. Williams. 1971. Cerebral atrophy in young cannabis smokers. *Lancet* 2: 1219–1224.

Rumbaugh, C. L., R. T. Bergeron, H. C. H. Fang, and R. McCormick. 1971. Cerebral angiographic changes in the drug abuse patient. *Radiology.* 101: 335–344.

Sher, J. Personal communication from Kings County Hospital, Department of Pathology.

Tenner, M. S., and G. Wodraska. 1975. *Diagnostic Ultrasound in Neurology.* John Wiley & Sons, New York.

Tenner, M. S., G. Wodraska, and B. Adapon. 1974. Newer ultrasound techniques in the evaluation of neurologic disorders. *Radiologic Clinics of North America* 12: 283–295.

Valkeakari, T. 1973. Analysis of serial echoencephalograms in healthy newborn infants during the first week of life. *Acta Paediatrica Scandinavica* 242 (Suppl.)

Von Zerssen, D., K. Fliege, and M. Wolf. 1970. Cerebral atrophy in drug addicts (letter). *Lancet.* 2: 313.

Tissue Responses to Addictive Drugs
© 1976, Spectrum Publications, Inc.

Prenatal Studies of Infants In Methadone Maintained Women

GEORGE I. SOLISH
RITA G. HARPER
ELLEN FEINGOLD

Department of Obstetrics and Gynecology
State University of New York
Downstate Medical Center
From the Division of Perinatal Medicine and the
Departments of Pediatrics and Obstetrics and Gynecology
North Shore University Hospital
Manhasset, New York
and
The Departments of Pediatrics and
Obstetrics and Gynecology
Cornell University Medical College
New York, New York

Early in 1971, an increasing incidence of narcotic withdrawal was noted among newborn infants at the State University of New York—Kings County Hospital Center. As a consequence of this and in an effort to prevent the multiple medical and social problems associated with addiction and pregnancy, the Departments of Obstetrics, Pediatrics, and Psychiatry at this medical center jointly organized a Family and Maternity Care Program (FMCP) for the care of pregnant addicts and their spouses (Harper et al., 1974).

The development of the FMCP provided a unique opportunity to administer proper prenatal care to a class of pregnant women, who in the past were usually seen for the first time by an obstetrician when well along in active labor or suffering from some severe complication of pregnancy. As more women registered in methadone programs, it soon became apparent, as others have also noted (Wallach et al., 1969), that women who enroll in methadone maintenance programs may display improved nutritional habits, improved social behavior, greater concern for personal hygiene and health and, indeed, may improve their fertility and increase their desire to carry pregnancies to term.

In the first year of FMCP operation, more than 25% of the 51 women delivered in the FMCP were treated for syphilis, about 10% received treatment for hepatitis during the prenatal period. Other diseases such as hypertension, asthma, kidney disease, diabetes, hyperthyroidism, epilepsy, thrombophlebitis, as well as the obstetric complications of pre-eclampsia, *hyperemisis gravidarum*, and third trimester bleeding were also treated antinatally. This small group of women might otherwise not have been seen at all prenatally, or seen too late, were it not for the FMCP. About 85% of the women remained in the FMCP at this or another related program in the city for at least a year after enrollment.

The many advantages of methadone maintenance for the pregnant woman have led to its acceptance as the standard method of treatment for narcotic addicted pregnant women. However, the effects on the fetus *in utero* of the methadone administered to mothers are not as clear cut nor has this aspect of the pregnancy been adequately investigated to date. In the FMCP, of the 51 infants delivered in the first year of the program, withdrawal symptoms were observed in all but 3. (Three other infants, one with meningitis, one with a diaphragmatic hernia, and one with meconium aspiration could not be evaluated for withdrawal because of their coexisting medical illness). The results of this small study again emphasized the high incidence of medical complications among addicted pregnant women and their infants over and above the problem of withdrawal.

Despite the earlier reports (Wallach et al., 1974) of "no apparent effect" of maternally administered methadone to the fetus, newborn and child, subsequent experience has shown that withdrawal symptoms do occur and that these symptoms may in fact be more severe and more frequent than those of infants of heroin addicted mothers (Felson et al., 1973). Only recently have suspicions been raised that the infant methadone withdrawal syndrome may differ in important respects from withdrawal seen after morphine or heroin. It was these suspicions that prompted the present study. For, if we are to continue to prescribe methadone for the pregnant addict it is essential that we learn more about the effect of this drug on the growth and development of the fetus *in utero*, as well as the long term effects on the child and its growth and development in later years.

For this study 30 pregnant women were selected from the same community matched for age, parity and ethnic origin. Both groups have been followed prospectively with periodic observations, examinations and collection of biological specimens for testing the hypothesis that the administration of methadone to pregnant women is no more damaging to the fetus *in utero* than is the nonadministration of this drug.

Every precaution was taken to obtain a pure sample of addicted and normal pregnant women. Periodic examination of urine specimens from both groups for evidence of drug abuse were made regularly. However, present methods of methadone detection do not quantitate the amount of methadone ingested and, therefore, supplementation of the prescribed dosage of methadone with "street methadone" goes undetected. That there are other weaknesses in the surveillance system has been recognized and will, of course, need to be evaluated in the final analysis of the present study. Medical and obstetrical complications of pregnancy, prematurity, as well as illicit drug abuse were grounds for elimination of patients from this study. The overall plan was to evaluate the fetus *in utero* by several presently available techniques and to compare the well being of the fetus of a methadone mother with that of the fetus of a control mother.

The first phase of our research program in drug addiction and pregnancy dealt with the identification and management of the pregnant addict with the aid of methadone maintenance and detoxification approaches to therapy. The second phase of our studies centers about detecting the effects of the inadvertent addiction of the fetus in utero of methadone maintained and detoxified mothers. The third phase, it is proposed, will attempt to study the long term effects of *in utero* addiction on the children of methadone addicted mothers. The chapter will deal with some aspects of the studies of the fetus in the uteri of methadone maintained mothers, i.e., the second phase of the overall program.

FETAL STUDIES

Studies that are in varying stages of completion are as follows:
1) Serum heat stable alkaline phosphatase levels in methadone-maintained pregnancies compared to levels in normal controls
2) Chromosome studies of methadone-maintained women and their newborn infants
3) Cellular content of DNA and RNA of placentas of methadone-maintained addicts
4) Quantitation of methadone in body fluids of methadone-main-

tained pregnant women and their infants by gas-liquid chromatography

5) Dermatoglyphic studies of infants of methadone-maintained women

6) Quantitation of IgG and IgM in cord blood of infants born to methadone-maintained women

7) Plasma estriol and estetrol levels in methadone-maintained pregnancies.

8) Ultrasonographic studies of the fetus in utero of methadone treated women

These studies are in varying stages of completion at this time. In a few instances, the results obtained have reached a stage where some discussion of the data are possible.

HEAT STABLE ALKALINE PHOSPHATASE

Alkaline phosphatases have been defined as a group of enzymes with low substrate specificity that catalyze the hydrolysis of phosphate esters at an alkaline pH (Posen, 1967). These enzymes are referred to as isoenzymes because they catalyze the same reaction, are found in the same organism or species, but differ in certain physicochemical properties. Alkaline phosphatases are found in bone, kidney, liver, intestine, white blood cells, and placentae. Their physiologic function is unknown but they are thought to be involved in active membrane transport because of their localization to cell membranes (Posen et al., 1969).

Placental alkaline phosphatase (HSAP) is the most heat stable of the human alkaline phosphatases and can be readily identified in serum because its resistance to heating to 56°C - 60°C for 30 minutes or more (Fishman and Ghosh, 1967). The enzyme arises from the syncytiotrophoblastic layer of the placenta (Wachstern et al., 1963). The level of HSAP rises gradually in the serum during the third trimester of pregnancy to levels four times higher than that seen in normal nonpregnant women (Zuckerman et al., 1965). There are indications that under some conditions of stress the placenta increases its production of HSAP (Benster, 1970; Merrit and Hunter, 1973; Lee and Lewis, 1963; Bagga et al., 1969). However, HSAP in serum has been shown to have no definite relation to maternal age, parity, maternal surface area, ABO blood group (Fishman et al., 1972; Kitchener et al., 1965), urinary estriol (Iyengar and Srikantia, 1970; Curzen and Hensel, 1972), urinary pregnanediol, crude birthweights, fetal sex, and crude placental weight (Pirani et al., 1972). Conflicting findings have been reported concerning the serum

1

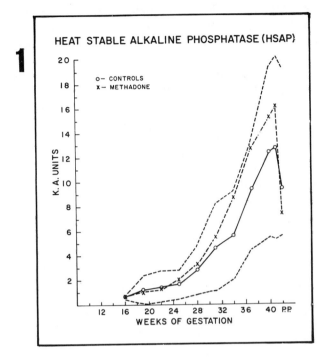

levels of placental alkaline phosphatase and their relationship to placental dysfunction and toxemia of pregnancy.

Since rising levels may reflect subtle placental damage and since the technique of measuring this enzyme is uncomplicated, measurements of this enzyme were made at periodic intervals throughout the pregnancies of three groups of pregnant women—the methadone maintained women, the detoxified (or "drug free" women), and the normal controls.

Blood was collected in vacutainers by venipuncture. The samples were centrifuged after clotting and the serum separated and heated to 56°C for one hour in a water bath. Alkaline phosphatase determinations were made by Hansen's (1966) modification of the method of Kind and King.

There were 22 mothers on methadone maintenance, 5 on "drug free" detoxification, and 15 controls for whom at least 3 or more serial determinations of HSAP in blood were made. The mean values of HSAP for each week of gestation of the three groups of women, methadone-maintained, drug free, and controls, are shown plotted in Figure 1.

The mean level of HSAP rose gradually through pregnancy but particularly from the twenty-eighth week to term, dropping rapidly after delivery. (The half life of HSAP has been reported to be seven days (Kaplin, 1972).

The mean level of HSAP of methadone-maintained women also rose with age of gestation and at each point was uniformly higher than control levels. Because of the large variance (dashed lines without x's in Figure 1), however, the differences are not statistically significant in this small group. In addition, there seems to be a relationship of the methadone dosage level and the level of serum HSAP but this has not been adequately tested statistically.

The mean level of HSAP among women maintained on a daily dose of 60 mgm of methadone or more seem to be significantly higher than those of the control women compared to women maintained on doses lower than 60 mgm of methadone daily. If these trends continue in the more formal statistical analyses of these data, it would suggest that methadone during pregnancy may affect the maternal-placental-fetal unit in more subtle ways than have previously been considered.

ESTRIOL AND ESTETROL

In the search for parameters to assess the state of fetal well being in high risk obstetrical patients, estriol (E_3) determinations have become well established as one of the better indices of feto-placental unit function. The dramatic rise in total estrogens with pregnancy was one of the exciting discoveries in obstetrics in the early part of this century. As early as 1928, Ascheim and Zondek by bioassay of urine observed rising levels of estrogenic activity during the course of pregnancy and rapid disappearance following delivery. Smith and Smith (1933) developed normal curves of urinary estrogen levels during pregnancy and in 1947, Finkelstein et al. described a practical method of measuring estriol levels. This was later shown to be a more precise method of evaluating the course of pregnancy than was the bioassay of total estrogens. With the development of more refined and sensitive techniques and particularly with the advent of radioactive immunoassays, estriol measurements have become a valuable aid in the assessment and management of high risk pregnancies. Estriol levels were noted to be significantly lower than normal controls in cases of fetal distress, anencephaly, and fetal death in utero (Natchtigall et al., 1966). Some controversy exists regarding the value of estriol in some complications of pregnancy, such as Rh immunization and diabetes but in general, a successive fall in estriol levels particularly in the latter weeks of pregnancy is cause for great concern for the life of the fetus. Alterations in estriol excretion in maternal urine have been reported to occur in glycosuria, proteinuria, maternal renal disease, and following ingestion of drugs such as ampicillin, cortisone, prednisone, dexamethasone, mandelamine, and a variety of diuretics (Pulkkinen and Willman, 1973).

Northrop et al. (1972), showed in eight narcotic-addicted women maintained on methadone, persistent low urinary excretion levels of estriol. Following withdrawal of these patients from narcotic drugs, urinary estriol levels rapidly rose toward average values expected for their period of gestation.

Recently another estrogen, 15 alpha hydroxyestriol or estetrol (E_4) has been described (Fishman and Guzik, 1972). This estrogen is primarily the product of fetal estradiol metabolism and its biosynthetic pathway is distinct from that of estriol of pregnancy. The unique fetal origin and route of biosynthesis suggested that the concentration of E_4 in pregnancy urine may be an even better index of fetal well being than estriol (E_3). During uncomplicated pregnancies, the concentration of E_4 rises in maternal serum and urine as pregnancy proceeds. The rate of increase of E_4 has been reported to be relatively greater than the increase of E_3 during the last weeks of pregnancy.

It seemed appropriate to explore the estriol and estetrol levels of methadone maintained pregnant women for evidence of placental or fetal changes as a consequence of prolonged methadone administration. The E_3 and E_4 levels in the plasma of 25 pregnant women maintained on different doses of methadone, 5 women who had become "drug free," and 19 normal pregnant controls were, therefore, measured. A minimum of 3 successive determinations were made in each patient. Two hundred fifty-two E_3 and an equal number of E_4 determinations were made at approximately 2 week intervals through the second and third trimester of the pregnancies of methadone patients. One hundred sixty-seven determinations each of E_3 and E_4 were made in the 19 normal pregnant controls and a total of 80 each of E_3 and E_4 were measured in the 5 "drug free" women. The results were averaged for each week of pregnancy and the means obtained (see Figures 2 and 3).

RESULTS

E_3 plasma levels rose progressively with weeks of gestation. The E_3 levels of methadone patients are lower than those of the control women while the levels for drug free women were scattered. Although the differences do not seem to be statistically significant, the suggestion is that estriol excretion in maternal plasma is decreased by chronic

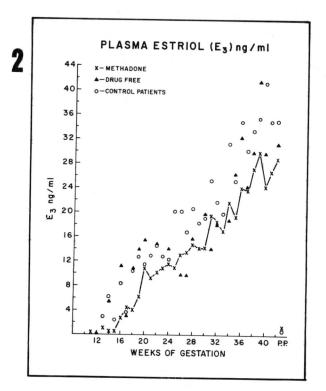

2

PLASMA ESTRIOL (E₃) ng / ml

X — METHADONE
▲ — DRUG FREE
O — CONTROL PATIENTS

methadone administration as suggested by the report of Northrop et al. (1972).

The results of E₄ measurement are not as clear cut. Here the suggestion is that levels of E₄ in methadone users are lower than those of controls. The levels of E₄ among detoxified women who are now drug free are in between those of methadone users and normal controls.

It is obvious that these data need to be much more completely analyzed and more work needs to be done before definite statements can be made about the effect of methadone maintenance on E₃ and E₄ metabolism. It is also important to know what the implications are of low estriol and estetrol plasma levels in terms of the well being and future prognosis of the fetus of a methadone addicted mother.

METHADONE QUANTIFICATION BY GAS-LIQUID CHROMATOGRAPHY

The higher incidence of withdrawal among newborn infants of methadone-maintained mothers than that of infants of heroin-addicted

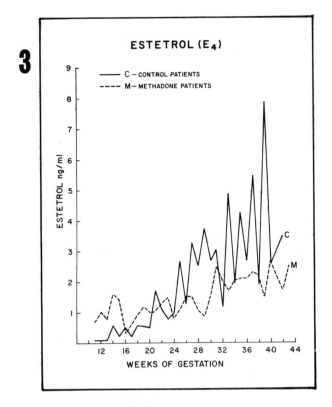

3

ESTETROL (E₄)

mothers has been the source of much concern regarding the advisability of continued usage of this drug even though it is the only one presently available for treatment of pregnant addicts. Other bits of information suggest that methadone addiction differs substantially from heroin addiction in the newborn. The delayed onset of symptoms, the severity of withdrawal, and the apparent unpredictability and lack of correlation of severity of withdrawal with maternal drug dosage indicate not only probable differences in effect of methadone versus heroin on the newborn, but also differences in metabolism of the two drugs which is inherent in their basic structures and functions..

The unique mode of administration of methadone to the fetus *in utero* may account for some of peculiarities noted. It has been shown by Inturrisi et al. (1973), and by Blinick et al. (1975) that methadone is found in the amniotic fluid of methadone-maintained mothers. However, the relationship of methadone levels in mother's blood, mother's urine, cord blood, amniotic fluid, and infant urine to the severity of withdrawal symptoms is not a simple one.

It is our hypothesis that the recirculation of fetal urine in amniotic fluid i.e., that varying amounts of unchanged methadone eliminated in fetal urine and subsequently swallowed by the fetus, according to the known circulation of amniotic fluid, may account for differing dosages of methadone the fetus receives, and thus, results in different degrees of severity of withdrawal among newborns irrespective of maternal methadone dosage. The reports of Anggard et al. (1974), Beckett et al. (1972) and Baselt and Casarett (1972) that significant amounts of unchanged methadone are found in the urine of adults taking methadone suggests that unmetabolized or partially metabolized methadone may similarly appear in the urine of the unborn fetus. In other words, the fetus may through swallowing amniotic fluid receive methadone obtained not only directly from the maternal circulation but also from its own urine recirculated into the amniotic fluid. Immature fetal metabolic facilities may significantly supplement the methadone levels the fetus gets through the placenta. This could result in prolonged fetal exposure to methadone even after the mother became drug free.

To test this possibility, simultaneous measurements of methadone in various body fluids of mother and infant and amniotic fluid are currently being studied. Measurements of methadone levels are being made by gas-liquid chromatography after the method of Inturrissi and Verebely (1972).

SUMMARY

Although the concept of methadone maintenance has been a significant stride forward in the management of pregnant narcotic addicted women, the effect of maternally administered methadone on the unborn child is suspect. The incidence of withdrawal among newborns of methadone-maintained mothers is high and the symptoms can be very severe. The effects of methadone on the fetus have not been adequately studied and if methadone maintenance is to continue to be the main method of management of the addicted pregnant women, investigation of the effects on the infant are mandatory.

This study at the State University of New York - Kings County Hospital Center and North Shore University Hospital is attempting to define any adverse effects of methadone to the fetus in utero. Heat stable alkaline phosphatase, plasma estriol, and estetrol determinations suggest that methadone may be producing very subtle biochemical changes in the fetal-placental unit that may effect the long term well being, growth and development of the child.

Current measurements of methadone levels in the body fluids of mother and infant may help to define the mechanism of methadone metabolism in the fetus and perhaps account for the high incidence and severity of symptoms of withdrawal in babies of methadone-maintained mothers. Long term studies of the effects of chronic methadone administration on fetal development and the consequences of infant methadone withdrawal on later mental and behavioral development must be done if the basic principle of all medical treatment is to continue to be *primum non nocere*.

REFERENCES

Anggard, E., L. M. Gunne, J. Holmstrand, R. E. McMahon, C. G. Sandberg, and H. R. Sullivan. 1975. Disposition of methadone in methadone maintenance. *Clin. Pharmacol. Ther.* 17: 258–266.

Ascheim, S., and B. Zondek. 1928. Die schwangerschaftsdiagnose aus dem harn durch nachweis des hypophysen vorder lappen hormons. *Klin. Wschr.* 7: 1453–1457.

Bagga, O. P., V. Dutt Mullick, P. Madan, and S. Dewan. 1969. Total serum alkaline phosphate and its isoenzymes in normal and toxemic pregnancies. *Am. J. Obstet. Gynecol.* 104: 850.855.

Baselt, R. C., and L. J. Casarett. 1972. Urinary excretion of methadone in man. *Clin. Pharmacol. Ther.* 13: 64–70.

Beckett, A. H. 1969. Distribution and metabolism in man of some narcotic analgesics and some "amphetamines." In H. Steinberg, Ed. *Scientific Basis of Drug Dependence.* J and A Churchill, Ltd., London, pp. 129–148.

Benster, B. 1970. Serum heat-stable alkaline phosphatase in pregnancy complicated by hypertension. *J. Obstet. Gynaecol. Br. Commonw.* 77: 990–993.

Blinick, G., C. E. Inturrisi, J. Eulogio, and R. C. Wallach. 1975. Methadone assays in pregnant women and progeny. *Am. J. Obstet. Gynecol.* 121: 617–621.

Curzen, P., and H. Hensel. 1972. Serum heat-stable alkaline phosphatase and its relationship to urinary oestrogen output, fetal and placental weight and placental enzyme content. *J. Obstet. Gynaecol. Br. Commonw.* 79: 23–28.

Finkelstein, M., S. Hestrin, and W. Koch. 1947. Estimation of steroid estrogens by fluorimetry. *Proc. Soc. Exp. Biol. Med.* 64: 64–71.

Fishman, J., and H. Guzik. 1972. Radioimmunoassay of 15 alpha-hydroxyestriol in pregnancy plasma. *J. Clin. Endoc. Metab.* 35: 892–896.

Fishman, W. H., W. A. Bardawil, H. G. Habib, et al. 1972. The placental isoenzymes of alkaline phosphatase in sera of normal pregnancy. *Am. J. Clin. Pathol.* 57: 65-74.

Fishman, W. H., and N. K. Ghosh. 1967. Isoenzymes of human alkaline phosphatase. *Adv. Clin. Chem.* 10: 255–370.

Hansen, P. W. 1966. A simplification of Kind and King's method for determination of serum phosphatase. *Scand. J. Clin. Lab. Invest.* 18: 353–356.

Harper, R. G., G. I. Solish, H. M. Purow, E. Sang, and W. C. Panepinto. 1974. The effect of a methadone treatment program upon pregnant heroin addicts and their newborn infants. *Pediatrics* 54: 300–311.

Inturrisi, C. E., and G. Blinick. 1973. The quantitation of methadone in human aminotic fluid. *Res. Commun. Pathol. & Pharmacol.* 6: 353–356.

Inturrisi, C. E., and K. Verebely. 1972. A gas-liquid chromatographic method for the quantitative determination of methadone in human plasma and urine. *J. Chromatogr.* 65: 361–369.

Iyengar, L., and S. G. Srikantia. 1970. Serum alkaline phosphatase in pregnancy. *Am. J. Clin. Nutr.* 23: 68–72.

Kaplan, M. M. 1972. Alkaline phosphatase. *New Eng. J. Med.* 286: 200–202.

Kitchener, P. N., F. C. Neale, S. Psen et al., 1965. Alkaline phosphatase in maternal and fetal sera at term and during the puerperium. *Am. J. Clin. Pathol.* 44: 654–661.

Lee, A. B., and P. L. Lewis. 1963. Alkaline phosphatase activity in normal and toxemic pregnancies. *Am. J. Obstet. Gynecol.* 87: 1071–1073.

Merrett, J. D., and R. J. Hunter. 1973. Serum heat-stable alkaline phosphatase levels in normal and abnormal pregnancies. *J. Obstet. Gynecol. Br. Commonw.* 80: 957–965.

Natchtigall, L., M. Basset, U. Hogsander, S. Slagle, and M. Levitz. 1966. A rapid method for the assay of plasma estriol in pregnancy. *J. Clin. Endo.* 26: 941–948.

Northrop, G., J. Ditzler, W. G. Ryan, and G. D. Wilbanks. 1972. Estriol excretion profiles in narcotic-addicted pregnant women. *Am. J. Obstet. Gynecol.* 112: 704–712.

Pirani, B. B. K., I. MacGillivray, and R. O. Duncan. 1972. Serum heat-stable alkaline phosphatase in normal pregnancy and its relationship to urinary oestriol and pregnanediol excretion, placental weight and baby weight. *J. Obstet. Gynaecol. Br. Commonw.* 79: 127–132.

Posen, S. 1967. Alkaline phosphatase. *Ann. Intern. Med.* 67: 183–203.

Pulkkinen, M. O., and K. Willman. 1973. Reduction of maternal estrogen excretion by neomycin. *Am. J. Obstet. Gynecol.* 115: 1153.

Smith, G. V. S., and O. W. Smith. 1933. Excessive anterior-pituitary-like hormone and variations in oestrin in the toxemias of late pregnancy. *Proc. Soc. Exp. Biol. Med.* 30: 918–919.

Wachstern, M., J. G. Meagher, and J. Otiz. 1963. Enzymatic histochemistry of the term human placenta. *Am. J. Obstet. Gynecol.* 87: 13–26.

Wallach, R. C., E. Jerez, and G. Blinick. 1969. Pregnancy and menstrual function in narcotics addicts treated with methadone: The methadone maintenance treatment program. *Amer. J. Obstet. Gynecol.* 105: 1226–1229.

Zelson, C., S. J. Lee, and M. Casalino. 1973. Neonatal narcotic addiction: Comparative effect of maternal intake of heroin and methadone. *New Eng. J. Med.* 289: 1216–1220.

Zuckerman, H., E. Sadovsky, and B. Kallner. 1965. Serum alkaline phosphatase in pregnancy and puerperium. *Obstet. Gynecol.* 25: 819–824.

Tissue Responses to Addictive Drugs
© 1976, Spectrum Publications, Inc.

Effects of Morphine, Narcotic Agonists and Antagonists on Single Neurons in the Brain Stem

PHILIP B. BRADLEY
Department of Pharmacology
The Medical School
Birmingham, England

There have been many experimental studies of the pharmacological actions of morphine and other narcotic analgesics in an endeavour to elucidate the mechanisms and site of action in the central nervous system through which these drugs produce analgesia. However, none of the studies to date have yielded any conclusive information. There are indications, however, from some reports, that morphine may exert at least part of its antinociceptive effect through an action on the brain stem. Thus, (1) localised perfusion of the cerebral ventricles with morphine resulted in antinociception developing when the drug was able to reach the anterior part of the fourth ventricle, but not when it was confined to the third or lateral ventricles (Herz et al., 1970); (2) local injections of morphine in the vicinity of the lateral reticular nucleus produced analgesia (Pert and Yaksh, 1974); (3) nociceptive-sensitive neurons have been found in the region of the hypoglossal nerve in the rat medulla (Benjamin, 1970); (4) analgesia has been elicited

667

by electrical stimulation of the periacqueductal gray in the cat (Liebeskind et al., 1973); and (5) this region appears to be one of the areas where opiate receptor binding sites are concentrated (Kuhar et al., 1973). At the time we started our own investigations no information was available on the effects of morphine, or of other opiate analgesic drugs, on single neurons in the brain. It therefore seemed appropriate to examine the effects of morphine and of other related drugs, both agonists and antagonists, on the activity of single neurons in the brain stem. For this purpose we used the technique of microiontophoresis which, although it has been used mainly for studies of the effects of putative neurotransmitters, has proved valuable for examining effects of centrally active drugs at the neuronal level (Bradley, 1968). The experimental techniques for microiontophoretic studies of single neurons on urethane-anaesthetised rats, which were also used in the present investigation, have been described in detail elsewhere (Bradley and Dray, 1973). The cells studied were located in the reticular formation and the majority were identified histologically by staining with Pontamine Blue (Boakes et al., 1974). Since the actions of morphine have been linked with those of various neurotransmitters in brain and since responses to certain neurotransmitters had been demonstrated for brain stem neurons (Bradley, 1968), we also examined the interactions between morphine and three transmitter substances, acetylcholine (ACh), noradrenaline (NA) and 5-hydroxytryptamine (5-HT), all applied iontophoretically to single, spontaneously active neurons.

METHODS AND DISCUSSION

In the first series of experiments, it was found that morphine, applied with iontophoretic currents of between 10 and 50 nA from 1% (0.03M; pH 4.0–5.0) solutions, modified the activity of approximately 65% of the neurons tested. The application time varied between 60 sec at a current of 50 nA to 5 min at 10 nA. In the early experiments two types of responses of neuronal activity were observed, the firing rate of the neurone being either increased (43%) or decreased (22%). Measurements of the transport number for morphine, using *in vitro* release of radiolabeled morphine from micropipettes identical to those used in the *in vivo* experiments and with similar current and time parameters, showed this to be low (0.051) which suggested that this substance is very potent in modifying neuronal activity (Bradley and Dray, 1974a). The morphine-sensitive cells were found to be grouped around the hypoglossal nerve in the n. reticularis paramedianus and n. reticularis gigantocellularis (Boakes et al., 1974). In more recent experiments

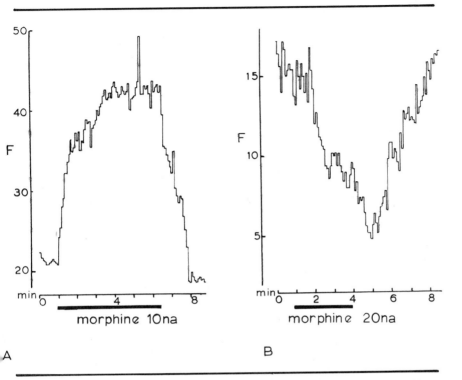

1 The effects of microiontophoretic applications of morphine on the activity of spontaneously firing brain stem neurons. The mean firing frequency (f, impulses sec^{-1}) in successive 5 sec epochs is plotted against the time (min). Iontophoretic applications are indicated by the horizontal bars and the ejecting currents are also shown. A: Excitation of a neuron by prolonged application of morphine (10 nA); B: inhibition of a neuron by morphine (20 nA) (from Bradley, P. B. and A. Dray, 1974a).

(Bramwell and Bradley, 1974), a third type of response which consisted of initial excitation, followed by depression, i.e. biphasic, was sometimes seen, although the number of neurons which responded in this way to morphine application was relatively small (5% of the total studied). The excitatory response to morphine was often slow to develop, usually commencing 10–70 sec after switching on the iontophoretic current, but also recovering within 30 sec of terminating the application (see Figure 1a). Depression also developed slowly (see Figure 1b) and in some cases outlasted the application by several minutes. This was also true of the depressant phase of the biphasic response. In some cases a

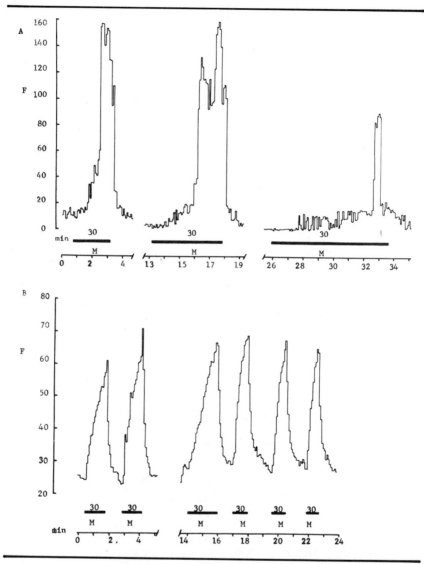

2 Excitatory responses to repeated microiontophoretic application of morphine (M) to the same neuron. A: Reduction of the excitatory response with consecutive applications of morphine (M); B: a neuron showing no desensitization to repeated morphine applications (from Bradley, P.B. and A. Dray, 1974a).

shortlasting depression was observed but as this usually paralleled the iontophoretic current in its time course, it was thought to be non-specific. Desensitization of tachyphyllaxis was sometimes observed with morphine-induced excitation. Thus, repeated applications of morphine to the same neuron resulted in a progressive reduction in the amplitude of the excitatory response, or a more prolonged application of morphine was needed to maintain the response at the same level (see Figure 2a). This desensitisation was never observed with morphine-induced depression and a significant number of neurons showed consistent excitatory responses (see Figure 2b), i.e. even with repeated morphine applications. Furthermore, all these effects were observed without any changes in spike height or shape occurring, although with more concentrated solutions of morphine in the micropipettes (e.g. 10%), or with prolonged application, a reduction in spike height and/or distortion of the action potentials could sometimes be seen (Bradley and Dray, 1974a).

Comparison of the effects of iontophoretically applied morphine with those of acetylcholine, noradrenaline or 5-hydroxytryptamine showed little correlation although neurons excited by morphine were almost always excited by ACh, and sometimes by 5-HT as well (Bradley and Dray, 1974a). However, only a proportion (<50%) of cells excited by ACh were also excited by morphine. Both potentiation and antagonism by morphine of the effects of ACh, NA and 5-HT were observed (Bradley and Dray, 1974a), but such effects were not consistent and no evidence of any correlation between these effects was seen. Thus, although most morphine-sensitive cells were found to be cholinoceptive (Bramwell and Bradley, 1974), potentiation of the effects of ACh by morphine, as has been reported for Renshaw cells (Davies and Duggan, 1974) did not occur consistently. Furthermore, when the effects of acetyl-β-methylcholine, applied to morphine-sensitive cells, were compared with those of ACh, no consistent effects were observed (Bradley and Bramwell, 1975a). Thus, if a cholinergic receptor is involved in morphine-induced excitation of neuronal activity in the brain stem, it is unlikely to be exclusively muscarinic.

Studies in animals in which dependence had been induced by chronic administration of morphine revealed remarkably few changes in neuronal activity and responses to iontophoretically applied morphine and the neurotransmitters, as compared with control untreated animals (Bradley and Dray, 1974b). Dependence was induced by administering morphine in the drinking water in doses of 0.5 mg/ml, 1.0 mg/ml and 2.0 mg/ml over successive 7 day periods. In some animals the morphine pretreatment was stopped 24 hours before the recording experi-

ment in order to induce symptoms of withdrawal. No significant differences were found in the initial spontaneous neuronal firing rates or in the
qualitative or quantitative effects of iontophoretically applied ACh, NA,
or 5-HT, when morphine-dependent animals were compared with controls. However, in the dependent animals, significantly fewer neurons
were excited by iontophoretically applied morphine and more neurons
were unaffected. The number of neurons inhibited by morphine was not
affected.

In a further series of experiments (Bramwell and Bradley, 1974;
Bradley and Bramwell, 1975) we have attempted to analyze the pharmacology of morphine-induced excitation and depression of brain stem
neurones and to determine the susceptibility of these two actions to
antagonism by the narcotic antagonist naloxone and the agonist-antagonist, nalorphine. In addition, the effects of another narcotic analgesic,
levorphanol were compared with those of morphine, as well as the
effects of its nonnarcotic isomer, dextrorphan. Morphine-induced depression of neuronal firing was selectively antagonized by both nalorphine
and naloxone (see Figure 3). This antagonism could be demonstrated in
two ways: firstly, nalorphine or naloxone application caused a return
to control firing rate, when applied during a period of morphine-induced
depression; and secondly, the antagonist reduced or completely blocked
the depressant response to a subsequent application of morphine. Morphine-induced excitation was never observed to be antagonised by
either nalorphine or naloxone but in some cases potentiation of the
excitatory effects of morphine was seen (see Figure 4). In the case of
the small number of neurons showing biphasic responses to morphine,
only the depressant phase was antagonised by naloxone. Thus, the individual components of the biphasic response showed the same susceptibility towards antagonism by naloxone as did simple depression or excitation and an application of morphine after naloxone produced only
the excitatory component of the response (see Figure 5). Both nalorphine
and naloxone had effects of their own on neuronal activity. In the case
of nalorphine only depression was observed and this mimicked morphine-
induced shortlasting depression, suggesting that it might represent a
nonspecific effect. Naloxone, on the other hand, excited some cells and
depressed others. However, these effects did not correlate in any way
with those of morphine and the one consistent effect observed with both
nalorphine and naloxone was antagonism of morphine-induced depression.

When levorphanol was applied to brain stem neurons, it was found
to exert effects similar to morphine. The response of these neurons
to levorphanol also tended to parallel their response to morphine. Thus,

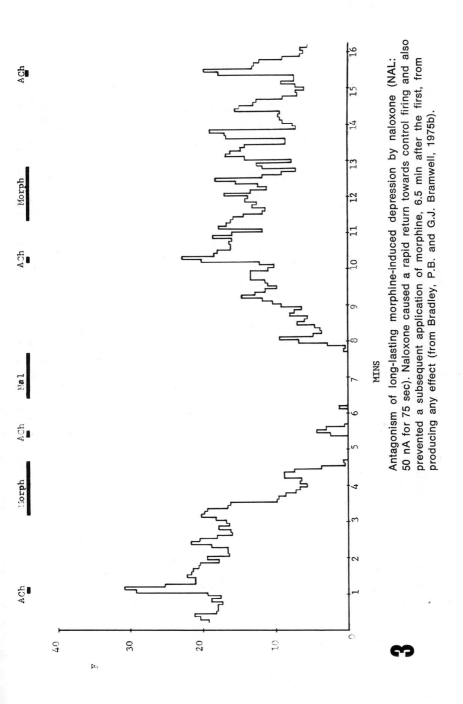

ACh ▬   Morph ▬▬▬   ACh ▬   Nal ▬▬▬   ACh ▬   Morph ▬▬▬   ACh ▬

MINS

Antagonism of long-lasting morphine-induced depression by naloxone (NAL: 50 nA for 75 sec). Naloxone caused a rapid return towards control firing and also prevented a subsequent application of morphine, 6.5 min after the first, from producing any effect (from Bradley, P.B. and G.J. Bramwell, 1975b).

3

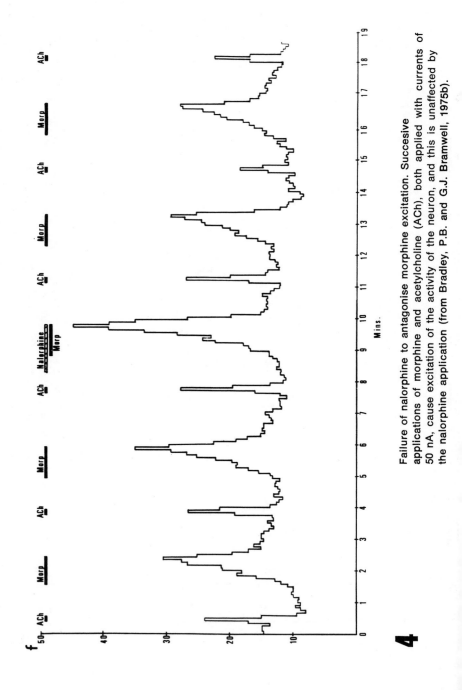

Failure of nalorphine to antagonise morphine excitation. Succesive applications of morphine and acetylcholine (ACh), both applied with currents of 50 nA, cause excitation of the activity of the neuron, and this is unaffected by the nalorphine application (from Bradley, P.B. and G.J. Bramwell, 1975b).

674

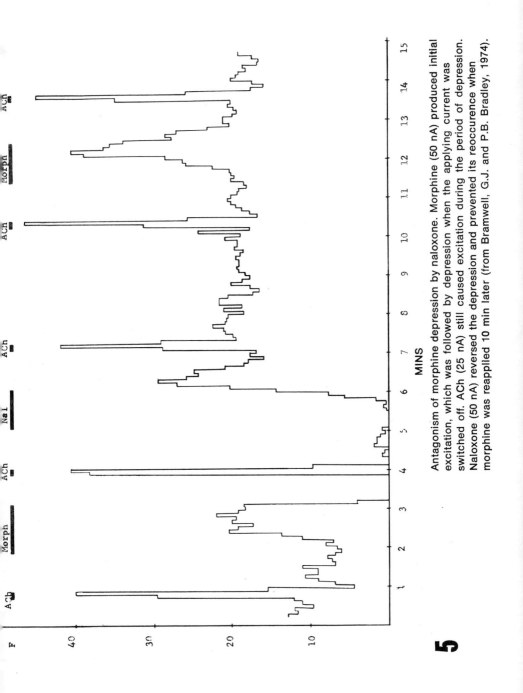

Antagonism of morphine depression by naloxone. Morphine (50 nA) produced initial
excitation, which was followed by depression when the applying current was
switched off. ACh (25 nA) still caused excitation during the period of depression.
Naloxone (50 nA) reversed the depression and prevented its reoccurence when
morphine was reapplied 10 min later (from Bramwell, G.J. and P.B. Bradley, 1974).

675

no cell responded to morphine and levorphanol in opposite ways. though more neurons were excited by morphine than by levorphanol Furthermore, levorphanol-induced changes in neuronal firing showed the same susceptibility towards antagonism by naloxone as did the equivalent morphine effect; thus levorphanol-induced depressions were consistently antagonised by naloxone.

In contrast, dextrorphan did not cause longlasting depression, nor excitation followed by depression, though it did excite some neurons. Instead, dextrorphan produced shortlasting depression, which was not antagonised by naloxone, on several occasions. In addition, the responses of these cells to dextrorphan did not parallel their responses to morphine, for not only did dextrorphan excite fewer neurons than morphine, but occasionally dextrorphan was inhibitory when morphine was excitatory. These shortlasting depressions usually outlasted the application. It is possible that they represent an extreme example of a local anaesthetic effect, since ACh excitation was often greatly reduced following short-lasting depression. In addition, morphine-induced excitation was some-times reduced following a dextrorphan application, which itself had no effect on spike height or firing rate.

During the study with levorphanol and dextrorphan, it was found that a relatively large proportion of the neurons underwent a reduction in spike height and/or a broadening of spikes during applications of these compounds, when otherwise showing no change in firing rate. This effect did not occur with morphine using twice the molar concen-tration, or at twice the applying current. It must be assumed, therefore, that both levorphanol and dextrorphan exerted significant local anaes-thetic effects when applied locally to neurones, and that these may have masked many specific interactions.

CONCLUSIONS

In conclusion, it appears from the results presented here that mor-phine-induced depression of neuronal activity in the brain stem, which is sensitive to naloxone antagonism (at low currents and using dilute solutions), represents a stereospecific narcotic action, shared by the nar-cotic agonist levorphanol, but not by the nonnarcotic isomer, dextror-phan. On the other hand, morphine-induced excitation of brain stem neurons represents an action shared by morphine, levorphanol and possibly also by dextrorphan, but since this effect was not antagonised by either nalorphine or naloxone, but could even be potentiated, it is unlikely to be a stereospecific effect. It therefore seems reasonable to propose that morphine-induced neuronal excitation and depression may be mediated by morphine acting at two different receptors, differing in stereospecificity. Furthermore, since it is the receptor which is responsible for the depressant response which shows the greatest stereospecificity, we should like to suggest that it is this receptor which mediates the analgesic action. A similar antagonism by naloxone of morphine-induced changes in neuronal firing in the cerebral cortex has recently been reported (Satoh et al., 1974). On the other hand, on the Renshaw cell in the cat, morphine-induced excitation was found to be antagonised by naloxone (Davies and Duggan, 1974).

The demonstration of a stereospecific morphine effect in the brain stem is in keeping with reports of stereospecific binding of levorphanol in this region of the mouse brain (Goldstein et al., 1971), of naloxone in the rat brain (Pert and Snyder, 1973), and of dihydromorphine in the human and monkey brain (Kuhar et al., 1973). The failure to demonstrate any correlation between morphine-induced depression of brain stem neurons and the sensitivity of such neurons to various neurotransmitters probably explains why no correlation has been found between the distribution of stereospecific binding and putative neurotransmitter systems (Kuhar et al., 1973). It is possible that morphine-induced excitation of neuronal activity may be mediated through ACh receptors since all neurons excited by morphine were cholinoceptive.

In view of the lack of stereospecificity shown by morphine-induced excitation of neuronal activity in the brain stem, it would be easy to dismiss this effect as nonspecific. However, the fact that this response sometimes showed tachyphyllaxis led us to suggest (Bradley and Dray, 1974a) that it might be associated with tolerance and this idea is supported by the finding that in morphine-tolerant animals, significantly fewer neurons were excited by morphine (Bradley and Dray, 1974b).

ACKNOWLEDGMENTS

I am grateful to Drs. G. J. Bramwell and A. Dray for their collaboration.

REFERENCES

Benjamin, R. M. 1970. Single neurons in rat medulla responsive to nociceptive stimulation. *Brain Research* 24: 525–529.

Boakes, R. J., G. J. Bramwell, I. Briggs, J. M. Candy, and E. Tempesta. 1974. Localisation with Pontamine Sky Blue of neurones in the brain stem responding to microiontophoretically applied compounds. *Neuropharmacology* 13: 475–479.

Bradley, P. B. 1968. Synaptic transmission in the central nervous system and its relevance for drug action. *Int. Rev. Neurobiol.* 11: 1–56.

Bradley, P. B., and G. J. Bramwell. 1975. A stereospecific action of morphine on brain stem neuronal activity: A microiontophoretic study. *Br. J. Pharmac.* 53: 462P.

Bradley, P. B. and A. Dray. 1973. Modification of the responses of brain stem neurones to transmitter substances by anaesthetic agents. *Br. J. Pharmac.* 48: 212–224.

Bradley, P. B., and A. Dray. 1974a. Morphine and neurotransmitter substances: Microiontophoretic study in the rat brain stem. *Br. J. Pharmac.* 50: 47–55.

Bradley, P. B., and A. Dray. 1974b. Effects of microiontophoretically applied morphine and transmitter substances in rats in chronic treatment and after withdrawal from morphine. *Br. J. Pharmac.* 51: 104–106.

Bramwell, G. J., and P. B. Bradley. 1974. Actions and interactions of narcotic agonists and antagonists on brain stem neurons. *Brain Research* 73: 167–170.

Davies, J., and A. W. Duggan. 1974. Opiate agonist-antagonist effects on Renshaw cells and spinal interneurons. *Nature* (London) 250: 70–71.

Goldstein, A., L. I. Lowney, and B. K. Pal. 1971. Stereospecific and non-specific interactions of the morphine congener levorphanol in subcellular fractions of mouse brain. *Proc. Nat. Acad. Sci.* 68: 1742–1747.

Herz, A., K. Albus, J. Metys, P. Schubert, and H. Teschemacher. 1970. On the central sites for the antinociceptive action of morphine and Fentanyl. *Neuropharmacology* 9: 539–551.

Kuhar, M. J., C. B. Pert, and S. H. Snyder. 1973. Regional distribution of opiate receptor binding in monkey and human brain. *Nature* 245: 447–450.

Liebeskind, J. C., G. Guilbaud, J-M. Besson, and J-L Oliveras. 1973. Analgesia from electrical stimulation of the periacqueductal grey matter in the cat: Behavioral observations and inhibitory effects on spinal cord interneurons. *Brain Research* 50: 441–446.

Pert, C. B., and S. H. Snyder. 1973. Opiate receptor: Demonstration in nervous tissue. *Science* 179: 1011–1014.

Pert, A., and T. Yaksh. 1974. Sites of morphine induced analgesia in the primate brain: Relation to pain pathways. *Brain Research* 80: 135–140.

Satoh, M., W. Zieglgansberger, W. Fries, and A. Herz. 1974. Opiate agonist-antagonist interaction at cortical neurones of naive and tolerance rats. *Brain Research* 82: 378–382.

Concluding Remarks

Since one purpose of a conference such as this is to provide a forum for exchange of ideas and presentation of data which may be controversial and lead to discussion not obtained through publication in existing journals, it is useful to review what has been said and determine if new, useful and provocative information has been presented which will be of value to newcomers in the field of study as well as to those with a greater experience.

Braude commented with some pertinence on the current situation at the NIDA in relation to support of research. While funds are available, competition is high and there are more worthwhile promising proposals submitted than can be funded, which puts considerable pressure on the review panel. Thus, one should prepare his proposal very carefully and avoid what might appear to be unnecessary expenditures.

In an excellent review of the physiological disposition of some narcotic drugs within the CNS, Misra discussed the significance of the Blood-Brain Barrier in relation to drug uptake, as well as the blood-CSF relationships which could influence the distribution of a narcotic to the CNS. He then further considered the physicochemical factors which could influence the rate of drug penetration into the brain, all of which in a sense contribute to what is considered the BBB phenomenon. Before describing the distribution of a wide variety of narcotic agonists and the antagonists naloxone and nalorphine, Misra briefly reminded us of the tertiary nitrogen possessed by most narcotic drugs, the significance of the aromatic ring and the stereochemical activities of the enantiomorphs, and concluded with comments on metabolism and excretion. Finally, he surveyed the distribution of morphine, heroin, methadone, pethidine, thebaine, levorphanol, dextrorphan, alpha-acetyl methadol, naloxone and nalorphine in the CNS, and factors which influence their distribution, accumulation and effectiveness, such as the development of tolerance.

Several contributors considered the localization of drugs in the CNS and other tissues. Pertschuk and Sher and their collaborators presented a new approach to localizing methadone and morphine in the CNS by an immunofluorescent technique. By this procedure, Pertschuk described neurons and occasionally glia which were immunofluorescently positive to methadone in many areas of the CNS, with a predominance in the components of the limbic system in the rat. The response was observed to be intracellular and not associated with the cell membrane. However, he was unable to demonstrate a similar response when rats, guinea pigs, mice or rabbits were injected with morphine. Sher observed a similar pattern of immunofluorescent neurons in human addicts who had died from an overdose of methadone. She was also able to demonstrate neurons which were positive after washing the sections with the antimorphine rabbit serum in subjects who had overdosed with heroin. The failure to demonstrate positive responding neurons in rats treated with morphine as compared to methadone may reflect on the greater lipid solubility of methadone or on the amount of drug in the cells. Further, the positive responses obtained from heroin addicts may be due to the much greater lipid solubility of heroin and 6-mono-acetyl morphine as compared to morphine, which could facilitate drug entry and intracellular localization in a manner not possible with the less lipid soluble morphine. As was indicated in the discussion, the response may be nonspecific and further studies with the d and l isomers of methadone are needed to determine stereospecificity. Despite this problem, the technique offers unique possibilities in studying the brains of addicts who have died from an overdose of drugs. Further, the degree of conformity in the distribution of cells which were positive with the localizations of pharmacologically active receptors is very close. It was also observed that there were some immunofluorescent granule cells in the cerebellum, which so far has demonstrated a much lower concentration of pharmacologically active receptors.

Watanabe and colleagues, using the elegant autoradiographic technique developed by Roth and Stumpf, described the distribution of ^{3}H-morphine in the brain following parenteral injection in pharmacological doses. They observed a nonspecific distribution of radio-activity with higher concentrations in the cortical gray matter, medulla, spinal cord, and in areas beneath the pia mater. Except for the optic tract, areas of white matter contained very little radioactivity. The ventromedial hypothalamic nucleus and the medial thalamic nucleus both contained higher levels of radioactivity than the surrounding areas. Activity was also observed in the ganglionic cells of the adrenal medulla. Using similar techniques, Diab and colleagues demonstrated ^{3}H-morphine accumulation in neuronal supporting elements of the myenteric plexus in the guinea pig illeum. The association of the drug with these satellite elements or the nerve ending impinging on these cells suggested that the site of action of morphine in the ileum might be on these supporting cellular elements rather than on the ganglion cells. They also noted an intense adrenergic fluorescence which was associated with the nerve fibers impinging on these supporting cells, correlating the localization of the amine with the narcotic drug. The above investigations provide anatomical evidence as to sites of drug localization, but not necessarily of function. Radioautographic observations made by Pert et al. using a technique described by Appleton, demonstrated the presence of radioactivity in the zona compacta of the substantia nigra, in the lateral edge of the medial habenular nucleus, in the locus coeruleus and in the caudate nucleus in the rat after intravenous injection of ^{3}H-diprenorphine. Similar autographic studies of cerebellar tissue and the pyriform cortex were essentially negative. Pasternak et al. presented their findings concerning an endogenous morphine-like factor found in the brains of rats and calves. This agonistic ligand has been shown to have a molecular weight of 1000, to be a peptide, and to bind specifically to the opiate receptors. It was localized to the synpatosomal fraction and found to be released by osmotic lysis. The data suggested that it may be a neurotransmitter. While information about this ligand is preliminary, extension of data in the present direction could lead to a considerable change in our concepts about the physiological perception of pain.

The chapter presented by Jacquet and Lajtha wherein micro-injections of morphine were made into different brain areas demonstrated that the periaqueductal gray matter is involved in the analgesia produced by morphine injection.

Berkowitz and co-workers considered the disposition of naloxone, a pure antagonist of opiate drugs, and pentazocine, a widely used analgesic drug with weak narcotic antagonistic activity. Pentazocine entered the brain rapidly and its pharmacological action was closely correlated with the plasma levels. Since little free pentazocine was excreted and since its metabolites have little activity, the metabolism of the drug and its distribution appear the primary factors limiting its action. Naloxone entered the brain very rapidly, reaching peak levels within 15 minutes. By 60 minutes, brain naloxone levels had declined by 50%. Berkowitz and co-workers concluded that the high brain-serum ratio of naloxone contribute to its potency, whereas its rapid efflux from the brain contribute to its short period of activity. Pentazocine appeared to have no effect on brain serotonin, but had marked effects on catecholamines, both norepinephrine and dopamine being lowered in concentration by the drug. It is believed that these amines play a role in the analgesia produced by pentazocine, which may be mediated by its effect on calcium movement. Naloxone, on the other hand, has not been observed to alter brain catecholamine biochemistry. However, naloxone can prevent the release or depletion of brain dopamine elicited by pentazocine, which could be explained by assuming that naloxone competes with pentazocine for the specific receptor, as it does with morphine.

Iontophoretic studies by Bradley on the excitation of single neurons indicated that the morphine-induced depression of neuronal activity in the brainstem was sensitive to naloxone and represented a stereospecific narcotic action shared by levorphanol, but not by dextrophan. Morphine-induced excitation of brainstem neurons represented an action shared by both levorphanol and dextrorphan which was not antagonized by naloxone or nalorphine (and may even be potentiated). Thus, this response was neither pharmacologically nor stereologically specific. Morphine induced depression and excitation of neurons seem to be mediated by two different receptors. Bradley suggests that the receptor which induced depression and appeared to be stereospecific is responsible for analgesia. Bradley further suggested that the morphine-excited neurons might be associated with tolerance because in morphine-tolerant animals there were significantly less neurons that are excited by morphine.

Musacchio and colleagues commented on the action of cationic local anesthetics and drugs of similar structure which competitively inhibit the stereospecific binding of opiates to mouse brain narcotic receptors. They suggest that the inhibition is achieved through a similarity in stereoconfiguration such that the aromatic portion of these drugs fits onto the flat surface of the narcotic receptor and the amino group fits the anionic site. On the other hand, noncationic local anesthetics, which produce a noncompetitive inhibition of opiate binding may do so by disrupting the structure of the opiate receptor.

While the primary action of narcotic drugs is still not clear, it is evident from the literature and from the observations made at this conference that dopamine, norepinephrine, serotonin, and acetylcholine all appear to play some role in the secondary responses to opiates. Dewey, Domino, Lal, Musacchio, Ordy, Wajda, Ho, and Way all contributed to this area of discussion. Lal observed that both morphine and haloperidol produce a dose-dependent increase in striatal dopamine turnover without altering steady state concentrations, which coincides with their effect in inducing catalepsy. Naloxone blocked the effect on striatal dopamine produced by morphine, but not by haloperidol. Wajda also noted that acute treatment with morphine increased dopamine turnover, but without marked effects on striatal content of the transmitter after short time intervals. However, if measurements were made of striatal dopamine 2 and 4 hours after injection of morphine, DA levels rose significantly above normal. Tyrosine hydroxylase activity did not change during this period. Norepinephrine levels tended to be decreased (with marked fluctuations) to about 40% of normal levels in this study, while acetylcholine levels increased.

The observations of Ho et al. indicated that morphine appeared to inhibit the uptake of ^{3}H-NE and was additive to a similar effect caused by reserpine. However, since the dose response curve of reserpine on ^{3}H-NE uptake was not displaced in either direction by the presence of morphine, their findings may imply different sites of action of the two drugs. While the mechanism of action of reserpine in relation to morphine analgesia is obscure, the results from the reserpine and morphine studies indicate an interaction of morphine with chatecholamines at synaptic junctions.

An increase in acetylcholine (ACh) levels in some brain areas after narcotic drugs has been suggested and presumed to be due to a decreased release from nerve terminals. Inasmuch as the alteration in brain ACh levels precedes the changes in DA, and can be correlated with the disturbances in motor activity after morphine-treatment, Wajda concluded that the cholinergic system plays a monitoring role in activating neural activity in the striatum. However, as pointed out by Dewey, few workers have observed increases in brain ACh with doses of less than 50 mg/kg. Further, Dewey was unable to observe changes in brain ACh in rats treated chronically with increasing doses of morphine reaching 200 mg/day. Finally, ACh and other cholinergic agents seem to have an antinociceptive action similar to opiates, which appears to be mediated by central muscarinic systems. A wide range of narcotic antagonists block this effect of ACh. Dewey concluded that the evidence obtained support the hypothesis that central cholinergic mechanisms are involved in the analgesic action of morphine and other narcotic analgesics.

Way also agreed that doses of morphine which produce analgesia fail to alter brain levels of ACh, while only much higher doses will significantly increase brain ACh. Finally, ACh appears to play some role in withdrawal symptoms and the expression of abstinence, although the mechanisms are not understood. In animals subjected to naloxone-precipitated withdrawal, ACh levels were significantly decreased, while choline levels were unchanged. Further, manipulation of brain ACh levels by pharmacological manipulation influences morphine effects in different ways. None of these experimental models influenced the development of tolerance or dependence. Way concluded, therefore, that none of the receptors mediating central cholinergic responses are primarily concerned with development of tolerance or dependence, though they may play an indirect role.

Not all observations in relation to receptors and transmitters are restricted to amines and ACh. Thus, Ehrenpreis and co-workers concluded that prostaglandins E play a role in the mediation of the ACh effect in the guinea pig ileum and presumably also in brain. They believe that their results are compatible with the "postulate that a prostaglandin system is directly involved with the release of ACh in the ileum; opiates act as prostaglandin receptor inhibitors; and such receptor inhibition results in blockade of prostaglandin modulatory function and reduced ACh output." They did not feel that the adenylate cyclase system was involved in this mechanism. Thus, they differ from Collier and Roy (1971) who observed that the prostaglandins E stimulation of adenylate cyclase in rat brain homogenates was inhibited by morphine. In this framework then, prostaglandins is considered in the mode of a transmitter. However, as indicated by Clouet (chapter 19), there is no predictable pattern of response in the brain of the adenylate cyclase system to morphine. In their own study, Clouet and Iwatsubo observed that transient fluctuations in cAMP and adenylate cyclase did occur in the brain, which could account for the contradictions in the literature. They further observed that opiates did not inhibit basal adenylate cyclase activity in shocked nerve ending preparations when the drugs were added to the assay medium. More importantly, the dopamine-sensitive adenylate cyclase isolated in striatal nerve ending preparations was inhibited by haloperidol; it was not inhibited by opiates, indicating that the opiates do not act directly on the postsynaptic dopamine receptor, as neuroleptics do.

In the observations reported by Lal, systemic injection of either morphine or haloperidol stimulated adenylate cyclase activity, while chronic administration of morphine significantly increased the response of adenylate cyclase activity to the stimulating effect of dopamine. Lal concluded that in relation to dopamine, their work, in conjunction with others, suggests that acute narcotic treatment inhibits the central dopaminergic activity and that chronic treatment induces a latent dopamine receptor supersensitivity. To a degree, certainly, these observations are at variance with those of Collier and Francis (Nature 235:159, 1975) who suggested that the neuronal cyclic AMP mechanism was held in check by opiates, but that adenylate cyclase activity was increased during withdrawal from morphine.

Domino et al. observed that morphine has a biphasic effect on locomotor activity and ACh utilization. A dose of 1.0 mg/kg s.c. enhanced both locomotion and ACh utilization, while a dose of 10 mg/kg caused an initial depression and a subsequent stimulation in both measures. Tolerance developed to both the depressant and stimulant effects of morphine on locomotion and ACh utilization. Further, both components of the biphasic response were antagonized by naloxone. Since dissociation occurred between the locomotor and ACh effect after using benzomorphans (UM747 and cyclazocine both increased locomotor activity without effecting ACh utilization), it may be that the two responses are mediated by different receptors. However, dissociation may be more apparent than real, because sensitivity of one measure may be greater than the other [editorial comment]. The possibility of there being more than one kind of opiate receptor was also suggested by Mulé and by Smith (this text) from the view that there may be receptors which are not involved in the pharmacological responses to opiates but which mediate other biochemical responses.

In the normal anatomical framework of the CNS organization, one would proceed from presynaptic to the postsynaptic ending. In this instance the component of the postsynaptic membrane of special interest is of course the receptor. Clearly from the observations made in this volume there are believed to be special narcotic receptors on synaptic membranes which may be either pre- or postsynaptic. These would appear to be in addition to alpha, beta, nicotinic or muscarinic receptors normally associated with norepinephrine or ACh. Further, there appear to be stereospecific receptors for opiates which are significant in providing for the pharmacological response to the drugs. These responses can be blocked by antagonists such as naloxone or nalorphine. However, as suggested by Mulé and Smith, there may be other receptors which may be important in the effects on protein and RNA synthesis observed with morphine. Further, the receptors mediating a pharmacological response may not necessarily be the receptors concerned with the development of tolerance and dependence. Such receptors may be intracellular and may not demonstrate stereospecificity. The immunofluorescent studies demonstrating intracellular and intranuclear localization for morphine and methadone, as noted by Sher and Pertschuk, may depend on some such opiate receptor which is not associated with surface membranes. Such an observation would fit with those of Levi et al. who noted an inhibition of protein synthesis in the cerebellum of equal magnitude to that observed in the hypothalamus. Since the cerebellum appears to have fewer pharmacologically active receptors than other brain areas (or at least only a few are occupied by either agonist or antagonist), one might presume that this response depends on an interaction of morphine with some other type of receptor.

To review briefly, apparently there is a close correlation between the affinity for opiate receptor binding sites and the ability of opiate agonists and antagonists to influence electrically induced contractions of the guinea pig ileum (Creese and Synder). Inasmuch as the response of the guinea pig ileum to opiate drugs is generally believed to parallel the CNS responses, this observation would also presumably be true in the brain. Hiller and Simon observed that it was possible to detect reproducible differences in opiate receptor distribution between brains of animal species whose primary reaction to opiates is depression from those whose primary response is excitation. They and Creese and Snyder both commented on the role of Na$^+$ ions in conformational changes in the opiate receptor wherein sodium enhances the binding of antagonists and inhibits the binding of agonists. The work from both laboratories as well as others reflect the need for developing techniques to further isolate the drug receptor, as distinct from other receptors and better characterize its structure. It was generally agreed by all that a thorough understanding of the opiate receptor and its interactions with endogenous and exogenous ligands is essential to view the mechanisms of opiate action. Mulé and colleagues, using ^{3}H-etorphine demonstrated clear pharmacological or stereospecific binding of an opiate in the CNS, with specific areas of accumulation in midbrain, hypothalamus and striatum. The number of stereospecific sites for ^{3}H-etorphine in the synaptic membranes of the rat was very similar to the number of pharmacologically active sites in the same membrane fraction. Mulé also observed that there appears to be many opiate binding or receptor sites which do not need to be occupied for a pharmacological response to occur.

Cox et al. contributed further observations in relation to opiate receptors by discussing their utilization of the technique of photoaffinity labeling to identify the receptor and investigated the possibility that synthetic opiate analogues might be induced to form covalent complexes with opiate receptors. N-β-(p-azidophenyl) (α-^{3}H) ethylnorlevorphanol (APL) demonstrated low stereospecific binding while the quaternary derivative of APL, N-methyl-N-β-(p-azidophenyl) (α-^{3}H) ethylnor-levorphanol (MAPL) achieved opiate receptor binding despite a lower receptor affinity.

Loh and Cho investigated the possibility that cerebroside sulfate constituted a good molecular model of a structure present in neuronal membranes which could serve as an opiate receptor. They proposed that the analgesic action of opiates may be attributed to the dehydration of the surface membrane by the analgesic through the formation of intimate ion pairs between the pronated nitrogen of the opiate agonist and the anionic site of the receptor. Such receptors could contain either protein, lipid or carbohydrate. This proposal explains why antagonists cannot produce an analgesic effect, inasmuch as they form mainly hydrated ion pairs with receptors, not dehydrated ion pairs. Partial agonists are analgesic at low concentrations, but behave like antagonists at high concentrations. Presumably the receptor considered by Loh and Cho is only the pharmacologically active one as it seems to preclude the possibility of receptors, such as might be concerned with protein synthesis.

Wong and Horng also commented on the effect of sodium in relation to binding of naloxone and dihydromorphine to receptors in the brain. Uptake of both drugs was highest in the corpus striatum, midbrain and hypothalamus; intermediate in pons + medulla and cerebral cortex and lowest in the cerebellum, again supporting the concept that there are fewer pharmacologically active receptors in the cerebellum. The addition of 20 mM NaCl doubled the binding of naloxone in all regions except the cerebellum while reducing the binding of dihydromorphine by about 50%. Increasing the NaCl to 100 mM virtually eliminated binding of the agonist. Naloxone appeared to have only one binding component, while the opiate had both a high and a low affinity component. The high affinity component was reduced by NaCl at 20 mM, while the low affinity component was virtually lost at the higher sodium concentrations. The low level of accumulation of either naloxone or dihydromorphine in the cerebellum further supports the concept that there are few pharmacologically active agonist binding sites in this area, but does not discount the possibility of binding to other drug acceptor components either on the surface membranes or within the cells which relate to other responses. Finally, the observations of Smith et al. suggested that the analgesic, respiratory depression, cataractogenic, and growth-inhibiting responses to opiate drugs are each mediated by receptors differing on the basis of the degree of tolerance development in each of the four parameters. A question which might be subsequently raised is: does the development of dependence necessitate some interaction with four such receptors, or is there yet another mechanism associated with this phenomena?

Mushlin and Cochin concluded from their studies that agonists and antagonists both bind at the same receptor site and that the various responses to opiates are mediated by a single type of receptor. Antagonist blockade of the agonist responses prevent development of tolerance to or dependence on the agonist. Their data did not lead to the conclusion that chronic administration of antagonists leads to an expansion in the number of available receptor sites, as postulated by some investigators. They further concluded that an interaction with a receptor site is necessary for the development of tolerance and dependence and that there is a threshold dose below which dependence and tolerance are not initiated. They also found that the expression of a pharmacologic response was not necessary for the development of tolerance.

While alcohol is not an opiate and it is not clear that there are receptors in the same sense as there are for opiates, it is a drug to which dependence and tolerance develops, and alcoholics deprived of alcohol demonstrate a withdrawal symptomatology. Further, alcohol administration is known to depress protein synthesis, respiration, and reflex activity. Ho and Kissen noted that the development of alcohol preference in rats depends on some interaction between serotonin and ACh and that adrenergic mechanisms may also be involved. From their studies on brain excitability in rats treated with alcohol, Porjesz et al. suggested that complex modifications in CNS responsivity occur during the addiction process. They suggested that these changes could be considered as a form of long-term memory, "an addiction memory," which normally lies dormant in an individual who had been previously exposed to alcohol which can then become reactivated on renewed exposure to an addictive substance. Such a concept might equally be applied to opiate addiction. If such a hypothesis is true, then the effects of alcohol, or any other addictive substance, could last far longer than the time during which the drug is available and present in the CNS.

Despite the current preoccupation with receptors and transmitters, there still appear to be many reasons for continuing research on the effect of opiates in relation to synthesis of macromolecules in the CNS. Narcotic effects have not as yet been associated with the synthesis of a new protein in brain. Numerous investigations in the past decade have demonstrated that morphine administration inhibits the incorporation of labeled amino acid into brain protein. Levi (using Wistar male rats) and Ford (using Sprague Dawley rats) have both demonstrated that morphine injected into intact unanesthetized animals via indwelling cannulas markedly depressed ^{3}H-l-lysine incorporation into brain protein. A comparison of the curves from the two reports (two strains) demonstrated a significantly higher accumulation of lysine into brain protein from the Sprague Dawley animals, as well as a difference in degree of response to morphine, suggesting a strain difference. This difference in response is disturbing in view of the variations in animal strain, suppliers and species utilized in different laboratories. The extent to which strain differences may influence our interpretation of results was indicated by Shuster et al. in a 1975 Federation paper wherein they reported differences in the amount of opiate receptors and analgesic responses in seven recombinant-inbred strains derived from the F_2 generation from an original mating between C57B1/6By with BALB/cBy mice. These problems in data which arise from using different strains of a species have also been reported by several other laboratories. Thus, it is clear that each laboratory must evaluate overt responses as well as neurochemical findings between various strains of a specific species as well as between species.

Levi noted that 24 hours after injection of morphine lysine accumulation into brain protein had returned to normal. Ford reported that morphinization of rats caused a decrease in incorporation of lysine into plasma proteins. Both Levi and Ford noted an increase in the levels of free total lysine in the plasma after morphine, which may have some clinical significance in view of the pathological effects associated with congenital hyperlyseinemia. In Ford's, chapter an attempt was made to measure the combined effect of morphine and naloxone on ^{3}H-l-lysine incorporation into brain protein. Unexpectedly, the naloxone (10 mg/kg dose) had a stimulatory effect on incorporation of lysine into brain protein which was about equal in magnitude to the inhibition caused by morphine. This is of particular interest since high doses of naloxone have also been reported to have a stimulatory effect on behavior. Thus, at present it is difficult to know if the protection against morphine-induced depression of protein synthesis is due to blockage of the effect or simply because it produces an opposite effect in and of itself.

In a study with addicts, Joshi was able to detect two protein bands by acrylamide gel electrophoresis in CSF from known heroin addicts which did not appear in the CSF of control patients or patients on the methadone maintenance program. The molecular weight of the faster moving protein was determined to be close to 45,000. The source of this protein, which was not observed in the plasma obtained from the same patient, remains to be determined.

During the last few years it has become increasingly clear that opiate drug abuse is associated with varying degrees of alteration in pituitary function. Earlier, Sawyer and colleagues showed that ovulation was inhibited in rats by morphine treatment. George and Kokka observed that acute treatment with morphine has an effect on adenohypophyseal function, as indicated by measurements of plasma hormone levels, which is dose related. Low doses were observed to increase the secretion of GH and to inhibit TSH secretion. High doses increased both GH and corticosteroid plasma levels while inhibiting TSH secretion. Pretreatment with blocking doses of naloxone completely blocked the rise in plasma corticosteroids while enhancing the GH releasing effect. Chronic administration of the opiate caused hypertrophy of the adrenals, while plasma corticosteroid levels return to normal. TSH secretion remained below normal in these animals, while the increase in GH secretion persisted. Abstinence or naloxone precipitated withdrawal was then observed to cause an elevation of plasma corticosteroid levels while lowering TSH and GH levels.

Zimmerman and Pang extended the discussion on morphine effects on pituitary function to include the effects on gonadotrophins. Their observations confirmed the earlier findings of Barraclough and Sawyer (1955) and demonstrated that large doses of morphine block spontaneous ovulation in the rat by preventing the ovulatory surge of LH and FSH. They also observed that morphine inhibited the tonic elevation of gonodotrophins which follows ovariectomy. They further noted that morphine stimulates the release of prolactin, possibly accounting for the galactorrhea observed in female heroin addicts. It seems reasonable that these effects of morphine are mediatd through the hypothalamus and probably also the limbic system.

With the rather marked response of the hypophyseal-pituitary system to morphine-treatment and previous observations by Ford and colleagues (1974) that there are changes in neurons of the median arcuate area of the hypothalamus after morphine, it seemed reasonable to conclude that there could also be anatomical correlates in the anterior lobe of the pituitary which might be revealed by electron microscopy. Preliminary observations by Cramer demonstrated that there is a decrease in secretory droplets in the somatotrophs after morphine-treatment. This might be expected in view of the report by George and Kokka. Since an increased level of GH persisted during chronic treatment, the decrease in secretory granules observed by Cramer could possibly be associated with both an elevation in synthetic activity and secretion within these cells. The latter might be revealed, as Cramer suggested, by electronmicroscopic autoradiography. Cramer further observed an apparent increase in lipid droplets in somatotrophs and in luteotrophic cells. No definitive changes were observed in the gonadectomy cells by morphine treatment. Conceivably, here, too, EM autoradiography would be useful in determining in which cells an alteration in biochemical activity is influenced by the opiate drug.

Numerous reports in the clinical literature have indicated that children born of mothers taking opiate drugs are born dependent to the same class of drugs. Further, they demonstrate withdrawal unless remedial measures are undertaken. Beyond these clinical observations, there are a few reports in the research literature which suggest that there may be some problems in growth and development in offspring from opiate-treated mothers. The degree to which this is a serious socio-clinical problem is still uncertain. The data on the effects of such drugs as morphine and methadone is fragmentary with a difficulty in disassociating drug from nutritional effects. Sonderegger and Zimmerman and McGinty and Ford presented two aspects of this problem.

In the Sonderegger study, treatment of rat pups with morphine commenced after birth. Certain long-lasting effects in the offspring were observed. The body weights were lower, which was of variable duration and followed by a rebound after ceasing treatment. There were no differences in the acquisition of appetitive responses, but there was a failure in one group to acquire normal "emotional" response. In open field behavior studies there was evidence that early morphine treatment caused some qualitative differences between the different groups. There was protracted tolerance to analgesia as a result of induction of dependence just after birth as well as to the pituitary-adrenal stimulating effect of morphine.

In the study by McGinty and Ford rats were exposed to morphine or methadone prenatally. Since opiate ingestion by pregnant females decreased food consumption, one control group was pair-fed with an amount of food equivalent to that eaten by the morphine-treated mothers. Another control group was fed ad libitum. The offspring of the methadone-treated mothers were the least healthy, with a 50% mortality at birth and a 100% mortality of male offspring by weaning. The offspring of the morphine-treated mothers were minimally different from the pair-fed controls. The development of reflex pattern responses lagged behind those of controls in the drug-treated rats and was most apparent after methadone.

Both Sonderegger and McGinty have presented what are preliminary investigations into the serious problem of the effects of narcotics on the young of mammals. While the experimental design of the two studies differ, they both suggest some impairment in postnatal development. In both instances, there appears to be a problem in distinguishing between drug and nutritional effects, which should be resolved.

There have been several model systems suggested for the study of opiate action on cells. Cardasis and Schuel examined opiate effects on the sea urchin egg. Both morphine and methadone inhibited the release of secretory granules from the eggs. Naloxone had a biphasic effect, depending on its concentration.

Two reports were presented at the conference pertaining to observations in a patient population at the Downstate-Kings County Medical Center. Tenner et al. noted that there is a greater degree of cerebral ventricular enlargement among a group of adult methadone patients than in the general population, 70% being larger than the expected size. The offspring of methadone-treated mothers, while showing a lesser percentage of increase in ventricular size, had ventricles which were larger than those in the normal population. They concluded that the findings may indicate a mild degree of brain atrophy or that there is a mild increase in CSF pressure. In neonates undergoing withdrawal, there was evidence of ventricular compression, which was usually on the left side. Follow-up studies demonstrated that this compression was transient.

Other observations made by Solish et al. on infants subjected to methadone in utero while their mothers were treated on a methadone-maintenance program suggested that subtle changes may be occurring in the fetal-placental unit as evidence by changes in heat stable alkaline phosphatase and in the estriol and estetrol levels. These changes could well reflect changes in fetal support which could influence the long range growth and development of the child.

Vast strides have been made in the last few years in understanding the basic mechanisms of opiate action. Some of the evidence has been presented at this conference. The initial interaction between drug and nervous tissue is presumably the establishment of a drug:membrane opiate receptor bond. Some data pertaining to the nature of the opiate receptor, whether it is of one or more than one type throughout the CNS, whether agonists and antagonists bind at the same sites with the same number of attachments, etc. have been discussed. However, the chemical nature of the receptor and of the "natural ligand" remain to be demonstrated. The secondary responses to the initial drug:receptor interaction seem to involve neurotransmitters, the adenylate cyclase system, and prostaglandins; in other words, all of the modulators of synaptic transmission. Whether there are secondary intracellular binding sites for narcotics is open to exploration, although some hints (from opiate histochemical localization and their effects on macromolecular synthesis) suggest that this is a possibility.

The interaction between scientists of various disciplines (anatomy, physiology, biochemistry, pharmacology and endocrinology) with varying degrees of experience (established investigators, students) has been fruitful. Final proof of the value of meetings such as this will come when progress in these research areas is reported in future conferences.

D. H. Ford
D. H. Clouet

Subject Index